Community Health
and **Wellness 4**

Primary Health Care in Practice

Dedication

For my children and the special girls who energise my life and keep me curious about the world and its people — Kate, Emily, Nina, Bianca and Lara — may you always live in good health, happiness and harmony with your communities.

Anne McMurray September 2010

For my husband and children — Gordon, Ben and Sally — who have patiently carried on with life while I have been writing this book with Anne, and for the communities I have worked with and lived in over the years that provide the inspiration to continue this work.

Jill Clendon September 2010

Community Health
and **Wellness 4**
Primary Health Care in Practice

Anne McMurray
Jill Clendon

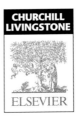

CHURCHILL
LIVINGSTONE

ELSEVIER

Sydney   Edinburgh   London   New York   Philadelphia   St Louis
Toronto

Mosby
is an imprint of Elsevier

Elsevier Australia. ACN 001 002 357
(a division of Reed International Books Australia Pty Ltd)
Tower 1, 475 Victoria Avenue, Chatswood, NSW 2067

National Library of Australia Cataloguing-in-Publication Data

McMurray, Anne

    Community health & wellness: primary health care in
    practice/Anne McMurray; Jill Clendon.

    4th ed.

    9780729539548 (pbk.)

    Includes index.

    Public health--Social aspects--Australia.

    Health promotion--Social aspects--Australia.

    Social medicine--Australia.

    Clendon, Jill.

362.120994

Publisher: Libby Houston
Developmental Editor: Larissa Norrie
Publishing Services Manager: Helena Klijn
Project Coordinator: Natalie Hamad
Edited and indexed by Forsyth Publishing Services
Proofread by Pam Dunne
Cover and internal design by Lisa Petroff
Typeset by TNQ Books and Journals
Printed in China by 1010 Printing International Limited

Contents

About the authors   xv
Preface   xvii
Acknowledgements   xix
Reviewers   xix

Section 1 Healthy people, healthy places
Introduction to the section   2

Chapter 1 Health as a socio-ecological concept   **5**
  Introduction   5
  What is health?   7
  Health and wellness   7
  Defining 'community' and 'community health'   9
  Community health and wellness   9
  Social determinants of health   11
  The role of communities in intergenerational health   13
  Social capital   14
  Sustainable community health   15
  Community development: helping communities change   16
    Health literacy   17
  Research to practice   20
  Case study: meet the Millers   22
  Reflecting on the big issues   22
  Reflective questions: how would I use this knowledge in practice? 23
  Research-informed practice: intergenerational health   24

Chapter 2 Primary health care: principles and practices   **28**
  Introduction   28
  Clarification of terms   29
    Primary health care (PHC)   29
    Primary, secondary and tertiary prevention   30
    Primary care   30
  Public health, population health and primary health care: a brief history 32
    Population health   32
    Primary health care and the Declaration of Alma Ata   33
    Problems with the 'old public health' era   33
  PHC and the social gradient   34
  PHC and the health promotion charters   34
  PHC principles   36
    Accessibility: a case of equity and social justice   36
    Appropriate technology   37
      The ethics of appropriate technologies   38
    Increased emphasis on health promotion   39
    Health education   40
    Cultural sensitivity, cultural safety   41

Intersectoral collaboration 42
Public participation 43
Community health promotion: the Ottawa Charter for Health Promotion 44
Implications for community health promotion 46
Leadership, professionalism and citizenship 47
Case study 48
Reflecting on the big issues 48
Reflective questions: how would I use this knowledge in practice? 48
Research-informed practice 49

Chapter 3 Promoting health in an era of globalisation **53**
Introduction 53
Globalisation 53
The pros and cons of globalisation 55
Globalisation as a health promotion variable 57
Health promotion strategies for global health 58
Health as security 59
Health as development 59
Health as a global public good 61
Health as a human right 62
Building the evidence base: the population approach 62
The global burden of disease project 63
The epidemiology of health and ill health 64
Social epidemiology 66
Health and place 66
Healthy cities 68
The Healthy Cities Movement 69
Health promotion planning: diarrhoea and dirt to community activism 69
Community-wide health promotion and the 'new health education' 70
Community assessment: health planning for the enabling community 72
Phase one: the lay of the land 74
Phase two: mapping resources 75
Phase three: who will help? 75
Phase four: people, place, health and gatekeepers 75
Phase five: strengths, weaknesses, opportunities, threats 75
Helping people change 76
Case study 78
Reflecting on the big issues 78
Reflective questions: how would I use this knowledge in practice? 79
Research-informed practice 79

Chapter 4 Enabling health and wellness: practice roles and models of care **83**
Introduction 83
The role of nurses and midwives in promoting social justice 83
Nurse practitioners and advanced practice: models of practice 85
Experiences in the UK: public health, population health and role development 87
Primary health care roles: specialist or generalist? 89
Practice nursing: Australia 90
Practice and primary health care nursing: New Zealand 91
Managing chronic conditions in the community 92
Child health nursing practice 94
School health nursing 95

Rural and remote area nursing practice 99
Paramedic practice in the community 102
Community mental health nursing practice 103
Occupational health nursing 105
Collaborative models of nursing and midwifery in the community 108
Case study 110
Reflecting on the big issues 110
Reflective questions: how would I use this knowledge in practice? 111
Research-informed practice 111

Section 2 Sustainable health for the family and the individual

Introduction to the section 121
Chapter 5 Healthy families **123**
Introduction 123
The family, community and society 123
Defining the family 125
Family functions 125
Family developmental pathways 126
Changing families, changing partners, changing roles 127
Fertility, child bearing and population trends 130
Families and work 131
Casualisation, part-time work and parental leave 132
Work and stress 132
Gender issues and work 133
Fly-in fly-out families 134
Couple relationships 136
Social influences on couple relationships 137
Relationship satisfaction 137
Healthy couples, healthy families: communication and resilience 138
Communication and power 139
Communication and change 139
Adaptation and resilience 140
Marriage, separation, divorce and parenting 140
Divorce and parenting 141
Divorce and the blended family 142
The impact of divorce on parents 142
Non-resident parenting 142
Parenting and child support 143
Divorce and the rights of the child 143
Violence in the family 144
Intimate partner violence 145
IPV and the children 146
Migrant families and health 147
Migration and family life 147
Migrants, refugees, stress and coping 147
Families dealing with illness 148
Family caregiving issues 149
Caring for children with disabilities 150
Caregiver stress 150
Rural families 151
Social determinants of the health of rural families 152
Family life in the 21st century 152
Goals for healthy families 153

Building healthy public policy 153
  Marriage policies 153
  Parental and children's rights policies 154
  Policies protecting human rights and non-violence 154
  Inclusive policies 155
  Policies for vulnerable families 155
  Policies protecting the community 156
Creating supportive environments 156
  Parent groups 156
  Culturally inclusive support 157
Strengthening community action 157
  Supporting family decision-making 158
  Family support in the workplace 158
  Family advocacy 158
Developing personal skills 159
  Supporting civic participation 159
  Supporting family relationship skills 159
Reorienting health services 160
  Assessment and screening 160
  Family-centred care 161
  Health professionals 161
  Evidence-based practice 161
Case study 162
Reflecting on the big issues 162
Reflective questions: how would I use this knowledge in practice? 163
Research-informed practice 163

Chapter 6 Healthy children **170**
Introduction 170
The healthy child 171
Biological embedding and childhood stress 172
Socio-economic factors and childhood stress 172
Global child health, disadvantage and poverty 173
Children and homelessness 175
Indicators of child health in Australia and New Zealand 175
Health indicators for Indigenous children 176
Chronic illnesses in childhood 176
Nutrition, physical activity and the social determinants of child health 177
  Breastfeeding 178
  Healthy pregnancy 179
  Antenatal care 180
  Childbirth 180
  Postnatal depression 181
Children's psychosocial wellbeing 182
  Mental ill health 183
  Learning readiness and social development 183
Resilience 184
Parenting patterns and children's health outcomes 185
Family lifestyle practices 186
  Obesogenic environments 187
Keeping children safe 188
Critical pathways to child health 189
  Goals for child health 190

Building healthy public policy 191
  Collaborative policy development 192
Creating supportive environments 194
Strengthening community action 196
Developing personal skills 197
Reorienting health services 197
Case study 199
Reflecting on the big issues 199
Reflective questions: how would I use this knowledge in practice? 200
Research-informed practice 200

Chapter 7 Healthy adolescents **207**
Introduction 207
The development of social competence 208
Social determinants of adolescent health, risk and potential 209
  Identity and body image: weight management and eating disorders 209
  Eating disorders and family life 211
  Risky sexual behaviours 211
  Compounding risk: alcohol, drug use and tobacco smoking 213
  Depression, self-harm and suicide 214
  Recognising the risk of suicide 215
Adolescent life in the community context 216
Adolescent life in the school context 218
School, home and social networking 218
Risk, resilience and decision-making 220
Hope and self-esteem 220
Countering risk: healthy adolescence 222
  Goals for adolescent health 222
Building healthy public policy 222
  Harm minimisation policies 223
Creating supportive environments 223
  Supporting parenting 225
Strengthening community action 226
Developing personal skills 227
Reorienting health services 228
  Electronic media, risk and support 229
Case study 233
Reflecting on the big issues 233
Reflective questions: how would I use this knowledge in practice? 233
Research-informed practice 234

Chapter 8 Healthy adults **239**
Introduction 239
The healthy adult 239
Risks to health 240
Adult morbidities 241
Stress in adult life 242
Lifestyle and chronic disease 242
Rural lifestyle risks 245
Stress, mental health and the social determinants of health 246
Positive mental health and wellbeing 247
Social exclusion and mental ill health 248
Family stress 249

Stress in the workplace 249
Other workplace health and safety issues 251
Stressful working conditions 252
Environmental factors affecting adult health 254
Healthy adulthood 255
Goals for adult health 255
Building healthy public policy 256
Creating supportive environments 257
Strengthening community action 258
Developing personal skills 259
Reorienting health services 260
Case study 261
Reflecting on the big issues 262
Reflective questions: how would I use this knowledge in practice? 262
Research-informed practice 263

Chapter 9 Healthy ageing **269**
Introduction 269
Ageing and society 269
Population ageing 271
Global ageing perspectives 271
Risk and potential in older persons 273
Weight and mobility in older age 275
Physical activity and ageing 275
Mental health issues 276
Health and place 277
Safe environments for ageing 279
Elder abuse 280
Social and spiritual support 280
Maintaining dignity in coping 281
Critical pathways to ageing 282
Transitions: challenges and opportunities 283
Workplace and retirement transitions 283
Transitions to single ageing or widowhood 283
Transitions in intimacy and sexuality 284
Transitions to the end of life 285
Resilience and health in older age 286
Goals for healthy ageing 287
Building healthy public policy 287
Creating supportive environments 288
Strengthening community action 289
Developing personal skills 290
Reorienting health services 290
Case study 292
Reflecting on the big issues 292
Reflective questions: how would I use this knowledge in practice? 293
Research-informed practice 293

Section 3 Inclusive communities and societies
Introduction to the section 299
Chapter 10 Health and gender: healthy women, healthy men **301**
Introduction 301
Inequality, social exclusion and gender 302

Empowerment 303
Women's health issues 304
Women and social disadvantage 307
Intimate partner violence and empowerment 308
Men's health issues 310
Men's lifestyles and health 311
Men's health risks 312
Masculinity, behaviour and the men's health movement 313
The need for men's and women's health policies 314
Men, women and intimacy 314
Gender issues among sexually diverse populations 315
Gendering society: goals for the health of men and women 316
Building healthy public policy 317
Creating supportive environments 318
Strengthening community action 319
Developing personal skills 320
Reorienting health services 321
Case study 323
Reflecting on the big issues 323
Reflective questions: how would I use this knowledge in practice? 324
Research-informed practice 324

Chapter 11 Cultural inclusiveness: safe cultures, healthy Indigenous people **329**
Introduction 329
Culture and health 330
Culture conflict 331
Cultural safety 332
Multiculturalism 333
Ethnocentrism to racism 333
Aboriginality, culture and health 335
Indigenous people's relationships between health and place 335
Colonisation and disconnection between health and place 336
Culture blindness and the Stolen Generations 338
The health of Indigenous people throughout the world 338
The health of Australian Indigenous people 339
The health of New Zealand Māori 341
Behavioural risk factors 342
Mental health and healing 343
Injury and family violence 345
Addressing the problems through healing and empowerment 346
Building capacity and social capital 346
Goals for Indigenous health 348
Building healthy public policy 348
Creating supportive environments 351
Strengthening community action 352
Developing personal skills 353
Reorienting health services 355
Case study 356
Reflecting on the big issues 357
Reflective questions: how would I use this knowledge in practice? 357
Research-informed practice 357

Chapter 12 Building the evidence base: research to practice   **363**

Introduction   363
Global community health research   364
Social determinants of health and the research agenda   366
Conducting research for policy and practice   367
  Evidence-based practice   368
  Systematic reviews, literature reviews, integrative reviews and
      meta-analysis   368
  Randomised controlled trials   369
  Sources of evidence   370
  Translational research   371
    Community-based research partnerships   373
    Action research   373
  Participatory action research   374
Researching the community: paradigms and strategies   375
  Mixed methods   375
Case study research   375
Researching culture   377
  Researching with Indigenous people   378
Researching the future   381
Getting started: from research question to solution   384
  The question   385
  The argument   385
  Conceptual framework   385
  Method   385
    Research ethics   386
    Findings/results   386
    Discussion   386
Case study   387
Reflecting on the big issues   387
Reflective questions: how would I use this knowledge in practice?   388
Research-informed practice   388

Chapter 13 Inclusive policies, equitable health care systems   **392**

Introduction   392
Politics, policy-making and health care   393
Health services policies and the social determinants of health   395
  Rural health policies   395
  Health promotion policies   395
  Community development policies   396
Policy-making and primary health care   396
Policy action at the national level: think global, act local   397
The need for policy integration: lessons from mental health   397
  Social policies and family life   398
The New Zealand health care system   400
The Australian health care system   403
  Health sector reform in Australia   405
  Recommendations for change   406
Health care: building a better system   407
Best practice in health care systems   408
Concluding comments   409
Case study   410
Reflecting on the big issues   410

Reflective questions: how would I use this knowledge in practice?   410
Research-informed practice   411

Appendices   **415**
Appendix A Symbols used in a genogram   417
Appendix B Jakarta Declaration on Leading Health
   Promotion into the 21st Century   419
Appendix C People's Health Charter   421
Appendix D The Bangkok Charter for Health Promotion in a
   Globalized World   429
Appendix E Chart for community assessment   433
Appendix F Transforming Australia for our children's future:
   making prevention work   435
Appendix G HEEADSSS assessment tool for use with adolescents   439
Appendix H Ecomap   443
Index   **444**

About the authors

Anne McMurray is a registered nurse, a Fellow of the Royal College of Nursing Australia and a member of Sigma Theta Tau International. She is an Adjunct Professor in the School of Nursing and Midwifery, Griffith University, Gold Coast Queensland, and Emeritus Professor, Faculty of Health Sciences, Murdoch University, Perth. Anne has practised in a range of nursing and community health settings in Canada and Australia, and is actively involved in research and research supervision, publishing, mentoring and leadership programs in the academic environment. She is an Expert Advisor on Primary Health Care to the International Council of Nurses. Anne was made a Member of the Order of Australia in the 2006 Queen's Birthday honours list for services to nursing, particularly in the development of nurse education and community health practices, and as a contributor to professional publications.

Jill Clendon is a registered nurse currently working as a nursing policy advisor and researcher for the New Zealand Nurses Organisation. Jill spent the 12 years previous to her current position in nursing education, teaching at both undergraduate and post graduate levels with a specific interest in primary health care and child and family health. Jill's research has examined the efficacy of community-based nurse-led clinics, and the historical and contemporary context of community-based well child care in New Zealand. Jill holds a PhD in Nursing and a Masters of Philosophy in Nursing from Massey University and a Bachelor of Arts in Political Studies from Auckland University. She is a member of the Nelson Bays Primary Health Care Nurse Advisory Group, and a member of the Nelson Bays Primary Health Organisation Clinical Governance Board. Jill has a background in public health nursing and in her spare time, maintains her clinical skills by working in the Special Care Baby Unit and paediatrics at Nelson Hospital.

Preface

This book represents the culmination of our knowledge of what makes a community healthy, and how nurses and midwives can support community health and wellbeing. In preparing the text, we have attempted to combine global insights with those that emerge from our trans-Tasman knowledge base to form a common yet distinctive foundation for practice with communities of the 21st century. Throughout the book, community health is conceptualised as a socio-ecological construct. Although the study of ecology is not new, seeing health as an ecological concept broadens our understanding of health by situating it within the physical, cultural, social, spiritual and employment settings of daily life. People are influenced by their *environments*: anywhere they work, play, study or live; their home, work and/or school, recreational settings, cities, towns, villages and camps; and places they go to receive or provide assistance, enact their religious beliefs, and negotiate and transact the exchanges of daily life. This is also *reciprocal*. When people interact with their environments, the environments themselves are energised, revitalised, and often changed. These reciprocal influences on health are most evident in the family and community, where the social determinants of health create an interplay of factors that have a profound effect across the life span. This text examines the inter-relatedness of the social determinants of health throughout the various chapters, indicating appropriate areas for nursing and midwifery intervention and health promotion.

Interaction is central to the ecological view of health. So too are the notions of *place* and *participation*; both of which are integral to community health. Nurses and midwives working with families and communities play an important role in supporting and nurturing people. They also play a vital role in helping ensure that the community itself is viable and sustainable, and that it has the resources to support people in their quest for good health. In this respect, the role of nurses and midwives is multidimensional. This means that there are two areas of focus: the community itself and those who live there. Nursing and midwifery practice 'in the community' involves all actions that are undertaken to support people's health and wellbeing. Nursing 'the community' means caring for the community itself. To meet both of these important goals nurses and midwives bring to families and communities an evidence base of knowledge that includes understanding physical and psychological health, the social and cultural determinants that support or impinge on health, and features of the community that support health. The latter includes the physical environment, health and social services, and the infrastructure that supports health.

The penultimate goal of community health is community competence. This is a developmental process integral to community health, which situates nursing and midwifery practice within strategic partnerships rather than patronage. Working cooperatively and in partnership with family and community advocates, we can function as enablers and facilitators of community health, encouraging community participation in all aspects of community life.

Another perspective threaded throughout this book is the link between global and local conditions, often seen in the expression *think global, act local.* Our global connections provide information about newly discovered illnesses and mutations of causative agents springing up around us, perhaps because of the state of the world, perhaps because of our expertise in surveillance and detection, perhaps both. At the same time, there is a widening gap between those with the opportunity to avail themselves of advice and support for their choices and pathways to health and wellbeing, and those who are marginalised from the mainstream. Sadly, it is often those most disadvantaged by distance from services or the means to access them who are most vulnerable to ill health. Their situation may also be compounded by genetic endowment, impoverished lifestyles, and the kind of political decisions that keep them in a perpetual cycle of despair. Some years ago, a popular view was that if populations were given the opportunity to create wealth, their health status would improve. However, today we have come to realise that, despite many nations having greater wealth, knowledge and health expertise, health services do not always get to those most in need. This is called 'Modernity's Paradox'; the situation where, despite the relative wealth of a society there remains an ever-widening gap between rich and poor. The disparity between the health of the rich and poor has become even more problematic with the global financial crisis having disproportionately affected those already living in poverty. For those societies also living with civil strife and conflict, community health often seems like an untenable goal.

Our knowledge base for helping communities become and stay healthy has evolved dramatically over the past decades. We have a greater understanding of the structural and social determinants of health. We also know with some certainty that what occurs in early life can set the stage for whether or not a person will become a healthy adult and experience good health during ageing. This is called a 'pathways' approach to health. Along a person's life pathway from birth to death lie a vast number of risks to good health, as well as opportunities for intervention. It is helpful for nurses and midwives promoting health to know the points of critical development and age-appropriate interventions. We outline some of these in Section 2 of the book, which addresses healthy families, healthy children, healthy adolescents, healthy adults and older persons. After nearly a quarter of a century, the Ottawa Charter is still the most useful guide for strategic health promotion planning with each of these groups. The Charter guides intersectoral collaborations for community empowerment, where citizens work in partnership with health professionals to achieve access, equity and self-determination in establishing health goals and appropriate processes for achieving them. We use the symbol of the Ottawa Charter in each chapter in Section 2 to signal that the discussion is moving towards the challenges and solutions in assisting people to work towards healthy public policies, creating supportive environments, strengthening community action, developing personal skills and reorienting health services.

The rapid expansion of research knowledge also indicates that states of health and illness can be passed on through different generations, either by biological factors such as genetic endowment, or through the transmission of similar or worsening social circumstances, or a combination of these factors. We therefore add an intergenerational approach to working with individuals, families and communities, considering the future outcomes that may result from current circumstances.

Community participation is a cornerstone of community health. Maintaining an attitude of *inclusiveness* is one way we can encourage community members to become authentic partners in securing and shaping their health and the health of their community. Inclusive communities are the main focus of Section 3. Within the chapters of this section we suggest approaches that promote cultural safety and sensitivity in helping Indigenous people and others disadvantaged or discriminated against, to develop their capacity for change. To accomplish this we need to use knowledge wisely, which means that we need evidence and innovation for all of our activities. Clearly, our professional expertise rests on becoming research literate and developing leadership skills for both personal and community capacity development. Using both sets of skills courageously has the potential to assist communities to reach towards greater levels of health, vibrancy and sustainability for the future. To illustrate, we explain a variety a sample of community health research approaches that convey the essential notion that practice is based on knowledge and research evidence. Section 3 also addresses the research and policy interface, emphasising the importance of evidence-based and evidence-informed practice to develop policies that promote and sustain health and wellbeing.

Throughout the book we accompany 'the Miller family', as they experience community life with its challenges and potential. The Millers are an extended family of Australian and New Zealand residents, some of whom reside in Sydney, others in a rural town on the South Island of New Zealand. We follow the journey of the Millers as they experience childbirth, child care, adult health issues, and some of the threats to their communities. We hope you enjoy working with them during their journey, and develop a deeper sense of their family development through a series of genograms each time new members join the family. At various stages of the chapters we have added 'points to ponder' and interactive activities to stimulate your thoughts on community health. We also urge you to be thinking of the 'big issues', which will be outlined in the reflective section at the end of each chapter.

Acknowledgements

We would like to acknowledge those who helped shape our thinking during the contemplation and writing of this book: students, colleagues and friends, who continue to provide stimulating ideas. Our thanks go to Melanie Coates for her help in searching the literature, to Maureen Ward, Lisa Panozzo and the School Nurses of Victoria and Western Australia, who generously shared their thoughts and visions for school health, and to Loretta Baker and Debbie Tillitzki for sharing their experiences in developing the Coachstop Caravan Park program. Jill would like to thank Kim Powell, Dayne, Liam and Danielle Saina, Matt Dunlop, Lorraine Rosser, Heather Clendon, and Thomas Smale for being willing participants in her search for appropriate photos. We are grateful to our reviewers who helped strengthen the book, and the entire team at Elsevier, particularly Larissa Norrie and Natalie Hamad who provided invaluable assistance in producing this work. Bringing a trans-Tasman perspective to the book has been both challenging and rewarding. Being able to bounce ideas off one another and melding together the various perspectives we bring has been both inspirational and enjoyable. We hope that communities on both sides of the Tasman will benefit from the insights that working together has brought. We would also like to thank our families for their support and patience.

Reviewers

Paul N Bennett
RN PhD MHSM MRCNA
Associate Professor, Graduate Programs Coordinator, School of Nursing and Midwifery, Flinders University of South Australia, Australia

Ailsa Munns
RN, RM, Cert Child Health, Bach Sc (Nursing), Master of Nursing, FRCNA
Lecturer, Course Coordinator, Postgraduate Child and Adolescent Health Program
School of Nursing and Midwifery, Curtin University, Australia

Heather Latham
M.N, B.Soc.Sci, DNE, RN, RM, Paed Cert, MRCNA
Undergraduate Courses Manager, School of Nursing, Midwifery and Indigenous Health
Charles Sturt University, Bathurst, Australia

Diana Guzys
RN, RM, BPubHlth, GradDipEd, GradDipAdolsntHlthWelf
Lecturer in Nursing, LaTrobe University, Bendigo, Australia

Judy Yarwood
RN, MA (Hons), Dip Tchg (Tertiary), FCNA (NZ)
Principal lecturer, School of Nursing and Human Services
Christchurch Polytechnic Institute of Technology, New Zealand

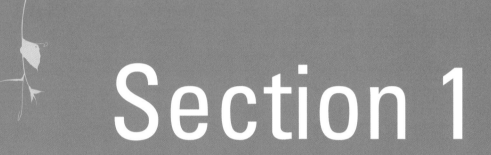

Section 1

Healthy people, healthy places

Chapter 1 **Health as a socio-ecological concept**
Chapter 2 **Primary health care: principles and practices**
Chapter 3 **Promoting health in an era of globalisation**
Chapter 4 **Enabling health and wellness: practice roles and models of care**

INTRODUCTION TO THE SECTION

The four chapters that introduce this text provide a foundation to help frame what we understand about communities in contemporary society, and how community health and wellness is achieved and maintained. Chapter 1 explains health as a socio-ecological concept; that is, how health and well-being is shaped through their interactions in the environments of people's lives. We also examine the integral concepts of community participation in creating and maintaining health, and the importance of *place* in health. A large part of nursing and midwifery work with communities is framed within our knowledge of the *social determinants of health* (SDOH). The chapters in Section 1 provide an in-depth examination of the SDOH, which is a major theme elaborated throughout the book.

As we outline in Chapter 2, for those of us advocating for community health, the principles of *primary health care* (PHC) continue to guide our activities. The PHC principles situate people's aspirations for health within an ethos of *social justice*. The challenge of PHC lies in promoting conditions that would provide *equity* and *access* to supports, care and services for all members of a community or a population. The strategies for achieving this are intersectoral collaboration, appropriate use of technology, and cultural sensitivity. These strategies are explained further in Chapter 2, as a way of promoting health in the settings of people's lives; healthy neighbourhoods, healthy schools, healthy workplaces and places of worship, healthy villages, cities and communities. Health promotion is aimed at developing *inclusive* communities, which are able to develop their capacity. Nurses and midwives assist this process using a *comprehensive primary health care* approach, which supports all aspects of community life, helping to conserve what is special and helpful, and assisting them in countering what is not. Other activities are aimed at *selective primary health care*, which is a more targeted approach, where specific groups or issues are given priority attention. The chapter also includes an explanation of other terms related to PHC, including primary care, and primary, secondary and tertiary *levels* of care, all of which are linked, but separate concepts.

Two critical, inter-related concepts are fundamental to inclusive communities: *empowerment* and *health literacy*. Community empowerment is possible when members of a community have genuine opportunities and support for health decision-making. Such decisions are informed by adequate, appropriate and useful knowledge; that is, health literacy. A health literate community is one where people are not only aware of the things that keep them healthy, but they feel confident and comfortable making choices that influence their health, and they are comfortable working with health professionals to improve their health and the health of their community.

Health literacy and community empowerment are illustrated throughout the section, and throughout the text, as central themes in health promotion. If people have a functional understanding of the reasons they are being urged to create a smoke-free environment, grow healthy foods for consumption, and lobby their local government for space to engage in a physically and socially vibrant lifestyle, they are more likely to participate in these aspects of healthy lifestyles. If they are able to access appropriate and accurate information on the internet to help alleviate any health problems, this can also be helpful. And when they are in the process of recovery from illness or rehabilitation, health literacy can help allay fears and anxieties by providing greater predictability in their pathway to better health. Importantly, members of health literate communities can become a resource for others who may need a greater understanding of the structural and SDOH as a basis for making appropriate choices for good health.

Chapter 3 extends the discussion of health promotion to the global community. Included is an examination of health information and the health issues that unite nurses and midwives across the world. In this era of rapid communication through technology, we hear much about the perils of the internet, and the constant texting and emails that enslave many of us in our daily work life. However, these tools have also brought us closer to the global community. We see examples on the internet of what works elsewhere in achieving health. The information we share across the globe also provides those of us in research with better tools, stronger evidence for health care, and a connection with like-minded people who also spend their lives nurturing communities. This can be professionally empowering, particularly if our interventions are based on research findings. Various aspects of electronic communications technology have a direct effect on health. For example, text messaging is currently being used for appointment reminders and as prompts for taking medications and other treatments. The technology is also a way of social connectedness, letting people know they are not alone, and where opportunities exist to socialise with others. However, there is also a downside to having so much information. Every day, people are bombarded by media advice, some of which they seek out, other which arrives in their lives surreptitiously or because it is a part of the kaleidoscope of community life. In the face of an information overload, people rely heavily on professional advice to guide them as they sift through the onslaught of messages, trying to make sense of information related to their health and lifestyle. As it is often said, we have too much information, not enough knowledge.

Certain aspects of contemporary life such as international travel have clearly entrenched the notion that we are all members of the global community, and this is also explored in Chapter 3. Those who seek novelty in far-off horizons quickly learn that community health is not only multidimensional, but *unique* in each setting. Being mindful of global health issues also helps us benchmark the health of our community in terms of PHC goals. Interactions within and between communities helps us understand the dynamics of global health risks such as those created by global warming. The effects of a warming planet have wreaked havoc on some communities, displacing people from their homes and exacerbating existing inequities. Knowing how these and other weather events can impinge on health heightens our awareness of the need to be globally inclusive, to work towards addressing the needs of the marginalised and vulnerable among us and those beyond our shores. Accepting the responsibility of nurses and midwives to promote health through political activism is a crucial and necessary response to the inequities caused by globalisation.

The path to achieving and enhancing community health also extends the 'think global, act local' catchcry of the last century, to the Millennium Development Goals, which urge us to counter poverty and ignorance, to feed, clothe and educate the vulnerable among us and to help eradicate the modern plagues, such as HIV/AIDS, malaria and other diseases. Such lofty initiatives compel us towards economy of effort; to plan strategically for health promotion and services to assist those most in need. Because there is such wide variability among people and the environments that shape their lives, our services must not only be multi-dimensional, but flexible and adaptable. In all communities, health is a careful balance between the capabilities, aspirations and health-related needs and goals of individuals, various groups of people, and the whole population. Given that these dynamic features of community health are intertwined within a myriad of contextual features, our work should be designed to help people manage their own lives. As Chapter 4 explains, we can become fully engaged with our community some of the time, and sit as a 'guide on the side' at other times, but always using our expertise and our evidence as resources to their efforts.

Healthy communities are dynamic, constantly changing as people respond to the circumstances of their life and their environments, and as they make decisions that help develop their community's health capacity. Positive interactions change environments, conserving what is precious, rejecting influences that could be destructive. In a perfect world, there would be no need for health professionals to meddle in these interactions, but we all live in situations that could be improved. As health professionals we can help inform community members about the political, economic and cultural conditions within which health can be developed. Our role in the community also involves acting as a resource, using our scientific knowledge to help promote and preserve health and treat illness. Chapter 4 also explores the advocacy role of nurses and midwives, suggesting that it is an ever-changing role, as we argue for service improvements, or for environmental and social changes that will help individuals flourish and grow.

Because PHC has become integral to professional practice in both Australia and New Zealand we examine the PHC roles in the context of various models of practice. Since 2001, New Zealand has been leading the world in policies and practices that embed PHC as a national strategy to promote population health. More recently, the combined nursing and midwifery organisations in Australia and findings from a number of national reviews have developed a consensus position that PHC is, in fact, the way to approach health improvements across demographic groups and across health service settings. In providing exemplars of good and best practice we provide a template for others to innovate and implement strategies to help communities reach their potential. Our new and existing roles and models of care are constantly shaped by the circumstances of community life. Competent enactment of our roles requires attention to these contexts and situations to establish a pathway towards excellence in enabling health and wellness through a holistic, partnership approach with the community.

Chapter 1

Health as a socio-ecological concept

INTRODUCTION

For most people, the notion of 'community' is a friendly term, conjuring up a sense of place, a sense of belonging. Healthy communities are those places where belonging is valued, where the connections between individuals, families and the environments of their lives are as important as the life forces within. This is essentially an ecological relationship. Ecology embodies the idea that everything is connected to everything else. Health is both a social and ecological phenomenon, in that it is created and maintained in the context of community life. Although as individuals we can experience relative states of health or ill health because of our biological makeup, these are manifest within the social ecology of a community. Health is therefore dynamic, changing as a function of the myriad interactions between biology and our genetic predispositions, and the psychological, social, cultural, spiritual and physical environments that surround us.

As health professionals our role spans across the health–illness continuum. The role of any community nurse, midwife, or other health professional ranges from preventing illness to protecting people from harm or worsening health once they have experienced illness, to recovery and rehabilitation. Community practice also involves a parallel role to protect communities from harm or stagnation, to help community citizens build capacity for future development, and to work in partnership with the population to restore their viability following any difficult times. Community health activities are therefore undertaken on many levels, for individuals, families, groups and entire communities.

> ### Point to ponder
> Health is dynamic — constantly changing as our biology and genetic predispositions interact with the psychological, social, cultural, spiritual and physical environments that we live in.

They include educating communities and governments on the structures and supports conducive to good health, minimising risks to ill health or injury, and guidance to support recovery and sustainable health. The basis for this type of work is a combination of foundational knowledge, having the intellectual curiosity to seek out and, in some cases, generate research evidence for interventions, and social engagement with the community. Together these equip the nurse, midwife or other health practitioner with the skills for ongoing surveillance and monitoring, intervention and evaluation strategies, and political advocacy to lobby for family and community resources and supports.

Promoting the health of any community is therefore a multifaceted role. It is based on the *holistic*, *socio-ecological* perspective of health. Its philosophical foundation is entrenched in the World Health Organization's (WHO) definition of health, where it is not seen as one-half of a dichotomy of health and illness, but 'a state of complete physical, mental and social wellbeing and not merely the absence of disease or infirmity' (WHO 1974:1). This definition of health also reflects the growing body of research evidence outlining the importance of the *social determinants of health* (SDOH). Researchers have found that the SDOH are even more influential on the health of the population than medical care, with studies showing the greatest health gains in the population over the past two centuries from changes in broad economic and social conditions (Commission on the Social Determinants of Health [CSDH] 2008; Graham 2004; Link & Phelan 2005). This chapter will examine the various SDOH, and some of the ways they influence the health of communities and the people who live in them. It will also address the important issue of health literacy. Health literacy is a major goal for practitioners working in community health.

Point to ponder
The World Health Organization defines health as 'a state of complete physical, mental and social wellbeing and not merely the absence of disease'.

A well-informed, health literate population can participate fully in making health-related decisions that affect their personal health and the health of their community. The chapter culminates in a discussion of the research base for good and best practice in working effectively with communities.

Research is an important element in planning to improve and maintain the health of any community, particularly research into the SDOH. Although some community practitioners are new to researching the basis of their interventions, nurses, midwives and others have been systematically collecting and using research data for centuries. As early as the 19th century Florence Nightingale carefully documented various factors associated with outbreaks of illness in her community. Years later, scholars from psychology, sociology and other scientific disciplines, joined medical, nursing, and other health professions in seeking to explain and theorise about health (Syme 2005). As health scholars around the world expanded their research knowledge, their studies became circumscribed by what is now called the 'McKeown thesis'. McKeown (1979) argued that medical care and technology were not responsible for improving health; the major improvements were due to social, environmental and economic changes, smaller family size, better nutrition, a healthier physical environment and a greater emphasis on

preventive care. However, there is little evidence on how these factors interact to influence health in particular communities. Clearly, research evidence on the SDOH is needed to underpin community interventions. Throughout this and other chapters in this book, we provide examples of a wide range of research studies to guide these interventions. By committing ourselves to this scholarly approach to practice it is possible that over time, many of the compromises to community health may be overcome, and new, effective strategies developed for the benefit of society and communities everywhere.

Point to ponder
We know that the major improvements in health over the past century are due to changes in social, environmental and economic conditions as well as smaller family size, better nutrition and a greater emphasis on preventive care. However, we need more research to demonstrate how these factors interact to influence health in communities.

At the end of this and other chapters, we provide an example of a research study into an issue relevant to community health. This is designed to provoke your thinking about the evidence base for practice, and how research can be used to optimise health. The case study for this chapter also introduces 'The Millers'. We'll ask you to complete a genogram of the family and ask that you consider their particular strengths and needs in the context of reflecting on the main issues covered in the chapter.

Objectives

By the end of this chapter you will be able to:

1 explain health, wellness, and community health as socio-ecological concepts
2 identify the social determinants and structures of health and wellness
3 examine the intergenerational factors that influence health
4 analyse the concept of social capital and its contribution to community health
5 examine the factors that influence community sustainability
6 explain the importance of health literacy in enhancing individual and community health capacity
7 investigate the role of research and evidence-based practice in promoting community health.

WHAT IS HEALTH?

As mentioned previously, health is a product of reciprocal interactions between individuals and their environments. Each of us brings to our environmental interactions a number of factors unique to us alone. These include the following:

- a personal history
- our biology as it has been established by heredity and moulded by early environments
- previous events that have affected our health, including past illnesses or injuries
- our nutritional status as it is currently, and its adequacy in early infancy
- stressors; both good and bad events in our lives that may have caused us to respond in various ways.

Clearly, health is multifaceted. Becoming and staying healthy 'depends on our ability to understand and manage the interaction between human activities and the physical and biological environment' (WHO 1992: 409).

Biological factors provide the foundation for an individual to develop as a relatively healthy person, which is an adaptive process. From birth, individuals are programmed to develop certain biologically preset behaviours (bio-behaviours) at critical and sensitive developmental periods. This 'biological embedding' influences how people interact with the genetic, social and economic contexts of their lives (Best et al 2003). However, the environments or *conditions* of a person's life shape biological factors and the way individuals respond to the world around them (Hertzman 2001; Hertzman & Power 2006). These include family and community characteristics, and aspects of the wider society that create opportunities or threats to health.

> **Point to ponder**
> Although biological factors provide the foundation for an individual to develop into a healthy person, the environment or conditions of a person's life shape these biological factors.

Social conditions are particularly important, because social environments provide the context for interactions in all other environments. When the social environment is supportive, creating a climate of trust and mutual respect a person is more likely to be *empowered*, in control of their life, and therefore their health. On the other hand, if their social situation is plagued by civil strife, an oppressive political regime, crime, poverty, unemployment, violence, discrimination, food insecurity, diseases or a lack of access to health and social support services they may be *disempowered*, leaving them less likely to become healthy or recover from illness when it occurs. These issues that arise from power imbalances and unfair societal structures create inequalities in health (Edwards & MacLean Davison 2008; Marmot 2006). This is because people who are living in disadvantaged or disempowered situations are unable to access the same resources for health as those who live in more privileged situations.

> **Point to ponder**
> When a social environment is supportive, a person will feel empowered. If a social environment is affected by such things as war, crime, unemployment or poor access to health services a person may feel disempowered.

HEALTH AND WELLNESS

Healthy people's lives are characterised by *balance* and *potential*. In a balanced state of health there is harmony between the physical, emotional, social and spiritual. When they are part of a healthy community there are opportunities for them to reach and maintain high levels of health or *wellness*. Wellness, as originally described by Dunn (1959) extends beyond health. In the community context, it reflects the dynamic relationship between people and their environment that arises when individuals use that environment to maintain balance and purposeful direction. This underlines the ecological nature of health and wellness. Contemporary definitions of health acknowledge the connectivity between people and the environment in two ways: first, health is dynamic rather than static, and second, the environment or context of people's lives influences the extent to which they can reach their health potential. For example, people feel they have lifestyle choices, and if they choose, they will be able to exercise or relax in safe spaces. They have access to nutritious foods; students balance study with recreation; young families immunise their children and have time out from work to socialise, and older people have opportunities to stay active and socialise with others.

Eckersley et al (2005) explain that optimism, trust, self-respect and autonomy make us happy and therefore create feelings of wellbeing. The importance of happiness has been acknowledged by many health scholars, who are now expanding their research agenda to explore the relationship between happiness and health (Baum 2009). This type of research can be linked back to the proposal in the 1970s by the King of Bhutan that instead of focusing only on gross domestic product (GDP), nations should be concerned with the ultimate purpose in life, which is happiness. He proposed a gross national happiness (GNH) index comprised of psychological wellbeing, the use of time, community vitality, culture, health, education, environmental diversity, living standard and governance (online www.grossnationalhappiness.cm/gnhIndex /introductionGNH.aspx 2). Since then, many initiatives have been developed to try to bring this balanced perspective of health into mainstream thinking. The Happy Planet Index, developed in the United Kingdom refocused wellbeing on the criteria of average life expectancy, life satisfaction and ecological footprint (Marks et al 2006). The Canadian Index of Wellbeing has also adopted this approach, computing measures of quality of life into social, economic and environmental trends in Canadian cities (Hancock 2009). All of these measures address social health, and they are based on the knowledge that happiness and wellbeing increase longevity and make immune systems more robust, which in many cases, improves health (Layard 2005).

The pursuit of happiness from a social perspective lies in contrast to the consumerism in society today that fosters and exploits a restless, insatiable expectation that we need more and more. Although most of us enjoy having something to strive for, consumer goods offer hollow outcomes. Instead, we may find higher levels of wellness in communities that allow people to live in a stable, democratic society, to enjoy the company of family and friends, to have rewarding work that yields sufficient income, to feel personal happiness with the ability to address any mental health problems, to set goals related to common values, and to have some means of attaining guidance, purpose and meaning (Diener & Seligman 2004). This illustrates a clear link between personal and community wellness; in other words, a level of harmony between health and place.

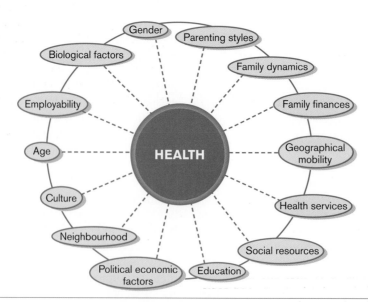

Figure 1.1 Interactions between factors affecting health

DEFINING 'COMMUNITY' AND 'COMMUNITY HEALTH'

In the most basic terms, the word *community* simply means that which is common. We often think of a community as the physical or geographical place we share with others, or the place from which care is delivered (Crooks & Andrews 2009). However, an *ecological* view focuses on the community as an *interdependent* group of plants and animals inhabiting a common space. People depending on one another, interacting with each other and with aspects of their environment, distinguish a living community from a collection of inanimate objects. Communities are thus dynamic entities that pulsate with the actions and interactions of people, the spaces they inhabit and the resources they use. Healthy communities are the *synthesis* or product of people interacting with their environments. This is an evolutionary concept, in that community health is 'a dynamic and evolving process' (Baisch 2009:2467). It is created by people working collaboratively to shape and develop the community in a way that will help them achieve positive health outcomes. A 'healthy community' is one of those positive outcomes. Community health is defined as follows:

> Community health is grounded in philosophical beliefs of social justice and empowerment. Dynamic and contextual, community health is achieved through participatory, community development processes based on ecological models that address broad determinants of health.
>
> (Baisch 2009:2472)

Point to ponder

An ecological definition of community focuses on a community as a group of people who are dependent on one another and who inhabit a common space.

Healthy communities have a number of common qualities as outlined in Box 1.1.

COMMUNITY HEALTH AND WELLNESS

Community wellness (or wellbeing) refers to an optimal quality of community life, one that meets people's needs and that creates harmony and social justice within a vibrant, sustainable community

BOX 1.1 QUALITIES OF A HEALTHY COMMUNITY

1 Clean and safe physical environment.
2 Peace, equity and social justice.
3 Adequate access to food, water, shelter, income, safety, work and recreation for all.
4 Adequate access to health care services.
5 Opportunities for learning and skill development.
6 Strong, mutually supportive relationships and networks.
7 Workplaces that are supportive of individual and family wellbeing.
8 Wide participation of residents in decision-making.
9 Strong local cultural and spiritual heritage.
10 Diverse and vital economy.
11 Protection of the natural environment.
12 Responsible use of resources to ensure long term sustainability.

(Online: http://www.ohcc-ccso.ca/en//what-makes-a-healthy-community)

(Rural Assist Information Network [RAIN] 2009; The Ian Potter Foundation 2009). The Government of Victoria (2009) identifies a number of priorities that promote community wellbeing. These include having governments that are responsive to the needs of new communities, building community capacity through a sense of belonging, working towards economic developments to sustain the population, and creating safe environments with opportunities for healthy activity, recreation and social interaction. These are essential characteristics of community health.

As members of a community, our lives are closely interwoven with the lives of others, some

Point to ponder

The essential characteristics of community health include having governments that are responsive to the needs of communities, building capacity through a sense of belonging, providing for economic development to sustain the population, and creating safe environments that encourage healthy activity, recreation and social interaction.

of whom live in close proximity to us; others who share common characteristics but do not inhabit our geographical space.

We also hold membership in various population groups on the basis of gender, age, physical capacity or culture. In the context of all of these group memberships, we interact with a moveable feast of other richly diverse communities. To these interactions we bring our own individuality; the combination of genetic predispositions, history, knowledge, attitudes, preferences and perceptions of capacity. Each community, in turn, brings to each of its members a set of distinct environments: physical, psychological, social, spiritual and cultural. Our socio-ecological interactions shape a characteristic community character, which determines the extent to which community members will become a cohesive entity. Each of these interactions, whether with our families, social groups or our physical environment, transforms the community as well as its residents. Bandura (1977) called this *reciprocal determinism*. By reciprocal determinism he meant that both the behaviours of people and the characteristics of their environments are determined by the set of dynamic exchanges between them.

Ecological exchange can yield both constraints and enhancements to personal and community health. Some of the more familiar constraints on health and wellbeing arise from the effects of contaminants in the physical environment, such as air and water pollution, infectious diseases and/or injury. Some degree of risk to health and wellbeing is also present in the social environment; in the workplace, school and neighbourhood. Interactions with our environment in recreation, education and social interchange present opportunities for achieving higher levels of health and wellbeing. Interactions between community members and the health care system are also imbued with challenges and opportunities for illness prevention and health improvements. For those of us whose role involves helping people achieve and maintain good health and protection from illness or injury, it is important to understand the effects of these interactions.

Point to ponder

Reciprocal determinism is simply the combination of what an individual brings to a community, what a community brings to the individual, and how these interact.

Like individuals, communities are open to a variety of interpretations. If you were to ask 'How healthy is the community in which I live?' a number of issues might come up. To gain at least a cursory view of the community you could look around at the geography. You might find yourself in a small town with plenty of vegetable gardens, well-kept houses, playgrounds and sporting fields, a community centre complete with child-minding facilities, a mix of healthy looking young and older people on the streets, none of whom are smoking, and public transportation. A very different picture may emerge if you cast your gaze to an inner-city neighbourhood where children play on the streets between parked cars, ramshackle buildings loom skyward with broken windows punctuating the places where people live, cars hoon around the corners, no older people walk the streets, and children seem to be tending to younger children with no adults supervising their activities. A vastly different community might emerge the further you get from the city. Depending on which continent you were in, you might find starving babies suffering from rampant disease, or Indigenous people smoking around a campfire, or an isolated farmer, too poor to either heat his frozen house or cool a sweltering one, reacting to his frustration by abusing his wife and children. Or, you might find happy, contented families, enjoying the fruits of their toils, whether on the land or in the city.

In each of the situations mentioned above, you could jump to a number of conclusions about the way the physical environment enhanced or impeded the health of the community. But in each community, a set of unseen influences lies just below the physical surface. For example, the small town may be comfortably situated in a place where everyone wanting employment has a job, because of a political decision taken some time previously to relocate a manufacturing company there. The playgrounds and sporting fields may be a product of a community development program and a workplace policy that provides flexible working hours so parents can take their children to sports. A local non-denominational church may have been built to double as a respite centre for carers, or a mothers group, or some other activity that keeps adults connected with one another. The schools may be well resourced because a government body has decreed that children should not be disadvantaged irrespective of where they live. In contrast, the inner-city neighbourhood may be neglected by government policies, with inadequate educational facilities. Young mothers raising children alone may be working swing shifts, leaving young children in the care of other children. Vandals may be receiving no deterrents because of a lack of funding for social policies, perhaps because military spending takes precedence over social services and local policing. In the rural area, a farming community may be suffering from the lack of markets for their produce, or have no chance of fertilising their lands to grow produce in the first place because of conservation policies. They may also be disadvantaged by natural disasters such as drought, or be vulnerable to mortgage lenders, substandard places to shelter, or unemployment. These aspects of community life are considered SDOH.

> **What's your opinion?**
> How healthy is the community you live in? What factors make it healthy? What factors make it less healthy?

SOCIAL DETERMINANTS OF HEALTH

The SDOH consist of a number of overlapping factors that determine health and wellbeing. These include factors that begin at birth, such as biology and genetic characteristics, gender, culture and various family influences on healthy child development. Family influences include having socio-economic resources for parents to provide for their child, parenting knowledge and skills, a peaceful family life and adequate support systems. Social support networks that are inclusive across genders, cultures and educational opportunities are also social determinants.

> **Point to ponder**
> The SDOH are a number of overlapping social and physical factors that contribute to health and wellbeing.

Support systems influence a person's ability to cope with life's stressors, and to make decisions about personal health practices that either prevent illness or maintain health. Other social determinants are a function of interactions between the individual, family and community, such as having a healthy and supportive neighbourhood, with adequate transportation and spaces for recreation, being able to access food and water, and services

for health and child care when they're needed, and having employment opportunities with good working conditions and sufficient income. Many of these determinants are embedded in the political and economic environment, where policy decisions affecting community life are made.

Within the SDOH are a number of structural conditions. For example, a community's social development needs structures to create employment opportunities, and a physical environment that supports healthy lifestyles and personal health practices. People need access to clean air, water and nutritious foods at a reasonable cost. They also need to have reasonable working conditions so that they can achieve a work–life balance. Other structures in the social environment that support health and wellbeing include health and social support services such as hospitals, medical practitioners, nurses and other allied health professionals who are accessible where and when they are needed. Structural supports for health also include government services that provide income protection in the case of unemployment, infrastructure such as safe roads and public transportation, and schools, playgrounds and adult recreational facilities that offer the opportunity for holistic health and wellbeing. Socio-political structures include equitable systems of governance over the community and society, to ensure preservation of resources through wise economic choices and a commitment to conservation; fairness in allocating resources across all groups in the population, and systems that protect people from harm or disempowerment.

The diagram in Figure 1.2 illustrates the social and structural determinants of health from a socio-ecological perspective. The metaphor of a cascade of bubbles is used to show the dynamic interaction between factors (Wilcox 2007). Each bubble interfaces with many others, and if one bubble is displaced or happens to pop, there is a cascade effect, where the surface tension and connectivity of the others are changed. One bubble may be directly influenced by an adjacent bubble, but it is also indirectly influenced by that bubble's connections to other surfaces. The bubbles may also merge and increase or decrease in size or in relation to one another. If there are changes in the wider environment, such as policy changes or a major environmental change, all bubbles may be affected or even disappear. In terms of the metaphor it would be like blowing air across the entire cascade or changing the water flow (Wilcox 2007).

The 'social determinants' approach to health resonates with the notion of human rights and social justice. Social justice refers to the 'fair distribution of society's benefits, responsibilities and their consequences' (Edwards & MacLean Davison 2008:130). This means that as health professionals, we have an obligation to identify unfairness or inequities, and their underlying determinants, advocating for human rights, and working towards just economic, social and political institutions (Edwards & MacLean Davison 2008; Whitehead 2007).

> **Point to ponder**
> Social justice occurs when the benefits, responsibilities and consequences of society are equally and fairly distributed between people.

Equitable, socially just conditions in our communities and society are a matter of life and death, affecting the way people live, their chances of becoming ill or their risk of premature death (CSDH 2008). In 2005, recognising the human rights implications of good health and the role of social determinants in supporting health and wellbeing, the WHO assembled an international Commission on Social Determinants of Health (CSDH). The Commission represents 19 countries, including Australia. After gathering information for 3 years, members met to consider global progress on eliminating disparities in health and how to encourage a more equitable social world.

The commissioners were united in three concerns: their passion for social justice, their respect for evidence and their frustration with a lack of progress on global responses to the SDOH (CSDH 2008). They recommended that governments everywhere take up the challenge of working with health and other organisations to improve health for the world's citizens. This involves reframing health services in terms of primary health care (PHC), ensuring sufficient health professionals to provide care, addressing economic issues, overcoming inequitable, exploitative, unhealthy and dangerous working conditions, including restoration of work–life balance for families, and providing social protection for all people across the life course (CSDH 2008). These overarching goals urge us to act in concert with members of our communities, igniting our passion for health and social justice and combining it with research that will build better understanding of what works, where, for what populations, with what outcomes.

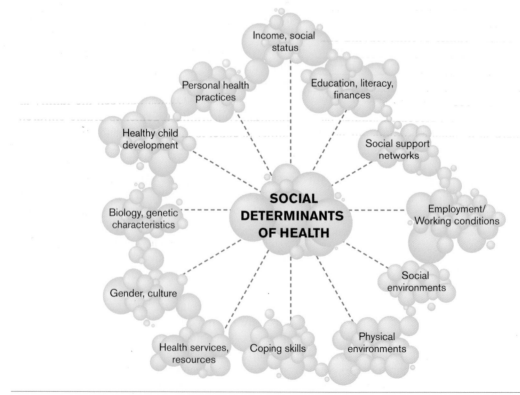

Figure 1.2 Social and structural determinants of health

Point to ponder
Governments worldwide are starting to recognise the importance of the SDOH in achieving health for all people.

THE ROLE OF COMMUNITIES IN INTERGENERATIONAL HEALTH

The quality of community health often changes dramatically over time to influence the way people grow and develop. For some, an ideal mix of conditions can create a positive start to life that becomes sustained into adulthood and throughout ageing. This is a 'life course' approach to understanding health. Improvements to the SDOH (housing, employment opportunities, transportation or social services) can provide optimal conditions in which all family members flourish and maintain good health over time. For others, a disadvantaged start to life may not be overcome by sufficient changes in any of the environments affecting their lives. So changing circumstances can create either threats or opportunities to health and well-being. For example, some physical environments have become transformed by global warming and droughts, creating natural disasters such as flooding, fires and other weather events, leaving entire families at risk of homelessness. For those already disadvantaged by poverty, discrimination or a lack of social support this can perpetuate ill health.

The family's socio-economic status is an important determinant of health. Research studies have shown that there is a 'social gradient' in health, whereby those employed at successively higher levels have better health than those on lower levels (Navarro 2009; Hertzman & Power 2006). This creates disadvantage from birth for some children. A child born into a lower socio-economic family for example, may be destined for an impoverished life, creating intergenerational ill health. This child lives in a situation of 'double-jeopardy', where interactions between the SDOH conspire against good health. Without external community supports the family may spiral into worsening circumstances, affecting their child's opportunities for the future. This is the case for many Indigenous people, whose parents have not had access to adequate employment or community supports that would sustain their own health, much less that of their children. They become caught in a cycle of vulnerability where the SDOH interact in a way that creates disempowerment across generations. Political decisions governing employment opportunities may hamper the parents' ability to improve finances.

Point to ponder
A 'social gradient' exists in health. That is, those who are employed or earn income at successively higher levels have better health than those who are unemployed or have lower levels of income.

A less than optimal physical environment may deprive both parents and the child of a chance to access social groups or gatherings. There may be few opportunities for education, health care or transportation to access services. Parenting skills may be absent for a range of reasons, including younger age, the lack of role modelling, geographic disadvantage or illness. Discrimination in the immediate environment can worsen the effects of any of these factors.

Alternatively, families who are able to garner sufficient resources and external supports to cope with difficulties or traumas may be able to overcome multiple challenges throughout their lifetime, creating a more optimistic outlook for their child's health. This can be accomplished within empowering partnerships between the family and community working together to cradle children's ability to cope, to grow and to learn (Li et al 2008). Clearly, the presence and adequacy of community services and supports are a matter of concern to all members of society, not just those who are parenting a child. Health professionals can help by promoting *civic engagement*, working in partnership with community members to lobby for fairness and democratic participation in economic and political decisions.

Point to ponder
Interventions that promote health across generations such as education, nurturing and anticipatory guidance can help overcome the hazards of being born into relatively deprived situations.

Throughout the world, nurses, midwives and other health professionals have begun to draw attention to the issues of intergenerational health. Researchers are now investigating how influences such as education, nurturing and anticipatory guidance can help overcome the health hazards of being born into a relatively deprived social situation (Hertzman & Power 2006; Laperriere 2008; Osberg & Sharpe 2006). There is also a growing body of knowledge suggesting a range of beneficial outcomes for individuals who participate in community programs that foster greater connectedness between the generations (Fujiwara et al 2009; Chung 2009; de Souza & Grundy 2007). With greater understanding, societies will be better equipped to make decisions that will support and sustain good health, even for those who are disadvantaged from birth. This is integral to the notion of social capital.

SOCIAL CAPITAL

When the health of the community is defined from a social perspective we acknowledge its *social capital*. Like *economic capital,* social capital is an accumulation of wealth, but it is the kind of wealth that draws people together as a cohesive force in a climate of trust and mutual respect (Putnam 2005). Putnam (1995) first described the value of social capital in terms of developing civic engagement, trust, and norms of reciprocity among community members. Communities become strong when people are connected through networks, associations, and any other means of sharing information and a sense of purpose. Information flows through the community in many directions, people are compelled to help others for mutual benefit, and they are more likely to participate in democratic institutions, thereby improving their accountability. When this type of climate pervades community life there is a greater likelihood of people realising shared goals and bonding together to become resilient to economic, social and environmental changes (Ontario Health Communities Coalition [OHCC] 2009).

Point to ponder

Social capital exists when a sense of trust, engagement, participation and a sense of belonging is present in a community.

Social capital is therefore a mechanism to help communities cope with adversity and limitations, as well as to build a positive sense of place. It is not just connecting people so they will be pressured into participating in healthy lifestyles or a common set of behaviours, but promoting a sense of cohesiveness, a network of social support and a sense of belonging (Nakhaie et al 2007). This can be empowering, creating equality of opportunities, regardless of age, gender, culture or other aspects of birthright. It can also shift people's expectations of their lives, improving mental health as well as the overall quality of community life (Baum et al 2000; Ziersch et al 2005).

A community may have the disadvantage of isolation, or few natural resources conducive to health, yet community attitudes and actions that bring people together can help strengthen *health capacity* (Aston et al 2009). Community health capacity can also be supported by organisational structures, such as schools, workplaces and community planning mechanisms that include participatory decision-making. Together, members of the community can use their collective voice to lobby for services such as health care, transportation, family-friendly education and job re-training, opportunities for physical activities, and community policing. With each successful action, there is a greater likelihood of building the capacity for subsequent developments. In this way communities can work from the ground up to respond to the SDOH, addressing inequalities and working towards a more inclusive society (CSDH 2008; Raphael et al 2008).

Examples of programs that help build social capital are those that unite people in developing opportunities, those that galvanise community action to preserve the environment, to undertake participatory school reform, or bring local businesses together to take steps to end discrimination. When communities draw members together to pursue these types of goals they develop community vitality, a capacity to thrive and change, and greater respect and inclusiveness. This is the key to empowerment (OHCC 2009). It is based on the premise that if people are prepared for events or circumstances with both information and community support systems, they can control their destiny by participating in decision-making and developing appropriate conditions for living and working (Aston et al 2009; Green et al 2004).

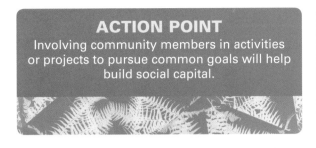

ACTION POINT
Involving community members in activities or projects to pursue common goals will help build social capital.

Point to ponder
A sustainable community is one that is bound by a common commitment to conserve the physical, social and cultural resources that exist within the community.

SUSTAINABLE COMMUNITY HEALTH

In those communities where there is a relatively healthy environment, and a sense of connectedness, or social capital, people tend to work together towards making the community sustainable. *Sustainable communities* are those that work towards *conservation* and *diversity* of personal and physical resources. This means that the community is bound by a common commitment to conserve not only its natural habitat, but all aspects of its diverse physical, social and cultural environment. There are several ways people can be encouraged to focus on community sustainability. One approach is to collaborate with local education, health, recreation, sporting and business groups to ensure that the younger generation develops an affinity with their physical and social environments. This involves ensuring that all citizens are aware of the strengths and resources particular to their community. Another measure is to use the broader systems that govern the community to advocate for public participation in creating and sustaining health. This can be as simple as voting, or as time consuming as spearheading a community action movement to ensure equitable distribution of natural, economic and social resources in a way that does not compromise the ability of future generations to meet their own needs (Kickbusch 2008). Community action may also involve becoming sufficiently informed to participate in scientific debates surrounding water, food and energy use; for example through libraries or websites such as those listed at the end of the chapter. Other ecological activities include such things as lobbying local, state or federal governments for initiatives to conserve the physical environment (such as recycling systems), or using the media to communicate to the local community the impact of local conservation (or destruction) to the wider arena.

Newspapers, magazines and the electronic media provide access to deliberations taking place at the major environmental meetings, including international summits sponsored by the United Nations (UN), the WHO, or scientific meetings on implementing strategies to preserve local environments. Because not all members of a community have access to or an interest in reading about global initiatives, it may be up to health care professionals to provide information and awareness on these issues. This extends conservation and diversity to the local social agendas. Community action in this context may range from drawing public attention to the links between poverty and health, lobbying for all educational facilities to have equal resources, to advocating for programs that acknowledge the contribution of diverse cultural groups to community life.

Sustainability in community health can be taken to mean that the community has a type of health–illness *carrying capacity*; that is, all the health resources it needs and the capacity to respond to all the illness it produces (Lowe 1994). This represents an ideal, as yet an unattainable goal, as no one country has been able to produce all the goods and services it needs to sustain its people. There is global recognition of the need to preserve the planet, and many people are aware that as the world's population continues to increase rapidly, our natural resources are becoming seriously degraded (Howat & Ritchie 2004). Global warming is the top issue on the global environment agenda, and the scientific community believes that climate change will lead to irreparable damage of the earth's ecosystems (McMichael 2005). It is ironic that people are living longer these days because of economic and technological developments, yet it is these very developments that have exploited, and thus degraded the environment so necessary to their survival (Howat & Ritchie 2004). In 2008, the WHO convened a group of eminent health researchers, practitioners, donors and representatives of global agencies to identify the research agenda for the immediate future. This group generated six key themes to be addressed as a matter of urgency (see Box 1.2).

What's your opinion?
Economic and technological developments have led to people living longer, healthier lives in many countries; however these developments have also led to global warming and damage to the earth's ecosystems. How do we balance these things to create sustainability?

Clearly there is a role for intervention and sustainability research at both the local and global levels. Just as land and water shortages have caused forced migration, wars, urbanisation and poverty have driven people all over the world to assimilate into foreign cultures. As a result, the world has lost languages and culturally diverse elements that have historically maintained cohesion and trust. In some cases, the fear of protecting borders from refugees and other migrants has had the effect of disempowering some cultures. This in itself is a health hazard, as the disappearance of cultures and traditional ways of life have left whole communities without an understandable means

BOX 1.2 URGENT AREAS OF ENVIRONMENTAL RESEARCH

1 Place climate change on the health agenda in terms of health equity to reduce the burden of climate-sensitive health outcomes, such as infectious diseases and air pollution.

2 Develop studies of policy-relevant risk assessment to inform strategies to help vulnerable populations that have been displaced by environmental hazards such as degradation of water supplies.

3 Evaluate the cost-effectiveness of protective measures.

4 Investigate intersectoral decisions, and how mechanisms such as carbon pricing, and household conservation efforts such as use of wastewater affect health.

5 Improve surveillance to enhance operational effectiveness of various measures.

6 Study the economic outcomes of proposed mitigation and adaptation measures (Campbell-Lendrum et al 2009).

of sustaining health or avenues for communicating with others. Their cultural disempowerment is therefore an important factor in determining the extent to which the communities in which they live will be able to develop health capacity.

The political landscape of the past two decades has ruthlessly favoured economic development over social development, and rendered many of our communities unsustainable. The outcomes of this are evident in urban communities where cities stretch endlessly along coastlines and borderlines, swallowing up small communities and economic migrants with inadequate infrastructure to support them (Howat & Ritchie 2004).

Point to ponder
Political emphasis on economic development over social development has rendered many communities unsustainable.

In some of these new, hastily formed communities, untenable lifestyle choices bombard young people with confusing choices. The global financial crisis of 2009 made their choices more intense, as young, urban families throughout the world have had to confront unemployment. Farming communities suffered from increased petrol taxes and lower profits. And charitable agencies found it more difficult to raise funds to help them. Communities of the future will have to work out ways to reverse the destruction of their physical and social resources to survive (Howat & Ritchie 2004). The key to overcoming these risks lies in greater empowerment of community members to find local, sustainable solutions and a sense of control to participate in successful, collective political action for community development (Bruni et al 2008). This includes helping people value their sense of 'place', which 'moulds people through their histories and geographies', integrating their collective histories, cultures, capital, economics, ethnicity, religion and other social factors (Tunstall et al 2004:7).

COMMUNITY DEVELOPMENT: HELPING COMMUNITIES CHANGE

Five key principles are instrumental in community development, as indicated in Box 1.3.

BOX 1.3 PRINCIPLES IN COMMUNITY DEVELOPMENT

1 Ensuring services are empowering; that is, applied with dignity and cultural sensitivity.

2 Using connective processes to ensure the basic goal is a caring, purposeful group.

3 Organisational actions should be focused on altering structural conditions to prevent isolation and/or self-blame among community members.

4 Collaborative strategies are employed to help clarify the task and empower the community in terms of their purpose and vision of the community.

5 Advocacy means challenging the status quo to help people become empowered even when there are conflicts or ambiguous issues (Labonte 2005).

Each of these principles is grounded in our human rights and social justice agenda. Together, they reflect a set of values that include the expectation that people will learn and change, and in the inherent value of community participation. One of the challenges of community development is to ensure that health professionals do not impose their agenda on the community. Instead, members of the community should decide what they wish to change, what services they need to assist change, and what support mechanisms are required to maintain the change. The role of the health professional is to provide information and opportunities for dialogue with others so that the community can take a leadership role in developmental planning (Aston et al 2009). The ultimate objective is to foster *community competence*. This places us as health professionals in an advocacy role, helping communities construct pathways to change on different levels. As social advocates, we adopt a respectful and culturally sensitive approach, shifting the balance of power to the community. As political advocates, we bring knowledge about the health and welfare systems to the table and help link people together to access resources. As professional advocates, we have an obligation to stay abreast of new knowledge and strategies that will help us maintain professional competence as well as solidarity with others. These processes are developmental in that by working together, people's skills, knowledge and self-confidence are developed, ultimately empowering them to go on to the next undertaking.

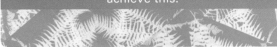

ACTION POINT

For communities to be able to take a leadership role in their own development, the health professional must provide information and opportunities for the community to achieve this.

Facilitating and enabling this type of change in communities also helps develop the skills of the health professional. Each community and the strategies it uses for capacity development is unique, so every opportunity to work with a community yields new information that the health professional can use to consolidate and refine health promotion skills. In this respect, advocacy is reciprocally determined; a deliberate two-way process of mutual development where knowledge is shared freely. One of the most important outcomes of sharing knowledge is the development of health literacy.

Health literacy

Health literacy is the ability to make sound health decisions in everyday life. Some decisions may be related to health care, but others may be lifestyle choices, decisions that improve quality of life, or that help in understanding civic responsibilities or opportunities. Health literacy is an important element in addressing health inequities, as those at the lower levels of health literacy are often the ones who live in socio-economically disadvantaged communities. Being unaware of information relevant to improving their health, or how to access health resources creates higher levels of disadvantage. For some people, a lack of education and the health literacy that would flow from education prevents them from becoming empowered at any time during their lives. For many women especially, low health literacy prevents them from adequate personal health and from ensuring their family's access to good nutrition, freedom from illness and exercising their own potential.

Point to ponder

Health literacy is the ability to make sound health decisions in everyday life.

A health literate person is able to participate in both public and private dialogues about health, medicine, scientific knowledge and their relation to society and culture (Zarcadoolas et al 2005). It is empowering to be able to make decisions that provide greater control, that help people interact as full participants in clinical situations and preventative care, and navigate the health care system (Coulter et al 2008; Kickbusch 2008; White 2008). Since health literacy became part of our research agenda in the 1990s, studies have found strong links between literacy and overall health and wellbeing (Kickbusch 2008). A concept analysis of health literacy revealed that it includes not only cognitive abilities such as problem-solving and decision-making, but social and cultural skills (Mancuso 2008). Health literate people are able to gather, analyse and evaluate health information when they have the capacity, comprehension and communication skills to make informed choices, reduce health risks, and increase the quality of their lives (Mancuso 2008). Researchers have also found an association between low literacy and health inequalities, with those having low levels of literacy experiencing poorer health and higher rates of hospitalisation than those with higher literacy (Coulter et al 2008; White 2008).

Having adequate health literacy promotes people's engagement in health care and other aspects of social life, which has clinical and economic benefits to society (Coulter et al 2008). Clinical benefits include smoother encounters in the processes of diagnosis and treatment of illness, better adherence to prescribed treatments and medications, and better understanding of instructions given by health providers. When people are engaged with their health services they tend to undertake more self-care and management, select appropriate treatments, and are better at monitoring their health and safety issues (Coulter et al 2008). Understanding how to navigate the health care system provides insight into bureaucratic processes associated with health insurance, admission to or discharge from hospital, and knowing the types of care they can expect to receive from a range of practitioners. Because health literate people tend to have healthier lifestyles they are more likely to engage in preventative activities, which not only improve their quality of life but reduce health care costs (Coulter et al 2008; White 2008). In this respect health literacy is a resource for living; a personal, community and societal asset that is integral to capacity building, citizenship and feelings of self-worth (Green et al 2007; Nutbeam 2008; Peerson & Saunders 2009).

Point to ponder
People with low levels of literacy experience poorer health and higher rates of hospitalisation than those with higher levels of literacy.

Three levels of health literacy have been identified by Nutbeam (2000) (see Table 1.1). *Functional health literacy* means that individuals have received sufficient factual information on health risks and health services, which they also understand, and which allows them to function effectively in a health context (Coulter et al 2008; Nutbeam 2000). They need to be able to read consent forms, medicine labels, and other written health care information. They also need to be able to understand and act on both verbal and written instructions from health care practitioners, pharmacists and insurers (Kickbusch 2001). At a second level, *communicative* or *interactive health literacy* develops personal skills to the extent that community members participate in community life, influencing social norms and helping others develop their personal health capacity. This involves understanding how organisations work, and communicating with others in the context of self-help or other support groups, as well as knowing how to get the services they need.

The third level of literacy, *critical health literacy* is where people use cognitive skills to improve individual resilience to social and economic adversity. This paves the way for community leadership structures to support community action and to facilitate community development (Nutbeam 2000). At a personal level critical health literacy is an enabling factor, developing capacity for confident, empowered interactions with others, including members of the health professions (Nutbeam 2008).

Point to ponder
The three levels of health literacy are functional, communicative (or interactive) and critical.

The fundamental element in critical health literacy is the community members' commitment to

Table 1.1 Health literacy: a continuum of knowledge and skill development

Functional	Communicative/ interactive	Critical	Civic
Knowledge to choose	Ability to influence	Skills for action	Capable of community action

working together to overcome structural barriers to health, which recognises the role of health literacy in creating awareness of the SDOH (Coulter et al 2008; Nutbeam 2008). Examples of outcomes include workers exerting pressure on workplaces to reduce hazardous risks, or lobby groups gathering support for environmental preservation, or supportive resources for parenting practices or health services. In each of these examples, the community is demonstrating critical health literacy. In some respects, this is also *civic literacy* in that community members actively participate in community life to find collective solutions to health problems. This emphasises the importance of the context for communication (Nutbeam 2008). Progression between the three levels of health literacy depends on a person's cognitive development, exposure to different forms of communication and the content (Nutbeam 2008).

The key objectives of health literacy interventions are to provide information and education, to encourage appropriate and effective use of health resources, to engage people in health decision-making, and to tackle health inequalities through empowerment (Coulter et al 2008; Peerson & Saunders 2009). To help people read, understand, evaluate and use health information requires an understanding of how people learn. This varies according to age, class, cultural group, gender, beliefs, preferences and coping strategies, and experience with the health system. Some differences also emerge as a function of their general literacy level, first language, skills and abilities (Coulter et al 2008). Health professionals can help people who may be only minimally health literate by understanding the scope of the problem. Those with low levels of literacy don't always reveal this, as they may be ashamed at their lack of understanding or reading skills. For this reason, health teaching should be sensitive to those who may have lesser understanding than others. Yet current research shows that printed health materials remain difficult for many people to understand (Shieh & Hosei 2008).

Anticipating people's needs at specific decision-making milestones is also important. Information should be not only appropriate, but timely, relevant and reliable, especially the type of material a person might access in a health care setting (Coulter et al 2008). Written health information tailored to individual needs has been found to help reinforce professionals' explanations of health problems, but used alone, it is not always understood. Computer-based information may be more helpful than written instructions, as it is more readily tailored to different needs. However, access to computers can be a problem for disadvantaged people (Coulter et al 2008). A review of the research has found that when they do have access, those from disadvantaged groups tend to benefit more from computer-based support interventions (Coulter et al 2008).

To date, there is a growing awareness of the need for health literacy throughout the world (Nutbeam 2008). South Australia has taken the lead in Australia by forming a Health Literacy Alliance comprised of health and social service personnel, including educators, librarians, representatives from the refugee network, and WorkCover (Kickbusch 2008).

ACTION POINT

People with low levels of health literacy may not reveal this to the health professional. It is important to ensure accurate assessment of a person's level of health literacy before providing any health teaching.

Their goal is to provide leadership and support for achieving equity through health literacy. Kickbusch (2008) also suggests that health literacy become a key indicator of good hospital care and general practice. This would see hospitals and clinics develop self-assessment skills in communicating health information and making their environments literacy-friendly. She also suggests strengthening health literacy in school education programs, to the extent of granting educational credits for health literacy. Her recommendations also include special attention to the needs of Indigenous people and migrant groups who often have greater vulnerability because of language and literacy problems (Kickbusch 2008). The New South Wales Clinical Excellence Commission also advocates including health literacy in the health research agenda (Smith & McCaffery 2010). Some work has already been undertaken to develop a screening tool that will help identify and measure the level of difficulty people may be having in understanding health information such as food labelling information (Smith & McCaffery 2010). This type of research will be extended in future to provide greater clarification of an individual's specific information needs. As nurses and midwives our responsibility also lies in filtering information for people seeking our assistance. For the internet-savvy population in our 'googlised' society, we need to develop more sophisticated approaches, as a large component of the information found on the internet often lacks moral guidance (Ratzan 2002, 2007). To encourage community participation people need to know that their health professionals value their knowledge and decisions, and will help ensure the accuracy of health information by keeping abreast of new research findings. Figure 1.3 provides a set of strategies recommended by the US Department of Health and Human Services for promoting health literacy.

Health literacy research is still in its infancy, although the area is now attracting growing attention with measures of health literacy being developed in the US, Canada and the UK (Nutbeam 2008). Some have focused on improving health literacy through interactive television, audio-tapes, text-messages and web-based information, with mixed results, but these media have been found to have the advantage of improving confidence and ability to participate in decision-making (Coulter et al 2008; Nutbeam 2008). American researchers have undertaken the first national study of health literacy as a basis for health promotion and disease prevention (White 2008). This has created the impetus for further studies to investigate health literacy across different contexts, different groups, and different baseline levels. There remains an important need for further research to generate a body of robust evidence to support patient decision-making. Coulter et al (2008) report that this work is continuing

with more than 500 evidence-based tools available internationally. These patient-friendly tools use a variety of media and help patients review the evidence on different treatments, so they can work out their preferences and make appropriate decisions (Ottawa Health Research Institute Online. Available: www.ohri.ca/decisionaid/ accessed 8 July 2009).

RESEARCH TO PRACTICE

The need for ongoing, systematic research as a foundation for practice has never been more acute. The world is changing, and as health professionals we need to investigate the way to help communities access information and resources that will do the most good in sustaining their future. This was acknowledged in an international meeting of government and research groups held in 2008, to discuss how research could help advance population health (McKee 2008). Those attending the meeting put forward a collective request for countries throughout the world to allocate at least 2% of their annual budgets on health research. The objective of this was to advance the notion that policies, practices and decisions at all levels of society should be based on research evidence (McKee 2008). This aspiration may not eventuate, especially in poorer countries, but it does signal a coming of age of the evidence-based practice (EBP) agenda. At the global level health research can help us better understand environmental changes such as the effects of global warming on the planet, and how shortages of water, food and space affect community life.

The EBP movement is based on the notion that providing research evidence for all activities in the health professions ensures accountability to the population for clinical decision-making and interventions (McMurray 2004). Research evidence collected according to the rules of EBP is typically used as a basis for justifying or changing practice, and we discuss this further in Chapter 12. Although objective, scientific evidence is important it can also obscure the subjective elements that are part of human enquiry (Morrison et al 2008).

Point to ponder
Ongoing, systematic health research as a foundation for practice in primary health care is vital to creating sustainable communities.

1 Improve the usability of health information

- Identify the intended user of the health information and services; for example, know their profile including demographics, behaviour, culture, attitude, literacy skills, language, socio-economic status, access to services, language preferences, health practices.
- Decide which channel and format of sharing information is most appropriate.
- Evaluate users' understanding *before* (formative), *during* (process) and *after* (outcome) the introduction of materials.
- Acknowledge cultural differences and practise respect.
- Use plain language; for example, use simple language and define technical terms, use the active voice, break down complex information into understandable pieces, organise information so the most important points come first.
- Speak clearly and listen carefully; use a medically trained interpreter where necessary, ask open-ended questions, have the person restate the information in their own words — the 'teach-back' method.
- Improve usability of internet information; for example, plain language, large font, white space, simple graphics.

2 Improve the usability of health services

- Improve the usability of health forms and instructions. Revise forms to ensure clarity and simplicity, test forms with intended users, offer assistance with completing forms.
- Improve the accessibility of the physical environment. Include universal symbols and clear signage in multiple languages.

3 Build knowledge to improve decision-making

- Improve access to accurate and appropriate health information; for example, partner with educators to improve health curricula.
- Identify new methods for information dissemination e.g. cell phones, palm pilots, personalised and interactive content, information kiosks, talking prescription bottles, etc.
- Facilitate healthy decision-making; for example, use short documents that present 'bottom-line' information, step-by-step instructions, and visual cues that highlight the most important information.

4 Advocate for improved health literacy

- Make the case for improving health literacy; for example, target key leaders with health literacy information.
- Incorporate health literacy in mission and planning; for example, include health literacy statements in strategic plans, program plans and educational initiatives.
- Establish accountability for health literacy activities; for example, include health literacy improvement criteria in program evaluation.

Figure 1.3 Strategies for promoting health literacy (Adapted from the US Department of Health and Human Services Office of Disease Prevention and Health Promotion Health Communication Activities web page 2009: http://www.health.gov/communication/literacy/powerpoint/)

Objective information can help demonstrate that the practice of nursing and midwifery is based on scientific evidence rather than historical reasons. The mounting evidence base for practice is persuasive, particularly in demonstrating the value of interventions such as wound management, falls prevention, post-surgical outcomes, infection control, and a variety of acute care outcomes that also include measures of efficiency and cost-effectiveness (Dall et al 2009). However, practice in the community is ultimately linked to the overarching goals of health care. These include equity, access, public participation in decision-making, health promotion, appropriate use of our tools and technologies, and collaboration between all public sectors and services of society.

In working with communities, the rules for scientific studies often fail to take into account the complexities of community life and the value of tacit, subjective knowledge that is gained from community engagement. This type of knowledge must be contextualised, accounting for holistic understandings of family and community life, complete with cultural, spiritual and environmental knowledge (McMurray 2004).

Throughout this text we will be presenting a series of research studies that help inform practice in the community. Many of these are aimed at seeking in-depth situational knowledge that illustrates good and best practice in advancing community health and wellness. Some studies are specific to various cultures, and their particular needs, an important aspect of ensuring cultural relevance for practice. Others are situation specific, providing a research foundation for planning or interventions with various communities. All are examples of the type of information that helps us recognise diversity, foster community competence, engage in meaningful relationships with our communities and make practice defensible.

Point to ponder

Research in the community must be a balance of objective, scientific evidence combined with the subjective knowledge that represents people's experiences.

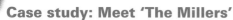

Case study: Meet 'The Millers'

Anna and *Dominic*, aged 60 and 64 respectively, met and married in Torino, Italy. Their daughter Maria was born in 1975 and immigrated to Australia when she met her husband, Jim, on a backpackers' holiday in 2000. She was 25 and Jim was 28. They now live in Sydney.

Jim (now aged 38) was born in the UK but moved with his parents *Harold* (aged 59) and *Millie* (aged 62) to Auckland in 1980 when he was just 8 years old. Harold and Millie still live in New Zealand, but are now in a small rural town on the South Island, some one and a half hours from the nearest hospital. Maria and Jim have had two children in the past 10 years: *Lily* (aged 6) and *Samantha* (aged 3). They are both in child care as Maria and Jim both have full-time jobs; Maria in a bank and Jim in sales.

We'll be following the Millers as the family changes and their communities expand across the Tasman. We hope you enjoy the journey and find them a stimulating learning experience.

REFLECTING ON THE BIG ISSUES
- Health is a state of balance between individual, social and environmental factors; the social determinants of health.
- Being healthy includes wellbeing and happiness.
- Sustaining health requires attention to intergenerational factors.
- The health of a community is dependent on the interactions between different

people who live there as well as equity in health policies and services.

- Social capital is created when people feel connected with others, developing mutuality and trust.
- Health literacy is vital to achieving equity in community health.
- Research is an essential part of helping communities develop.

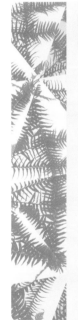

Reflective questions: how would I use this knowledge in practice?

1 Explain the difference between 'nursing in the community' and 'nursing the community'.

2 Construct a genogram of the Miller family (see Box 1.4 and Appendix A).

3 Identify some of the major social determinants of the Millers' health and wellbeing.

4 What aspects of the community surrounding Maria and Jim would facilitate their family life? Which might be considered constraining factors on family life? How would these community influences differ from that of their parents?

5 Outline the main elements you would include in promoting health literacy to Maria and Jim for their parenting needs.

6 How could a nurse working in the community help build social capital?

7 Identify one research question that would help inform your work with Maria and Jim.

BOX 1.4 THE GENOGRAM

A genogram is a graphic representation of a family tree. It displays the interactions of generations, allowing the user to analyse family members and their relationships to one another. In a standard genogram the male is drawn as a square, and the female as a circle. There are three different types of children depicted in a genogram: a biological child, adopted child or foster child (see Appendix A). A triangle is used to represent a pregnancy, miscarriage or abortion. Where there has been a miscarriage or abortion, a diagonal cross is drawn on top of the triangle to symbolise death. Abortions have an additional horizontal line. A still-birth is displayed by the gender symbol, with a diagonal cross the same size but a half-size gender symbol. For multiple births the child links are joined together.

(Online:http://www.genopro.com/genogram/symbols. Accessed 24 August 2009)

Research-informed practice: intergenerational health

Clendon (2007, 2009) conducted a study of how New Zealand mothers use their children's health and development record book (Plunket book) as a basis for subsequent mother–daughter interactions. Using an oral history approach, she explored the experiences of 34 women and one man as they used the child health and development record book at varying times throughout their lives. The study tracked the historical development of the book in relation to social change, examined how the Plunket book has been used to strengthen intergenerational relationships within families, and how it has helped facilitate and build relationships between nurses and mothers. Clendon found that mothers have consistently used the book as a tool to link past with present, to maintain kinship ties across generations, to deal with change intergenerationally, and in a manner that contributes to their self-identity as woman and mother. Although mothers were able to use the book to affirm their own knowledge and that of their mothers, a medically dominated discourse persisted in the book. Despite this, Clendon found that the child health and development record book is an effective clinical tool for nurses, midwives and other health professionals to use in their work with families. She recommends that nurses, midwives and other health professionals continue to use the book in practice but to be mindful of the fact that the book remains in use beyond the health professional's immediate involvement with the mother and child, playing an important role in the context of the family across generations. Clendon suggests that health professionals use the book to build on the strengths and abilities of a mother as she cares for her child. This reaffirms her role and identity as a mother, not only when her children are younger but as they grow and become parents themselves.

References

Aston M, Meagher-Stewart D, Edwards N, Young L 2009 Public health nurses' primary health care practice: strategies for fostering citizen participation. Journal of Community Health Nursing 26:24–34

Baisch M 2009 Community health: an evolutionary concept analysis. Journal of Advanced Nursing 65(11):2464–76

Bandura A 1977 Self-efficacy: toward a unifying theory of behavioral change. Psychological Review 84:191–215

Baum F 2009 Envisioning a healthy and sustainable future: essential to closing the gap in a generation. Global Health Promotion 1757–9759 Supp (1):72–80

Baum F, Bush R, Modra C, Murray C, Cox E, Alexander K, Potter R 2000 Epidemiology of participation. Journal of Epidemiology & Community Health 54:414–23

Best A, Stokols D, Green L, Leischow S, Holmes B, Bucholz K 2003 An integrative framework for community partnering to translate theory into effective health promotion strategy. American Journal of Health Promotion 18(2):168–76

Bruni R, Laupacis A, Martin D 2008 Public engagement in setting priorities in health care. Canadian Medical Association Journal 179(1): 15–18

Campbell-Lendrum D, Bertollini R, Neira M, Ebi K, McMichael A 2009 Health and climate change: a roadmap for applied research. The Lancet 373(9676):1663–5

Chung J 2009 An intergenerational reminiscence programme for older adults with early dementia and youth volunteers: values and challenges. Scandinavian Journal of Caring Sciences 23:259–64

Clendon J 2007 Mother/daughter intergenerational interviews: insights into qualitative interviewing. Contemporary Nurse 23(2):243–51

Clendon J 2009 Motherhood and the Plunket book: a social history. Unpublished doctoral thesis. New Zealand, Massey University

Commission on the Social Determinants of Health (CSDH) 2008 Closing the gap in a generation. Health equity through action on the social determinants of health, Final report of the Commission on the Social Determinants of Health. WHO, Geneva

Coulter A, Parsons S, Ashkham J 2008 Where are the Patients in Decision-Making About Their Own Care? Policy Brief, 'WHO and WHO European Observatory on Health Systems and Policies'. Copenhagen, Regional Office for Europe

Crooks V, Andrews G 2009 Community, equity, access: core geographic concepts in primary health care. Primary Health Care Research & Development 10:270–3

Dall T, Chen Y, Yaozhu J, Seifert R, Maddox P, Hogan P 2009 The economic value of professional nursing. Medical Care 47(1):97–104

De Souza E M, Grundy E 2007 Intergenerational interaction, social capital and health: results from a randomized controlled trial in Brazil. Social Science and Medicine 65:1397–409

Diener E, Seligman M 2004 Beyond money: toward an economy of wellbeing. Psychological Science in the Public Interest 5(1):1–31

Dunn H 1959 High-level wellness for man and society. American Journal of Public Health 49:789

Eckersley R, Wierenga A, Wyn J 2005 Life in a time of uncertainty: optimising the health and wellbeing of young Australians. Medical Journal of Australia, 183(8):402–5

Edwards N, MacLean Davison C 2008 Social justice and core competencies for public health. Improving the fit. Canadian Journal of Public Health 99(2):130–2

Fujiwara Y, Sakuma N, Ohba H 2009 Effects of an intergenerational health promotion program for older adults in Japan. Journal of Intergenerational Relationships 7(1): 17–39

Government of Victoria 2009 Community wellbeing. Online. Available: http://www.sustainablecommunity rating.com/cs/Satellite?c=VPage&cid=11915651675 (accessed 7 July 2009)

Graham H 2004 Social determinants and their unequal distribution: clarifying policy understandings. The Milbank Quarterly 82(1):101–24

Green J 2007 Health literacy: terminology and trends in making and communicating health-related information. Health Issues 92:11–14

Green S, Parkinson L, Bonevski B, Considine R 2004 Community health needs assessment for health service planning: realising consumer participation in the health service setting. Health Promotion Journal of Australia 15(2):142–50

Gross National Happiness Index. Online. Available: www.grossnationalhappiness.cm/gnhIndex/introductionGNH.aspx (accessed 2 July 2009)

Hancock T 2009 Act Locally: Community-based population health. Report for The Senate Sub-Committee on Population Health, Victoria BC

Canada. Online. Available: http://www.parl.gc.ca/40/2/parlbus/commbus/senate/com-e/popu-e/rep-e/appendixBjun09-e.pdf (accessed 17 July 2009)

Hertzman C 2001 Health and human society. American Scientist 89(6):538–44

Hertzman C, Power C 2006 A life course approach to health and human development. In: Heymann J, Hertzman C, Barer M, Evans R (eds) Healthier Societies: From Analysis to Action, Blackwell, Oxford, pp 83–106

Howat P, Ritchie J 2004 Sustainable population growth — implications for health promotion. Health Promotion Journal of Australia 15(2):103–8

Kickbusch I 2001 Health literacy: addressing the health and education divide. Health Promotion International 16(30):289–97

—— 2008 Healthy Societies: Addressing 21st Century Health Challenges. Government of South Australia, Department of the Premier and Cabinet, Adelaide

Labonte R 2005 Community Health Centres and Community Development. Toronto: Centre for Social Justice

Laperriere H 2008 Developing professional autonomy in advanced nursing practice: the critical analysis of socio-political variables. International Journal of Nursing Practice 14:391–7

Layard R 2005 Happiness. Penguin Books, London

Li J, McMurray A, Stanley F 2008 Modernity's paradox and the structural determinants of child health and wellbeing. Health Sociology Review 17(1):64–78

Link B, Phelan J 2005 Fundamental sources of health inequalities. In: Robert Wood Johnson Foundation Policy Challenges in Modern Health Care, Robert Wood Johnson Foundation, Princeton, NH, pp 71–84

Lowe I 1994 Priorities for a sustainable future. In: Chu C, Simpson R (eds) Ecological Public Health: from Vision to Practice. Griffith University, Institute for Applied Environmental Research, Brisbane, pp. vii–viii

Mancuso J 2008 Health literacy: a concept/dimensional analysis. Nursing and Health Sciences 10:248–55

Marks N, Abdallah S, Simms A, Thompson S 2006 The (un)Happy Planet Index: An index of human wellbeing and ecological impact. New Economic Foundation (NEF), London. Online. Available: www.happyplanetindex.org (accessed 15 June 2010)

Marmot M 2006 Health in an unequal world. The Lancet 368 (9552):2081–94

McKee M 2008 Global research for health. Editorial, British Medical Journal 337(2733):1–3

McKeown T 1979 The Role of Medicine: Dream, Mirage or Nemesis? (2nd edn). Blackwell, Oxford

McMichael A 2005 Climate Change and Human Health: Global and Local Consequences. The Western Australian Greenhouse Unit, Perth

McMurray A 2004 Culturally sensitive evidence-based practice. Collegian 11(4):14–18

Morrison I, Stosz L, Clift S 2008 An evidence base for mental health promotion through supported education: a practical application of Antonovsky's salutogenic model of health. International Journal of Health Promotion & Education 46(1):11–20

Nakhaie M, Smylie L, Arnold R 2007 Social inequalities, social capital, and health of Canadians. Review of Radical Political Economics 39(4):562–85

Navarro V 2009 What we mean by social determinants of health. International Journal of Health Services 39(3):423–41

Nutbeam D 2000 Health literacy as a public health goal: a challenge for contemporary health education and communication strategies into the 21st century. Health Promotion International 15(3):259–67

—— 2008 The evolving concept of health literacy. Social Science & Medicine 67:2072–8

Ontario Healthy Communities Coalition (OHCC). What Makes a Healthy Community. Online. Available: http://www.ohcc-ccso.ca/en//what-makes-a-healthy-community (accessed 6 July 2009)

—— 2009 Social Capital. Online. Available: http://www,ohcc-ccso.ca/en/social-capital (accessed 6 July 2009)

Osberg L, Sharpe A 2006 Comparison of Trends in GDP and Economic Wellbeing: The Impact of Social Capital. The Department of Economics, Dalhousie University, Halifax

Oswald A 2007 Commentary: human wellbeing and causality in social epidemiology. International Journal of Epidemiology 36:1253–4

Ottawa Health Research Institute 2009 Patient decision aids. Online. Available: http://www.ohri.ca/decisionaid/ (accessed 8 July 2009)

Peerson A, Saunders M 2009 Health literacy revisited: what do we mean and why does it matter? Health Promotion International 24(3):285–96

Putnam R 1995 Bowling alone: America's declining social capital. Journal of Democracy 6(1):65–78

Putnam R 2005 Civic Renewal and Social Capital. Round Table Discussion, Alcoa Research Centre for Stronger Communities, Curtin University, Perth

Raphael D, Curry-Stevens A, Bryant T 2008 Barriers to addressing the social determinants of health: insights from the Canadian experience. Health Policy 88(2/3):222–35

Ratzan S 2002 The plural of anecdote is not evidence. Journal of Health Communication 7:169–70

Ratzan S 2007 An informed patient — an oxymoron in an information restricted society. Journal of Health Communication 12:101–3

Rural Assist Information Network (RAIN) 2009 Community wellbeing. Online. Available: http://www.rain.net.au/community_wellbeing.htm (accessed 7 July 2009)

Shieh C, Hosei B 2008 Printed health information materials: evaluation of readability and suitability. Journal of Community Health Nursing 25:73–90

Smith S, McCaffery K 2010 Health Literacy: a Brief Literature Review. NSW Clinical Excellence Commission, Sydney

Syme S 2005 Historical perspective: The social determinants of disease — some roots of the movement. Epidemiologic Perspectives & Innovations 2(2):1–7. Online. Available: http://www.epi-perspectives.com/content/2/1/2 (accessed 22 May 2010)

The Ian Potter Foundation 2009 Improving community wellbeing through prevention and innovation. Online. Available: http://foundation.ianpotter.org.au/community_wellbeing.html (accessed 7 July 2009)

Tunstall H, Shaw M, Dorling D 2004 Places and health. Journal of Epidemiology Community Health 58:6–10

White S 2008 Assessing the Nation's Health Literacy. AMA Foundation, Washington

Whitehead M 2007 A typology of actions to tackle social inequalities in health. Journal of Epidemiology Community Health 61:473–8

Wilcox L 2007 Onions and bubbles: models of the social determinants of health, CDC, Preventing chronic disease. Online. Available: http://www.cdc.gov/pcd/issues/2007/oct07_0126.htm (accessed 24 September 2007)

World Health Organization (WHO) 1974 Basic Documents (36th ed). Geneva, WHO

—— 1992 Health and the environment: a global challenge. Bulletin of the World Health Organization 70(4):409–13

World Health Organization-Health and Welfare Canada-CPHA 1986 Ottawa Charter for Health Promotion. Canadian Journal of Public Health 77(12):425–30

Zarcadoolas C, Pleasant A, Greer D 2005 Understanding health literacy: an expanded model. Health Promotion International 20(2):195–203

Ziersch A, Baum F, MacDougall C, Putland C 2005 Neighbourhood life and social capital: the implications for health. Social Science & Medicine 60:71–86

Useful websites

http://www.euro.who.int/HEN/policybriefs/ — WHO health evidence network for decision-makers

http://www.who.int/entity/social_determinants/en/ — WHO social determinants of health

http://www.who.int/social_determinants/knowledge_networks/exclusion/en/index.html — WHO social exclusion and social determinants of health

http://www.un.org/millenniumgoals/ — MDGs

http://www2.ids.ac.uk/ghen/about/index.html — UK Gender and Health equity network

http://www.euro.who.int/hen — WHO health evidence network

http://www.euro.who.int/observatory — WHO European Observatory on Health Systems and Policies

http://www.SDOH@YORKU.CA — International website and archives on social determinants of health

http://www.healthinsite.gov.au/topics/Health_and_Wellbeing — Australian government site for all health topics

http://www.nphp.gov.au/ — Australian National Public Health Partnerships

http://www.rain.net.au/community_wellbeing.htm — Australian Rural Assist Information Network

http://nrha.ruralhealth.org.au — Australian National Rural Health Alliance

http://www.serviceseeker.com.au/ — Australian Infoxchange community directories

http://www.ihca.com.au/ — Australian Institute for Healthy Communities

http://www.canberra.edu.au/centres/sustainable-communities — Australian Institute for Sustainable Communities

http://www.health.nsw.gov.au/pubs/2000/pdf/capbuild.pdf or http://www.health.nsw.gov.au/pubs/2000/capbuild.html — Indicators to help with Capacity Building, NSW Health

http://www.nafhc.org/about/ — US National Alliance for Healthy Communities

http://www.ohcc-ccso.ca/ — Ontario Healthy Communities Coalition

http://www.nlm.nih.gov/pubs/cbm/healthliteracybarriers.html — American health literacy bibliography to 2003

http://www.nifl.gov/mailman/listinfo/Healthliteracy — Health and Literacy Discussion List

http://www.hsph.harvard.edu/healthliteracy/— Harvard School of Public Health, Health and Literacy Website

http://www.centreforliteracy.qc.ca/health/healthlt.htm — Canadian Care for Research Briefs on Health Literacy

http://www.nzliteracyportal.org.nz/ — New Zealand literacy portal

http://www.healthnavigator.org.nz/centre-for-clinical-excellence/health-literacy — New Zealand health literacy information

Chapter 2

Primary health care: principles and practices

INTRODUCTION

Primary health care (PHC) is a pathway to achieving basic human rights, which is essentially social justice. Since the Declaration of Alma Ata in 1978, PHC has been both a philosophy and organising framework for nurses, midwives and other health professionals. As a framework, PHC circumscribes nursing and midwifery activities in terms of illness prevention, health promotion, and structural and environmental modifications that support health and wellness. This does not exclude the important work in caring for those experiencing illness or disability. It does, however, shift the caring agenda to the social determinants of health (SDOH), in primary care settings such as general practice, in critical or acute care, home care, rehabilitation settings, residential care, or in working to modify the community itself. As we mentioned in Chapter 1, health, illness prevention, and recovery from illness and injury, are socially determined; that is, created and maintained in the social environments and settings where people live, play, work, are educated, worship and interact with others.

> ### Point to ponder
> PHC is both a philosophy of care and an organising framework for nurses, midwives and other health professionals.

The overarching principles embodied in PHC guide us to work towards equitable social circumstances, equal access to health care, and community empowerment through public participation in all aspects of life. This approach includes being culturally sensitive to diversity in people's lifestyles, preferences and situations. PHC is focused on promoting healthy social and structural conditions for good health. These conditions include health literacy and citizen participation so that people are empowered to make informed choices to develop their personal and community capacity.

For individuals, developing health capacity means becoming health literate, knowing where and how to access and maintain health knowledge and skills, feeling comfortable in participating in discussions or activities about health, and having supportive, sustainable resources to support empowered health and lifestyle choices.

Working with community networks and organisations committed to capacity building development demonstrates nurses' and midwives' accountability to the community and to partnerships for good health. The outcome of community partnerships should be better health, equity, justice, and good governance in health services, including appropriate, effective, and efficient use of available technologies. To guide this work, we use the Ottawa Charter for Health Promotion (World Health Organization, Health and Welfare Canada & CPHA 1986). The Charter is a framework that encapsulates the goals of PHC, and we outline how this can be helpful in practice throughout the chapter. Because the principles of PHC are not uniformly understood, this chapter also provides an explanation of the PHC principles and how they fit with community health promotion. This is aimed at encouraging common understandings and a common framework for working with communities. We also explain the relevant historical moments in health promotion, to illustrate how our thinking has been shaped by new knowledge and new understandings of communities. In this discussion we will also revisit the SDOH, particularly those which either foster or compromise social justice and community empowerment.

> ### Point to ponder
> The Ottawa Charter for Health Promotion provides a framework for health promotion that health professionals can use to enact the goals of PHC.

Objectives

By the end of this chapter you will be able to:

1 explain the terms 'primary health care', 'primary care', 'primary, secondary and tertiary prevention'

2 analyse the principles of PHC in relation to community health and wellness

3 identify primary, secondary and tertiary prevention activities in promoting community health

4 explain the difference between health promotion and health education and the significance of each in community health

5 discuss the application of PHC principles to the strategies of the Ottawa Charter for Health Promotion

6 devise a strategic plan to address population health in a given community using the Ottawa Charter as a guide.

CLARIFICATION OF TERMS

PHC is a term that is sometimes confused with other, similar terms, such as primary care and primary prevention, so to ensure clarity, this chapter begins with some definitions of terms.

Primary health care (PHC)

PHC encompasses a broad spectrum of activities to encourage health and wellbeing. These can include primary (initial) care and include follow-up activities for promoting the health of the community, protecting community members from harm, and/or preventing illness or injury. Importantly, the ultimate goal of PHC is to build community capacity to enable sustainable health and wellbeing. Community capacity building is based on the fundamental values of equity, community participation and self-determination, which embody human rights and shared social expectations (WHO 2008).

Point to ponder

Primary health care is a philosophy of care intended to redress inequities in health by recognising that wellbeing is dependent on a broad range of social, political, economic and environmental factors.

Two types of PHC have been described in the literature. 'Selective primary health care' is a term that emerged in the 1980s under neoliberal economic policies that emphasised medical and technical solutions to health problems (Baum 2007; deVos et al 2009). Health was seen as an investment, and selective PHC was aimed at 'best investments in health'; ensuring that the health care system funded programs that would have a significant effect on certain groups in the population. The language of selective PHC was typical of the economic policies of the time. Certain population groups were seen as 'targets'. Health care was 'outcome focused'. Health planning was 'target oriented', and success was defined in terms of concrete health improvements linked to specific expenditures (deVos et al 2009:122). Selective PHC did not build sustainable communities, but led to fragmentation of services, draining expertise and resources (Baum 2007). However, today, selective PHC is seen as focusing on a specific group with high priority needs within the broader context of comprehensive PHC (Baum et al 2009).

'Comprehensive primary health care' adopts a community development approach, which is more closely aligned with the social justice agenda. Comprehensive PHC revolves around an empowerment framework, where community members work in partnership with health professionals to participate fully in health decision-making (Baum 2007; Baum et al 2009; deVos; et al 2009). This shifts the agenda from professional control over decisions about priorities and resources, to one where community empowerment is the main objective. Members of the community are not beneficiaries of health services, but rather have the power to control resources and how they are distributed, which is aimed at creating equitable conditions (Baum 2007; deVos et al 2009). Throughout this text PHC will refer to comprehensive PHC.

> **Point to ponder**
> Primary prevention is aimed at maintaining health and preventing illness, secondary prevention is aimed at treating and limiting illness or injury, and tertiary prevention is aimed at rehabilitative or restorative actions.

Primary, secondary and tertiary prevention

As mentioned previously, prevention is a major focus of PHC. Leavell and Clark's (1965) three levels of prevention are widely accepted as encompassing the range of activities involved in preventing illness or injury. These levels, primary prevention, secondary prevention and tertiary prevention, distinguish between strategies aimed at maintaining health and wellbeing and preventing illness (primary), treating and limiting illness or injury (secondary), and rehabilitative or restorative actions (tertiary). The aim of primary prevention is to promote health by removing the precipitating causes and determinants of ill health or injury. This can include vaccinating children against communicable diseases, health education and promotion of healthy lifestyles in areas such as personal nutrition, rest, exercise and companionship, and protecting the physical, social and cultural environments. Secondary prevention usually refers to steps taken to recover from illness, to guard against any deterioration in health, screening for early detection and treatment of disease, and any measures to limit disability. Tertiary prevention is restorative. Programs revolve around rehabilitation, transitions to community care and education for industry support programs (Leavell & Clark 1965).

Conceptualising health professionals' activities across these three levels indicates a holistic, PHC approach that can be applied across the life span. The metaphor of a waterfall illustrates. Primary prevention activities at the community level are 'upstream' actions, such as developing educational materials to portray the benefits of nutrition or regular exercise to help individuals stay healthy. Besides offering encouragement for healthy lifestyles, primary prevention includes lobbying the local council or government agencies to create the conditions that support community health and development. This type of activity might include helping secure cost-effective foods or safe spaces for children to play. Secondary, or 'midstream', prevention includes such preventative activities as screening for skin cancer, conducting mammography clinics, or establishing drop-in centres for adolescents or isolated older people. Tertiary prevention occurs 'downstream' and typically involves providing assistance or information to help people cope with a potentially disabling condition. This could involve the establishment of walking programs for those who have had a cardiac incident, support groups for family members coping with a loss, or any measure that helps ensure continuity of care and health literacy, such as access to timely health advice (see Figure 2.1).

Primary care

When people require health care because of injury or illness, the first line of care is primary. So primary care is the initial decision as to what must be done and it usually guides the subsequent management of a person's condition or needs. Primary care may involve only one intervention, or treatment over an extended period of time, but it is still primary, in that it is aimed at helping people with whatever problem required care in the first place. Physicians, nurses, paramedics, dentists, physiotherapists, complementary therapists and a range of other health professionals may provide the initial care.

An ambulance officer or paramedic may be first on the scene to deal with a road accident or injury; a physical education teacher, trainer or school nurse may be the first line of care in the recreational setting. Each would provide care and then would likely refer the person needing assistance to a physician who would assume the role of primary care provider. Paramedics, by nature of their role in responding to emergencies are quite often the primary care providers, usually in a life-saving capacity.

> **Point to ponder**
> Primary care is the first line of care when a person is sick or injured.

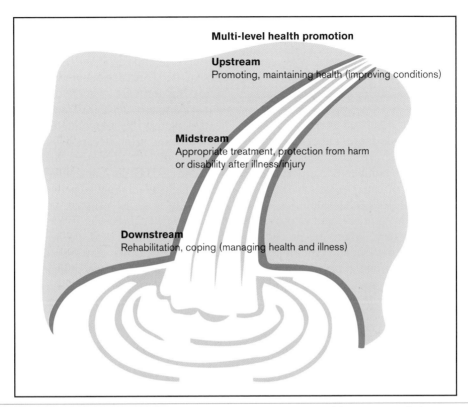

Figure 2.1 Primary, secondary, tertiary prevention: upstream, midstream and downstream interventions

Similarly, nurses in a hospital emergency department or in a community clinic may provide initial treatment for an emergency, then either refer the patient to the local medical practitioner to manage the condition, or manage it themselves, depending on the situation. In the latter case, the nurse would be acting as a primary care provider. This role is often enacted by nurses and nurse practitioners in remote locations where there is no medical practitioner. There is also some discussion internationally regarding an expanded paramedic role. Given that paramedics often follow up primary care by providing care in a person's home, there is growing acceptance of reframing the role of the 'paramedic practitioner' who provides a brief initial intervention and then appropriate referral (Stirling et al 2007; Woollard 2006).

Another situation where someone other than a medical practitioner acts as primary care provider is in the workplace. Many manufacturing and mining companies, for example, employ nurses or other health professionals to manage occupational health and safety. For some workplace-based problems, the occupational health professional

may be the most appropriate and available person to provide primary care. However, in addition to primary care, this role differs from the paramedic role in that it extends beyond 'nursing in the community' to 'nursing the community', as we mentioned in Chapter 1. Whereas the paramedic or other emergency personnel provide acute and sometimes ongoing care 'in the community', the occupational health nurse provides care of the occupational environment as well, which is 'nursing the community'. This role will be elaborated on further in Chapter 4.

The model of primary care most people encounter is that of general practice. Most general practitioners (GPs) provide primary care and variable levels of follow-up of patients and families, depending on many factors. These factors include the time pressures of the practice, especially where there are staff shortages, demand and preferences of the practice clients, and the health care system in which the practice operates. In some countries such as Australia and Canada, general practice operates on a 'fee-for-service' basis, with reimbursement from Medicare for episodes of care.

Point to ponder
The model of primary care most people in Australia and New Zealand encounter is general practice.

This system has been described as creating a perverse incentive to provide more, rather than more comprehensive services, because the financial rewards flow from the number of care episodes rather than the quality of care (Australian Nursing Federation [ANF] 2009). In other countries, such as the United Kingdom, primary care is provided under a 'capitation' system, where the practice is paid on the basis of the number and type of people enrolled in a practice, or group of practices. In New Zealand, primary care is provided under a mixed system with 'capitation' covering most services but with many general practices still charging a fee-for-service to cover the shortfall in capitation funding. As in Australia, general practice in New Zealand is still largely run under a business model and fees for service vary widely. However, when funding is provided on a 'per capita' or population basis, as it is in New Zealand, there is a greater likelihood of comprehensive, multidisciplinary, integrated PHC. For this reason, the worldwide trend towards PHC is gradually creating an impetus for general practice to change to this system (Martin 2008; WHO 2008).

Point to ponder
New Zealand was one of the first countries in the world to make a strategic commitment to implementing PHC at a national level.

Nurses and midwives in Australia and New Zealand play an important role in the PHC movement. New Zealand was one of the first countries to make a national commitment to PHC (Ministry of Health New Zealand [MOHNZ] 2001), and New Zealand nurses worked hard to ensure their role was clearly identified as crucial to enactment of the new strategy. Evaluation of nursing developments since implementation demonstrate that, despite a range of barriers, there has been substantial growth in some nursing roles and capability in PHC (Finlayson et al 2009). As New Zealand nurses seek out opportunities for improving population health under the PHC strategy's new funding streams, New Zealand is slowly seeing increasing

numbers of nurse-led initiatives in PHC. These include a shift to name all nurses working in PHC 'primary health care nurses', increasing numbers of nurse practitioners working in PHC and increasing numbers of nurse-led clinics.

In Australia, recent government policy changes have recognised the important role of practice nurses in broadening primary care to PHC (Halcomb et al 2008). Similar examples of this trend are evident in countries such as Canada, with models of collaborative general practice between GPs and nurses effectively 'infusing primary care principles in the delivery of PHC' (Besner 2004:356). These initiatives are consonant with the recommendations of the WHO (2008) that care should be brought closer to people, relocating entry points from hospitals and specialist services to generalist, primary care centres aimed at improving coordination of care.

PUBLIC HEALTH, POPULATION HEALTH AND PRIMARY HEALTH CARE: A BRIEF HISTORY

Public health is aimed at preventing disease and promoting the health of populations. Public health initiatives are based on population-level data and typically involve measurement and surveillance, and development of evidence-based strategies to either prevent or overcome diseases. This involves collecting and analysing epidemiological information on the distribution and determinants of health and ill health in a particular community or country, and linking this information to what is known in other populations. One of the problems with this approach is that by aggregating this type of information, the assumption is made that all community members develop or behave in similar ways, thereby creating stereotypes of communities that are actually diverse and changing (Abbott et al 2008).

Population health
Population health is similar to public health in that it is:

The organized response by society to protect and promote health, and so prevent illness, injury, disability and early mortality. The programs, services and institutions of population health emphasise the prevention of disease and the health needs of the population as a whole.

(Commonwealth Department of Health and Ageing. Online. http://www.health.gov.au/internet/main/publishing.nsf/ Content/health-pubhlth-about)

Primary health care and the Declaration of Alma Ata

Public health and population health approaches can be differentiated from PHC, which is defined in the Declaration of Alma Ata as:

> Essential health care based on practical, scientifically sound and socially acceptable methods and technology made universally accessible to individuals and families in the community through their full participation and at a cost that the community and country can afford to maintain at every stage of their development in the spirit of self-reliance and self-determination. It is the first level of contact with individuals, the family and community with the national health systems bringing health care as close as possible to where people live and work and constitutes the first element of a continuing care process.
>
> (WHO & UNICEF 1978:6)

The distinctions between public health, population health and PHC illustrate how the ideas of health planners and policy-makers have changed over time. Although the focus of public health has always been to ensure the highest level of health for the greatest number of the population, historically, public health has been about illness, not health. From the 19th century, public health authorities adopted a regulatory approach of surveillance and control to overcome infectious diseases. They tracked epidemics or potential epidemics, and ensured that government regulations were in place for monitoring illness in the population and responding quickly when it was required.

Point to ponder
Public health was historically focused on surveillance and tracking infectious disease. This is still an important focus but now public health also includes examining the SDOH and how these affect population health.

Public health was therefore defined according to a biomedical model where the emphasis was on understanding the causes of illness in order to apportion resources appropriately. In the biomedical model the public health focus is on midstream (interventions) and downstream (rehabilitation) activities to manage epidemics and protect people, rather than promote health. This resulted in concentrating resources in hospitals and acute-sector services (Bernier 2005). However, the current focus revolves around the SDOH and how these affect the population. This approach has become incorporated into social epidemiological models of health planning, which will be further explained in Chapter 3.

Problems with the 'old public health era'

In the biomedical public health era, public health experts were guided by current medical knowledge, political factors and the availability of financial and personal resources. So, for example, in those parts of the world where health personnel and resources were plentiful, people were expected to have higher levels of health. Where vaccines were available and where the politics of the day encouraged medical research through generous funding schemes, diseases should be curtailed. Members of the public rarely questioned the medical experts on any of these public health matters. Yet, no relationship was found between good health and the provision of services. Clearly, there was a need to look for a broader set of criteria for good health.

In 1978 an important international meeting among members of 189 countries culminated in the Declaration of Alma Ata, named after the city in the former USSR where the meeting took place. The Declaration was the first global proclamation that a broader perspective of health was needed to galvanise the efforts of health planners around the world to meet current and future challenges. PHC was declared as the roadmap to achieving better health for all populations. The architects of the Declaration found no opposition to this approach among health professionals.

Point to ponder
The Declaration of Alma Ata made the first global assertion that a broader view of health was needed to address health needs. PHC was declared as the vehicle through which better health would be achieved.

Four years earlier, the *Lalonde Report* in Canada had suggested a more socially contextualised definition of health, including strategies for achieving health that placed less onus on individuals and more emphasis on creating the right conditions in their environments (Lalonde 1974). PHC embodied this idea. It was not only a vision for health, it was seen as a philosophy permeating the entire health system, a strategy for organising care, a level of care (primary or 'first line' of care) and a set of activities (Chamberlain & Beckingham 1987).

The Declaration of Alma Ata represented a watershed in public health. Its focus was on empowering people to have control over decisions that affected health in their own families and communities. The PHC approach conceptualised health as a fundamental right, an individual and collective responsibility, an equal opportunity concept and an essential element of socio-economic development (Holzemer 1992). This represented a stark contrast to the historical 'top-down' approach to planning for public health in that people at the grassroots level of societies were now to have a greater say in planning from the 'bottom-up', or 'inside out' instead of 'outside in' (Courtney 1995). The PHC approach has been described as keeping health professionals on tap rather than on top; acting as a resource to the community (Baum 2007).

PHC AND THE SOCIAL GRADIENT

As the Declaration of Alma Ata became integrated into health strategies throughout the world, in 1980 the UK government published the *Black Report on Inequalities in Health* (UK Department of Health and Social Services 1980). The report illustrated the extent to which ill health and mortality were distributed unequally among the social classes in the UK. It showed a widening gap between rich and poor, providing clear evidence that health was associated with income, education, diet, housing, employment and other conditions of work. This work was subsequently extended in the 'Whitehall studies', which investigated different levels of health among British bus drivers as a function of their level of employment (Marmot 1993; Marmot & Shipley 1996; Marmot et al 1984, 1987). The researchers concluded that people's health status is better with each successive step up a socio-economic gradient, now called the 'social gradients' finding (Hertzman 1999, 2001).

Throughout the 1980s and 1990s health policies in many countries, including Australia and New Zealand, focused on programs that create, maintain and protect health and wellbeing, through income security, a good education system, a clean environment, adequate social housing and community services (Baum 2002; MOHNZ 2001). In the

Point to ponder

The 'social gradients' finding shows that a person's health is better with each successive step up a socio-economic gradient. In other words, the more you earn, the better your income and the safer your housing, the better your health will be.

21st century, there is global support for PHC and research evidence into the reasons for the social gradients continues to influence both the policy and research agenda, as we outline in Chapters 12 and 13 (Commission on the Social Determinants of Health [CSDH] 2008).

PHC AND THE HEALTH PROMOTION CHARTERS

The Lalonde Report, the Declaration of Alma Ata and the Black Report, were all important milestones in our evolving policy and research agenda, collectively signalling a shift in thinking from the 'old public health', wherein health professionals decided what was best for the community, to a 'new public health', where communities themselves decide priorities and preferences for health from where people live, work and play. This PHC vision placed collective action by the community at the centre of health decision-making, with health professionals working as partners to help the community build health capacity. Another significant shift has been the focus on health promotion. This can be linked back to the leadership of Ilona Kickbusch, then Head of Canada's Health Promotion Directorate, who convened the first WHO International Conference on Health Promotion, in 1986 in Ottawa, Canada. The conference embodied PHC as the new public health, focusing the health promotion discussions on lifestyle factors, living conditions and the environments where people lived rather than health services with the objective of providing health for all (Kickbusch 2003).

Point to ponder

A series of WHO sponsored conferences on health promotion have provided strategic direction for development in health promotion for over 20 years.

The Second International Conference on Health Promotion was hosted by Australia in 1988, with an emphasis on healthy public policy. The Third International Conference on Health Promotion was held in Sundsvall, Sweden in 1991, focusing on supportive environments for health. The fourth took place in Jakarta, Indonesia in 1997, culminating in the Jakarta Declaration on Leading Health Promotion into the 21st Century (see Appendix B). By this time, the influence of economic rationalism had shaped global politics, and the Indonesian meeting focused on health promotion as an investment in overcoming poverty as a major cause of ill health. The Fifth Global Conference on Health Promotion, in Mexico City in 2000 was called 'Bridging the Equity Gap'. The recommendations from this conference revolved around positioning health promotion as a fundamental political priority in all countries, across all sectors, with information shared freely between nations (Catford 2000). At the end of 2000, eight non-government groups came together in Bangladesh as the First People's Health Assembly. The meeting culminated in the People's Health Charter (see Appendix C), which demanded that the WHO eliminate their links with the corporate interests of economic globalisation that had influenced its activities, and focus instead on comprehensive PHC and protection of the natural environment (Baum 2007). Following this, the Bangkok Charter (see Appendix D) arose from the Sixth Global Conference on Health Promotion in Bangkok, Thailand. The conference's discussions sought to highlight the global development agenda as a core responsibility for all governments, focusing on communities and civil society and the need for good corporate practices (Wilson 2005).

The basis of the original Declaration of Alma Ata and the Jakarta, Bangkok and People's Health Charters have drawn global attention to the health effects of widespread inequalities (unequal distribution of health resources) and inequities (the moral aspect of health inequality in terms of decisions taken on health care and the distribution of resources) (Asada 2005; Baum 2007; Raphael 2009). These important statements and those from subsequent international meetings and policy deliberations have been unequivocal in their goal to address the SDOH, and they have been extremely powerful in shaping PHC thinking today. In the 21st century, mainstream thinking in the promotion of health takes the view that without equal access to education, health care, transportation, nutritious food and social support, the world will never have health for all.

Point to ponder
The WHO health promotion conferences have drawn global attention to the health effects of unequal distribution of health resources (inequities in health).

From its inception in the 1970s, the PHC agenda has created a legacy to communities of the 21st century, where members of the community, rather than the experts, are squarely positioned at the centre of health care. People in communities, health professionals, educators, engineers, service workers and parents alike are now considered partners and full participants in creating and sustaining health, rather than being recipients of health services (Aston et al 2009; Coulter et al 2008). This renders the notion of 'consumer' (the public) and 'provider' (the health professional) outdated. Greater sharing of health knowledge, along with enhanced transparency of decision-making represents a more democratised approach to health, one that embodies current thinking in promoting health, that is, comprehensive PHC.

In 2008 the WHO (2008) commemorated the 30th anniversary of the Declaration of Alma Ata by recommitting its PHC agenda in its annual report: 'Primary health care — now more than ever' (WHO 2008). 'Now more than ever' refers to the state of global health care, which continues to be plagued by inequitable access, impoverishing costs and erosion of trust. Together, these constitute a threat to social stability. The report underlines the need for PHC at a time when the global financial crisis is compromising people's quality of life, and when our failure to create an equitable world is impinging on human rights (WHO 2008).

Many health professionals are working to embed PHC principles into their practice. Nurses, pharmacists, social workers, nurse practitioners, Plunket nurses, advanced practice and/or remote area nurses and other allied health professionals have a broad, PHC scope of practice, participating with communities to help define their needs and advocate for changes to the social and structural environments. Their roles vary, but their commitment to PHC is a common bond. In a variety of contexts they are promoting equitable access to their services, adopting inclusive practices, fostering public participation and community empowerment, using appropriate technology, collaborating beyond health services to ensure that other sectors of society are contributing to health, and focusing their practice on health promotion as well as appropriate illness care. These are the principles of PHC.

Point to ponder
The principles of PHC are accessible health care, appropriate technology, health promotion, intersectoral collaboration, community participation and cultural sensitivity.

PHC PRINCIPLES

PHC is guided by the principles of accessible health care, appropriate technology, health promotion, cultural sensitivity, intersectoral collaboration and community participation. The literature on PHC includes cultural inclusiveness as a common thread in each of these principles. However, we include cultural sensitivity as a separate principle. This acknowledges the important work on cultural safety that has been done over the past two decades in New Zealand. Being culturally sensitive and enabling culturally appropriate health care that protects cultural safety is one of the most important factors in achieving PHC. The principles are interconnected, but they are examined separately below to underline the importance of each to the overall philosophy of PHC.

ACCESSIBILITY: A CASE OF EQUITY AND SOCIAL JUSTICE

As described above the PHC movement that began with Alma Ata was based on the need for social justice, to redress 'politically, socially and economically unacceptable health inequalities in all countries' (WHO 2008:xii). More than three decades after Alma Ata many inequities persist. Globally, some progress has been made in reducing mortality and providing access to health care, but there has been a widening gap in income, with increasing health disparities in the most fragile countries of the world, especially sub-Saharan Africa (WHO 2008). Many African families continue to find access to vaccination difficult. Childbirth care and unsafe abortions continue to be problematic, with little access to qualified health care providers. Northern Africa, Asia (including India) and Latin America have had impressive gains, particularly in life expectancy. However, countries such as the Russian Federation and Newly Independent States have seen life expectancy either stagnate or decline, due to widespread poverty and the commercialisation of clinical services (WHO 2008).

The link between poverty and health is now clearly evident in studies on health outcomes. Poverty is a product of the social environment, linked to political decisions (Schrecker 2008). When people live below the 'poverty line' of having less than $US2 per day it is called *absolute poverty*. Being poor in relation to the rest of society is called *relative poverty*. Many developing countries experience high rates of absolute poverty. Absolute poverty is usually accompanied by high child and adult mortality rates, lower investments in human and physical resources, higher inflation and less trade, less effective disease prevention, and worse educational outcomes and other risk factors that threaten health (Ruger & Kim 2006).

Point to ponder
The link between poverty and health is clearly evident in studies on health outcomes. Many developing countries experience *absolute poverty* while many developed countries experience *relative poverty*.

Despite networks of PHC facilities provided by the United Nations (UN), many refugees and people displaced by war and conflicts are among the most impoverished and disadvantaged, experiencing absolute poverty in refugee camps (UN 2009).

In many countries of the world, including those considered highly developed, there is a widening gap in access to health services between genders, cultures, Indigenous and non-Indigenous people, and those living in urban and rural or remote areas (WHO 2008). These factors cause relative poverty or a state of *disparity* between rich and poor. Other outcomes of disparities include declining health status, exposure to communicable diseases, a lack of opportunity, escalating rates of violent trauma and substance abuse, and a lack of access to PHC (Kendall 2008). In some cases, policy decisions can cause health disparities. For example, since the election of a conservative National government in New Zealand in 2008, health targets that had included improving nutrition, physical activity and reducing obesity (MOHNZ 2008) have been refocused to shorter stays in emergency departments and improved access to elective surgery (MOHNZ 2009). This creates a disparity between those with and those without access to health resources and supports.

The major objective of providing equity of access is to eliminate disadvantage, whether it is related to social, economic or environmental factors. Barriers to access include such things as unemployment, lack of education and health literacy, age, gender, functional capacity, and cultural or language difficulties.

> **Point to ponder**
> The greater the gap between the rich and poor in a country (income inequality) the worse the health status of the whole population in that country.

These factors prevent an individual from developing personal capacity. Barriers to community capacity include geographical features that isolate people from services or opportunities, civil conflict, or a lack of structures and services that support human endeavour.

> **Point to ponder**
> Inequity of access to health services creates disadvantage. Addressing barriers to access such as unemployment, lack of education or poor health literacy will help eliminate disadvantage.

As the WHO reports (2008), a plethora of research evidence has shown that in any country, the greater the gap between the incomes of the rich and poor, the worse the health status of its citizens. This occurs unevenly, as health is distributed differently among different groups. Various interactions among influences also produce different levels of health and illness, and there is also differential progression across the generations (Starfield 2006). Some inequities also affect the community

itself. Global warming, overpopulation, the destruction of forests and the harmful effects of globalised industrial processes all add insult to the injurious effects of social policies that keep the wealth at the top of the hierarchy. Decisions for community health should therefore involve awareness of simultaneous assessment of the impact on other people and communities, future generations and the global community.

Global and intergenerational issues should be included in our community health promotion strategies to unravel the pathways to health for all of society. This suggests the need for health impact assessment in assessing all community development initiatives. It is also an indication that part of our civic responsibility as nurses and midwives is to maintain a critical political and social consciousness to be responsive to the needs of everyone. This is where the notion of social justice permeates all PHC activities. Social justice, or equitable access for all, must supersede individual goals, so that the least advantaged people in a community receive equal opportunity, education, care and service to those who are advantaged by virtue of both tangible (finances) and intangible (knowledge) resources. A commitment to PHC dictates ongoing awareness of the health needs and disparities in both local and global communities (CSDH 2008). This 'think global and act local' approach can be used as a rallying cry for political activism, to disseminate information and work towards political changes (Falk-Rafael 2006; Hancock 2009).

APPROPRIATE TECHNOLOGY

To some extent, the failure of our health care systems to address inequities in health over the past decades is due to the use of inappropriate technologies in health care. PHC requires efficiency and effectiveness, that is, 'the right care provided to the right people by the right provider, in the right setting and using the most suitable and cost-effective technology' (Besner 2004:352). In the community this often requires a multidisciplinary workforce (Martin 2008). Although progress has been made in community management of chronic diseases, health systems continue to revolve around services with a medical–technical focus. This has not only distanced care from the community, but its focus on secondary and tertiary care has depleted primary preventive services (Starfield 2006). The magnitude of spending on hospital care is staggering. Medical equipment budgets have grown 10% per year globally, with the United States, Europe and Japan spending more than $US250 billion annually on equipment. The pharmaceutical industry has accumulated a major share of the global economy, expanding rapidly each year, with expenditures of $US745 billion in 2008. Pharmaceutical and equipment markets rely on health systems like those in the US and Japan, that are funded on the basis of hospital and specialist care.

Point to ponder

Inappropriate application of technology in health care leads to inequities in the distribution of health care.

These two countries have 5–8 times more magnetic resonance imaging (MRI) units per million inhabitants than countries such as Canada and the Netherlands, with their public systems of health care. For computerised tomography (CT) scanners, this is even more pronounced, with Japan having 20 times as many as the Netherlands. The use of these technologies is rapidly expanding, at the expense of investments in PHC (WHO 2008).

Ageing, urbanisation and globalisation have accelerated worldwide transmission of communicable diseases and increased the burden of chronic and non-communicable disorders (WHO 2008). Yet, instead of allocating resources to the communities where people live with these conditions, there has been a lack of community or geographically based planning for 'distributional equity' (Crooks & Andrews 2009:271). This has continued the fragmentation of services on the basis of single, short-term priorities; treating single diseases, or single population groups instead of the whole-of-community. Priorities have become overshadowed by shrinking health care budgets with many hands competing for scarce resources. The WHO (2008), concerned about these trends, has identified five common shortcomings of health care delivery (Box 2.1).

At the point of care, appropriate technologies are not always used, and this creates inequities that arise from the ethical issues embedded in resource use. We have the technology to keep very small birth-weight (VSB) infants alive, yet should we do so at the expense of others? Similarly, is it appropriate use of technology to sustain the life of the very oldest people? Is it appropriate to provide

BOX 2.1 PROBLEMS IN HEALTH SERVICES

1 Inverse care — those with greater means consume more care.

2 Impoverishing care — those with no social protection, such as that provided in universal health care systems, become poor from health care costs.

3 Fragmentation of care — excessive specialisation of care has discouraged holistic care and the need for continuity of care.

4 Unsafe care — poor system design has led to hospital-acquired infections and adverse events.

5 Misdirected care — resources have been allocated to curative care rather than primary prevention and health promotion. The health sector has failed to integrate care with other sectors or mitigate the adverse effects on health of the activities of other sectors (WHO 2008).

access to technologically advanced medicine for very old or very young people only if, by chance or geographic proximity to clinical trials, they are able to test the devices? Is it fair to deny access to the type of health care provided in big cities to those who live in rural areas? Should fertility treatment be allocated on the basis of gender or age equity, or on the basis of human desire for a child regardless of overpopulation problems? Other questions loom as dramatic developments in stem cell research are made.

What's your opinion?

Do you think spending by developed countries on health technology is equitable or appropriate? Why or why not?

The ethics of appropriate technologies

In the research, legal and political arenas there have been debates as to whether medical scientists should be allowed to harvest organs or clone body parts to repair damaged bodies, or provide fertility treatments that would lead to greater selectivity or 'designer babies'. Most embryonic stem cells are removed from embryos created by in vitro fertilisation (IVF). Those opposed to embryonic stem cell research argue that embryonic stem cells, like any substance designed to become human tissue should be granted the same protection as a human embryo. Those opposed to the use of these cells do not support the idea that in the future embryos will be created purposefully for treatment of existing disease states. Among this group are those who have been alarmed that scientists plan to fertilise an ovum with synthetic sperm.

Advocates on the other side of the argument consider embryos slated for disposal in fertility clinics a wasted resource unless they are used to heal and support human life. This issue, like the abortion debates that have raged on for many years, remains unresolved. Scientific advances show that adult stem cells either from discarded IVF embryos or therapeutic cloning may be able to create new cells and even enhance existing cells in the bodies of those suffering from a wide range of diseases.

Point to ponder

New and emerging health technologies will generate as many questions as they will answers.

From each new development, questions of social justice arise. Who will be the beneficiaries of technology? Who is in danger of being excluded? To what extent will community members be involved in decision-making related to technological innovations? What strategies will be included to ensure informed choices can be made? Are new developments achievable at a cost the community and the country can afford? What will be the opportunity costs involved; in other words, where will the funding be decreased in favour of funding new technologies?

Technological developments have had an impact on health for many years. For example, when the refrigerator was invented, it represented the single most important device to prevent illness by guarding against contamination of foods. Refrigerators were, however, accessible only to those who could afford them and the public health authorities did not consider providing refrigerators for all people. Today, partly because of global communication and increased consumer sophistication, new technologies have become part of the public interest. It is important for nurses and midwives to participate

in these discussions to remain abreast of the issues and help ensure that community members are also informed about health care decision-making.

INCREASED EMPHASIS ON HEALTH PROMOTION

Health promotion is essentially a political, ecological and capacity building process, aimed at arranging the social and structural determinants of health in a way that facilitates health. It is the combination of circumstances that enable people to increase control over and improve their health (WHO, Health and Welfare Canada & CPHA 1986). Health promotion activities include global initiatives as well as local community planning activities that develop participative, capacity building structures for community development (Whitehead 2009). At the local level, strategies may involve working with intersectoral groups to lobby the government for better roads or more parklands, or helping to institute measures to ensure healthy school lunches or access to workplace-based health services. At the global level, health promotion may involve becoming personally aware of the problems of other countries and making sure their health issues are understood and publicised.

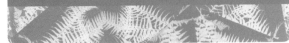

ACTION POINT

The role of the health professional in community health promotion activities is to assess the factors associated with health and ill health in the community and combine this with local knowledge and understanding of the community's health goals.

The role of nurses and midwives in promoting community health is to unravel available information on the factors involved in health and ill health, together with local knowledge and understanding of the community's health goals. Central to this type of analysis is assessing the interplay of social and structural determinants, how these are interacting with the environment in the local context, and what influences are exerting pressures on the community and its residents along their social, cultural and developmental pathways. This is a more inclusive, comprehensive view of health promotion than simply seeing the community in terms of a single issue at a discrete moment in time. It sees the community as a 'crucible' for the SDOH; where people live, learn, work and play (Hancock 2009:B6). Health promotion should be focused on the community's assets and strengths rather than risks and weaknesses (Hancock 2009). It is intended to examine how to enable people to thrive and build resilience rather than just coping with their lives (Hancock 2009). Health promotion activities may be aimed at different population subgroups, such as creating day care centres for the elderly to prevent them from being socially isolated, or working with new parents to ensure they have the informal support system they need. What these have in common is a commitment to capacity building through participation, empowerment and health literacy.

HEALTH EDUCATION

Health education is intended to assist people develop health literacy. It is generally considered to include any planned educational intervention that is aimed at the voluntary actions people can take to look after their health or the health of others (Green & Kreuter 2005). As one aspect of health promotion, health education can provide people with substantive information and processes for accessing health knowledge. This can include access to information on health issues and the structures and processes that help them use this knowledge for self-management (functional health literacy).

> **Point to ponder**
> Health education is any planned educational intervention aimed at increasing a person's ability to look after their own health. Health education assists people to develop health literacy.

Health education can also provide people with helpful techniques for influencing determinants in the local community and society (communicative health literacy), skills and mechanisms for developing coalitions and networks for change (critical health literacy), and political skills to engage in community action and work with others for health capacity building.

Successful health education programs play an essential role in raising people's awareness of healthy lifestyle choices such as physical activity, smoking cessation, food and alcohol consumption, and access to healthy environments (Barter-Godfrey et al 2007; Choi et al 2005). Knowledge of these factors is the starting point for securing conditions in their environment that could support healthy lifestyles. It begins with knowledge of the local context, and includes understanding policies such as those that promote accessible healthy foods, neighbourhood supports for exercising, community safety, income protection and risk reduction policies such as tobacco taxes and limiting exposure to tobacco smoke and other pollutants. Engaging with people to make lifestyle changes first must address the tensions between education and providing enabling opportunities. Barter-Godfrey et al (2007:346) suggest that health education be conceptualised in terms of 'agency' and 'structure'. *Agency* refers to individual capacity, a person's disposition and preference for health behaviours, while *structure* includes the context, resources and social factors that contour these choices.

Nurses, midwives and other health professionals provide health education but they also work towards modifying the environments for health (Barter-Godfrey et al 2007). Health education is therefore an important aspect of community engagement strategies without placing the onus on individuals to adopt health promoting behaviours. Educating people seeks to enable health by providing access to expertise, research evidence, and contextual information that will assist people in making healthy choices and finding the resources they need. One of the important ways health professionals assist community members is in acting as a filter for the large volume of information they may be exposed to in the electronic media (Ratzan 2007). However, health communication flows both ways.

> **Point to ponder**
> One of the most important health education strategies a health professional can employ is to help people to filter and understand the large volume of health information available on the internet.

Health professionals need to understand the barriers and facilitating factors that exist in the community, as well as personal and psychological factors that may be influencing personal choices. Recognising that work, study, child care or safety fears may be discouraging people from participating in lifestyle improvements is as important as knowing where people can access affordable venues, programs, information and other resources that facilitate participation (Barter-Godfrey et al 2007). Understanding people's social and cultural supports and any factors that impinge on their lifestyles is also critical information in assessing their education needs (Wainwright et al 2007).

Facilities such as neighbourhood PHC centres, where people can access many types of health-related information and services, can make health education more efficient (ANF 2009; MOHNZ 2001). Another avenue for health education is in the context of illness care, where hospitals include health education and continuity of care as part of a more holistic partnership with the community (Whitehead 2005). Irrespective of the setting, appropriate communication is the key to effective interactions (Hancock 2009). This means communicating the right information at the right time, in the right situation, with the right point of entry for guidance. The message conveyed should be transparent and aimed at empowerment and capacity development. Interactions should communicate trust, respect, participation by all involved and have realistic expectations. Where change is expected, evaluation strategies help to provide mutual feedback to all involved so that barriers and facilitating factors are identified, as well as whatever lessons can be taken away from one situation and applied to another.

CULTURAL SENSITIVITY, CULTURAL SAFETY

Culture is the accumulation of beliefs, values and knowledge that are inherited from one generation to another and that determine social behaviour. *Cultural sensitivity* means being responsive to the way an individual or group's cultural mores and lifestyle habits shape health and health behaviours. *Cultural safety* is a concept that refers to exploring, reflecting on and understanding one's own culture and how it relates to other cultures. This is a form of cultural relativism, which is concerned with how culture shapes power relations within the social world of the community. It is designed to enable safe spaces for the interaction of all cultural groups and their understanding of cultural identity.

In a culturally safe environment no one culture has dominance over another. It is not the nurse, midwife or other health practitioner who determines whether practice is culturally safe, but the recipient of care (Richardson & Carryer 2005). Cultural safety is an important aspect of PHC, given its focus on maintaining equity and empowerment, and we will revisit this in depth in Chapter 11.

> ### Point to ponder
> Cultural sensitivity means being aware of the way an individual or group's actions and lifestyle practices may shape their health behaviours. Cultural safety refers to exploring, reflecting on and understanding one's own culture and how it relates to other cultures.

Some examples of cultural differences in health behaviours stand out clearly; for example, the way some ethnic groups use hot and cold foods to overcome various illnesses, and their reliance on kinship ties to support one another during rehabilitation. Others are subtle, for example, the way certain spiritual beliefs contribute to mind–body–spiritual harmony. Still others are linked to popular folklore, through expressions perpetrated in the media as 'youth culture' or 'urban culture'. These refer to a perception of common values, behaviours and lifestyles that may or may not be characteristic of a particular group. Presumptions of similarity or commonality can be insensitive to those who only selectively adopt the behaviours or lifestyles associated with certain cultures. This can be a cross-generational problem when older members of migrant families, for example, may adhere closely to certain cultural practices, while younger members may change to become more closely aligned with their new culture. A sensitive, 'critical multicultural' approach (Culley 2006) involves ascertaining what people think, value and choose rather than making pre-emptive judgements of people on the basis of cultural membership.

Cultural sensitivity requires *cultural literacy*. This is developed through openness to people's interpretation of their cultural identity and how their expressions of culture shape their behaviour. Careful assessment can help unravel the various interactions between culture, societal structures and social inequalities (McMurray

& Param 2008). In this way, culture is framed within the relevant structural and political structures (Whitehead 2007). Cultural sensitivity also requires attention to the way language is used to describe members of different cultures. This can be problematic, as sometimes medical jargon can be disempowering. Being vigilant about language and communication may be as basic as reviewing seemingly innocuous expressions such as describing someone 'at risk' of certain behaviours, reframing descriptions in terms of being 'at promise', which shifts the description to one of potential rather than liability (Barry et al 2007). On the other hand, describing Indigenous people in relation to non-Indigenous benchmarks may be denigrating. Similarly, describing the experience of all refugees as if they were a homogenous group without close attention to their experiences may have a detrimental effect on their health and healing.

As health professionals, we have an obligation to adopt a receptive attitude towards cultures, to learn about culturally diverse practices and how they affect health behaviours for different members of the culture across different situations. For example, in some African countries, it is a cultural expectation for breastfeeding mothers to abstain from sexual relations.

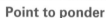

> ### Point to ponder
> Understanding our own culture and being openly receptive to differences in other cultures enables health professionals to provide more effective health care.

It is also customary and a highly valued family tradition, that breastfeeding continues for at least 2 years. To preserve the sanctity of the mother–child relationship there is also tolerance for the perceived need of males to satisfy their sexual needs outside the family during this time. Since the HIV/AIDS infection has devastated whole populations in African countries, these cultural norms have come under the microscope, especially when many African males hold entrenched beliefs that prevent them from using protection during sexual intercourse. The dilemma is at once cultural, social and public health related: how does the community strike a balance between cultural sensitivity, community empowerment and saving lives? The answer lies in careful assessment of individuals

and groups, assisting them as members of the community to address issues of access (for example, to information) and equity, including for the unborn; and working towards community empowerment, to develop self-determined changes without overriding cultural norms. One of the ways these issues can be approached is by casting beyond the immediate problem to the wider environment and enlisting the help of others in non-health sectors of society.

INTERSECTORAL COLLABORATION

Intersectoral collaboration requires cooperation between different community sectors, including (but not limited to) those managing health, education, social services, housing, transportation, environmental planning and local government. Tapping into the expertise of different sectors and different alliances can respond to certain needs in a more flexible and collaborative way. Non-health sectors include housing, education, agriculture, water resources and environmental management as well as health and social welfare agencies (ANF 2009). Tobacco control provides a good example of this type of collaboration, where legislators and policy-makers have developed non-smoking and quit-smoking initiatives, and enlisted the business, education and management sectors in reinforcing these strategies.

> ### Point to ponder
> Intersectoral collaboration is the cooperation or working together of all sectors who are involved in improving health.

Another advantage of intersectoral collaboration is the increased likelihood of widespread acceptance of the need for a health initiative when all parties involved work together for its success. Collaborative alliances also encourage efficient and effective use of resources, with economies achieved from including a range of specialists who, as a collective, may have an interest in long-term continuity of various interventions (Talbot & Verrinder 2010). For many public employees, working across sectors represents a major change, given their propensity to work in organisational silos (Martin 2008). A PHC collaboration can help shift this style of working, and focus more on cooperative efforts to help build the community's capacity for change.

Some collaborations have a finite existence, while other alliances may be longer term. Various initiatives can have an 'all-in' approach, an 'all-at-once' approach, or be comprised of a series of stages where smaller subgroups collaborate to achieve small gains that will contribute to larger solutions. For example, members of an Indigenous community may decide to institute a culturally appropriate campaign to examine family health issues. They may begin by convening an intersectoral planning group, involving the spiritual elders first. With cultural input the group may then decide to develop a plan to promote health literacy among adults and young people. This could involve a series of forums for bringing people together (transportation), enlisting the assistance of workers and teachers in the workplaces and schools (teachers, employers), arranging child care (child care workers, women's networks), and communicating with local and national political leaders to secure resources (council and legislative members). The group could invite local community health professionals to act as a resource to their initiative, and to provide substantive information that would help inform their program and evaluate its effectiveness.

Another collaboration might take place in an urban community where there may be a high prevalence of chronic disease. Intersectoral collaboration could involve occupational screening for diabetes and cardiovascular disease, liaison with local supermarkets to promote healthy foods, working with the local council for greener spaces and provision of bicycle racks throughout the community (Choi et al 2005). Schools, businesses and the media may also be involved to provide support for healthy behaviours.

> ### ACTION POINT
> Intersectoral collaboration takes many forms. Different approaches to working together will have different outcomes. Be open to exploring new ways of working together with other organisations to achieve health equity.

Health professionals would again act as partners to help members of non-health sectors develop communicative health literacy and to recognise the value of adding health to their operations.

They may contribute to the education industry by integrating health issues into the curriculum, or contribute to the environment and transportation industry by providing information on pollution hazards and road safety, or, with members of the recreation and fitness industries, propound the merits of corporate health programs for private or public industry which, in turn, has a 'value added' effect of reducing absenteeism.

At a broader level, intersectoral collaboration is an intensely political activity, especially where there is a need to allocate economic resources to health budgets. The essential elements for successful intersectoral collaboration at this level include national PHC policies that support decentralised control, and this is relatively easier in countries such as New Zealand, where there is a single, national Ministry of Health. In other countries, the complications of federal governments and state health authorities make this more difficult, especially when there may be differing political views between state governments and national government policy-makers. Further compromises to collaborative agreements come from powerful lobby groups, which may have their own vision of health care. For example, in Australia, the Australian Medical Association (AMA) has, for many years, defended its sole right to seek reimbursement from Medicare for treatments, which has effectively precluded other health professions from providing services to under-served communities unless they are under direct medical control. This has only recently changed, with reimbursement now allowed for some activities of practice nurses and nurse practitioners (ANF 2009). The ideal situation would be full participation by members of the community, who would have the right to choose their health professional, which is not yet a reality.

PUBLIC PARTICIPATION

Community participation is one of the central tenets of PHC. It is also part of a worldwide trend towards client-centred care (Coulter et al 2008; Robinson et al 2008; Wiggins 2008). This partnership model, as described previously, sees the health care professional and members of the community having equal status, control and reciprocal responsibility for health (Aston et al 2009). Community engagement is empowering for the community, building on existing assets and strengths for decision-making based on local knowledge and experience (Aston et al 2009). It also exemplifies capacity for developing social capital with mutual trust and reciprocity as well as cooperative networks for better health. However, the major goal of community participation is empowerment itself.

Point to ponder

Community participation is one of the central tenets of PHC. Community engagement empowers individuals, families and communities to achieve health.

This is a community development approach wherein community members are mobilised to participate in health decision-making, not just to improve local service delivery, but to develop mastery and control over the key processes that influence their lives (deVos et al 2009). In this respect, community participation creates a more socially just environment where people develop the skills to challenge non-responsive or oppressive institutions to redress power imbalances (deVos et al 2009).

Every encounter with the health care system is an opportunity to encourage community engagement. Having fully-engaged citizens increases the visibility of community strengths and needs as well as developing citizens' leadership capacity for change. This includes addressing social circumstances such as living and working conditions, access to health and other services, and consideration of the policies that maintain these circumstances.

ACTION POINT

Community engagement is a priority role for health professionals. Work with communities to facilitate their involvement in health projects.

With input from the community, health professionals will be able to move away from 'deficit models' to recognising community assets and capabilities (Whitehead 2007:474). As mentioned previously, some people are excluded from taking part in society because of social inequalities. For many, self-determination seems an untenable goal. By creating a climate that fosters vertical and horizontal linkages it is more likely that people will interact on different levels (vertically) and across different situations (horizontally). This fosters solidarity and inclusiveness, which are themselves major milestones in health capacity building (Whitehead 2007). Community solidarity and inclusiveness can, in turn, help members of the community develop intergenerational approaches to problem-solving, sharing strengths and experiences. This is described as an *enabling* community. The overarching goal of community participation is to channel society's resources towards support for better health equity, eliminating exclusion, reframing services around people's needs and expectations, and developing public policies that recognise the need for citizen engagement, sustainability and quality improvement (WHO 2008).

Nutbeam (2008), who has undertaken significant work in the area of health literacy, has developed a conceptual framework for practice, education and research that revolves around the notion of health literacy as an asset. This conceptual model is presented as an example of community participation and empowerment in health promotion. The value of this model will lie in its application across settings and across different population groups, including those with different starting points in progressing through the various levels of health literacy (see Figure 2.2).

COMMUNITY HEALTH PROMOTION: THE OTTAWA CHARTER FOR HEALTH PROMOTION

The Ottawa Charter for Health Promotion emphasises the importance of promoting health at a global level and identifies the fundamental conditions and resources for community health. These include peace, shelter, education, food, income, a stable ecosystem, sustainable resources, social justice and equity (WHO, Health and Welfare Canada & CPHA 1986). Five major strategies for health promotion are circumscribed within the public health activities of disease control and resource allocation, yet activities are guided by the PHC approach of grassroots community development and an ecological view of health. The five strategies are as follows:

1 Build healthy public policy

   This strategy is aimed at encouraging all those involved in health care to ensure that health becomes incorporated into all public policy decisions. The Charter suggests intersectoral collaboration where there is mutual recognition that

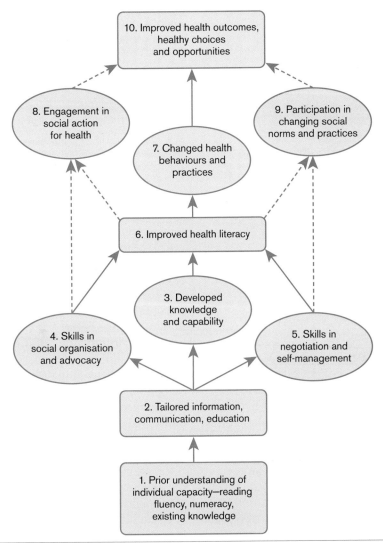

Figure 2.2 Conceptual model of health literacy as an asset (Source: Nutbeam D 2008 The evolving concept of health literacy. Social Science & Medicine 67)

the policies of other sectors, such as education, housing, industry, social welfare and environmental planning, also affect and are affected by, those that guide the health of our communities.

2 Create supportive environments

This strategy embodies the socio-ecological approach to health. The Charter encourages all people to recognise the importance of conserving and capitalising on those resources that enable people to maintain health, including physical or social resources.

3 Strengthen community action

Information and learning opportunities are seen as the focus for empowering communities to make informed choices for better health. This type of community action exemplifies what is meant by community capacity development.

4 Develop personal skills

This strategy guides communities to provide adequate and appropriate education and opportunities for skills development so that people can influence their communities to make local decisions for effective use of resources in order to attain health.

5 Reorient health services

Those involved in decisions affecting community health should operate from a base of evidence on what best works to foster the health of people. Included in this strategy is the need for research and the dissemination of knowledge

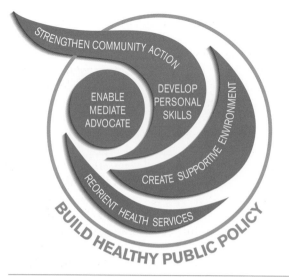

Figure 2.3 The Ottawa Charter for Health Promotion (WHO, Health and Welfare Canada & CPHA 1986)

from the multiple perspectives of those concerned with social, political, economic and physical resources as well as health.

The strategies of the Ottawa Charter have been endorsed by all countries involved in international conferences on health promotion and in 1997 were extended to focus on economic issues and alleviation of poverty through the Jakarta Declaration on Health Promotion Into the 21st Century (WHO 1997). In 2005, the Bangkok Charter for Health Promotion in a Globalized World was developed to chart a more global course in health promotion (WHO 2005). The rhetoric of the Bangkok Charter refocuses attention on new opportunities to counter the social changes that have affected working conditions, learning environments, family patterns and the culture and social fabric of communities. These are important issues, but the Charter is also supposed to embody a global pledge to work towards good governance, a civil society and good corporate practices, including world trade and financing (WHO 2005) (see Figure 2.3).

IMPLICATIONS FOR COMMUNITY HEALTH PROMOTION

Effective health promotion requires access to information and some very unique skills. It is almost impossible to become knowledgeable in all health matters or to keep up to date on all of the latest research results. However, the internet has made it possible to access current information on a wide range of health-related topics almost instantaneously. This has significantly enhanced the ability of health professionals to assist communities, but it has also created disparity between those people with internet access and those without. Health professionals should be aware of this inequity and ensure that information is accessible in appropriate ways. Appropriate use of technology means that the relevant technologies are used to support people in achieving health literacy and eliminating inequities.

Besides information, the most important elements in helping people achieve better health are a broad understanding of human development and behaviour, the ability to communicate well, and a PHC philosophy of community empowerment and participation. These three characteristics are fundamental to the role of a health advocate. To work with a community requires a sensitive approach to different people's needs at different stages of their development, and accountable governance at both community and societal levels (Hancock 2009).

To enable and facilitate the development of community health also requires a commitment to the SDOH. We are primarily social creatures who live in communal environments. We energise and are energised by those environments, which are constructed on foundations layered by historical, personal and situational events. Within this framework, health is not given to people, but generated by them. Our role is therefore one of mediating, enabling and facilitating the processes, people and systems that can be mobilised to achieve health goals. This requires leadership, citizenship and professionalism.

Point to ponder

The five strategies of the Ottawa Charter for Health Promotion are: build healthy public policy, create supportive environments, strengthen community action, develop personal skills and reorient health services.

Point to ponder

Health is not given to people but generated by them. The role of the health professional is to mediate, enable, facilitate and mobilise communities to achieve health goals.

Leadership, professionalism and citizenship

Leadership has been described as 'the capacity of a human community to shape its future' (Senge 2002:13). Accepting the mantle of leadership can help nurses, midwives and other health professionals create an avenue for influencing the way members of a community develop and sustain their common goals. Good leaders help develop this capacity by combining their innate skills and abilities with deliberate efforts to challenge, inspire, empower and act as a role model for others. For some, this is embellished with artistic flair and charisma. For others it is a deliberate, conscientious and committed progression towards excellence, achieved through careful assessment and rational planning. The best leaders are able to balance both sides of the coin (or the brain) sometimes simultaneously, sometimes sequentially. A charismatic personality, which draws on personal charm, can be helpful, but it must be accompanied by the substance of strategic thinking, change management skills, personal strength, confidence, negotiation skills, knowledge management and willingness to form strategic alliances (Jooste 2004).

The ideal image of a good leader epitomises courage. Courageous leaders practise with their eye and their intellect on the big picture, however they also create cycles of personal and professional affirmation and confidence that are fuelled by small, incremental successes. This is where professionalism is paramount. In working as part of a team, the leader must become adept at articulating the contribution of everyone working with the community, as well as articulating the broader range of community perspectives.

Point to ponder

Promoting community health requires nurses, midwives and other health professionals to take a leadership role.

This requires strong communication skills and an attitude of reflective humility. Being attentive and receptive to the range and breadth of voices in the community creates a meaningful understanding of how culture is captured in the language used by others (Gray 2009). This same type of reflective attitude applies to co-workers and members of the many networks that converge on the community's agenda. When the team has clear communication it is easier to form effective collaborations that are able to gather information, share its implications and engage in forward planning without dissent. One of the most challenging leadership issues lies in fostering genuine collaboration among all members of the team. This requires complementary skills, commitment to a common purpose and goals, and mutual accountability (Javellana-Anunciado 2007). For the team leader, successful collaborations make visible their acceptance of the leadership role, attracts support from those around them, and inspires others to become leaders.

Accepting a leadership role does not always come easily to nurses or midwives, especially when their practice experience has been predominantly in a rigid, hierarchical environment such as a hospital or other institution.

Point to ponder

Leaders in community health role-model good citizenship by becoming part of the community.

This type of organisational culture often prohibits self-development and creative thinking, although this is beginning to change with the pressure to increase nurses' and midwives' satisfaction to promote greater retention of the workforce. Another barrier to the development of leadership behaviours lies within the health professionals themselves. The motivation to develop leadership capacity can sometimes be sabotaged by our propensity to bypass, downplay or devalue our work. This creates misunderstandings about the importance of nursing and midwifery where it is most vital, that is, in the community. It also perpetuates the myth that practising nurses are virtuous, meek and self-sacrificing (Miller et al 2008). This couldn't be further from the reality of contemporary nursing practice, especially in the context of today's significant financial constraints and the pressure to manage effectively and efficiently, while continuing to advocate for personal, professional and community empowerment. The advocacy role is directed towards creating alliances and networks; flattening and reshaping hierarchies into community coalitions. Networking is therefore a critical, fundamental element of good leadership (Borbasi & Gaston 2002).

Embracing the leadership role is a sign of citizenship, a commitment to social capital and the development of trust among community members. Strong leaders embrace this role willingly, understanding that successful advocacy and lobbying for change will help grow their own as well as others' strengths (Graetz 2000; Porter O'Grady & Malloch 2003). Leaders role, model good citizenship by becoming part of the community as 'boundary crossers' (Kilpatrick et al 2009).

Instead of keeping their distance, as is often the case in formal client–professional relationships, working with communities involves becoming part of the community to see through the lens of a community member to identify needs and resources. This provides a basis for influencing people, advocating for their empowerment and planning strategically for the future. We provide an illustration of this type of leadership in Chapter 4, where nurses working with residents of a caravan park used their initiative and in-depth knowledge to instigate health improvements in that community.

Case study

In this chapter we see the Millers as community members with a range of needs, given their different ages and work pressures. The children are involved in recreational activities, with Samantha starting swimming lessons and Lily joining the soccer team. Samantha has had two bouts of wheezing and the family GP is considering further tests for the possibility of childhood asthma. Maria attends the school parents' group as often as she can, except when the bank is busy with audits and she has to work overtime. Lily has been using a computer for 2 years, despite the fact that she is only 6, and there is some pressure on the family to purchase a computer for home. The school-based health promotion program has provided hearing and sight screening for Lily, and she is learning about good nutrition in her health class. Her class is also going on an excursion to the local park to plant trees. The local GP, who sees all family members, recently sent Jim a text message reminder of his upcoming appointment as part of the practice's new program to screen all local men for testicular cancer. Maria and Jim are generally well, but worried about school fees, and the global financial crisis, especially with some of their work colleagues being laid off.

REFLECTING ON THE BIG ISSUES

- Being healthy in any community means having equitable access to resources, empowerment, cultural inclusiveness, healthy environments, and participation in decision-making.
- Health professionals undertake primary, secondary and tertiary prevention, using health promotion, appropriate technology and intersectoral collaboration.
- Health promotion is a combination of health education and helping people arrange the social and structural circumstances of their lives to maintain health.
- PHC principles focus on capacity building and empowerment of communities and those who reside in them.
- Leadership, professionalism and citizenship are integral to community advocacy.

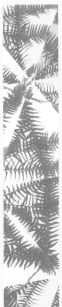

Reflective questions: how would I use this knowledge in practice?

1 What are the some of the most important needs the Millers might experience as the year progresses?

2 What primary, secondary and tertiary prevention strategies could the school nurse use to help the family?

3 How would intersectoral collaboration be used to promote the family's health and that of their community?

4 How would you use the Ottawa Charter for Health Promotion as a guide to helping build community capacity for families like the Millers?

5 What type of information would each member of the Millers need to develop health literacy? To what extent would this differ between members of the family?

6 Think of a community nurse or midwife you have encountered in community practice. What leadership skills were evident in their work?

7 To what extent do you think intersectoral collaboration can be achieved?

Research-informed practice

Read the article by Whitehead (2005) 'The health-promoting school: what role for nursing?'

• How does the research evidence add value to your nursing engagement with the Millers?

• To what extent do you think school nurses have been a victim of selective PHC practices by their employers?

• What are some of the constraints on school nurses in planning health promotion?

• How would the school nurse work with other health professionals and members of other sectors to help the Miller family maintain their health?

References

Abbott S, Bickerton J, Daly M, Procter S 2008 Evidence-based primary health care and local research: a necessary but problematic partnership. Primary Health Care Research & Development 9:191–8

Asada Y 2005 A framework for measuring health inequity. Journal of Epidemiology and Community Health 59:700–5

Aston M, Meagher-Stewart D, Edwards N, Young L 2009 Public health nurses' primary health care practice: strategies for fostering citizen participation. Journal of Community Health Nursing 26:24–34

Australian Nursing Federation 2009 Primary Health Care in Australia. A Nursing and Midwifery Consensus View. ANF, Canberra

Barry C, Gordon S, Lange B 2007 The usefulness of the community nursing practice model in grounding practice and research: narratives from the United States and Africa. Research and Theory for Nursing Practice: An International Journal 21(3):174–84

Barter-Godfrey S, Taket A, Rowlands G 2007 Evaluating a community lifestyle intervention: adherence and the role of perceived support. Primary Health Care Research & Development 8:345–54

Baum F 2002 The New Public Health: an Australian Perspective (2nd edn). Oxford University Press, Melbourne
—— 2007 Health for all now! Reviving the spirit of Alma Ata in the twenty-first century: an introduction to the Alma Ata Declaration. Social Medicine 2(1):34–41

Baum F, Begin M, Houweling T, Taylor S 2009 Changes not for the fainthearted: reorienting health care systems toward health equity through action on the social determinants of health. American Journal of Public Health 99(11):1967–74

Bernier N 2005 Public Health Policy and the New Public Health: Approaches to Improving the Population's Health in Canada. Conference presentation, 'The price of life: Welfare systems, social nets and economic growth', June 17–18, Catania, Italy

Besner J 2004 Nurses' role in advancing primary health care: a call to action. Primary Health Care Research & Development 5:351–8

Borbasi S, Gaston C 2002 Nursing and the 21st century: what's happened to leadership? Collegian 19(1):31–5

Catford J 2000 Mexico ministerial statement for the promotion of health: from ideas to action. Health Promotion International 15(4):275–6

Chamberlain M, Beckingham A 1987 Primary health care in Canada: in praise of the nurse? International Nursing Review 34(6):158–60

Choi B, Hunter D, Tsou W, Sainsbury P 2005 diseases of comfort: primary cause of death in the 22nd century. Journal of Epidemiology & Community Health 59:1030–4

Commission on the Social Determinants of Health (CSDH) 2008 Closing the Gap in a Generation. Health Equity Through Action on the Social Determinants of Health. Final report of the Commission on the Social Determinants of Health. WHO, Geneva

Commonwealth Department of Health and Ageing, Population Health. Online. Available: http://www.health.gov.au/internet/main/publishing.nsf/Content/health-pubhlth-about (accessed 13 July 2009)

Coulter A, Parsons S, Ashkham J 2008 Where are the patients in decision-making about their own care? Policy Brief, WHO and WHO European Observatory on Health Systems and Policies. Regional Office for Europe, Copenhagen

Courtney R 1995 Community partnership primary care: a new paradigm for primary care. Public Health Nursing 12(6):366–73

Crooks V, Andrews G 2009 Community, equity, access: core geographic concepts in primary health care. Primary Health Care Research & Development 10:270–3

Culley L 2006 Transcending transculturalism? Race, ethnicity and health-care. Nursing Inquiry 13(20):144–53

deVos P, Malaise G, De Ceukelaire W, Perez D, Lefevre P, Van der Stuyft P 2009 Participation and empowerment in primary health care: from Alma Ata to the era of globalization. Social Medicine 4(2):121–7

Falk-Rafael A 2006 Globalization and global health: toward nursing praxis in the global community. Advances in Nursing Science 29(1):2–14

Finlayson M, Sheridan N, Cumming J 2009 Nursing developments in primary health care 2001–2007. Health Services Research Centre, Victoria University of Wellington, Wellington, New Zealand

Graetz F 2000 Strategic change leadership. Management Decision 38 (8):550–62

Gray M 2009 Public health leadership: creating the culture for the twenty-first century. Journal of Public Health 31(2):208–9

Green L, Kreuter M 2005 Health Promotion Planning: An Educational and Ecological Approach. McGraw-Hill, New York

Halcomb E, Davidson P, Patterson E 2008 Promoting leadership and management in Australian general practice nursing: what will it take? Journal of Nursing Management 16:846–52

Hancock T 2009 Act Locally: Community-based Population Health. Report for The Senate Sub-Committee on Population Health, Victoria BC Canada. Online. Available: http://www.parl.gc.ca/40/2/parlbus/commbus/senate/com-e/popu-e/rep-e/appendixBjun09-e.pdf (accessed 17 July 2009)

Hertzman C 1999 Population health and human development. In: Keating D, Hertzman C (eds) Developmental Health and the Wealth of Nations. Guildford Press, New York
—— 2001 Health and human society. American Scientist 89(6):538–544

Holzemer W 1992 Linking primary health care and self care through management. International Nursing Review 39(3):83–9

Javellana-Anunciado C 2007 Effective team building. In: Kelly P (ed.) Nursing Leadership and Management (2nd edn). Thomson Delmar Learning, Clifton Park NY, pp 246–58

Jooste K 2004 Leadership: a new perspective. Journal of Nursing Management 12:217–23

Kendall S 2008 How has primary health care progressed? Some observations since Alma Ata. Editorial. Primary Health Care Research & Development 9:169–71

Kickbusch I 2003 The contribution of the World Health Organization to a new public health and health promotion. American Journal of Public Health 93(3):383–8

Kilpatrick S, Cheers B, Gilles M, Taylor J 2009 Boundary crossers, communities, and health: exploring the role of rural health professionals. Health & Place 15:284–90

Lalonde M 1974 A New Perspective on the Health of Canadians: A Working Paper. Government of Canada, Ottawa

Leavell H, Clarke A 1965 Preventive Medicine for the Doctor in his Community (3rd edn). McGraw-Hill, New York

Marmot M 1993 Explaining Socio-economic Differences in Sickness Absence: the Whitehall 11 Study. Toronto, Canadian Institute for Advanced Research

—— 2005 Social determinants of health inequalities. The Lancet 365(9464):1099–104

Marmot M, Rose G, Shipley M, Hamilton M 1987 Employment grade and coronary heart disease in British civil servants. Journal of Epidemiology & Community Health 32:244–9

Marmot M, Shipley M 1996 Do socio-economic differences in mortality persist after retirement? 25 year follow-up of civil servants from the first Whitehall study. BioMedical Journal 313(7066):1177–80

Marmot M, Shipley M, Rose G 1984 Inequalities in death-specific explanations of a general pattern. The Lancet I:1003–6

Martin C 2008 Addressing health inequities. A case for implementing primary health care. Canadian Family Physician 54(11):1515–17

McMurray A, Param R 2008 Culture-specific care for Indigenous people: a primary health care perspective. Contemporary Nurse 28(1–2):165–72

Miller T, Maloney R, Maloney P 2008 Power. In: Kelly P (ed.) Nursing Leadership and Management (2nd edn). Thomson Delmar Learning, Clifton Park NY, pp 259–68

Ministry of Health New Zealand (MOHNZ) 2001 The Primary Health Care Strategy. MOHNZ, Wellington

—— 2008 Health Targets: Moving Towards Healthier Futures2008/09 — The Results. MOHNZ, Wellington

—— 2009 Health targets. MOHNZ, Wellington. Online. Available: http://www.moh.govt.nz/moh.nsf/indexmh/healthtargets-targets (accessed 25 May 2010)

Nutbeam D 2008 The evolving concept of health literacy. Social Science & Medicine 67:2072–8

Porter O'Grady T, Malloch K 2003 Quantum Leadership: a Textbook of New Leadership. Jones and Bartlett, Toronto

Raphael D 2009 Poverty, human development, and health in Canada: research, practice, and advocacy dilemmas. Canadian Journal of Nursing Research 41(2):1–9

Ratzan S 2007 An informed patient — an oxymoron in an information restricted society. Journal of Health Communication 12:101–3

Richardson F, Carryer J 2005 Teaching cultural safety in a New Zealand nursing education program. Journal of Nursing Education 44(5): 201–8

Robinson J, Callister L, Berry J, Dearing K 2008 Patient-centered care and adherence: definitions and applications to improve outcomes. Journal of the American Academy of Nurse Practitioners 20:600–7

Ruger J, Kim H 2006 Global health inequalities: an international comparison. Journal of Epidemiology and Community Health 60:928–36

Schrecker T 2008 Denaturalizing scarcity: a strategy of enquiry for public health ethics. Bulletin of the World Health Organization 86:600–8

Senge 2002 Servant leadership: afterword. In: Spears L (ed.) Servant Leadership, a Journey into the Nature of Legitimate Power and Greatness (25th anniversary edn). Paulist Press, New York, pp 1–13

Starfield B 2006 Are social determinants of health the same as societal determinants of health? Health Promotion Journal of Australia 17(3):170–3

Stirling CM, O'Meara P, Pedler D, Tourle V, Walker J 2007 Engaging rural communities in health care through a paramedic expanded scope of practice. Rural and Remote Health 7(4):839

Talbot L, Verrinder G 2010 Promoting Health, the Primary Health Care Approach (4th edn). Elsevier, Sydney

United Kingdom Department of Health and Social Services (UKDHSS) 1980 Inequities in Health. Report of a Research Working Group Chaired by Sir Douglas Black. DHSS, London

United Nations 2009 Online. Available: http://www.un.org/unrwa/programmes/health/primary.html (accessed 15 July 2009)

Wainwright N, Surtees P, Welch A, Luben R, Khaw K, Bingham A 2007 Healthy lifestyle choices: could sense of coherence aid health promotion? Journal of Epidemiology and Community Health 61:871–6

Whitehead D 2003 Health promotion and health education viewed as symbiotic paradigms: bridging the theory and practice gap between them. Journal of Clinical Nursing 12:796–805

—— 2005 The health-promoting school: what role for nursing? Journal of Clinical Nursing 15:264–71

—— 2009 Reconciling the differences between health promotion in nursing and 'general' health promotion. International Journal of Nursing Studies 46:865–74

Whitehead M 2007 A typology of actions to tackle social inequalities in health. Journal of Epidemiology Community Health 61:473–8

Wiggins M 2008 The partnership care delivery model: an examination of the core concept and the need for a new model of care. Journal of Nursing Management 16:629–38

Wilson E 2005 6th Global Conference on Health Promotion. Canadian Journal of Public Health 96(5):324

Woollard M 2006 The role of the paramedic practitioner in the UK. Journal of Emergency Primary Health Care 4(1)

World Health Organization 1997 The Jakarta Declaration on Health Promotion Into the 21st Century. WHO, Geneva

—— 2005 The Bangkok Charter for Health Promotion in a Globalized World. WHO, Geneva. Online. Available: http://www.who.int/healthpromotion/conferences/6gchp/bangkok_charter/en/ (accessed 24 August 2005)

—— 2008 World Health Report 2008 Primary Health Care, Now More Than Ever. Online. Available: http://www.who.int/whr/2008/whr08_en.pdf (accessed 14 July 2009)

World Health Organization, Health and Welfare Canada & CPHA 1986 Ottawa Charter for Health Promotion. Canadian Journal of Public Health 77(12):425–30

World Health Organization & UNICEF 1978 Primary Health Care. WHO, Geneva

Useful websites

http://www.un.org/unrwa/programmes/health/primary.html — United Nations Primary Health Care Programmes

http://www.who.int/en/ — World Health Organization

http://www.un.org/en/rights/index.shtml — United Nations human rights organizations and issues

http://www.phmovement.org/en/resources/charters/peopleshealth — People's Health Charter

http://www.phmovement.org/en/node/798 — Cuenca Declaration, People's Health Movement

http://www.who.int/hpr/NPH/docs/ottawa_charter_hp.pdf — Ottawa Charter

http://www.who.int/healthpromotion/conferences/6gchp/bangkok_charter/en/ — Bangkok Charter

http://www.SDOH@YORKU.CA — Social Determinants of Health Website and archives

http://www.un.org/millenniumgoals/ — Millennium Development Goals

http://www.nlm.nih.gov/pubs/cbm/healthliteracybarriers.html — United States National Institutes of Health on Health Literacy

http://www.healthinfonet. — General health information

http://www.health.gov.au — Commonwealth Department of Health and Aged Care

http://www.healthinsite.gov.au — Health Insite (Commonwealth Government)

http://www.facs.gov.au/internet/facsinternet.nsf/ — Commonwealth Family and Community Services

http://www.aihw.gov.au — Australian Institute of Health and Welfare

http://www.phaa.net.au/ — Public Health Association of Australia

http://www.healthpromotion.org.au — Australian Health Promotion Association

http://www.hreoc.gov.au — Human Rights and Equal Opportunity Commission

http://www.ceh.org.au — Centre for Culture, Ethnicity and Health

http://www.ea.gov.au/esd/national/strategy/index.html — National Strategy for Ecologically Sustainable Development

http://www.health.gov.au/internet/main/publishing.nsf/content/ohp-environ-envstrat.htm or http://www.health.gov.au/internet/main/publishing.nsf/content/798726839F2B2FA6CA2572D40008D566/$File/enHealth%20NEHS%20final%20for%20web%20Nov%202007.pdf — National Environmental Health Strategy

http://www.nphp.gov.au/ — National Public Health Partnerships

http://www.health.nsw.gov.au/pubs/2000/pdf/capbuild.pdf or http://www.health.nsw.gov.au/pubs/2000/capbuild.html — Indicators to Help with Capacity Building, NSW Health

http://www.msd.govt.nz/about-msd-and-our-work/publications-resources/research/nz-families-today/ — New Zealand Families Today

http://www.plunket.org.nz — Royal New Zealand Plunket Society

http://www.moh.govt.nz — Manatu Hauora New Zealand Ministry of Health

http://www.nzhis.govt.nz — Te Parongo Hauora New Zealand Health Information Service

http://www.kidshealth.org.nz — New Zealand Child Health

http://www.hc-sc.gc.ca/hppb/phdd/pdf/perspective/pdf — A New Perspective on the Health of Canadians — the Lalonde Report

http://www.canadian-health-network.ca — Canadian health facts and figures

http://www.moh.govt.nz/hiasupportunit — New Zealand Ministry of Health — Health Impact Assessment Support Unit

http://www.hauora.co.nz — Health Promotion Forum of New Zealand

Chapter 3

Promoting health in an era of globalisation

INTRODUCTION

Health promotion is the central process involved in developing community capacity. As proposed in the Ottawa Charter, health promotion includes a comprehensive set of activities to build healthy public policy, create supportive environments, strengthen community action, develop personal skills and reorient health services. The framework of the Ottawa Charter has been accepted by those involved in promoting health for more than three decades, strengthened by a body of research and practice initiatives. The original tenets of the Ottawa Charter and the subsequent Bangkok and People's Charters have underlined the need to connect health promotion in local communities with the global health promotion agenda. The recommendations of all three charters reinforce the preeminence of primary health care (PHC) principles as the foundation of health promotion strategies throughout the world. They are also testimony to the heightened and persistent global awareness of the social and structural determinants of health across all contexts and populations.

> ### Point to ponder
> Health promotion is one of the most important strategies a health professional can use to develop community capacity.

Although the determinants of health may change according to the characteristics of any given community, the centrality of equity as a human rights issue remains constant. Equity is a product of the political environment. It is forged in the relations between governments, between different sectors of society, between cultures, neighbourhoods and families. Policy decisions determine the extent to which social justice can be achieved; whether people experience peace, shelter, education, food, income, a stable ecosystem and sustainable resources. These decisions reverberate down from the highest levels of government to the community level, dictating the creation and distribution of wealth, and the conditions and resources that will determine the extent to which individuals, families and communities will be able to achieve health. When the policy decisions engage civic participation at the grassroots level there is a greater chance of relevant, useful and effective health outcomes.

As health professionals in today's world we have an obligation to develop a sound knowledge base as well as an attitude of responsiveness to the features and occurrences of community life. Both are shaped by global knowledge and events as well as community characteristics. Health promotion pivots on the exchange of knowledge. By sharing knowledge in the context of interactions with the community our health promotion plans and objectives are strengthened and made relevant to their circumstances. In turn, the community gains health literacy and empowerment. This is health promotion in the 21st century. It is based on rational planning, responsiveness, inclusiveness, advocacy and community participation. It is creative, stimulating and professionally rewarding. Most importantly, it requires social and political activism based on global events, so this is where we will begin laying the foundation for promoting health in the community.

GLOBALISATION

Globalisation refers to the integration of the world economy over the past quarter century through the movement of goods and services, capital, technology and labour (Labonte & Schrecker 2007a). This integration has led to a situation where economic decisions affecting people in all corners of the world are influenced by global conditions. When we first encountered the notion of a globalised world in the 1980s it seemed a palatable idea. A globalised world held the promise of increased markets for goods, porous borders through which

Objectives

By the end of this chapter you will be able to:

1 explain globalisation and its role in contemporary health promotion
2 undertake a community assessment
3 plan a health promotion intervention
4 explain how knowledge of health and place can be used in promoting health
5 analyse the relevance of the Ottawa Charter and subsequent charters as a basis for health promotion
6 explain the difference between the risk factor approach to health promotion and the social determinants approach
7 develop a comprehensive strategy for promoting health in a particular community.

people could pass freely, greater sharing of cultures, and economies of scale where goods might become cheaper because they could be bought and sold efficiently by large business concerns. However, time has shown that globalisation has privileged only a few, the global elite, who have profited enormously from worldwide commercial endeavours at the expense of social, environmental and health concerns.

Point to ponder

Globalisation is the integration of the world economy through the movement of goods and services, capital, technology and labour.

The political environment that paved the way for globalisation was one that valued not only free trade between nations, but deregulation of financial markets and a host of other financial decisions that ultimately created the 2009 global financial crisis. This is neoliberal politics, which began in the mid-1970s with an intellectual blueprint that supported the virtues of free markets and private ownership (Labonte & Schrecker 2007a; Navarro 2009). The World Bank, the International Monetary Fund (IMF) and the World Trade Organization (WTO) have played a major role in globalisation by encouraging the commodification of such things as labour markets, health care, pharmaceuticals and public pension systems. Together, these three organisations have extraordinary power over global financial decisions and share markets worldwide. They are dominated by the wealthiest nations in the world, which control 48% of the

global economy and 49% of global trade (Labonte & Schrecker 2007a).

Global markets have been good for industrialised economies, but they have impoverished many countries, especially those who were already poor. In the 1980s, as globalisation gained momentum and the domestic markets of many developing countries declined, the IMF and the World Bank provided loans to those nations that agreed to adopt 'structural adjustment policies' in order to reorganise their economies. As nations this placed them in a precarious, disempowered position. Because the loans were also provided indiscriminately to political leaders who had no moral obligation to defend the legitimacy of their rule, many local communities were deprived of democratic participation in decision-making. This situation has continued to the present time as a number of despotic rulers maintain their leadership through repression (Labonte & Schrecker 2007b). Some African and Asian countries have experienced this for many years. People in Zimbabwe starve to death regularly. In Bangladesh, which is the poorest country in the world, only a fraction of the food aid reaches the poor, the majority of it being given to the government, which sells it at subsidised prices to the military, the police and middle-class families (Navarro 2009). This has led Navarro (2009:440) to declare that 'it is not *inequalities* that kill, but those who benefit from the inequalities that kill'.

Many governments attempting to respond to the globalised economy by becoming more 'business-friendly', have gradually relaxed their labour standards, health and safety regulations, and other social policy measures that may have provided greater income security (Labonte & Schrecker 2007b).

Point to ponder

Globalisation has arisen as a result of developed countries implementing free trade policies. This is called a neo-liberal approach to politics

To service international loans and to accommodate the lower price of imported goods from the global markets some adopted major policy changes. Newly developed policies on education, food subsidies, health, water, sewage, housing, employment and child care services actually had a deteriorating effect on the health of their populations, especially child health. The livelihoods of entire farming communities were destroyed by cheaper imported goods (Labonte & Schrecker 2007a, 2007b). Increased global imports of goods reduced the incomes of workers producing domestic products. Production of goods became fragmented and reorganised across borders in 'commodity chains' where each element is produced where it contributes most to financial returns, while reducing financial risk. For example, a number of products are now constructed where both labour and taxes are cheap. Various aspects of production are outsourced to companies with strong ties to the parent company, rather than local businesses. This maximises profits for the global company but erodes the local economy and its tax base that could have been used to fund infrastructure and support systems for health (Labonte & Schrecker 2007b).

Workers engaging in the new production processes became exposed to new workplace hazards and industrial pollution, which have been tolerated to increase labour market position. For many, increased casualisation of labour and excessive hours of work have become the norm. As casual, rather than permanent staff, they are readily open to exploitation by their employers. As a result, many workers in the developing countries have become deskilled, magnifying inequalities

Point to ponder

Globalisation has had a profound impact upon developing countries, resulting in an increase in health inequalities for many people already living in disadvantaged circumstances.

between rich and poor countries (Labonte & Schrecker 2007b).

A further layer of disadvantage has arisen by privatisation. Many countries have privatised what had previously been public services, and this has led to user fees for health care and education, which then became unaffordable. Some women have been forced into relying on 'survival sex' with its high risk of abuse and HIV/AIDS. Across entire populations, high external debts have increased personal income taxes. At the government level many currencies became devalued as interest rates to external banks increased. This occurred just as world prices were rising, when the economic elites became worried about tax increases and the threat of future devaluations. The result was an outflow of foreign loan repayments to safer, tax-free havens, which stripped the country producing goods of tax funding that may have been used to improve citizens' quality of life. With a financial crisis looming, internationally mobile investors tried to move their funds to safer ground. In some cases (in African countries) roughly 80% of all foreign loans flowed straight back out the same year (Labonte & Schrecker 2007b). Over the past decade, rich countries have offered some debt relief to various recipient countries, but the terms and conditions of this relief are so strict that many have not been seen as desperate enough to qualify, and three countries have actually seen debt increase over that time (Labonte & Schrecker 2007c).

THE PROS AND CONS OF GLOBALISATION

Clearly our globalised world has brought significant changes to community life, some more dramatic and far-reaching than others. In many circles, the very mention of 'globalisation' polarises opinion, attracting praise from some quarters and criticism from others. Globalisation optimists argue that economic arrangements since globalisation have added wealth to various nations, reducing absolute poverty (the total number of people living in poverty). Global technology has also enhanced knowledge for many people, providing instant electronic access to a wealth of information, including health information. Information disseminated throughout the world in this way has also connected ideas and research data, in some cases leading to greater collaboration in research and, ultimately, treatment strategies. It has also led to greater educational opportunities for some who would not have had the opportunity to study outside their countries.

Point to ponder

Globalisation has both pros and cons. Pros include improved access to information and greater educational opportunities. Cons include the feminisation of poverty and decreased accessibility to many health services.

Globalisation pessimists argue that the benefits are outweighed by the negative effects of a globalised world. Researchers cite the health effects of excluding some nations from the global market, particularly the developing countries, many of which are already suffering from communicable diseases such as HIV/AIDS, hepatitis and malaria (Huynen et al 2005). Falk-Rafael (2006) cites the colonising character of globalisation as contributing to the feminisation of poverty in such countries, which has seen poverty rates among women continuing to grow. Poverty, gender inequality, development policy and health sector reforms that have established user fees and reduced access to care have been linked to six million deaths per year from HIV/AIDS, tuberculosis and malaria (Labonte & Schrecker 2007a). The impact on accessibility of health services is profound. Many health services have become privatised, with increasing user fees. Multinational pharmaceutical companies dominate the trade in medicines, creating higher costs with no accountability to current and future generations in relation to local development or any social or environmental damage they may cause (Baum 2009; Labonte 2008; Labonte & Schrecker 2007a). Developing countries have also experienced an alarming brain-drain, with mass migration of health professionals stripping many countries of their workforce (Labonte & Schrecker 2007a). Africa, with 25% of the world's burden of disease and 3% of its workforce, loses 20 000 health professionals a year to migration (Robinson 2009). The net loss of these health workers has caused the near collapse of already fragile health systems.

These outcomes of the global marketplace have had a profound effect on nutrition, with certain countries being unable to produce their own food. The result has been a vicious circle of poor nutrition, forgone education and ongoing illness among the most disadvantaged in society (Navarro 2009).

Globalisation has also engendered concerns about losing cultural identities, languages and the right to choice in securing the best level of health for the most number of people. The reality is that as globalisation has progressed, there have been greater disparities between rich and poor countries, and between the rich and poor within most countries. The disparities are evident even in the United States (US), where multinational alliances between the automobile industry and the gasoline and oil industries are responsible for a failure to develop and maintain public transportation. A large proportion of the US population has no health insurance or are underinsured, often leading to family bankruptcy (Navarro 2009). For many, these disparities have led to declining health standards. Despite the promise of generating new wealth globalisation has failed to deliver equity in its distribution across populations.

What's your opinion?

Globalisation has had a significant impact on individuals, families, communities and nations. What negative and what positive impact has globalisation had on you as an individual, your family and your community?

After three decades there is greater understanding today of the perils of globalisation, yet it is escalating beyond all expectations. As all nations now trade more of their national income internationally, world trade has increased. This includes an increase in the illegal drug trade, which takes advantage of global finance systems, new information technologies and transportation. Migration has also increased, accompanied by a globalisation-induced increase in cultural tension and intolerance of others. As a result, the world is experiencing major social changes, manifest in increased individualism and social exclusion. Exclusion has created 'disintegration from common cultural processes, lack of participation in social activities, alienation from decision-making and civic participation, and barriers to employment and material sources', eroding social capital and creating fertile soil for conflict, violence, and increasing illegal trade in alcohol, firearms and drugs (Huynen et al 2005:7).

GLOBALISATION AS A HEALTH PROMOTION VARIABLE

As it has reverberated around the world, we have begun to understand globalisation as a comprehensive phenomenon, far beyond economic processes. In health promotion terms it has been called the quintessential *upstream variable* because it has created changes to the social determinants of health (SDOH) at the most fundamental level of daily life (Labonte & Schrecker 2007a:1).

Point to ponder
Proximal factors that influence health are those that directly cause disease or health gain (e.g. choosing a healthy diet). Distal factors that influence health are those that are a step removed from a person's life (e.g. a policy that ensures healthy food is available at an affordable price).

Its profound effects extend to both *proximal* and *distal* factors that influence health (Huynen et al 2005). Proximal factors are those that directly cause disease or health gain (health behaviour, a clean environment), whereas distal factors are a step removed from the person's life and are mediated by a number of other factors. For example, choosing a healthy diet is a proximal factor (closest to the person) influencing health. Distal factors that add other layers to that person's health choices can include the health policy that ensures access to healthy food at an affordable price, the economic environment that allows trade and marketing of certain foods, the socio-cultural environment that fosters knowledge and health literacy to assist food-related decisions, and the technology to store, supply and regulate the security of food.

Lifestyle choices for members of any given community are therefore dominated by global trade. Although technology and global policies can be used to discourage unhealthy behaviours by taxing unhealthy products (e.g. tobacco) the reverse is often the case. Many companies, especially in the fast-food industry, take advantage of opportunities for global marketing to promote diets high in fat, sugar and salt (Baum 2009). Some countries whose resource base leaves them unable to produce sufficient foods become 'food insecure' from being at the mercy of global markets. Multinational companies such as Monsanto and McDonald's, for example, have been responsible for extinguishing certain gene pools within developing countries' ecosystems (Falk-Rafael 2006).

Point to ponder
Lifestyle choices by any member of a community are dominated by globalisation.

The companies' quest for productivity (with bio-engineering and products heavily dependent on pesticides) and uniformity (McDonald's demand for only one variety of potato) effectively eliminate their capacity as growers (Falk-Rafael 2006).

Where this type of food insecurity is extreme, food aid can be advertised, but in many cases, food-insecure countries become vulnerable to shocks that reduce the global market, further impinging on their ability to purchase what they need. Even water is now traded on the global market as a commodity, and this has major health impacts both globally and locally. In Australia, for example, it has become commonplace to trade water rights, disrupting the ecosystem as well as the local rural economy.

Point to ponder
One of the most profound impacts of globalisation has been a growth in urbanisation and the subsequent detrimental effect on the environment.

In New Zealand the globalisation of milk production, which removed subsidies for the milk producers and deregulated the market conditions that kept milk affordable, has had a dramatic effect on milk consumption (Smith & Signal 2009). This has led to a situation where many low socio-economic families have difficulties in purchasing milk. The effects are profound. Nearly 10% of young New Zealanders do not consume milk, and one-third consume less than a glass per day, substituting the cheaper products of global producers which include soft drinks, cola and powdered fruit drinks (Smith & Signal 2009). Because of globalisation the mass media also have a greater 'reach' than in past decades.

Global promotion of certain brands of consumer goods such as Coca-Cola and McDonald's has contributed to dietary changes and subsequent health consequences throughout the world. These companies are also part of the globalisation of culture as their advertising pervades sports and culture as well as consumerism (Labonte 2008).

Although the effects of globalisation on the SDOH are asymmetrical, there have been some common trends. With rapid population growth there has been increasing urbanisation of populations throughout the world. This often creates further disadvantage as urban economies become less industrialised and more geared towards commerce and tourism, with the poor shifted to suburban or remote locations. This leaves many people having to rely on fewer support systems and inferior services, often with a lack of public transportation and protective services (Labonte & Schrecker 2007b). Urbanisation also disrupts the ecological footprint, with overconsumption, declining air and water quality, loss of biodiversity, chemical pollution and decline in living environments, especially for the poor (Baum 2009). This compromises environmental sustainability. Those who live in industrialised cities experience deterioration of the environment disproportionately as they tend to live energy-intensive lifestyles, consuming 75% of the world's energy, through excessive use of automobiles and other polluting devices. Cars not only make cities congested with high pollution levels, but they cut people off from social interactions (Baum 2009).

Urban dwellers often have exposure to a wider range of harmful environments than rural people. A case in point is the ground contamination caused by the production of orchard chemicals in one of the most picturesque regions of New Zealand. Attempts have been made over the past several years to clean up the contamination, and the local District Council has pronounced the area safe for redevelopment of commercial and residential interests. However, the ground will never again be entirely contaminant free and ongoing monitoring of soil and groundwater will continue indefinitely (Pattle Delamore Partners Ltd 2009). This example demonstrates that although some environmental effects may be 'cleaned up' the long-term impact industrial pollutants may have on the environment, on people and on places is immeasurable.

Global warming and the resultant natural disasters of rapidly changing climates, also exacerbate the health effects of urbanisation. The effects of a deteriorating physical, social and political environment because of climate changes can lead to exploitation and control over technology, finances, employment and a host of social and structural determinants that disadvantage women, the poor, Indigenous and other vulnerable people (Baum 2009; Robinson 2009). The impact of climate change is so important to health that an international alliance has been formed on climate justice, under the Global Humanitarian Forum chaired by Kofi Annan, the former Director-General of the United Nations (UN) (Robinson 2009). The major challenge lies not only in reducing emissions causing global warming, but ensuring that those disadvantaged by environmental degradation are able to achieve an adequate standard of living and the dignity to lead the lives they choose (Robinson 2009).

HEALTH PROMOTION STRATEGIES FOR GLOBAL HEALTH

Global health promotion is a central tenet of global development, and therefore a core responsibility of governments. It is also a key focus for communities and civil society, including the corporate and business world. Labonte (2008) suggests that promoting health at the global level requires two major changes in how we deal with globalisation. These include social risk management, which means aligning social protection with global realities. This would see households earn their keep, by smoothing their consumption patterns in response to external events, ranging from natural disasters to financial crises. Such an approach does not take into account how crises are created by global forces or the disproportionate effect on the most vulnerable. The second seeks to blunt the negative impact of the global marketplace through the actions outlined in Box 3.1.

The approach mentioned in Box 3.1 is closely aligned with PHC principles and responds to the SDOH. Labonte (2008) urges critical appraisal of the health problems that have become inherently global in cause and consequence. He outlines five different ways of conceptualising health in relation to globalisation: health as security, as development, as global public good, as commodity and as a human right. Health as commodity is a convoluted way to view health. It represents the worst of globalisation, in reducing health to goods (drugs, new technologies) and services (private health

- Recognition of access to resources as a human right.
- Reframing globalisation in terms of social obligations and new institutions for global governance (Labonte 2008).
- Regulating global market forces in a way that is people-centred rather than capital-driven.
- Public policy development based on a vision of the world that people matter and social justice is paramount.
- Developing a global contract where industrialised countries support contemporary welfare states (Labonte & Schrecker 2007c).

insurance, facilities or providers) with trade having the outcome of maximising profit rather than health. The other four concepts embody a type of 'transnational health activism' suggested by the Bangkok Charter's recommendation that health be central to the global development agenda (Labonte 2008:467).

Point to ponder
Fear of epidemics that may influence global trade, finance or travel has been used as a means of privileging high-income nations and in particular the industries that create drugs aimed at preventing or treating such epidemics.

Health as security

When health is seen as security it conjures up fear of bio-terrorism, terrorists, and the general inclination towards border protection, 'whether the invaders are pathogens or people' (Labonte 2008:468). This idea has given more political clout to public health measures, particularly with global epidemics, but it is also associated with 'repressive political measures', such as the rhetoric and actions of the war on terror (Labonte 2008:468). Instead of encouraging high-income nations to help those less fortunate it has privileged those diseases most likely to inconvenience global trade and finance or travel to wealthy countries. Fear of

epidemics such as avian flu or H1N1 (swine flu), has also proven a major windfall for the pharmaceutical industry, particularly Roche, the company that makes Tamiflu. Labonte (2008) suggests a shift from the national security approach to one of working towards human security. The latter is based on a core moral value of individual security, including income, health care, housing, education, environmental security and other essentials for life (Labonte 2008). This indicates the political nature of health promotion, and the need for vigilance, activism and community participation to shift ideas, attitudes, resources and power to focus on strengthening the health and wellbeing of the population (Sparks 2009).

Health as development

The Millennium Development Goals (MDGs) have been described as 'the most concentrated and collected global statement of development intent in human history' (Labonte 2008:470) (see Figure 3.1). MDGs clearly situate health as a development outcome. The MDGs, to be achieved by the year 2015, were defined at a UN summit of 191 nations to address the effects of poverty on health in the developing nations. They are aimed at addressing extreme poverty, hunger, disease, lack of adequate shelter and exclusion while promoting education, gender equality and environmental sustainability (Sachs 2005). The Millennium project, under the auspices of the Director-General of the UN, is based on the assumption that sound, proven, cost-effective interventions can ameliorate and often eliminate extreme poverty, especially where it is most needed, such as in the countries of sub-Saharan Africa. To achieve the goals requires investment of wealthy countries in the poorer nations to help develop capacity in education, the environment, health care, nutrition and social programs, especially those that foster equity.

The intention of the MDG project has been no less than to change the world. If the goals are met, 500 million people will be lifted out of extreme poverty. More than 300 million will no longer suffer from hunger.

Point to ponder
The Millennium Development Goals are a set of goals designed to address the effects of poverty on health in developing nations.

Millennium Development Goals
Eradicate extreme poverty and hunger — reduce by half, the proportion of people living on less than a dollar a day; reduce by half the proportion of people who suffer from hunger.
Achieve universal primary education — ensure that both boys and girls complete a full course of primary schooling.
Promote gender equality and empower women — eliminate gender disparity in primary and secondary education preferably by 2005 and at all levels by 2015.
Reduce child mortality — reduce by two-thirds the mortality rate among children under five.
Improve maternal health — reduce by three-quarters the maternal mortality ratio.
Combat HIV/AIDS, malaria and other diseases — halt and begin to reverse the spread of HIV/AIDS, halt and begin to reverse the incidence of malaria and other major diseases.
Ensure environmental sustainability — integrate the principles of sustainable development into country policies and programs; reverse the loss of environmental resources; reduce by half the proportion of people without sustainable access to safe drinking water.
Develop a global partnership for development — develop further an open trading and financial system that is rule-based, predictable and non-discriminatory. This includes a commitment to good governance, development and poverty reduction nationally and internationally. Address the least developed countries' special needs. This includes: tariff and quota-free access for their exports; enhanced debt relief for heavily indebted poor countries; cancellation of official bilateral debt; and more generous official development assistance for countries committed to poverty reduction. Address the special needs of landlocked and small island developing states. Deal comprehensively with developing countries' debt problems through national and international measures to make debt sustainable in the long term. In cooperation with the developing countries, develop decent and productive work for youth. In cooperation with pharmaceutical companies, provide access to affordable essential drugs in developing countries. In cooperation with the private sector, make available the benefits of new technologies — especially information and communications technologies.

Figure 3.1 The UN Millennium Development Goals

The lives of 30 million children and 2 million mothers will be saved. Hundreds of millions of people will have safe drinking water and basic sanitation. Hundreds of millions of women and girls will go to school, be able to access economic and political opportunities and be safer and more secure (Sachs 2005). Yet to date, there have been only modest gains in achieving the goals, although there has been a renewed Global Campaign for achieving the MDGs, which is centred around improving maternal health through innovative financing and better health services (http://www.un.org/News/briefings/docs/2008/08 0925_MDG_Health.doc.htm [accessed 15/07/09]). However, long-term trends show that progress has been slow. The ratio between the richest and poorest countries continues to increase significantly, and the number of people living in absolute poverty (less than $US2 per day) has also increased (Baum 2009). One billion people worldwide try to survive on less than $US1 per day while 35 000 of the world's children die (Mooney & Ataguba 2009).

Criticisms of the MDGs focus on the lack of equity and inclusiveness of the goals in terms of human development. The objective of human development is to try to ensure that everyone develops to their maximum potential as a human being (Hancock 2009). The UN Development Programme is based on the holistic nature of human development in terms of securing essential areas of choice, including political, economic and social opportunities for being creative and productive, and enjoying self-respect, empowerment and the sense of belonging to a community (Hancock 2009).

Point to ponder
Despite the potential for significant improvement in health outcomes for the world's poorest, progress in achieving the Millennium Development Goals has been slow. Critics argue that this is due in some part to the lack of equity and inclusiveness of the goals in terms of human development.

Because of the way the goals are cast, and their emphasis on economic goals it would be possible to meet their criteria by improving the health of the wealthy while worsening the health of the poor (Labonte 2008). The goals are also difficult to measure and do not identify the causes of the problems that need to be addressed (Labonte 2008). They are unambitious, setting only minimal standards (Baum 2009; Labonte 2008) and the target of Goal 8 to further an open trading and financial system may be at odds with the others, given the disadvantage created thus far by open markets (Labonte 2008). The MDGs have been lauded for their call to wealthy countries to support those at an economic disadvantage. However, even in this respect, there have been significant problems in relation to foreign aid. In general, with the exception of the Nordic countries, aid levels remain ungenerous (Labonte 2008). Aid given to Africa has not created economic development, but instead most has been lost to 'capital flight' (the removal of funds to wealthy countries). Some aid arrangements have been used to pressure poor recipient countries into trade treaties that favour wealthy, donor nations. Over 60% of the increase in donor aid between 2001 and 2004 has gone to Afghanistan, Iran and the conflict-ridden, mineral-rich Democratic Republic of the Congo, which together constitute less than 3% of the world's poor. This calls into question whether aid is protecting the interests of the givers or the recipients (Mooney & Ataguba 2009).

Point to ponder
With the exception of Nordic countries, humanitarian aid contributions by developed countries remain ungenerous.

Australia provides $A42 billion in aid, yet the funds are now tied to long-term anti-terrorism projects in the Asia–Pacific region, officially reoriented towards combating terrorism and promoting regional security (Mooney & Ataguba 2009). In New Zealand, election of a National government in 2008 has seen a re-orientation of New Zealand aid policy from a focus on social equity to one on sustainable economic growth (McCully 2009), resulting in a total redistribution of New Zealand's aid. This demonstrates how even within countries, differing government agendas can have a wide-ranging impact on global health (http://www.beehive.govt.nz/release/aid+increases+nzaid+changes+focus).

These outcomes suggest that the development agenda and the notion of 'aid' needs to be recast in terms of human potential through 'redistributive obligations' rather than market performance (Labonte 2008:473). This would help temper investments in health to distinguish the objective (human development) from the tool (economic growth). An alternative way of approaching global health is to see health as a public good.

Health as a global public good

One approach to promoting global health that has gained momentum since the 1990s is the notion that when wealthy nations provide health assistance to the less fortunate it is not only humanitarian aid, but a selfish investment in protecting health in their own population (Smith & MacKellar 2007). This conception of health is one that evokes community, where the emphasis is on the collective, and stable, sustainable systems that support health and nation building. Globally, this idea of sharing would see a broader perspective where all countries became concerned about risks (risk pooling) and worked towards developing common financial regulations to benefit everyone, not just those in positions of wealth and power (Baum 2009; Labonte 2008).

The Commission on the Social Determinants of Health (CSDH) has done some analysis of financial possibilities in relation to this type of aid, especially in the context of the 2009 global financial crisis. They agreed that it was important for the world's economies to prop up the financial systems of industrialised nations to prevent normal families from falling victim to the lack of credit, but the amount spent on the initial stimulus packages at the beginning of the crisis was beyond what was required. The commission estimated that for $100 billion, far less than what was spent in the stimulus packages in either the US or the United Kingdom (UK), the world's slums could have been upgraded (Marmot 2009). For one-ninth of what the banks received, every urban citizen of the world could have clean, running water, and every child could have free education (Marmot 2009). This leaves us to ponder the argument that even global institutions such as financial organisations must be based on global social justice and world citizenry, without a return to the open, competitive market system of the past (Mooney & Ataguba 2009).

Health as a human right

This view of health is that conveyed in the People's Health Movement, which has support from 40 countries. Its focus is on a bottom-up mobilisation of action through training, capacity building, documenting health rights violations, and lobbying governments for policy change. It has created the momentum for a global health ethic which would entrench rights, regulations, redistributive justice and a concern with the inequality of persistent poverty.

Point to ponder

Viewing health as a human right redirects the focus of addressing health issues from a top-down, government-directed approach, to a bottom-up, people-led approach, where addressing inequality between people and nations is seen as a priority.

Health promotion in this context is through global health diplomacy, based on the need for ethical, rights-based, public good, development, and security in the foreign policy of all governments (Labonte 2008). Baum (2009) uses the metaphor of a nutcracker, explaining that grassroots or bottom-up pressure is most effective when combined with top-down policy action to open up the issue for discussion.

Employment is absolutely critical to human rights. Mary Robinson, the former UN Commissioner for Human Rights argues that job creation must be the central objective for private companies as well as governments. This includes respecting core labour standards such as non-discrimination and workplace health and safety, promoting social protection by income security and supporting those who are ill, providing insurance for older persons, and promoting social dialogue between governments, employers and workers (Robinson 2009). Questions to ponder in relation to health promotion in an era of globalisation are listed in Box 3.2.

BUILDING THE EVIDENCE BASE: THE POPULATION APPROACH

Promoting health involves getting to know a community, its people, their resources and their goals, and developing an understanding of how this local

---

BOX 3.2 HEALTH PROMOTION QUESTIONS IN AN ERA OF GLOBALISATION

- How can knowledge of the global environment be used to promote health at the local level?
- What social, cultural and environmental conditions can be modified to create the conditions for health in a community?
- How can community members become engaged in civic participation to change the social and structural conditions that impinge on their health?
- What actions can health professionals take to participate in political processes that have an effect on health and wellbeing?
- How can health professionals help people develop health literacy, empowerment and health capacity?
- How can scientific knowledge be used to underpin health promotion strategies?
- What health promotion and health education strategies will achieve optimal results for which types of societies, communities and populations?

Point to ponder

Promoting health requires research, resourcefulness, information exchange, receptivity to new ideas and strategies, an attitude of inclusiveness, and a focus on the dual goals of equity and community empowerment.

knowledge can be linked with wider societal and global knowledge and aspirations. This requires research, resourcefulness, information exchange, receptivity to new ideas and strategies, an attitude of inclusiveness, and a focus on the dual goals of equity and community empowerment. The process begins by building the knowledge base, then using strategies that have been shown to be effective in facilitating better health for communities in the context of their local conditions while keeping an attitude of openness to new ideas and approaches.

Epidemiology is the traditional starting point for developing a base of evidence on health and its determinants in specified populations. Epidemiological studies are designed to gather sufficient data to monitor trends and inform planners and policy-makers on ways of improving health (Bezruchka 2006; Kawachi 2002). Until recently, epidemiology has been overly focused on uncovering the causal connections between exposure to risk factors and the development of disease, rather than health and wellbeing.

Point to ponder

Epidemiology is the study of factors that affect the health of populations.

Epidemiology as a discrete area of study, began with John Snow, an English physician who was concerned with the number of people dying of cholera. He plotted the incidence of deaths in a London neighbourhood, and found an association with the pump supplying the local drinking water by talking with local residents about their daily habits. Although he did not know the causative agent (a bacteria) he understood that the source of the problem was the water supply. He removed the pump handle and the death rate declined. His actions therefore controlled the epidemic.

John Snow had a major influence on epidemiology (www.ph.ucla.edu/epi/snow.html) yet his action-oriented approach, to follow up on epidemiological data is rarely included in accounts of epidemiological studies (Bezruchka 2006). Snow and others investigating the sources of diseases in the 19th century began to draw a connection between poverty and material disadvantage and ill health, which called into question whether dissecting single factors provided a viable base of evidence for intervention (Bezruchka 2006). Single risk factors are easy to measure and there are clear-cut statistical conventions for linking them to specific outcomes. However, the effects of culture, community trust and fairness, and the elements of social capital are more challenging. Yet the evidence base is incomplete without this knowledge, which is a missing link in the global research agenda.

THE GLOBAL BURDEN OF DISEASE PROJECT

To inform national and international health policies for prevention and control of disease and injury, in 1990, researchers from the Harvard School of Public Health, the World Bank, and the WHO began an epidemiological investigation into the worldwide burden of illness. This is called the global burden of disease (GBD) study (WHO 2005). The goal of the study was to draw on many sources of data to develop internally consistent estimates of incidence, health state prevalence, severity and duration, and mortality for over 130 major causes of disease. The original studies identified the major causes of death, disability and disease for various demographic groups in eight regions of the world (Murray & Lopez 1997a). The findings calculated the burden of disease (Murray & Lopez 1997b). Some 20 years later, the original findings have limited usefulness for health planning at the local level, partly because of the way data were aggregated to show an international picture, and also because of the time delay between collection and dissemination of the information. However, the GBD study has provided a template for calculating where each country fits on an international scale of health, how widespread some diseases are, particularly the lifestyle diseases such as cardiovascular disease and diabetes, and what trends are most likely to occur in the future. What is as yet unknown is how health service planners will use the data to persuade governments to develop population-wide strategies for better health, or to fund protective supports that will help people live healthier lives.

Point to ponder
The global burden of disease study investigated the worldwide incidence, prevalence, severity, duration and mortality of over 130 major causes of disease.

The other contribution of the GBD study has been the impetus for national measures of burden of disease as a basis for health promotion planning at the national level. Towards this end, national GBD data are collected by the health departments of many countries. This work has also been extended by other global studies conducted by the World Bank and the United Nations Development Programme to analyse inequities within countries and within demographic groups, and to compare these with other nations on the basis of World Development Indicators (Ruger & Kim 2006). New measures have been established, including the relative inequality index (RII) and the concentration index (CI), which are measures of cumulative population inequalities that are sensitive to demographic differences (Safaie 2007). The single indisputable finding from all of these studies continues to point to the health divide between rich and poor, which is not improving (Baum 2009; Hancock 2009; Oliver 2008; Ruger & Kim 2006; Safaie 2007). As we mentioned earlier in this text, this is 'modernity's paradox', the situation where, despite global prosperity, there are increasing inequalities in health and wellbeing (Keating & Hertzman 1999; Li et al 2008).

Point to ponder
Incidence is the measure of the number of new cases of a particular disease or health issue in a specific period of time. Prevalence is the total number of cases of a particular disease or health issue in a population at any one time.

THE EPIDEMIOLOGY OF HEALTH AND ILL HEALTH

The classic conceptual model of epidemiology has been to examine specific aspects of the host (biology), the agent (a causative factor) and environment (factors that exacerbate or moderate the effects of the agent on the host), to see how each of these affects the spread of a disease or ill health in the population. However, studying each of these in relative isolation is not helpful in measuring the effects of the SDOH.

The objective of epidemiological researchers is to collect data on the incidence of individuals 'at risk' of developing a particular disease in order to inform development of a vaccine or treatment for that disease. Data from epidemiological analyses are presented in terms of rates of incidence and prevalence. Incidence is calculated by dividing the number of new cases in a population by the population at risk, then multiplying this by a base number (1000 or 100 000). This provides an estimate of the likelihood that a condition would occur in the population. The prevalence of a certain condition is the number of new and existing cases divided by the population at risk multiplied by 1000 or 100 000 (see Box 3.3).

Point to ponder
Incidence and prevalence are useful measures for understanding the nature of groups who may be targeted in a health education or intervention program. For example, if the incidence of breast cancer were rising in a given population (i.e. there was an increase in new cases of breast cancer in a certain population), then it may be appropriate to target breast screening programs towards that group.

Epidemiological analysis provides this type of estimate (a crude rate) of what may occur in a given population, and this is helpful for public health planning. These rates can also be more specifically computed on the basis of different demographic groups according to such factors as age, gender or ethnicity, for example. This can be used to understand the groups who might be targeted in a health education or intervention program if certain health authorities were implementing this type of approach.

If we know that certain groups are more 'at risk' for developing influenza or cervical cancer, health planners can develop strategies around this information, such as promoting immunisation

BOX 3.3 EXAMPLE OF EPIDEMIOLOGICAL RATE

Rate:

$$\text{Incidence} = \frac{\text{No. of new cases}}{\text{Population at risk}}$$

$$\times\ 1000\ (\text{or } 100\,000)$$

$$\text{Prevalence} = \frac{\text{No. of existing cases (new and old)}}{\text{Population at risk}}$$

$$\times\ 1000\ (\text{or } 100\,000)$$

programs. Epidemiological data can also provide rates of incidence in relation to exposure to factors creating illness. If an occupational group is exposed to a certain toxic substance, a measure of the 'relative risk' of becoming ill from that exposure can be calculated by comparing a group (called a cohort) who were exposed to the hazard with a cohort who were not exposed. If the group exposed to the risk has a higher rate of the illness that hazard is declared a risk factor. To provide better understanding of the risk epidemiologists would then study the effect of the risk factor over a longer period of time in the entire population, which would provide a greater insight into its effect.

Traditional epidemiological measurements of an agent, host and environment are somewhat limited in terms of what we know about the causes of illness. For this reason an expanded model, the web of causation, which includes the interconnections between each of these factors, provides a more comprehensive basis for analysis (see Figure 3.2).

Further limitations of epidemiological measurements, including those in a web of causation, is that unless the people being studied (those at risk) have similar incomes, or education, or wealth, or status in society the researchers may not find the right solution to their illness or strategies for promoting health. Interventions targeting individuals and groups identified as at risk of certain outcomes can provoke feelings of exclusion and stigmatisation (Ridde 2007). Although large population studies can show a link between interventions and population outcomes (Rose 1985), such an approach fails to address persistent inequities among some groups, especially for child health, women's health and Indigenous populations (Baum 2009; Ridde 2007). Instead, economic, social, environmental and health services inadequacies continue to contribute to inequalities in child and adult health and mortality (Baum 2009; Ridde 2007; Ruger & Kim 2006). This major failure of health planning poses a question of whether the focus should be on individuals or populations.

We know from the growing body of research into the SDOH that the determinants of individual health are often different from the determinants of the health of a population (Kawachi

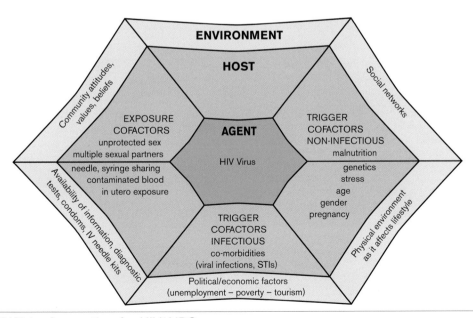

Figure 3.2 Web of causation for HIV/AIDS

2002). Traditional epidemiological studies of the link between a risk factor and individual outcomes may be used to inform someone of the need for behavioural change: to have a vaccination, reduce their alcohol intake, maintain a lean body weight or abstain from unprotected sex. But an alternative approach is to analyse epidemiological data at the population level, to explain why some societies might have high rates of alcohol abuse, hypertension, obesity and diabetes (Bezruchka 2006; Kawachi 2002). This helps track combinations of factors that affect health, to identify what those factors are, to analyse how they act together in a harmful or healthful way, and to understand how the combinations of factors are shaped by the environments of people's lives to either multiply or diminish the effect. Social epidemiology is a method of examining these effects (Kawachi 2002) (see Figure 3.3).

SOCIAL EPIDEMIOLOGY

Social epidemiology is a multidisciplinary approach to understanding health and ill health based on a broad understanding of the social and environmental circumstances of people's lives. Its goal is to conceptualise, operationalise and test associations between the social environment and population outcomes in order to intervene on social conditions (Kawachi 2002).

Point to ponder
Social epidemiology is the study of the relationship between the social environment and health outcomes.

Social epidemiological studies also gather information about people's behaviour, but not with the intention of blaming them personally for a certain health outcome (e.g. diabetes as a result of poor diet) but rather, to help them rearrange the circumstances of their lives so that healthy choices become easier. This can be illustrated in the context of health and place. As we reported in Chapter 1, there are significant differences in illness in communities where there is high inequality between rich and poor people (Wilkinson & Pickett 2006). However, this does not occur with uniformity, so it is important to study the social epidemiological base of each community, to peel back the layers of social life to investigate health and health choices in the context of that particular environment. This accentuates the relationship between health and place.

Health and place

The socio-ecological view of health embodies the fact that health is created in the settings where people live their lives. This is where the promise of

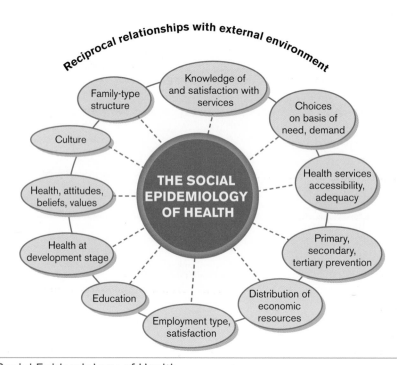

Figure 3.3 The Social Epidemiology of Health

health promotion lies, where people can be meaningfully engaged with one another and with the resources they need to develop health capacity (Hancock 2009). Communities are the most powerful settings for promoting health as they contain all other settings, especially the neighbourhoods where people learn, work, play and worship (Hancock 2009). Researchers have found that features of the built environment, such as the availability of open green spaces, have an effect on people's perceptions of health (Maas et al 2009). Public green spaces provide an opportunity for local exploration, group-based nature activities, social support and developing a sense of community connectedness (Maas et al 2009). These therapeutic landscapes can help foster a sense of belonging and social integration as well as a spirit of civic participation (Cattell et al 2008; Kilpatrick et al 2009).

Point to ponder
Health is created where people live. This makes communities the most powerful setting for promoting health.

Civic participation often occurs spontaneously in rural areas when there are challenges to community wellbeing such as during the threat of having services closed or when natural disasters are imminent (Kilpatrick et al 2009). The 2009 bushfires in Victorian rural communities, was a prime example of this type of community bonding. However, in today's urban environments, social isolation is a major problem as so many urban dwellers live alone. Having a geographically bounded 'community of place' where the people interact with others can help promote community attachment, cohesion and solidarity (Kilpatrick et al 2009:285). In such a setting children, older persons and those with few resources have a greater likelihood of developing feelings of health and wellbeing as well as the restorative benefits of place identity and residential satisfaction (Cattell et al 2008; Maas et al 2009). The community itself benefits from being seen as a place with high social capital, which in some cases, helps provide a buffer against adversity (Cattell et al 2008).

Neighbourhoods have been the focus of considerable research, particularly in linking the health effects of a poor neighbourhood to those already at a disadvantage (Kawachi & Kennedy 1999; Wainwright & Surtees 2003). In some cases people choose neighbourhoods according to the features they desire for their lifestyle, or because they wish to live close to people who are similar to them. However, the choices of those who can afford to be selective may leave the poor without similar choices, and they become marginalised in environmentally deprived cities (Kawachi 2002). Deprived environments contain more pollution, less green space, more derelict land and less bio-diversity, all of which create cycles of poorer health for those already at a disadvantage (Benn 2009).

Health promotion programs to create healthy settings such as 'healthy schools', 'healthy workplaces', 'healthy hospitals', and others have been committed to the principle of community empowerment and citizen participation. They have been developed in conjunction with local goals through community and health professional partnerships to ensure that information and technologies are shared, and that any initiatives developed enhance personal and community capacity. Ideally, this is achieved through 'deliberative democracy', a process wherein community governance is inclusive, and individuals from the community are given the autonomy to pursue their goals (Mooney 2008; Wise 2008). Citizens' juries, where community members are brought together to deliberate a certain health issue or initiative, are one way to promote greater involvement of community members in decision-making and priority setting in the community. Other strategies include consensus conferences, deliberative polling, focus groups, open meetings and forums, and population surveys (Mooney 2008).

Point to ponder
Living in a poor neighbourhood increases the risks of poor health for those already disadvantaged.

In New Zealand, District Health Boards (governing bodies overseeing the provision of public health services) are required to have elected community representation, as well as seek further community input into strategic planning and other major decisions (MOHNZ 2000). Commitment to this level of participation requires that health promotion principles become embedded in the agencies and settings where they have the best chance of sustaining community health. Where these programs have been successful they are guided by PHC principles to focus on the goal of creating the social capital (Hancock 2009). The most significant of these settings-based programs has been the Healthy Cities initiatives.

HEALTHY CITIES

Increasingly, <u>health promotion attention has been drawn to the challenge of helping those who live in</u> cities, whether through choice or the mass migration that has occurred because of globalisation. Migration to urban areas has also been precipitated by wars and civil strife as well as environmental degradation. In most parts of the world, the major cities are bulging at the seams, trying to accommodate the vast influx of rural and regional people, migrants seeking employment, and the homeless. In the city, the layered dimensions of life are played out in daily exchanges of social life and commerce, celebrations and exploitative acts, illness and wellness, birth and death.

Point to ponder
As cities try to cope with burgeoning population increases, health promotion attention has increasingly been focused on helping those who live in cities.

Urban life is a microcosm of the many relationships between health, social, cultural and environmental factors, portraying both visible and hidden aspects of family and community life. As population density increases in the cities, the effects of being both economically disadvantaged and vulnerable to illness and injury are evident.

To some extent, the hopelessness seen in impoverished city dwellers reflects the physical and social degradation of rural areas and the intractability of living in poverty away from any support systems, which many rural people experience. As the rich get richer, the divide between the 'haves' and the 'have nots' becomes more entrenched, eroding social capital (Hancock 2009; Kawachi & Kennedy 1999). For the 'have nots' life holds few expectations, given the drift of the wealthier citizens out of the city and into the suburbs, leaving an inflated housing market that is out of reach of many of the working poor. The wealthy also take with them the tax base that might have funded additional services in the core of many cities. Because of declining commerce and conditions in the heart of the city many economically disadvantaged people are relegated to lower paying jobs. At the same time, most urban societies have an unprecedented need to support older citizens and other family members, especially for migrant and refugee families. Many live their lives in substandard housing, which places all family members, particularly children, at risk of ill health.

Point to ponder
The complexity of the urban environment challenges many people: intricate transport systems, homelessness, the risk of violence in concealed spaces, overcrowding and motor vehicle accidents are just some of the difficulties faced.

For some, the vibrancy and energy of urban life serves as a life-sustaining force. For others, city life is a rat race without respite, refusing to soothe ageing or disabled needs or, for many workers, to counter the agitation of overwork. The influence of the built environment is more challenging in the city, primarily because of concerns about transportation and mobility and the risk of violence in well-concealed spaces. Cities are also complex systems where human interactions are dictated by streetscapes, and where travel to and from work involves difficult manoeuvres through crowded, regulated spaces.

Homelessness is a particular concern in most large cities, as inadequate shelters struggle to keep up with the demand for food, clothing or safety. Among these are a growing number of adolescent homeless and young families whose wages have not kept up with housing costs, a situation that has been worsened by the 2009 global financial crisis. Many of the homeless are mentally ill people who have been left on the streets by deinstitutionalisation and the inadequacy of mental health support services. <u>Risks and hazards of city living include crowding, violence, virus infections, motor ve</u>hicle accidents, substance abuse and any of the factors that cause ill health and injury as a result of being poor, including an increase in violence and having to breathe polluted air (Freudenberg 2000). Many of these factors are multiplied several times for those living in poverty. Homelessness is the ultimate visible marker of disadvantage and economic inequality, situated at the extreme end of a continuum of disadvantage and economic inequality.

THE HEALTHY CITIES MOVEMENT

The Healthy Cities initiatives have foregrounded the importance of 'place' in health (Hancock 2009). Supported by the WHO, since its beginnings in 1986 the Healthy Cities Movement has spanned the globe, drawing support from health professionals, representatives of recreation, police, social services, voluntary organisations and people of all ages. The model of Healthy Cities is to create awareness of the importance of place in achieving and maintaining health. Healthy Cities initiatives have instigated actions to reduce crime and environmental degradation, increase recreational spaces and promote connectedness between people for health, education and quality of life. The movement now incorporates thousands of cities worldwide, all with the common aim of using intersectoral collaboration and community participation to respond to the compromises to health that flow from people's everyday lives in the city, to promote a holistic view of health, and to inform policy (Hancock 2009; WHO 1998). A healthy city is one where people have choices that allow them to reach their maximum potential. The features of a healthy city are illustrated in Box 3.4.

Point to ponder
The Healthy Cities Movement is a WHO initiative that incorporates thousands of cities worldwide. A healthy city recognises the importance of place in achieving and maintaining health.

Like many other health promotion initiatives, the sustainability of Healthy Cities programs relies on continuing political commitment and support. This reflects a triad of priorities, which include equity, sustainability and health in all policies (Kickbusch 2008; Smith et al 2009). Some cities have been relatively successful in achieving this level of dialogue and health improvements, while others have become mired in inaction and intergovernmental conflicts. The most effective seem

BOX 3.4 FEATURES OF A HEALTHY CITY

- A clean, safe, high-quality physical environment, including adequate housing.
- A stable and sustainable ecosystem.
- Strong, mutually supportive and non-exploitative communities.
- Public participation in and control over decisions affecting one's life, health and wellbeing.
- Meeting basic needs for all, including food, water, shelter, income, safety and work.
- Access to a wide variety of experiences and resources within the possibility of multiple contacts, interaction and communication.
- A diverse, vital and innovative city economy.
- Encouragement of connectedness with the past, with the cultural and biological heritage, and with other groups and individuals.
- A city form that is compatible with and enhances the above parameters and behaviours.
- An optimum level of appropriate public health and sick care services accessible to all.
- High health status and low burden of disease for community residents (WHO 1998).

to be those linked to other Healthy Cities networks or municipalities, in a way that promotes citizen engagement and mutual support. These networks span the globe, involving municipal leaders in many countries who have pledged to reduce health inequalities and poverty, to promote citizen influence and address social exclusion (Hancock 2009).

HEALTH PROMOTION PLANNING: DIARRHOEA AND DIRT TO COMMUNITY ACTIVISM

The early days of health promotion were based on the type of epidemiological information collected by John Snow and his public health colleagues. This was followed by health education campaigns early in the 20th century oriented towards the scourges of 'diarrhoea, dirt, spitting and venereal disease' which emphasised propaganda and instruction (Green 2008:448). Over the next half-century research into the causes and consequences of diseases continued but created a growing awareness of the influence of behavioural, social and environmental influences on health. By the mid-1970s widespread criticism of the narrow, epidemiological focus had shifted the emphasis from disease to health and the need for research into multiple factors simultaneously. Around this time, the health promotion movement developed an unprecedented momentum and an almost evangelical zeal to persuade individuals to change their behaviour and adopt healthier lifestyles. Health promotion specialists borrowed strategies from marketing specialists to sell 'health' as a product, through what was called social marketing (Kotler 1975). The social marketing of health was based on a new 'healthism'; the notion that health was a product of voluntary behaviours with little acknowledgement of the fact that social and environmental circumstances may limit rationality and free choice (Green 2008). Health messages promoted in the mass media gave the impression that they were based on scientific, medical truth. This led many people to conclude that health solutions were beyond their control and in time health problems would be solved by scientists.

Point to ponder

Early health promotion campaigns focused on persuading individuals to change their behaviour without recognising that social and environmental circumstances may limit people's ability to achieve this.

COMMUNITY-WIDE HEALTH PROMOTION AND THE 'NEW HEALTH EDUCATION'

In the 1970s and 1980s, the number of community health promotion campaigns proliferated around the world, with several notable campaigns developing programs to evaluate their effectiveness. These included large-scale, longitudinal studies of health-related behaviour change in the US (Maccoby & Solomon 1981; Lasater et al 1988), Finland (McAlister 1981), Wales (Nutbeam & Catford 1987) and Australia (Egger et al 1983). Each of these studies reported substantial improvements in a range of lifestyle factors, with the largest gains evident in the extent to which community attitudes became more attuned towards health issues. As community-wide programs, each was impressive from the perspective of general population awareness. However, few were able

to demonstrate that the intervention effects were maintained beyond the post-intervention follow-up. Some contributed to positive changes such as the following:

- legislative change (e.g. compulsory wearing of seat belts)
- organisational change (e.g. parental leave for early child care)
- socio-cultural change (e.g. restricting smoking in public places)
- environmental change (e.g. reducing automobile emissions and pesticide use in food)
- behavioural change (e.g. promoting safe sexual practices)
- technological change (e.g. introduction of lead-free petrol)
- economic change (e.g. removing subsidies for tobacco producers).

(Sindall 1992)

Community-wide health promotion campaigns provided some important lessons for the future. In some cases, health education messages were developed in the expectation that behaviour change would occur as a result of mass media messages. Although heightening public awareness of health knowledge through information campaigns has been shown to improve health in certain populations, the outcomes are unevenly experienced. For example, in the US only 3% of the population responded positively to the national health education campaign urging people to follow the four health rules of non-smoking, normal weight, healthy diet, exercise (Choi et al 2005). In most cases, these campaigns 'preach to the converted', in that those who are already considering making lifestyle changes are the ones whose behaviour changes most effectively. When different levels of the population and different cultural groups are actually asked about their knowledge, it is evident that the 'reach' of the information and the uptake of the message have not been consistently received across the population (Dyer 2005). In other words, sending out information and then counting the various outcomes in terms of health indicators such as better nutrition, more activity and fewer diagnoses of lifestyle diseases shows that change occurs among only a select group in the population. Another outcome of this approach was 'victim blaming', where in many cases, people were made to feel that if they became ill it was because they failed to follow the advice of the experts.

Point to ponder

Health promotion campaigns that focus on heightening public awareness of health issues have been shown to improve health for those in middle and upper classes, while having little impact on those already disadvantaged.

The major conclusion from the approach of this era was that health promotion campaigns actually widen health disparities across broad population groups, because the messages tend to be better understood and have a greater uptake by the upper and middle classes in society (Green 2008). Many health professionals became involved in what were called the 'lifestyle campaigns', however there was considerable confusion as to the distinction between 'health education' and 'health promotion' and the respective goals of each.

Point to ponder

Health promotion is the combination of a broad range of strategies (such as those found in the Ottawa Charter) to improve health. Health education is a tool that health professionals can use to work with people to help them learn from their own experiences. Health education may be one of the strategies used to promote health.

The Ottawa Charter of 1986 focused the health promotion agenda on an advocacy and enabling role to promote supportive environments and policies, access to information, life skills and opportunities for making choices (Green 2008). Health education, on the other hand, was seen as the propaganda engine for persuading people to lead healthy lives. However, leaders in the field of health education such as Green and Kreuter (1991) influenced a shift in the way health education was conceptualised, emphasising the voluntary, rather than coercive nature of making health choices. Health promotion was seen to incorporate health education as part of creating the social, environmental and political conditions for within which those choices could be made. At the same time, the centrality of empowerment was recognised

in the rhetoric of PHC and among health promotion researchers. For example, Tones (1986, 2002) argued for a more radical model of community empowerment that would focus on communities having both knowledge of the fundamental causes of ill health and the capacity to address them. His work foreshadowed the move towards health literacy, and today health education is considered an essential component of health promotion programs (Green 2008).

The approach of knowledge plus capacity is the 'new health education', which is oriented towards empowerment rather than persuasion. It is more closely aligned with health promotion by addressing the way societies are best arranged to promote health and wellbeing rather than focusing on individuals' health-related behaviours (Baum 2009). The new health education focuses on social change, with interventions being planned around social justice for individuals, communities and society (Freudenberg 2006). It is based on the idea that people can be helped to learn from their own experience, and analyse the world in order to change it. Social change can be achieved through multidimensional strategies, with each intervention enhancing the contribution of the others, but it should be planned on the basis of what needs to be done and what resources can be helpful for short-term and long-term planning (Smith et al 2008). Depending on the population, the issue and the goals, this approach may integrate the activities of the mass media, canvassing, demonstrations, legal actions, lobbying or face-to-face counselling as well as educating health professionals (Freudenberg 2006).

Today there is widespread understanding that health promotion is inherently political, inviting community participation and activism (Sparks 2009; Whitehead 2004, 2009). Health education involves strategies that seek to influence people's values, beliefs, attitudes and motivations in relation to health, health risks and health behaviours (Whitehead 2003, 2004). Health promotion and health education are not interdependent, but they are interrelated (Whitehead 2006). This has become clearer with the increasing focus on health literacy (Nutbeam 2000). Health literacy is not an end in itself, but it provides a conceptual framework for empowerment and capacity building through the development of knowledge, confidence, participation and community activism. These characteristics are essential for promoting empowerment and social change (Nutbeam 2008; Peerson & Saunders 2009). The new health education is therefore a combination of information-giving and enabling (Green 2008; Whitehead 2004, 2009).

Point to ponder
Health promotion, health education and health literacy is a powerful combination for promoting empowerment and social change.

In Australia, health promotion programs have achieved considerable improvements over the past two decades, due to sustained investment, advocacy and government intervention (Wise 2008). As in other countries, the campaigns of the 1970s and 1980s failed to promote social justice, instead proving an inordinately expensive exercise yielding few returns. The interventions did not provide enabling environments for health, failing to encourage mass transit, maintain green spaces, purchase healthier foods or promote exercise (Choi et al 2005). However, there have been some reductions in injuries and mortality from road traffic accidents, a reduction in mortality from some cancers and cardiovascular disease and Sudden Infant Death Syndrome (SIDS), and limiting the spread of HIV and reducing deaths from AIDS and suicide. Some community-level improvements have been seen in Indigenous health, but with much yet to be achieved. There are safer cars, non-smoking pubs and clubs, bicycle lanes, socially supportive school environments, improved nutrition for Indigenous mothers and babies, changes in infant sleeping positions, and in the roles of police, retailers and advertisers (Wise 2008).

Point to ponder
Lessons from the health promotion efforts of the 1970s and 1980s in Australia and New Zealand have resulted in a reorientation of health promotion efforts to focus on social justice and equity among Indigenous and non-Indigenous groups.

In New Zealand, health promotion practice is underpinned by the 1840 Treaty of Waitangi (Te Tiriti o Waitangi — the founding document between Maori and the Crown) (the Treaty) and the Ottawa Charter. Key tenets of the Treaty are partnership (between the Crown and Maori), participation (by Maori in all aspects of society) and active protection (recognition that the Crown must actively work towards protecting the rights of Maori) (Waa et al 1998). The Treaty recognises the social and economic aspirations of Maori and non-Maori and can be used as a framework by both to exercise control over their health and wellbeing (Waa et al 1998). Despite the development of a range of effective health promotion initiatives for non-Maori in New Zealand, there remains considerable work to achieve equitable outcomes for Maori in many of these programs. For example, smoking prevalence in New Zealand has decreased from 32% in 1981 to 23.5% in 2006 but this decrease has not been consistent among all social, demographic and ethnic groups. Maori women continue to have one of the highest smoking rates in the world (Barnett et al 2009). Barnett et al argue that for smoking cessation initiatives to be effective for all New Zealanders, the focus must shift from individual interventions to a focus on the broader determinants of ethnic socio-economic inequality and the local environments in which people are situated.

Despite the need for continued work towards achieving health equity, New Zealand has the distinction of being ranked number one in the world on the Global Peace Index. This is an index developed by a group of international leaders called 'Vision of Humanity'. Included are such things as measures of non-violence, within and external to the country as well as any external or organised conflicts, relationships with neighbouring countries, respect for human rights, military spending and capability (http://www.visionofhumanity.org/gpi/results/rankings.php).

COMMUNITY ASSESSMENT: HEALTH PLANNING FOR THE ENABLING COMMUNITY

To be effective, health promotion programs must be developed on the basis of an inclusive, social justice, PHC approach to benefit all socio-economic levels and all cultural groups in the population. This underlines the importance of maintaining equity at the heart of health promotion (Ridde 2007). Health promotion planning should be based on research evidence from local evaluative information, which is changeable, so it cannot be taken for granted. Existing research findings can be helpful in health promotion planning, but they must be contextualised. Knowing that health is multidimensional and dynamic as a function of a changing social context, it is important to assess features of the social environment, while gathering input from members of the community and observing what is occurring in the environment. This can enhance the success of local health promotion programs and also provide a basis for studying the effectiveness of practical interventions, knowledge transfer, and the linkages between policy and practice (Smith et al 2009).

> Community assessment is a process for systematically collecting and analysing information about a community, as well as an opportunity to build the capacity of community members, by involving them integrally in the process.

Systematic collection of demographic and clinical information on the community can be done at arm's length; that is, using health and government service reports. This is an important part of community assessment, however, states of health and wellness are also a function of how people interpret their situation at any given time, and this can only be ascertained by interviewing people to gain their opinions. A friend asks 'How are you?' and you might reply 'not bad', 'pretty good', 'I have a cold', 'getting by, thank you', 'feeling better', or the old classic 'don't ask!' As a health professional this may be quite baffling, and you might jump to conclusions about what the person meant by their response; that is, their *perception* of health status, unless you have at least a brief history of their previous health history. For example, knowing their age, gender, where they live, their family history and current family situation, or that they recently had an illness or injury provides a deeper insight into their actual state of health at a certain moment in time.

As health professionals we sometimes make the mistake of trying to label and categorise people and their health status according to a checklist of assessment categories. So we may call someone 'deficient' in certain areas, or 'very comfortable' when we actually know little of how they benchmark health or personal comfort. This is problematic in many inventories and checklists, which tend to approach assessment from predetermined assumptions and run the risk of failing to document unexpected issues. In order to avoid the pitfalls of making predetermined assumptions about people and communities, it is important to involve community members at the outset of the community assessment process. This, in itself, can promote community capacity building.

> **ACTION POINT**
> When undertaking a community assessment, involving community members from the outset will help you avoid making assumptions about a community.

Community assessment is therefore a tool for finding out more about a community, but is also an opportunity to involve a community in working towards achieving health. In this context, we construe community assessment as a process similar to that of growing a tree. Just as a tree grows, we grow both our own knowledge of the community and the capacity of the community through the process of community assessment. This can be a complex process. The following categories are therefore presented as a simplified guide to community assessment with the opportunity in each area to gather community members' own descriptions of how they see their health and their community, and by definition, involve them in the community assessment process.

We use the analogy of the tree (see Figure 3.4) to represent each of the categories or phases in the community assessment process. Briefly, phase one, the lay of the land, provides information on people's perceptions of what forms the foundation of the community. It is the initial stage where we involve the community in the process, and this phase is likened to the roots of the tree. Phase two, mapping resources, provides information on what supports the community in terms of resources and political willingness. This is the lower, supportive trunk of the tree. Phase three, who will help, is the identification of the people who can support community health and start to spread the message, where the trunk of the tree starts to branch out. Phase four, people, place, health and gatekeepers,

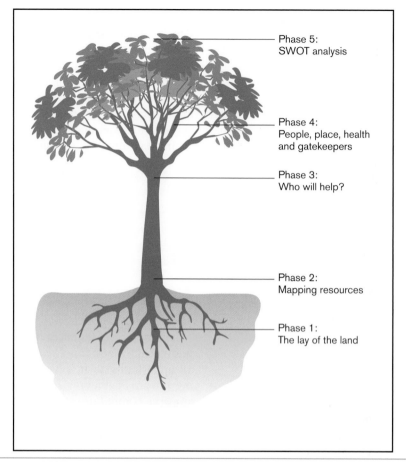

Figure 3.4 The community assessment tree

can be likened to the upper branches of the tree. Here, there are many branches that need to be analysed to provide an overview of the community, to identify who protects the community, and how people want to be involved in promoting health. Phase five is where the strengths, weaknesses, opportunities and threats to community health are revealed. This is where the canopy of the tree is both exposed to the elements, but also protects the tree.

Phase one: the lay of the land
Some of the questions to ask community members include the following:
- Are there large proportions of elderly or young families that will require particular health services either in the present or future?
- What is the cultural mix?
- How does the community see itself?
- What do people think of living in this community?
- Do they believe it is conducive to health for those with abilities and disabilities?
- What is the level of awareness of health and ecological issues?
- What are the environmental strengths?
- What do they think the community needs most?
- Is there access to transportation for those who need health services?
- What should be sustained?
- What structural features will be conducive to achieving health goals?
- What social processes will contribute to health planning?
- What notable differences in opinion exist?
- What is the level of volunteerism in the community?
- What community development initiatives are planned?
- Which initiatives have been successful? For what reasons?

This information needs to be integrated with how things 'work' in the community. Specifically:
- Who are the gatekeepers, or key funders of health?
- Are there adequate numbers and types of health professionals?
- What are their priorities for the short, medium and long term?
- In what way are these tied to political goals? What are the political goals?
- Who are the health-literate policy-makers?
- To what extent can they foster intersectoral knowledge, awareness and collaboration?

Phase two: mapping resources

All health programs require financial resources. Where a community has a visible problem that is high on the list of government health priorities, it is easier to argue for the necessary funds for an intervention program. However, many issues remain problematic to the community, yet they are often invisible to, or dismissed by, government funding agencies because of the need to justify return on investment. Because of the competition for resources, community assessment must be conducted within political and economic constraints and the wider health budgeting arena. Yet, few health promotion investments demonstrate return on investment in terms of either human or other resources within the timeframe of a political term, especially for outcomes that are difficult to quantify. Where there is competition for funds between programs, an immunisation program, for instance, is readily measurable within a fairly reasonable timeframe. A domestic violence program aimed at teaching young people about relationships is not. Sometimes this can be redressed by using a creative way of documenting assessment data within a practical framework. This should be informed by first conducting a scoping exercise or 'asset map' to lay a foundation for change based on what already exists.

Point to ponder
The five phases of community assessment are:
1 the lay of the land
2 mapping resources
3 who will help?
4 people, place, health and gatekeepers
5 SWOT analysis.

Phase three: who will help?

This step in community assessment is linked to identifying the key players within the community who will provide the ongoing support for any necessary changes to community health. The following questions should be asked:
- Who are the key health-literate players who will be willing to engage in serious resource dialogue to sustain both community health and economic viability?
- What networks and coalitions can be built?
- Who in the community are the opinion leaders?
- Who plays important roles in resource allocation?
- How does the community show its capacity for caring?
- What precedents have been set in previous planning exercises?

This line of questioning means addressing the issue of equity, but it also aims at making subtle aspects of the community transparent, so that the processes, as well as the structures of change can be made visible. Then programs can be developed which tap into the strengths of the community and acknowledge the constraints in the environment, whether these are personal, physical, social or financial constraints.

Phase four: people, place, health and gatekeepers

During this phase, a detailed analysis is prepared, describing the people and their contextual resources in relation to patterns of health and illness and any relevant information on getting initiatives underway. This includes knowing the gatekeepers, those who will protect the community, and especially those who will facilitate the wider access with community members. This phase is also where we identify how people want to be involved in promoting health.

Appendix E provides a chart for collecting and analysing this type of information in the community.

Phase five: strengths, weaknesses, opportunities, threats

The object of the exercise is to reveal the strengths, weaknesses, opportunities and threats (SWOT) to community health. Once that has been achieved, the information can be shared among members

People:
- people–place relationships
- networks for communication, volunteerism support systems, family and professional caregivers
- community leadership
- psychosocial factors
- cultural factors, ethnic mix
- demographic characteristics.

Place:
- geographic area
- natural resources
- development base, including taxation
- other structural features
- access to welfare, housing, transportation, schools
- land owners, non-land owners
- urban–rural–regional–remote.

Health patterns:
- local burden of disease and disability
- social determinants of health
- access, availability, affordability of health and disability services
- local patterns of service utilisation.

Gatekeepers:
- intersectoral coalitions
- local, state/provincial, national health policies and priorities
- financial resources
- competing political, development goals
- health professionals
- global factors.

Figure 3.5 Community assessment

of the community to help them look for acceptable solutions to existing problems and strategies for maintaining these over time. The health professional then acts as a community advocate; a resource person who mediates between people and those responsible for freeing up the resources they need, enables community groups to achieve their goals by helping to build coalitions for change and monitors their progress by collecting information to inform them of the benchmarks they achieve along the way and to help them revise their goals for the future. The key to accurate assessment is community participation. Planning for equitable, accessible and culturally sensitive and safe health services and resources in a community can only be achieved by incorporating local knowledge and insight into the risk factors and determinants of health that are peculiar to that community, then using this knowledge to inform future planning. Chapter 4 will explore models of implementing health promotion strategies based on this type of data. Appendix F provides a SWOT analysis framework for you to use to analyse your community assessment data.

HELPING PEOPLE CHANGE

Models are helpful as a guide to what needs to be done in managing health conditions, and often, in identifying the skills required for effectiveness. Some also indicate the general strategies nurses and midwives can use in helping people achieve the change they seek. A comprehensive, integrative approach can help connect individual or group change with the broader health promotion agenda. For example, to reduce tobacco smoking in the community, it is widely understood that legislation to ban smoking from public places, together with organisational and socio-cultural support for those seeking to quit smoking, and environmental and economic modifications are significant influences on change. Working towards modification of any of these conditions should be based on evidence. Using the assessment tool we introduced in Chapter 3 (Appendix E) the nurse or midwife would act as the 'change agent', developing an action plan based on the four phases of assessment, and the SWOT analysis of the community's strengths, weaknesses, opportunities and threats. This provides the change management plan with a strong foundation, linked to the context and local knowledge of the potential for change. Structured change management strategies are often helpful in working with groups. Talbot and Verrinder (2010) provide a number of useful strategies for health promotion in groups.

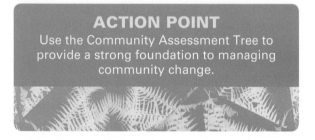

ACTION POINT
Use the Community Assessment Tree to provide a strong foundation to managing community change.

When change is managed in systematic steps with adequate evaluation and communication throughout the process, it is more likely to result in successful outcomes. This includes the need to identify the personal attitudes and concerns of those affected by a proposed change and to ensure that accurate information is collected and communicated at each step of the change process to promote understanding and garner support for the change. Lewin's (1951) model of unfreezing, changing and refreezing can be a useful guide to change. This involves first, identifying the driving and restraining forces that may be influencing group complacency or willingness to change as well as conditions in the environment that may present barriers to change. 'Unfreezing' is a process of ensuring there is accurate communication of the goals and expectations of the change, and what strategies are being suggested for improvement. The next stage, 'moving', creates awareness of shared understandings that people have about the change and its outcomes, identification of the key people who will take ownership of the change, and what information will be communicated throughout the implementation to ensure that the change is sustainable. Following implementation, the 'refreezing' stage is focused on communicating the impact of the change and how it will be evaluated and sustained over time (Lewin 1951). Clearly, communication is the key to success. Roger's (2003) Theory of the Diffusion of Innovations supports these steps, indicating that community members will be more likely to accept the change if they can see the relative advantage of the change, and its compatibility with their approach or goals. Changes will also be more

readily accepted if people can see its potential in meeting their needs, if they have a chance to try it out prior to full implementation, and if it can be customised to their environment or circumstances (Rogers 2003).

Among the biggest obstacles to change in organisations or groups is failure to articulate the change, its rationale, timeframe and individual implementation steps. Kotter (1995), one of the most influential leadership advocates from the Harvard Business School also advocates the need to establish a sense of urgency — motivating people to get outside their comfort zones and helping them become empowered through participation in a

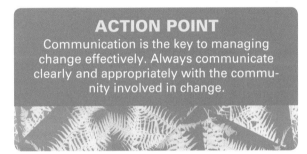

ACTION POINT
Communication is the key to managing change effectively. Always communicate clearly and appropriately with the community involved in change.

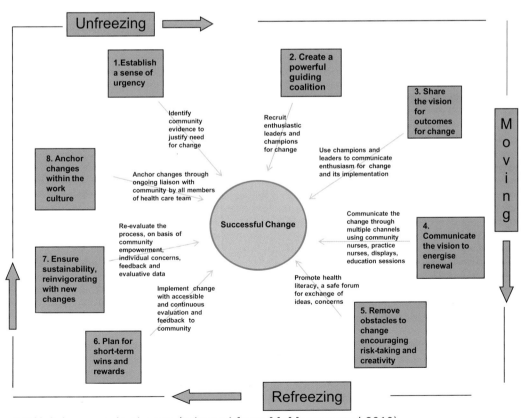

Figure 3.6 Helping people change (adapted from McMurray et al 2010)

powerful guiding coalition to oversee the change. The change agent then develops and communicates a vision for what the change will bring, encourages risk-taking and creative ideas, establishes plans for creating short-term wins, helps them create reward structures for those involved in implementing change, and ensures that victory is declared at the appropriate time and celebrated. This last stage should be accompanied by new ideas or projects that could extend the change and reinvigorate the process, anchoring the change in the local culture (Kotter 1995) (see Figure 3.6).

Case study

This chapter connects the circumstances of the Miller family with the wider agenda of globalisation. Although Maria and Jim are both employed they are only able to meet the family's financial needs by cutting costs wherever they can. Both Maria and Jim have tried to eliminate any extras other than necessities the family needs to get through the winter, however, they are determined to ensure that the children will live in a warm house. Although cold housing is not considered a significant health issue in Australia, it is a major public health issue in New Zealand and Jim is concerned about the health of his parents, Millie and Harold, who live in an old and inadequately insulated house in the South Island where winters can be bitter. There is important research evidence indicating improved health outcomes among children whose houses have had heating and insulation upgrades (Howden-Chapman et al 2008) and a current research program is examining the benefits of heating subsidies on the health of older people (http://www.uow.otago.ac.nz/academic /dph/research/housing/warmhomesforeldernewzealanders.html). The NZ government has allocated $323.3 million over four years for a campaign to fit homes with insulation and clean heating devices such as heat pumps and approved wood burners. The scheme, which is open to owners and occupiers of houses built before 2000, started on 1 July 2009 (Brownlee 2009), and Jim hopes his parents will benefit from this program.

Jim and Maria shop as carefully as possible, and are adamant that the children will have sufficient nutrition and clothing without having access to junk food or unnecessary consumer goods. The girls still experience peer pressure from child care and school friends, who spend long hours watching TV, including being exposed to junk food advertising. Maria has explained to her children the importance of healthy lifestyle habits for good dental and general health, and she is grateful that her messages are reinforced by their teachers. Maria has been approached by her local councillor, who is a nurse, to join a community movement to upgrade their local playground to meet safety standards. She is told by the nurse that a small group of concerned residents have begun to collect information on the number of children's accidents that have occurred in the playground.

REFLECTING ON THE BIG ISSUES

- Globalisation affects health at all levels of society.
- Social activism includes an attempt to influence governments to include health in all policies.
- Health promotion strategies must consider economic as well as environmental, social and cultural issues.
- Adopting a single solution to health challenges will be ineffective without building community capacity.
- Assessing the health of a community includes mapping resources and assets in relation to places and spaces where people can make healthy lifestyle choices.
- Community assessment should include community 'voices' to contextualise the information and lead to effective evaluation of the impact of health promotion strategies.

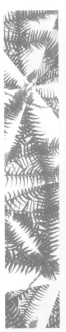

Reflective questions: how would I use this knowledge in practice?

1 Would your knowledge of the impact of globalisation cause you to change the way you promote health in the Millers' community?

2 What advice would you give Maria as she sets out to join the healthy playground initiative?

3 How would you assess the influence of health and place in the Millers' lives?

4 What health literacy needs would Jim and Maria need to ensure healthy nutrition for the family?

5 Could you help the family address nutrition as a separate issue from other health issues affecting the family?

6 How could Jim assist his parents in New Zealand to access funding for improving the heating in their house?

7 How would you use the Ottawa Charter guidelines to promote the health of the Millers' community?

8 Thinking about your experience in practice, consider an example of how globalisation has impacted on the health of the people you provide care for. What strategies could you implement to address this?

Research-informed practice

Read the article by Smith and Signal (2009) 'Global influences on milk purchasing in New Zealand — implications for health and inequities'.

• How does this information change the way you view social policies?

• Can you see the strengths and weaknesses of New Zealand making a decision to apply a goods and services tax on milk, when Australia refused to do so? How could you lobby to change this policy?

• How could your knowledge of globalisation be used to influence the Fonterra cooperative for the dairy market?

• What could be done to promote New Zealand children drinking more milk when soft drink is cheaper?

• What types of activities would you use to encourage members of the community to join the Healthy Eating–Healthy Action strategy?

References

Barnett R, Pearce J, Moon G 2009 Community inequality and smoking cessation in New Zealand, 1981–2006. Social Science & Medicine 68:876–84

Baum F 2009 Envisioning a healthy and sustainable future: essential to closing the gap in a generation. Global Health Promotion 1757–9759 Supp (1):72–80

Benn H 2009 The environmental determinants of health. Global Health Promotion 1757–9759 Supp (1):42–3

Bezruchka S 2006 Epidemiological approaches. In: Raphael D, Bryant T & Rioux M (eds) Staying Alive: Critical Perspectives on Health, Illness and Health Care, pp 13–33

Brownlee G 2009 Boost for Warmer, Drier, Healthier Kiwi Homes. Media release: Minister of Energy and Resources, Wellington New Zealand

Cattell V, Dines N, Gesler W, Curtis S 2008 Mingling, observing, and lingering: everyday public spaces and their implications for wellbeing and social relations. Health and Place 14:544–61

Choi B, Hunter D, Tsou W, Sainsbury P 2005 Diseases of comfort: primary cause of death in the 22nd century. Journal of Epidemiology and Community Health 59:1030–34

Dyer O 2005 Disparities in health widen between rich and poor in England. British Medical Journal 331:419

Egger G, Fitzgerald W, Frape G, Monaem A, Rubinstein P, Tyler C, Mackay B 1983 Results of a large scale media anti-smoking campaign in Australia: the North Coast Healthy Lifestyle Program. British Medical Journal 287:1125–87

Falk-Rafael A 2006 Globalization and global health. Advances in Nursing Science 29(1):2–14

Freudenberg N 2000 Health promotion in the city: a review of current practice and future prospects in the United States. Annual Review of Public Health 21:473–503

—— 2006 Training health educators for social change. International Quarterly of Community Health Education 25(1–2):63–77

Green J 2008 Health education — the case for rehabilitation. Critical Public Health 18(4):447–56

Green L, Kreuter M 1991 Health Promotion Planning: An Educational and Environmental Approach. Mayfield Publishing Company, Mountain View

Hancock T 2009 Act Locally: Community-based Population Health. Report for The Senate Sub-Committee on Population Health, Victoria BC Canada. Online. Available:

http://www.parl.gc.ca/40/2/parlbus/commbus/senate/com-e/popu-e/rep-e/appendixBjun09-e.pdf (accessed 17 July 2009)

Howden-Chapman P, Pierse N, Nicholls S, Gillespie-Bennett J, Viggers H, Cunningham M, Phipps R, Boulic M, Fjallstrom P, Free S, Chapman R, Lloyd B, Wickens K, Shields D, Baker M, Cunningham C, Woodward A, Bullen C, Crane J 2008 Effects of improved home heating on asthma in community dwelling children: randomized controlled trial. British Medical Journal 337:a1411

Huynen M, Martens P, Hilderink H 2005 The health impacts of globalization: a conceptual framework. Globalization and Health 1:14 doi 10.1186/1744-8603-1-14

Kawachi I 2002 Social epidemiology. Editorial, Social Science & Medicine 54:1739–41

Kawachi I, Kennedy B 1999 Income inequality and health: pathways and mechanisms. Health Services Research 34:215–27

Keating D, Hertzman C 1999 Developmental Health and the Wealth of Nations. Guildford Press, New York

Kickbusch I 2008 Healthy Societies: Addressing 21st Century Health Challenges. Government of South Australia, Department of the Premier and Cabinet, Adelaide

Kilpatrick S, Cheers B, Gilles M, Taylor J 2009 Boundary crossers, communities, and health: exploring the role of rural health professionals. Health & Place 15:284–90

Kotler P 1975 Marketing for Non-profit Organizations. Prentice-Hall, Englewood Cliffs, NJ

Labonte R 2008 Global health in public policy: finding the right frame? Critical Public Health 18(4):467–82

Labonte R, Schrecker T 2007a Globalization and social determinants of health: introduction and methodological background. Globalization and Health 3(5) doi:10.1186/1744-8603-3-5

—— 2007b Globalization and social determinants of health: the role of the global marketplace. Globalization and Health 3(6) doi:10.1186/1744-8603-3-6

—— 2007c Globalization and social determinants of health: promoting health equity in global governance. Globalization and Health 3(7) doi:10.1186/1744-8603-3-7

Lasater T, Carleton R, LeFebre R 1988 The Pawtucket heart health program: utilizing community resources for primary prevention. Rhode Island Medical Journal 71:63–7

Li J, McMurray A, Stanley F 2008 Modernity's paradox and the structural determinants of child health and wellbeing. Health Sociology Review 17(1):64–77

Maas J, van Dillen S, Verheij R, Groenewegen P 2009 Social contacts as a possible mechanism behind the relation between green space and health. Health and Place 15:586–95

Maccoby N, Solomon D 1981 The Stanford community studies in heart disease prevention. In: Rice R, Paisley W (eds) Public Communication Campaigns. Sage, Beverly Hills, LA

Marmot M 2009 Closing the health gap in a generation: the work of the Commission on Social Determinants of Health and its recommendations. Global Health Promotion 1757-9759 Supp (1):23–7

McAlister A 1981 Anti-smoking campaigns: progress in developing effective communications. In: Rice R, Paisley W (eds) Public Communication Campaigns. Sage, Beverly Hills, LA

McCully M 2009 Aid increases as NZAID changes focus: Press release. Online. Available: http://www.beehive.govt.nz/release/aid+increases+nzaid+changes+focus (accessed 18 June 2010)

McMurray A, Chaboyer W, Wallis M, Fetherston C 2010 Implementing Bedside Handover: Strategies for change management. Journal of Clinical Nursing 19(15): doi.10.1111/j1365-2702.2009.03033.X

Ministry of Health New Zealand (MOHNZ) 2000 New Zealand Health Strategy. MOHNZ, Wellington

Mooney G 2008 Involving communities in decision making. In: Sorensen R, Iedema R (eds) Managing Clinical Processes in Health Services. Elsevier, Sydney, pp 211–24

Mooney G, Ataguba J 2009 The global financial meltdown and the need for a political economy of health promotion. Health Promotion Journal of Australia 20(1):3–4

Murray C, Lopez A 1997a Mortality by cause for eight regions of the world: global burden of disease study. The Lancet 349(May 3):1269–76

—— 1997b Global mortality, disability, and the contribution of risk factors: global burden of disease study. The Lancet 349(May 17):1436–42

Navarro V 2009 What we mean by social determinants of health. International Journal of Health Services 39(3):423–41

Nutbeam D 2000 Health literacy as a public health goal: a challenge for contemporary health education and communication strategies into the 21st century. Health Promotion International 15(3):259–67

—— 2008 The evolving concept of health literacy. Social Science & Medicine 67:2072–8

Nutbeam D, Catford J 1987 The Welsh heart program evaluation strategy: progress, plans and possibilities. Health Promotion 2(1):5–18

Oliver A 2008 Reflections on the Development of Health Inequalities Policy in the United Kingdom. London School of Economics and Political Science Working paper No. 11/2008

Pattle Delamore Partners Ltd 2009 Audit of the remediation of the former Fruitgrowers Chemical Company site, Mapua. Pattle Delamore Partners Ltd, Wellington, New Zealand

Peerson A, Saunders M 2009 Health literacy revisited: what do we mean and why does it matter? Health Promotion International 24(3):285–96

Ridde V 2007 Reducing social inequalities in health: public health, community health or health promotion? Promotion & Education Vol XIV(2):63–7

Robinson M 2009 Equity, justice and the social determinants of health. Global Health Promotion 1757–9759 Supp (1):48–51

Rose G 1985 Sick individuals and sick populations. International Journal of Epidemiology 14(1):32–8

Ruger J, Kim H 2006 Global health inequalities: an international comparison. Journal of Epidemiology Community Health 60:928–36

Sachs J 2005 Investing in Development. A Practical Plan to Achieve the Millennium Development Goals. United Nations, New York

Safaie J 2007 Global income related health inequalities. Social Medicine 2(1):19–33

Sindall C 1992 Health promotion and community health in Australia: an overview of theory and practice. In: Baum F, Fry D, Lennie I (eds) Community Health Policy and Practice in Australia, pp 277–95

Smith B, Keleher H, Fry C 2008 Developing values, evidence and advocacy to address the social determinant of health. Health Promotion Journal of Australia 19(3):171–2

Smith J, Gleeson S, White I, Judd J, Jones-Roberts A, Hanzar T, Sparks M, Shilton T, Shand M 2009 Health promotion: essential to a national preventative health strategy. Health Promotion Journal of Australia 20(1):5–6

Smith M, Signal L 2009 Global influences on milk purchasing in New Zealand — implications for health and inequities. Globalization and Health 5(1) doi:10.1186/1744-8603-5-1

Smith R, MacKellar L 2007 Global public goods and the global health agenda: problems, priorities and potential. Globalization and Health 3(9) doi 10.1186/1744-8603-3-9

Sparks M 2009 Acting on the social determinants of health: health promotion needs to get more political. Editorial Health Promotion International 24(3):199–202

Tones B 1986 Health education and the health promotion ideology. Health Education Research 1(1): 3–12

—— 2002 Reveille for radicals! The paramount purpose of health education. Health Education Research 17:1–5

Waa A, Holibar F, Spinola F 1998 Planning and Doing Programme Evaluation: An Introductory Guide for Health Promotion. Auckland New Zealand Alcohol and Public Health Research Unit/Whariki, Runanga, Wananga, Hauora me te Paekaka

Wainwright N, Surtees P 2003 Places, people and their physical and mental functional health. Journal of Epidemiology Community Health 58:333–9

Whitehead D 2003 Health promotion and health education viewed as symbiotic paradigms: bridging the theory and practice gap between them. Journal of Clinical Nursing 12:796–805

—— 2004 Health promotion and health education: advancing the concepts. Journal of Advanced Nursing 47(3):311–20

—— 2006 Health promotion in the practice setting: findings from a review of clinical issues. Worldviews on Evidenced-Based Nursing 2:1–20

—— 2009 Reconciling the differences between health promotion in nursing and 'general' health promotion. International Journal of Nursing Studies 46:865–74

Wilkinson R 1996 Unhealthy societies: the afflictions of inequality. Routledge, London

Wilkinson R, Pickett K 2006 Income inequality and population health: a review and explanation of the evidence. Social Science & Medicine 62:1768–84

Wise M 2008 Health promotion in Australia: reviewing the past and looking to the future. Critical Public Health 18(4):497–508

World Health Organization (WHO) 1998 The Fifty-first World Health Assembly, Health Promotion. WHO, Geneva

—— 2005 Global Burden of Disease Study. WHO Geneva

Useful websites

http://www.everyhumanhasrights.org — International leaders working on Every Human Has Rights campaign

http://ph.ucla.edu/epi/snow.html — John Snow and his influence

http://www.inequality.org — An organisation dedicated to highlighting inequality

http://www.socialjustice.org — Canadian Centre for Social Justice

http://depts.washington.edu/eqhlth/ — Population Health Forum at University of Washington

http://www.visionof humanity.org/gpi/results/new-zealand/2009 — Global Peace Index

http://www.seattleglobaljustice.org/trade-justice/ — Community Alliance for Global Justice Trade Justice Project

http://www.phmovement.org/ — People's Health Movement

http://www.phmovement.org/cms/en/node/862#GHW2%20Overview — Global Health Watch

http://www.Inequality.org — information on all aspects of hierarchy

http://depts.washington.edu/eqhlth/pages/resources.html — University of Washington website for population health resources

http://www.stats.govt.nz — Tatauranga Aotearoa, New Zealand Department of Statistics — census data and community profiles

http://www.wnmeds.ac.nz/academic/dph/research/HIRP/index.html — Health Inequalities Research Programme at the Wellington School of Medicine, New Zealand

http://www.hpforum.org.nz — Runanga Whakapiki ake i te Hauora o Aotearoa — Health Promotion Forum of New Zealand — a collaboration of over 150 organisations committed to improving health in New Zealand

Chapter 4

Enabling health and wellness: practice roles and models of care

INTRODUCTION

This chapter is aimed at exploring the roles and strategies used by nurses, midwives and other health professionals to promote health and wellbeing in their communities. As you will see throughout the discussion, they use a wide variety of approaches to community health in the context of diverse and changing models of care. Despite the differences, initiatives to enable community health are guided by the primary health care (PHC) principles outlined in Chapter 2: accessible health care, appropriate technology, health promotion, cultural sensitivity, intersectoral collaboration, community participation and cultural safety.

Those responsible for developing community health capacity also have a common commitment to holistic practice, based on the understanding that health is a product of biological, psychological, social, cultural, environmental and political factors, as we have outlined in the previous chapters. Their practice is also based on the perception that health is created and maintained in the context of the settings of people's lives, where they work, play, study, worship, engage in recreational pursuits and access care. In each of these settings the community itself is at the centre of care, and members of the community are empowered by knowledge and the expectation that they will be full participants in health decision-making. Because the models and processes of care differ between settings and between different groups of people we describe both generalised and specialised practice. We outline the framework for various types of practice and explain the many ways practice is evolving to respond to changing needs and different contexts.

The chapter begins with a description of the changing nature of professional roles to respond to the global mandate for PHC. Although PHC and the goal of health for all people have been in place for the past three decades, in this second decade of the 21st century they are reaffirmed as lighthouse concepts, guiding the way towards global, national and local health promotion and illness prevention. The descriptions of current and potential practice provided in the sections to follow demonstrate how the social determinants of health are embedded in practice. The chapter concludes with a number of recommendations for strengthening the focus on communities, and exploration of various strategies for managing change in their populations.

> **Point to ponder**
> Although nurses, midwives and other health professionals use a variety of approaches to community health, all are guided by the principles of primary health care: accessible health care, appropriate technology, health promotion, intersectoral collaboration, community participation, cultural sensitivity and cultural safety.

THE ROLE OF NURSES AND MIDWIVES IN PROMOTING SOCIAL JUSTICE

As health professionals, many of us are aware that we hold enormous potential to change the world and help make it a fairer place. This is not blind ambition, but rather a moral imperative to help people change and develop in ways that would see them live the lives they choose (Sen 2000). We know that social inequalities exist in communities, but they also exist within health care systems and public health processes that sometimes constrain people's

Objectives

By the end of this chapter you will be able to:

1 describe the global re-orientation of practice roles towards primary health care
2 explore a variety of professional roles including those of nurses, nurse practitioners, midwives, paramedics and other specialised care providers working in communities
3 explain the importance of settings in the practice of child and family health, rural and remote area practice, community mental health, occupational health, and school health
4 outline the current and potential role of nurses in managing chronic disease in the community
5 identify appropriate approaches to intersectoral and interdisciplinary collaboration in practice.

abilities to achieve good health (Green et al 2007). Nurses and midwives are aware of their ability to facilitate community health, and they have been addressing health inequities and helping build community capacity for more than a century (Aston et al 2009).

Point to ponder

Nurses and midwives have been addressing health inequities and helping build community capacity for more than a century.

However, despite being the most numerically dominant groups in the health care system, nurses and midwives practise under a set of constraints imposed externally by the systems in which they are employed. A common inspiration held by these practitioners and many others in the health professions, comes from knowing their work can make a difference, especially from intervening 'for the collective good, using levers for change such as advocacy, policy change and social interventions' (Edwards & MacLean Davison 2008:130). At the level of community, many activities can improve the health of a community and those who reside there. These actions revolve around identifying inequities, their underlying determinants, and then helping people develop their capacity to maintain health or prevent illness, injury or disability.

Over the last century, there has been a professional focus on cultural considerations worldwide. This has created recognition of the health disparities between cultural groups, and the importance of working towards cultural competence across all nursing settings. Culturally

competent practice is based on being able to relate to people of different cultures in a way that recognises their values, ideas and identity, and how these are reflected in their health and wellbeing. Cultural safety is the goal of culturally competent practice. It is a process of exploring, reflecting on and understanding one's own culture, and how it relates to other cultures with a view towards promoting partnership, participation and cultural protection. These concepts will be elaborated further in Chapter 11.

Point to ponder

One of the unique aspects of practising in the community is that our understanding of the complexities of caring for people is grounded in the everyday reality of people's lives. Social equity and the impact of social gradients become increasingly visible.

Recognising the importance of culture has added to our growing understanding of the complexities of caring for those from diverse backgrounds. Practice experiences have also made visible other issues of social justice so evident in communities, particularly the escalating rates of chronic diseases and the impact of social gradients. A major role of nurses, particularly those practising in public health, is to help eliminate these inequities (Association of State and Territorial Directors of Nursing [ASTDN] 2009). In addition to cultural safety, essential aspects of nursing and midwifery roles include an emphasis on community strengths, advocacy and health promotion, all of which require strong leadership (ASTDN 2009). These

Table 4.1 Potential social justice core competencies for public health

Domain of core competencies	Potential competency reflecting social justice
Public health sciences	Describe role of public health in righting social injustices Understand relationship between social determinants of health and inequities
Assessment and analysis	Use data to differentiate inequities, inequalities Work with marginalised population for research-based action on inequities and disparities
Policy and program planning, implementation evaluation	Identify policy role in reducing or increasing inequities Recognise differential effects of interventions on population subgroups
Partnerships, collaboration, and advocacy	Support government and community partners to build just institutions Solicit input from individuals and institutions
Diversity and inclusiveness	Understand, apply Universal Declaration on Human Rights
Communication	Develop strategies for historically oppressed subpopulations
Leadership	Integrate social justice in organisational mission and strategic plans Identify how redistributing public health resources may alter or reinforce inequities

(Edwards & MacLean Davison 2008:131)

are also embedded in a set of core competencies developed by the Public Health Agency of Canada to reflect the global PHC focus of nursing roles. The competencies link the role to the attributes of social justice (see Table 4.1).

Most nurses working in the community undertake population-focused roles reflecting the type of activities and competencies illustrated in the public health model (in Table 4.1). Many are advanced practitioners, even though they use a range of titles and defining roles, some of which are outlined in the section to follow.

NURSE PRACTITIONERS AND ADVANCED PRACTICE: MODELS OF PRACTICE

Advanced nursing practice has been variously described as a specialist and generalist role, leading to some confusion about the role and how it is enacted in various contexts (Por 2008). Many advanced practice nurses are nurse practitioners (NPs) whose roles originally developed to improve PHC in under-served communities (Gardner et al 2007). Their roles have evolved over the past 40 years in the United States (US), and in the United Kingdom (UK), since the 1980s (Currie & Watterson 2009;

Duffield et al 2009). A review in 2005 indicated that nurses are working in advanced practice with some prescriptive authority in seven OECD countries (Buchan & Calman 2005). Canada has a long history of advanced practice nurses but it has only been since 2006 that Canadian NPs have had legislative approval to practise in all provinces and territories. Because Canada, like many other countries is engaged in PHC reform, most NPs in that country are PHC NPs. Their roles occur within a collaborative, consultative relationship with the family physician (DiCenso et al 2007). This model is similar to development of the NP role in New Zealand, the general practice nurse role in Australia, and some district nurses' roles in the UK, in that it represents an expanded scope of practice (Finlayson et al 2009; Thompson 2008).

There are numerous models of advanced practice throughout the world. Standardisation has been difficult because of the substantial diversity in the titles, definitions and scope of practice roles, educational preparation and credentialing, within and between various countries (Bonsall & Cheater 2007; Brookes; Davidson et al 2007; DiCenso et al 2007; Duffield et al 2009). Daly & Carnwell (2003) view advanced practice roles along a continuum from 'extension' to 'expansion' to advanced practice. Extension of practice is equivalent to Benner's 'novice' level, in her model of skills acquisition that progresses from novice to expert (Benner 1984). Role expansion is a step further along the continuum, reflecting what Benner would describe as competent practice (Daly & Carnwell 2003). Advanced practice is seen as equivalent to the proficient level in Benner's model, while the expert nurse, the advanced nurse practitioner or consultant still requires role clarification (Currie & Watterson 2009).

An alternative framework is used by Pearce and Marshman (2008) who also see advanced practice as progressing along a continuum from specialist, to nurse practitioner, to advanced nurse practitioner and consultant. But none of these models or frameworks fits all situations. Australian and New Zealand NPs have prescribing rights and conduct diagnostic tests within their area of specialty. The NP is not necessarily a step on the continuum of the practice nurse's professional development, but an option for those who seek this type of advanced role. For example, the Australian and New Zealand nurse consultant role can be undertaken by any specialist PHC nurse, whereas within Pearce and Marshman's (2008) framework places the consultant role as a step along the advanced practice continuum.

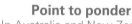

Point to ponder

In Australia and New Zealand, nurse practitioners (NPs) are both considered advanced nursing practice roles. New Zealand NPs have significant autonomy in practice, whereas Australian NPs are more limited in their scope.

In the reality of community PHC practice, the role is advanced, even though the title may differ. This is because community practice is dependent not only on nursing and midwifery skills, but the context, the regulatory environment, and historical policies that frame the needs of the employer.

In New Zealand, the Ministerial Taskforce on Nursing (MOHNZ 1998) was established to examine the obstacles that prevented nursing from contributing fully to health service delivery. Many of the recommendations from the Taskforce focused on PHC nursing practice with one of the key recommendations calling for the development of advanced nursing roles (MOHNZ 1998).

Point to ponder

Advanced nursing practice models have developed in many countries. Despite confusion over titles, it is generally understood that nurses working in advanced roles have formalised skills, experience and education to an advanced level in a specialised area of practice.

The first New Zealand Nurse Practitioner was approved for practice by the Nursing Council of New Zealand in 2001. The scope of practice for NPs was enshrined in legislation in New Zealand in 2003 with the passing of the *Health Practitioners Competence Assurance Act* (2003). A nurse practitioner in New Zealand has a Masters degree and at least four years working in their chosen clinical area. Registered nurses must meet Nursing Council of New Zealand assessment criteria and competencies before they can be recognised as an NP. At least 21 of the 77 NPs approved for practice by the Nursing Council of New Zealand since 2001 are approved for practice in PHC roles (College of Nurses Aotearoa 2010).

Since the New Zealand Primary Health Care Strategy was introduced in 2001 (MOHNZ 2001) further evolution of nursing and midwifery roles has led to a more integrated model of PHC in that country. Although few NPs work within the primary health organisations (PHOs) their role has the potential to develop innovative, nurse-led community programs and achieve greater access for under-served populations (Finlayson et al 2009). Apart from those nurses and midwives who are affiliated with PHOs, other New Zealand NPs working in PHC roles practise in wound care, diabetes, family planning, child and family nursing, youth health, rural health, older adult health and sexual health (College of Nurses Aotearoa 2010).

In Australia, the first NP was appointed in New South Wales in 2001, and by 2005 NPs had been appointed in every state and territory (Duffield et al 2009). The focus of the NP role is on health promotion, education and extended practice, including limited prescribing, initiation and interpretation of diagnostics, referral to medical specialists, and, in Victoria, admitting and discharging patients as well as approving absence from work certificates (Lee & Fitzgerald 2008). A growing number of NPs specialise in emergency nursing to help alleviate the pressure on emergency departments, and they have been found to improve efficiencies and quality of care in that setting (Searle 2007). Others work as gerontological NPs in residential or community settings, meeting the needs of under-served older persons (Caffrey 2005), and some NPs work in general practice settings.

Unlike New Zealand, which has a single health service and jurisdiction, Australian NPs, like their North American counterparts, have had a wide variety of roles and some inconsistencies in their educational preparation. These differences are due to varying state and territory accreditation requirements, health departments' employment criteria, and regional goals. As with NPs in New Zealand, all Australian NPs are required to have a Masters degree and a period of mentored experience in their specialised area of practice prior to their being granted NP status, which, in Australia, is granted by the state registration boards. In a move towards maintaining some consistency of the NP role a commissioned study jointly funded by the Australian Nursing and Midwifery Council (AMNC) and the Nursing Council of New Zealand (NCNZ) (Gardner et al 2004) has led to acceptance of a common trans-Tasman set of standards for education and practice (Duffield et al 2009). Development of a national regulatory body for accreditation of all nursing programs in 2010 is expected to achieve greater consistency for all practitioners across states and regions of Australia.

In many settings, especially in urban areas, there are few incentives and considerable resistance by medical practitioners to appoint NPs as collaborative practitioners. In Canada this is linked to the oversupply of medical practitioners (DiCenso et al 2007), but in Australia and New Zealand where serious shortages of both nurses and medical practitioners exist, it is often due to unfamiliarity with the role, dissonant philosophical positions, and lack of health system advocacy and funding for change. This has led to role ambiguity, where nurses find it difficult to describe and implement their role in the health care team. The lack of role clarity is exacerbated by insufficient research evidence for practice models that would provide exemplars of practice, and demonstrate effective outcomes from inter-and intra-professional interactions (Barry et al 2007; Brooks et al 2007b). Canada and New Zealand have been proactive in defining research as a key role of advanced practice nurses (Edwards & Macdonald 2009; Nursing Council of New Zealand 2008).

Other countries have yet to follow this mandate, which has implications for practice development as well as generating evidence for practice. The need for clarity and consistency in models of community health practice is especially important during times of role transition, which is the situation many nurses experience when they first adopt community nursing roles (Zurmehly 2007).

> **Point to ponder**
> Research is a key role of advanced practice nurses. Participating in, and leading research on their advanced practice roles, helps build the evidence that demonstrates effective health outcomes.

Nurses and midwives practising within a PHC model work on the principle that governance and control of community-based models of care should be vested in the community itself (Australian Nursing Federation [ANF] 2009). Examples of community-developed models of PHC practice include the original baby health centres in Australia and the Plunket clinics in New Zealand, women's health and reproductive services, gay and lesbian health services, community crisis and mental health services and services for refugees, immigrants and asylum seekers (ANF 2009:26). Many of these services have arisen from volunteer efforts in the communities themselves, subsequently becoming formalised through a variety of funding sources. However, some types of services are subject to transient funding opportunities which can lead to disempowerment if there is not sustainable leadership to guide community members through the funding application process. The model of care described below illustrates this type of situation where the impetus for change came from the community itself working in partnership with the community nurses (see Box 4.1).

EXPERIENCES IN THE UK: PUBLIC HEALTH, POPULATION HEALTH AND ROLE DEVELOPMENT

In the UK, general practice nurses are specialist practitioners who undertake population health roles and manage patients with chronic diseases within general practice (Robinson 2009). The model of PHC provision in the UK has also seen district

BOX 4.1 EXEMPLARY PRIMARY HEALTH CARE PRACTICE IN A CARAVAN PARK

The ANF (2009) review of PHC nursing services in Australia reports on an innovative outreach project at a caravan park in Maitland, New South Wales. A nurse-led clinic was developed to respond to the health needs of the caravan park's 150–200 residents, most of whom were living in serious disadvantaged conditions. The project was based on addressing their socially determined conditions of ill health and risk and aimed to provide equitable, accessible, empowered health services. Many residents had experienced transient living conditions, been homeless, imprisoned, refugees, former mental health patients, or were searching for affordable housing and health care. The high rate of referrals from the park to health services such as the local hospital emergency and obstetrics departments, the community health centre and children's services, was brought to the attention of the community health centre, where a child and family health nurse and a generalist community nurse developed a pilot project to provide a clinic operating from an onsite van. The nurses realised that those attending the van were severely disadvantaged, some relying solely on social benefits, some experiencing family violence or substance abuse, many being socially isolated, having poor functional health literacy, a high rate of Hepatitis C, poor school attendance, or experiencing abuse, neglect and poor self-esteem.

Equipped with meaningful data on the extent of the problems, the nurses successfully applied for two-year funding to develop a program based on the social determinants of health, focusing their efforts on advocacy and enablement. The key to its success has been community participation in decision-making, holistic, comprehensive, community-oriented services, and intersectoral collaboration. They have made changes to the environment (reducing needlestick injuries with a needle and syringe program), improved nutrition through better facilities for food storage, increased health literacy, strengthened community action and community activities, and fostered a greater sense of community in the park, which some would call social capital. Collaboration between health service providers, which have expanded the team to include mental health professionals and others, has not only met the community's needs but also helps provide the linkages between the outreach project and mainstream services.

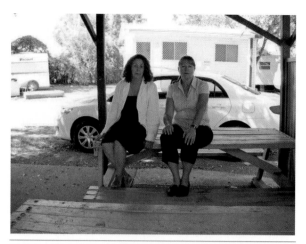

Figure 4.1 Generalist Community Nurses Loretta Baker and Debbie Tillitzki at their 'Coachstop Caravan Park' (*with permission*)

nurses attached to general practices and primary care trusts. However, district nurses have found it difficult to articulate the public health aspect of their role, especially when they are attached to medical practices with a traditional medical model of care (Toofany 2007). Other district nurses not attached to general practice have shaped their roles towards PHC more effectively, engaging in health promotion and education. For some however, resource and workload pressures results in them relegating health promotion activities to an 'after hours, leisure' activity (McMurray & Cheater 2004). This occurs despite the fact that their PHC role is clearly documented in government policy and the professional literature (Hayes 2005). Their impact on the health of the community remains poorly articulated, possibly due to extraordinary workloads. Like community nurses in Australia, New Zealand and other countries, district nurses' workloads have increased both in substance and complexity because of patients being discharged from hospital quickly with high-level needs, and because of the increased burden of chronic disease in the community (Baid et al 2009; Schroyen et al 2005). These increased demands have seen the district nurse's role expand to where advanced assessment skills, diagnostic and therapeutic interventions, and pharmacological knowledge are essential (Baid et al 2009). Even with this level of clinical expertise, and despite having been educated to take on a broader health promotion role, in some cases the district nurse continues to be seen as the 'nit nurse' (McMurray & Cheater 2004:46).

Derogatory labels and misperceptions of nurses as 'nit nurses' and 'tampon and bandaid distributors' are also common in New Zealand and Australia — particularly directed towards public health nurses — which leaves many feeling undervalued, neglected and unable to provide optimal care.

The role of the UK health visitor is more closely aligned with the North American public health nursing model, and many health visitors focus on health promotion in their geographic area of responsibility. In Ireland, integration of community and primary care services has created the impetus for an expanded, integrated nursing role (O'Neill & Cowman 2008).

Point to ponder

Nurses working in community roles in the UK have struggled to get the health promotion components of their work recognised in a meaningful way as they balance increasingly complex care of people with challenging organisational factors.

In Scotland, the health visitors' role has been re-titled as 'community health nurse' in preparation for a future PHC model of care (Thompson 2008; Wilson 2006). Other organisational factors present barriers to holistic, PHC practice for both health visitors and district nurses. These include a lack of clarity about models of delegation for such things as routine childhood screenings. Scottish nurses are also attempting to make greater use of telehealth and portable technologies for community care, and the need for interprofessional collaboration to create common understandings, service redesign and better administrative support (Swiadek 2009; Winters et al 2007).

Another model of care in the UK is the community matron role, which is a neighbourhood-based case management role (Chapman et al 2009; Downes & Pemberton 2009; Harrison & Lydon 2008). The community matron is a specialist in community care and inter-agency collaboration who focuses on personalised care planning for the most vulnerable in a community, including those with learning disabilities, travellers and people seeking asylum (Downes & Pemberton 2009; Harrison & Lydon 2008). The objective is to provide proactive patient care to promote health and minimise crises for those with complex, long-term conditions (UK Department of Health 2004).

The community matron is an advanced practitioner who provides patient education, facilitates self-management skills and monitors social needs (Chapman et al 2009). These activities fall within the realm of PHC, although, like the community health nurse and district nursing roles, there remains a lack of clear role definition (Chapman et al 2009; McMurray & Cheater 2004; Toofany 2007).

PRIMARY HEALTH CARE ROLES: SPECIALIST OR GENERALIST?

For many years, public health nurses have practised with a focus on individuals and families, rather than communities, providing child health clinics, immunisations and home visits as well as a number of other program-focused activities according to their organisational structures (Markham & Carney 2007; May et al 2003; McMurray & Cheater 2004; Wilson 2006; Winters et al 2007). With the growing trend towards population health and PHC, nurses incumbent in these roles are seeking to change their roles to be more closely aligned with a population-based approach. There is broad agreement on the goals of PHC, and the values underpinning practice (Barry et al 2007; Besner 2004). Many nurses are poised to act as community advocates, focusing on health promotion in integrated, generalist roles that allow them to work with the community as a whole rather than on a segmented system of predetermined public health priorities. However, the systems delivering public health care and the reporting mechanisms often work at cross-purposes to their achieving this goal. Programmatic approaches, with 'categorical' funding, where certain categories of activity (family planning, immunisation) dictate the role, because of funding arrangements thwart nurses' attempts to reframe their role from specialists to generalists (May et al 2003:252).

May et al (2009) argue that the specialist model inhibits a role that would see them working in partnership with the community, holistically, in an empowering way, having cultural relevance, and targeting primary, secondary and tertiary levels of prevention to improve population health. Yet, the trend towards specialised programs is occurring in many countries and health departments, as organisational cultures favour worker productivity instead of health promotion.

Point to ponder

Whether primary health care roles are categorised as generalist or specialist, retaining a focus on improving health equity will ensure a common goal for all nurses working in primary health care.

This trend also constrains nurses' attempts to enact an effective, generalist PHC role (May et al 2003; Toofany 2007). Besner (2004) and Thompson (2008) contend that this makes nursing work invisible, even in population-focused approaches to care. Nurses should be empowered to move beyond existing systems to develop systematic recording systems that document social, emotional, cultural and spiritual dimensions of health, as well as their contributions to care (Besner 2004). There is widespread agreement that advanced PHC roles have engendered high patient satisfaction, improved accessibility of care, effective communication, and some short-term outcomes (Bonsall & Cheater 2007). However, there is a dearth of research evidence for the efficacy of nurse-led systems or explicit findings indicating the nature or extent of long-term outcomes directly linked to the nurse or midwife's interventions (Bonsall & Cheater 2007).

Some nurse leaders have sought to clarify the specialist role rather than re-brand it as a generalist public health role. Fisher Robertson and Brandt Baldwin (2007) articulate such a role as an advanced community practitioner, a nurse who leads community initiatives for system-wide changes and health promotion through case management, project management, risk management, community advocacy and policy development, which is focused on high-level leadership. Lange (2006:E50) describes an alternative, the role of 'community nurse' who is a culture broker, liaison, advocate and activist rather than case manager or project manager. A literature review of the Australian community nursing role by Brooks et al (2004) indicated that there is still ambiguity between generalist/specialist, no role clarity, under-utilisation, underdeveloped models for professional education and research, and little power in decision-making. What all community scholars agree on, is the need for research and professional role development to provide rational arguments for changes, consistency in education and practice, and shared strategies for successful, high-quality community outcomes (Besner 2004; Bonsall & Cheater 2007; Markham & Carney

2007; Fisher Robertson & Brandt Baldwin 2007; Por 2008; Swearingen 2009).

PRACTICE NURSING: AUSTRALIA

As Australia responds to the international PHC agenda (WHO 2008) with its focus on general practice in the community, the role of the practice nurse (PN) is undergoing a renaissance (ANF 2009). The PN is not a protected title but it is a specialist PHC role (Halcomb et al 2005; Porritt 2007). However, because of the general practice focus on *primary care*, rather than the more comprehensive *PHC* agenda with its focus on community health promotion, most PN's roles are confined to primary care activities such as chronic illness management (Halcomb & Hickman 2010).

Point to ponder

Practice nurse roles in Australia are developing rapidly to meet the needs of an ageing population. However, funding, employment mechanisms, and a lack of research into practice nurse outcomes are inhibiting practice nurses' abilities to provide the care people need.

The Commonwealth government defines a practice nurse as a registered or enrolled nurse who is employed by, or whose services are otherwise retained by, a general practice (Commonwealth Department of Health and Ageing, in Walker 2010). Major changes in the Commonwealth policy environment over the first decade of this century have supported the development of the PN role, to respond to the needs of the population, shortages in the health workforce, community expectations, and rising health costs (Porritt 2007). Australian scholarships, funding and changes to the Medicare Benefit Schedule (MBS) to provide practice incentives have all had an impact on the role (Keleher et al 2007; Porritt 2007). Medicare funding and Practice Incentive Payments (PIP) have provided remuneration to GPs for PNs to undertake immunisations, provide wound care, cervical screening, assessments for older persons and management of conditions such as asthma, diabetes and mental health through the Chronic Disease Management Initiative (Halcomb et al 2005; Keleher et al 2007; Porritt 2007; Senior 2009).

Through the advocacy of the Australian Nurses Federation (ANF: www.anf.org.au/nurses_gp)

national competency standards have been developed for PNs (Keleher et al 2007; Porritt 2007). These reflect a rapidly evolving role which has changed from where PNs undertook simple tasks, to a complex, knowledge-based practice with many different contextual challenges (Walker 2010). Although teamwork is a major aspect of their role, PNs work under the supervision of a GP, and in many cases, roles are negotiated between the nurse and the practice (Keleher et al 2007). The scope of practice varies according to the nurse's expertise and experience, practice arrangements, the GP's understanding of the role and the needs of the local population (Halcomb et al 2005; Keleher et al 2007). In rural and remote areas, PN roles are rapidly expanding because of shortages of GPs (Halcomb et al 2005; Porritt 2007). As of 2007, 60% of Australian practices had employed at least one PN (Keleher et al 2007). In addition to the funding support for practices to employ a PN, establishment of a national professional PN association and increasing professional development opportunities, including national conferences, have all fostered rapid development of the role (Australian General Practice Network [AGPN] 2007).

Although there is no strong evidence yet on effectiveness, efficiency or outcomes of PN practice (Keleher et al 2007) the research agenda of PNs has been evolving over the past decade (Halcomb et al 2005; Mills & Fitzgerald 2009; Patterson & McMurray 2003; Phillips et al 2008; Senior 2009). The research agenda for practice nursing was outlined in a Delphi study conducted in 2009, which identified 53 areas for future PN studies, including clinical, educational and practice management issues (Halcomb & Hickman 2010). The PN research agenda will also be strengthened by the efforts of the national professional organisation (Australian Practice Nurses Association), and the Australian General Practice Network (AGPN). These two organisations, and the development of a mentoring network, are all helping to enhance the visibility of the role and establish its place in PHC (AGPN 2007; Mills et al 2009; Porritt 2007).

PRACTICE AND PRIMARY HEALTH CARE NURSING: NEW ZEALAND

Practice nursing in New Zealand is also growing in strength and numbers. When the New Zealand *Primary Health Care Strategy* was released in 2001, it was clearly indicated that nurses were seen

as crucial to its implementation (MOHNZ 2001). In 2003 the Expert Advisory Group on Primary Health Care Nursing created a framework for activating PHC nursing practice in New Zealand in order to realise the potential of nurses to achieve the goals of the PHC Strategy (Expert Advisory Group on Primary Health Care Nursing 2003).

> **Point to ponder**
>
> Practice nursing in New Zealand has developed significantly since publication of the *Primary Health Care Strategy* in 2001. A framework for developing primary health care nursing practice has enabled practice nurses to implement a number of new strategies to meet the needs of the population.

The framework provided a definition of PHC nursing and a set of corresponding goals. PHC nurses were defined as registered nurses with knowledge and expertise in PHC practice. They work autonomously and collaboratively to promote, improve, maintain and restore health, in roles that encompass population health, health promotion, disease prevention, wellness care, first-point-of-contact care and disease management across the life span. Their models of practice are determined by the setting and the ethnic and cultural grouping of their clientele. They practise in partnership with people — individuals, whānau, communities and populations — to achieve the shared goal of health for all, which is central to PHC nursing. The goals of practice therefore include aligning nursing practice with community need, innovative models of nursing practice, governance, leadership and career development (Expert Advisory Group on Primary Health Care Nursing 2003:9).

Many nurses practising in PHC settings have grasped the framework as a guide for developing their PHC nursing practice including district nurses, public health nurses and practice nurses. Practice nurses (PNs) in New Zealand were originally employed in the mid-1970s in GP practices, largely to provide support to GPs. Since that time, the role of the PN has evolved substantially. The Primary Health Care Strategy and subsequent framework for activating PHC nursing were seen as providing opportunities for PNs to demonstrate the impact they could have on population health. However, by 2007 the New Zealand Nurses Organisation and the College of Nurses (Aotearoa) suggested that significant work was still required to achieve the potential of PHC nursing in line with the original framework suggested by the Expert Advisory Group (New Zealand Nurses Organisation & the College of Nurses Aotearoa (NZ) Inc 2007).

Point to ponder

Despite significant developments in practice nursing in New Zealand, the same barriers facing Australian PNs exist for New Zealand PNs including inadequate funding mechanisms, hierarchical employment structures, and a lack of research into PN outcomes.

Evaluation data indicate that there are ongoing barriers to enacting the PN role, such as hierarchical employment structures, limited access to education and poor funding of nursing initiatives, all of which require urgent attention (New Zealand Nurses Organisation & the College of Nurses Aotearoa (NZ) Inc 2007). Professional development of PNs has largely been initiated and implemented by the New Zealand Nurses Organisation (NZNO). The organisation developed a strategic plan for PNs in 1996–1998, identifying a career pathway, a marketing plan to enhance the professional profile and adequate employment conditions. The College of Practice Nurses (a college under the NZNO) now offers a comprehensive accreditation program for PN members, a journal and various other publications and support processes (New Zealand Nurses Organisation, Online. Available: www.nzno.org.nz/groups/colleges/college_of_practice_nurses/about_us 23 February 2010). In 2010 the College of Practice Nurses is about to be reformed as the College of Primary Health Care Nurses broadening its membership base to include all nurses working in primary health care setting including district nurses, public health nurses school nurses and occupational nurses. Professional development programs for PNs are also becoming increasingly common, largely established within PHOs.

Formal evaluation of nursing developments in PHC in New Zealand from 2001 to 2007 demonstrated that the barriers identified by the NZNO and College of Nurses did indeed exist, and their recommendations included a need for leadership, mentoring, governance, and recruitment and retention of PNs (Finlayson et al 2009). Despite the barriers, the profession was able to demonstrate examples of excellence in practice nursing, including substantial growth in the development of nursing roles and capability within PHOs. Particular strengths of the PNs included the management of long-term conditions and, as mentioned above, working with under-served and vulnerable population groups (Finlayson et al 2009). Among these vulnerable populations are older persons in residential care settings, who too often are overlooked in the PHC agenda. This is being redressed through ongoing discussion of models of PHC in Australia and New Zealand, especially in the evolution of nurse practitioner roles. The care of older persons, like that of younger population groups, should be included in the PHC agenda, with appropriate needs assessment, care coordination, health promotion and disease management.

MANAGING CHRONIC CONDITIONS IN THE COMMUNITY

Because of population ageing and increasing rates of diseases such as cardiovascular disease and diabetes, the management of chronic conditions has become, and will continue to be, a major element of community health practice, especially for PNs. Most models of chronic condition management are based on the PHC principle that the client is the centre of the health care system. This places the emphasis on patient choice, shared decision-making and the psychosocial and health promotion aspects of care delivery (Commonwealth of Australia 2009; Forbes & While 2008). The WHO (2005) explains that the major goal of chronic disease management programs should be empowering people towards self-management. This is also incorporated into new models of care in the UK, such as the community matron role described above, which is intended to promote self-reliance among people living with chronic illness in the community (Harrison & Lydon 2008; Swiadek 2009). Self-management applies across the continuum from prevention and early risk identification to the way existing chronic conditions are managed, typically with a patient care plan tailored to individual needs. A variety of models have been developed for chronic condition management. All identify clear roles for nurses, placing the nurse as a manager or coordinator who works horizontally, to manage people through and between health systems, and vertically, providing preventative care, self-care support and education, case finding and identification, managing therapeutic interventions and complications, and case management (Forbes & While 2008). Health literacy features in all models as a cornerstone of health promotion.

Point to ponder

Chronic disease management is a major element of community health practice. Chronic disease management frameworks that guide nursing practice should be person-centred with the goal of empowering people towards self-management.

A major review of nurses' activities in managing chronic conditions in the community reveals that nurses are in fact, participating in this important element of practice, engaging with people holistically, targeting marginalised or excluded groups and leading a variety of interventions (Forbes & While 2008). In communities everywhere, nurses' health promotion activities at primary, secondary and tertiary levels have had significant impacts on people's lives and their capacity for self-management. Their role has helped bridge service gaps, brought interdisciplinary teams together, promoted access and appropriate use of technologies, and forged collaborative teams to address the care systems within which people deal with chronic conditions (Forbes & While 2008). Because of

the growing importance of chronic illness in the population, various models of care have been developed. One model for managing chronic illness in the community is the Chronic Disease Self-Management Program (CDSMP) that has been adapted by Queensland health professionals from an American model of chronic care (Catalano et al 2009). The CDSMP uses health professional leaders and peer leaders working together to provide self-management courses. The program provides a four-day leader training program for peer leaders who themselves have a chronic disease. They subsequently act as role models for other participants, under the guidance of the professional leaders in a type of 'expert patient' model. This has major potential for health education.

Another model widely used in community management of chronic illnesses is the 'Flinders Model' (Commonwealth of Australia 2009). This model identifies core skills for the PHC workforce in terms of promoting patient capabilities, fostering behaviour change and developing organisational and systems capabilities. Its focus on capabilities rather than competencies illustrates current benchmarking trends that move away from the procedural and technical focus of competencies to a broader, capabilities orientation, that may be comprised of many competencies (Gardner et al 2007). The model (see Table 4.2) also refrains from referring to chronic 'disease', instead expressing patients' needs in terms of chronic conditions.

The core skills identified above are aimed at developing community capabilities across all specialised PHC roles and settings. These settings and roles are described in the section to follow.

Table 4.2 Core skills for the PHC workforce to promote capabilities

Patient-centred	Behaviour change	Organisational/systems
Health promotion	Change management	Multidisciplinary learning and practice
Risk assessment	Motivational interviews	Information, communication systems
Communication skills	Collaborative problem defined	Organisational change techniques
Collaborative planning	Goal setting, achievement	Evidence-based knowledge
Peer support	Structured problem-solving	Practice research, quality improvement
Cultural awareness	Action planning	Awareness of community resources (psychosocial assessment, support)

(Commonwealth of Australia 2009)

CHILD HEALTH NURSING PRACTICE

Child health nursing is a specialised area of nursing in the community. In some areas, including different Australian states, the role is variously designated 'child health nurse', 'community health nurse', 'child and youth health nurse', 'maternal and child health nurse', 'child and family health nurse' or 'family and child health nurse' (Kruske et al 2006). Although all Australian child health nurses aspire to a PHC philosophy as prescribed by the Child and Family Health Nurses Association (CAFHNA 2000), confusion arises from the lack of consistent nomenclature and role description, which is influenced by the service structure within which they practise as well as different credentials and levels of preparation.

Most child health nurses in Australia consider themselves specialists. Many run child health clinics, and since the establishment by state health departments of universal home visiting, most nurses also conduct home visits (Briggs 2006–07). Some child health nurse specialists provide a range of PHC activities in primary schools, especially where there is no designated school nurse. These include student screening, health education for teachers and parents, and community engagement activities.

Point to ponder
Child health nurses in Australia and New Zealand provide a range of services, including child health clinics, home visits, student screening, health education, anticipatory guidance, parenting skills programs, and community engagement activities.

This PHC aspect of practice promotes the idea that the school should be seen as a resource for the community's health as well as its education. Another type of specialised child health practice involves acting as the expert resource person in special schools for children with disabilities. In this context, the nurse's health promotion activities extend from primary and secondary care of the child to ongoing tertiary care for the entire family. On occasion this includes hospital visiting and grief counselling for family members and fellow students.

Other child health nurses are attached to a variety of programs, some as part of comprehensive parenting or early learning centres that function as a referral point for parents. Others are part of outreach programs such as the Community Mothers program (in Western Australia) or the NSW Family Partnership Training program, both of which are aimed at developing parenting capacity. The model of child health care in these and other programs is comprehensive and enabling, in that nurses provide anticipatory guidance, education and skills development to parents simultaneously with their surveillance and monitoring of the child's health status (Munns et al 2004). In the Community Mothers model this is achieved through a partnership between the Western Australian Department of Health, child health specialists at Curtin University, a network of volunteer mothers and new mothers (Munns et al 2004). In other cases, child health nurses promote parenting capacity through group work and adopting a family advocacy role, where parents are put in touch with resources and community support systems (Carolan 2004–05). Groups include support networks following childbirth, some of which grow into important self-sustaining social networks for mothers in particular (Carolan 2004–05).

Point to ponder
'Plunket' nurses in New Zealand have been providing child health services since 1907.

Although there have been some studies of the scope of practice there remains a dearth of research into the impact of their roles. Kruske et al (2006) found that the role in New South Wales is diverse, even within that state, with some child health nurses emphasising the historical programmatic focus on growth assessment and monitoring, and others undertaking a 'strengths' based approach to supporting parenting (Kruske et al 2006:59). The latter indicated that the nurses worked in an egalitarian partnership with families, acknowledging their strengths and expertise, with the nurse seeking to play a facilitative, reinforcing role and providing psychosocial support (Briggs 2006–07, Kruske et al 2006). Other researchers have found that Australian child health nurses have a major impact on parenting capacity, through the support and guidance they provide (Barnes et al 2003; Rowe & Barnes 2006). Similarly, New Zealand child health nurses practising as 'Well Child' or 'Tamariki Ora' nurses or within the Royal

New Zealand Plunket Society (RNZPS) as 'Plunket' nurses provide family parenting support in home visits, and undertake an expanded, PHC role with families, particularly disadvantaged groups (Comino & Harris 2003; Yarwood 2008). Plunket nurses, Well Child and/or Tamariki Ora nurses are required to complete specialised postgraduate education in PHC nursing either prior to or on appointment to child health positions. The 'Parent Advisor Model' currently used by Plunket nurses in New Zealand and many health visitors in the UK has been demonstrated to improve the knowledge of helping and listening skills of nurses, improve outcomes for parents and children, and sensitise health visitors to the needs of families (Bidmead et al 2002). Research by Clendon (2009) suggests that it is the interaction between nurse and mother, rather than the information, that is the key element in determining the success of the relationship between the two.

In other countries, the child health role is broad-ranging and diffuse (Forbes et al 2007). Some practise in case management; for example, working with social workers and other disciplines to provide counselling, consultation and referrals for children in foster care (Schneiderman 2006). Many work as generalist public health nurses, rather than as specialists, focusing on health promotion and family guidance. In the UK midwives and health visitors provide this type of child and family orientation, also connecting their activities to community development work (Forbes et al 2007). In all cases, developing a sense of connectedness with the family is paramount, and this is typically based on a close and trusting relationship in which information is freely shared. This important role of child health nurses is aimed at fostering health literacy, therapeutic communication, preventative treatment and health education (Briggs 2006–07; Forbes et al 2007).

Telephone support lines for parents, currently available as a 24-hour service, have been an important vehicle for all of these aspects of the communication role in Australia, New Zealand and other countries. Both the Plunket Society and the New Zealand Ministry of Health provide telephone support lines for parents of young children (Online. Available: www.healthline.co.nz and www.Plunket.org.nz [accessed 23 August 2009]). Twenty-four hour telephone support is also available in all Australian states (Online. Available: www.cyh.com/SubContent/aspx?p=102 [accessed

13 August 2009]). In 2009 the Australian government announced a further extension of telephone support provided by child and family support nurses and midwives through a helpline for pregnant women and new mothers. The initiative is sponsored by four organisations: Post and Antenatal Depression Australia (PANDA), SIDS and Kids Australia, Stillbirth and Neonatal Death Support (SANDS) and the Bonnie Babes Foundation (Australian Labor Party media, Online. Available: www.alp.org.au/media/0709/msheag240.php [accessed 10 August 2009]). Telephone access provides immediate counselling for new parents with a range of needs, including breastfeeding, infant crying, sleeping and nutrition guidance, referrals and emotional support (Rowe & Barnes 2008; Sheehan & Barclay 1999). In 2007–2008 Plunket Society nurses answered 70 000 calls from parents and caregivers needing advice and support in areas such as breastfeeding, sleeping, nutrition and child behaviour (Plunket Society 2008).

SCHOOL HEALTH NURSING

The school nurse (SN) is a PHC practitioner who combines the roles of public health liaison or community nurse, child and family nurse, mental health nurse, occupational health nurse, case manager, and team coordinator (Brooks, Kendall et al 2007a; Journal of School Nursing [JOSN] 2008; NASN 2005; Smith & Firmin 2009). It is a specialised, advanced, complex practice role that revolves around promoting students' wellbeing, their academic success, normal development and lifelong achievement, as well as intervention for actual and potential health problems (Downie et al 2002; JOSN 2008). The way SNs' roles are organised depends on whether the SN is employed in a primary or secondary school, by the health service or the education department.

Point to ponder

School nurses have a complex practice role that revolves around promoting student wellbeing both at school and at home.

What all SNs have in common is a role as the 'navigator' who helps the child along the school journey (Brooks, Kendall et al 2007:226). The major focus of the role in primary school is to ensure students are safe, healthy and ready to learn. School nurses working in the primary school setting undertake developmental screening for conditions affecting learning, such as vision and hearing. They also respond to children's needs for support in relation to diet, behaviours at school, issues related to the home environment, and coping with stress, even in very young children. High school nurses tend to deal with student needs that revolve around adolescent 'acting out', problems with parental relationships and other issues that affect students' mental health. These can include issues related to sexuality, risky behaviours or other areas where peer pressure causes conflict between the young person's struggle for identity formation and family or group norms.

Contrary to popular perceptions, SN practice does not typically include dispensing bandaids or headache tablets. The role is multidimensional, requiring a wide breadth of activities and a current knowledge base that includes understanding clinical and technological developments affecting health, and maintaining current knowledge of health, education and professional policies (Barnes et al 2004a; Wainwright et al 2000). SNs in high schools have to maintain current knowledge of adolescent behaviours and the changing nature of their social world. For example, the immediacy of young people's communication tools means that the school day is extended through computers, texts, mobile phones and social networking. SNs know that this can translate into students coming to school with no respite from any of the previous day's troubling relationships. This type of insight is crucial to maintaining strong and trusting relationships with students.

SNs also need a working knowledge of education systems and the processes and protocols of their school. They often work towards maintaining a boundary between themselves and the teaching staff, but some find that they are more effective when they work as part of the school resource team, becoming an integral part of the school culture.

Point to ponder

School nurses must carefully balance the need to build effective relationships with students to promote health, responding quickly to any health needs arising in the school.

Within this culture SNs try to balance the proactive part of their role that focuses on relationships and student capacity development, with the need to respond quickly to any immediate health needs of students, teachers and school administrative staff. It can be a careful balancing act, one that requires strong leadership and management skills, as well as extensive networks for liaising with a wide range of personnel, family members and community resources (Smith & Firmin 2009). Most SNs practise relatively autonomously, but not in isolation from others. A major challenge is the immediacy of demands on their time because of unscheduled student access and the fact that many SNs work part-time (Smith & Firmin 2009).

Health promotion is a significant element of the SN role (Moses et al 2008; St Leger 1999). In this role SNs negotiate primary prevention initiatives on the basis of their understanding of the social determinants of health, promoting positive parenting, providing advice, support and counselling, and maintaining a student-centred, partnership approach (Brooks et al 2007a). Many see their role as helping young people become resilient adults by encouraging them to develop self awareness and the ability to find solutions and options to the issues that challenge them. This often requires the nurse to make the first overture towards students who seem to need support for a physical or emotional issue. Their approach is one of deliberate engagement, building trust, taking advantage of the 'teachable moments' and whatever opportunities arise to convey the message that they are there to help. One of the main challenges is the vast number of students, many of whom have multiple issues. In addition to counselling for students and staff with emotional health problems, some also engage with educational staff in planning and delivering health-related curriculum components (Barnes et al 2004a, 2004b; Green & Reffel 2009; JOSN 2008; NASN 2005; Wainwright et al 2000).

In many cases the health promotion role of SNs is poorly understood, with education authorities expecting a behavioural, healthy-lifestyle approach rather than a broader focus on school and student capacity building (Ryan 2008; Whitehead 2006a). The Health Promoting Schools (HPS) framework developed by the WHO in 1995 (WHO 1996) was intended to strengthen health promotion in schools at local, regional, national and global levels using a whole-of-school approach (St Leger 1999). The guidelines for health promotion were developed to address the school, its policies, social environment, community and health service relationships as well as personal health skills. In many cases the HPS model has been adopted as a guide to connecting the school community to the wider environment and its resources (Barnes et al 2004a, 2004b; Moses et al 2008; Victorian Government 2004). However, most HPS programs have retained the focus on changing students' behaviours rather than developing an empowering approach to promoting the health of schools and students. One exception is the development in the UK of the National Healthy School Standard (NHSS); a PHC framework aimed at reducing inequalities, promoting social inclusion and raising educational standards (DeBell 2006; Wicklander 2005). In this context, the SN has an important role in integrating services, coordinating activities and relationships, bridging health and education services, and promoting partnerships to build whole-of-school capacity as well as deliver programs with specific themes (Wicklander 2005). Another new initiative is the development in 2010 of professional practice standards for school nursing established by the Victorian School Nurses [VSN] 2010. The 12 standards, which are classified within the domains of professional practice, provision and coordination of care, collaborative and therapeutic practice, and critical thinking and analysis, are listed in Table 4.3.

Table 4.3 School Nursing Professional Practice Standards

Domain: professional practice	
Standard One	Demonstrates a comprehensive knowledge of school nursing incorporating child and adolescent health and development.
Standard Two	Practises within a professional and ethical nursing framework.
Standard Three	Practises in accordance with legislation related to school nursing practice and child and adolescent health care.
Standard Four	Advocates for and protects the rights of children and young people.
Standard Five	Effectively manages human and material resources.
Domain: provision and coordination of care	
Standard Six	Effectively addresses the health care needs of students and groups considering a whole-of-school-community approach.
Standard Seven	Coordinates, organises and provides health promotion considering a whole-of-school-community approach.
Standard Eight	Contributes to the maintenance of a healthy work and learning environment that is respectful, safe and supportive of students and the school community.
Domain: collaborative and therapeutic practice	
Standard Nine	Uses a range of effective communication skills.
Standard Ten	Engages in collaborative practice to provide comprehensive school nursing care.
Domain: critical thinking and analysis	
Standard Eleven	Participates in ongoing professional development of self and others.
Standard Twelve	Identifies the relevance of research in improving individual student and whole-of-school-community health outcomes.

(Victorian School Nurses (ANF, Vic Branch) Special Interest Group 2010:3, with permission)

Combining primary and secondary prevention, SNs typically maintain student health records and care plans for those with a range of conditions impacting on their health. They manage safety and protective strategies in the educational environment, which can include detecting infectious diseases and administering immunisations, treating, and where necessary, transporting sick and injured students, screening children for developmental and medical conditions, and environmental surveillance of the school community.

What's your opinion?
The Health Promoting Schools movement was developed to strengthen health promotion in schools using a whole-of-school approach. Unfortunately, many schools have continued to focus on changing student behaviour rather than developing an empowering approach to health promotion.

In some cases the nurse is the first person to provide early detection of children with developmental disabilities, which requires sensitive communication between parents, other health professionals and education staff (Wallis & Smith 2008). Where the school accommodates children with disabilities, the SN role extends to helping them with independent living needs and ensuring they have opportunities to participate in the educational experience, including field trips (NASN 2005). To achieve this, there is often a need to ensure educational staff as well as parents are fully apprised of the students' needs and potential, and help them plan for both the home and learning environment to accommodate their needs. Like the child health nurses mentioned previously, SNs working in schools where young people have disabilities often act as the mediator between the health and education systems. This includes liaising with teachers, parents, peers and others affected by the child's journey along the health and development continuum.

Research in the US indicates that up to 25% of school students have special needs, including asthma, diabetes, epilepsy or cancer, some of whom have the need for intermittent acute care and tertiary prevention (NASN 2005). In addition, many SNs are experiencing a rapid increase in helping students manage mental health issues and chronic conditions, particularly with growing rates of childhood obesity, stress-related illnesses and bullying (St Leger 1999; NASN 2005). Students can bring to school a wide range of vulnerabilities and social issues such as family crises, immigration or refugee-related problems, poverty and violence (Barnes et al 2004a; DeBell 2006; JOSN 2008). Adolescents in particular, can have serious mental health needs, sometimes requiring early detection of, and intervention for, substance abuse, family relationship challenges, adolescent pregnancy and/or sexually transmitted infections, or a risk of suicide (Brooks et al 2007a; JOSN 2008; NASN 2005; Tkaczyk & Edelson 2009).

Body image problems are a common issue, especially for girls, many of whom are overweight or obese. Other mental health interventions include the SNs' involvement in de-escalating reactive situations between students, school staff and parents (Weist et al 2009). Tertiary prevention may include periodic monitoring of a student or staff member's health condition or establishing a close engagement with groups or classes. The main objective of these relationships is empowerment, which requires the SN to bridge transitions between the family and school environment. This is done in an atmosphere of support and acceptance, a safe haven where young people can disclose their concerns, feel acknowledged and protected, receive non-judgemental help and build resilience (JOSN 2008; Smith & Firmin 2009). In many cases, administrators are unaware of students' need for rehabilitation and have little idea of the breadth of the SN role. This is because most activities are confidential and oriented towards building a trusting relationship with members of the school community (Green & Reffel 2009). School nurses need to be supportive of teachers, helping them deal with medically fragile students and their treatment requirements. Their support role with the school or education system is often expressed in bringing expert information to the school planning committee in areas such as emergency management and

Point to ponder
Adolescent mental health needs challenge school nurses to find effective ways of managing the impact of mental health issues on the student, on their school life and on their home life.

health protection (DeBell 2006; Green & Reffel 2009).

Documentation, planning and evaluation are important elements in helping to defend best practice and clarify SN outcomes (Wicklander 2005). Yet despite the wide range of initiatives, SNs have been relatively invisible and marginalised as participants in policy and planning agendas (Brooks et al 2007). To some extent this is because of insufficient research evidence for the effectiveness of their work (Brooks et al 2007; Wainwright et al 2000; Whitehead 2006a). School nurses in the UK have used the NHSS initiative to extend their research agenda. DeBell (2006) explains that, despite a commonly held view that SNs have overlooked the need for research, the problem is not that research data are absent from practice, but that they are highly dispersed in internal service reviews and a narrow range of journals. To heighten visibility of the role, there remains a need for research that would demonstrate the paradigm shift away from the exclusive focus on school health services, towards promoting health and its social determinants.

With a few exceptions (Barnes et al 2004a, 2004b; Downie et al 2002), little is published about the SN role in Australia, although SNs are obliged to submit reports of activities to employers in New South Wales and Victoria (Victorian Government 2004; Moses et al 2008). The NSW reports have developed a summary of the extent of SNs' roles, and common student concerns (School Nurses Association NSW, Online. Available: www.schoolnursesnse.asn.au/200.html [accessed 5 August 2009]). This followed an earlier publication which outlined the importance of the SN role in private boarding schools, where PHC extends across the spectrum of ages and needs (Armstrong 2004).

ACTION POINT

The invisibility of school nurses is inhibiting their ability to effectively advocate for the development of their role. Work toward undertaking and widely publishing high quality research into the role of the school nurse.

Further attention was drawn to the need for this type of report by the National Health and Hospitals Reform Commission reviewing Australian health services in 2009. The Commission reported that the lack of standardised data collection explains why little is known of the Australian SN role (Chiarella 2009). However, this may not be an accurate representation of the problem. Given the importance of SNs in PHC, it would be appropriate to develop a series of case studies identifying effective SN role enactment. Publishing this type of research would provide a greater insight into the potential of the role and how nurses are helping build school and student capacity throughout the country. It would also help validate their role within the broader scope of the nursing profession (Roberts 2009).

New Zealand SNs are similarly under-recognised and under-utilised in school settings. Of particular concern are funding and employment models that have frequently seen SNs paid on rates similar to administrative workers in schools. This devalues the work of the SN and contributes to the invisibility of the nurse as a key provider of health services to young people. Varying models of SN practice also exist with differing outcomes. Kool et al (2008) suggest that SNs utilising an embracing pattern of health care provision rather than a 'bandaid' pattern provide more effective school-based services. An example of the efficacy of an 'embracing' pattern of health care provision is in the improved health outcomes demonstrated among children attending a nurse-led clinic based in a primary school in Central Auckland (Krothe & Clendon 2006; Clendon 2004–05). An initial community assessment process and ongoing community involvement in the clinic have been integral to its success, demonstrating the importance of involving community members at the outset of any health project.

RURAL AND REMOTE AREA NURSING PRACTICE

Although the context may be different, practising in rural and remote areas holds common challenges for nurses and midwives around the world. Research conducted in the US in the late 1980s and 1990s by leaders in rural health such as Long and Weinert (1989) and Bushy (2000), established common understandings of the main challenges of rural nursing. As Long and Weinert (1989) declared, rural nursing is shaped by the way rural people perceive health, which is by being able to work and feel productive, carrying on their lives in the usual way. Rural people also have a common belief in the significance of their community, which is a type of cultural bond (Mills et al 2010). They are also typically more self-reliant and stoical than urban dwellers and tend to resist outside help, preferring to care for one another within the family unit.

Point to ponder

Rural and remote populations face unique health issues often compounded by a lack of geographic access to health care services. A lack of appropriately skilled health professionals to meet the needs of rural populations adds to the problem.

Other issues that pose challenges for rural populations include their higher morbidity and mortality rates; a growing number of residents who are ageing, many of whom have chronic diseases; the high levels of disadvantage because of restricted access to goods, services and opportunities for social interaction; the withdrawal of services as economic and infrastructure decline; limited educational, employment and recreational opportunities; limited choices for health care; and low levels of health literacy (Allan et al 2007; Burley & Greene 2007; Catalano et al 2009; Greenhill et al 2009; Wong & Regan 2009). In rural populations the lack of geographic access to services is often compounded by their lack of culturally appropriate care (Crooks & Andrews 2009). Shortages of health professionals are also a significant problem. Nurse shortages worldwide have compromised access to care for many people (Falk-Rafael 2006; WHO 2009), but this is more acute in rural settings.

Researchers describe a situation of 'distance decay' whereby there is lower service use with increased distance from the central health service (Wong & Regan 2009:2). This is exacerbated by the urban drift where families are moving to cities to seek employment, which causes declining quality of life for the remaining rural residents (Allan et al 2007). To date, services have been inadequate for rural people's needs, especially those with chronic conditions related to ageing (Allan et al 2007; Wong & Regan 2009). Instead rural services have been reactive, time limited, poorly coordinated and focused on either service providers or diseases, rather than being based on understanding

the rural context and culture, or the specific needs or assets of the community (Allan et al 2007). An alternative approach would see community capacity development; promoting health literacy to engage rural people in decisions about their treatment in the expectation of improving their quality of life and health outcomes (Allan et al 2007; Wong & Regan 2009).

Wong and Regan's research (2009) found that residents preferred staying in their community, content to trade off the specialist care they could access in cities. Participants in their study were more concerned about taking time off work, lost productivity and the cost and inconvenience of travel. This resonates with many rural residents who value the continuity and coherent management of their condition in their local community (Wong & Regan 2009).

Point to ponder

Geographic remoteness can present challenging issues for nurses working in rural and remote areas. Stress, isolation, longer working and on-call hours, and a lack of collegial support are among some of the concerns.

Caring for people in their rural and remote communities can also be enhanced by telehealth systems that improve connectedness and pave the way for diagnostic capabilities through telemedicine (Greenhill et al 2009). An added advantage of telehealth is the use of electronic health information systems by members of the community, which can be empowering for self-management of chronic disease as well as offering better system linkages (Wakerman 2009). Declining local services can also be mediated by appropriate transportation, social networks and the informal care of families, but these are not always freely available. Rural and remote area nurses and midwives understand this, and most work to support rural families within the context of country culture and its constraints. However, few non-rural nurses and midwives understand the complexity of working with rural and remote communities or the stress it can generate (Greenhill et al 2009; MacLeod et al 2004).

Geographically dispersed nurses report higher levels of work stress, few opportunities for replacement leave, longer working and on-call hours than nurses in urban areas, and a lack of support for new staff (Henwood et al 2009). Another difficulty is related to living in a community that may not be able to accommodate nurses and midwives who have family responsibilities. In many rural areas, school holiday programs are unavailable, making child care more difficult than in urban areas (Nankervis et al 2008). For remote area nurses (RANs) stress is a major issue because of the isolation and responsibilities, and the fact that they are too frequently subjected to violence in the community and workplace (Lenthall et al 2009). In addition, they spend a disproportionate amount of time on management tasks compared with their urban counterparts (Burley & Greene 2007; Hegney et al 1999). Another source of stress is that they are often the only way of providing a stable workforce given the disruption of medical practitioners rotating through the areas, and the unevenness and skill level of other health professionals (Searle 2007).

The advantages of rural and remote area nursing include feeling closely connected with the community on a social as well as professional level. Many nurses and midwives find this both personally and professionally rewarding, especially as community engagement is integral to the goals of PHC.

Point to ponder

Because of their close connection with the communities in which they live and work, rural and remote area nurses are in an ideal position to engage with communities, as they work towards achieving health equity.

In rural and remote settings, most nurses become 'boundary crossers' (Kilpatrick et al 2009:285), adept at fitting in to the community on multiple levels. As a member of a community of place, nurses and midwives can facilitate horizontal ties between people, groups and organisations such as hospital or district boards, community clinics and medical practices. Their relationships can be interdisciplinary, multi-institutional or intersectoral. As community residents as well as health professionals, they can also provide vertical ties between hospital and health departments and the wider society, to connect people with external resources and centres of power (Kilpatrick et al 2009). This tends to attract greater local public awareness of the potential of their role compared with public perceptions of nursing in non-rural communities.

Contemporary rural and remote nursing have four major areas of concern: maintaining excellence in practice, carrying major responsibilities, addressing the social determinants of health, and fitting in to the community (MacLeod et al 2004). Maintaining practice excellence often includes being prepared as a nurse practitioner, to provide the requisite skills to work as a sole practitioner having to deal with medical emergencies or families in crisis, mental health issues, first-aid and trauma management, palliative care and counselling, as well as health promotion and preventative activities (Burley & Greene 2007; Caffrey 2005). Rural and remote practitioners also have greater role diffusion than nurses working with non-rural populations, where the boundary between personal and professional life is porous (McCoy 2009). Some describe their lives as 'living their work', where maintaining relationships with colleagues outside of work has an effect on the work dynamic as well as social relationships (Mills et al 2010:33). This type of role diffusion has both negative and positive effects in that it can be difficult for the nurse or midwife to maintain anonymity in the community, which can lead to role strain. On the other hand, their closeness to the community may also make them more effective because of the level of trust they have established (McCoy 2009).

One of the major deterrents to rural and remote nursing is the lack of opportunities for continuing education and research, particularly in communities where electronic media are not functioning (McCoy 2009). It is difficult to feel that you have made a difference in the community, and can articulate that contribution if there are no evaluative data to demonstrate quality or effectiveness (Burley & Greene 2007). Rural researchers are attempting to address this with research into nurse-led models of remote area care (Burley & Greene 2007).

Point to ponder

Although research into rural nursing practice is increasing, this must continue if nurses are to demonstrate that nurse models of care in rural and remote settings improve health outcomes.

Their findings suggest that the role is influenced by contextual factors, including those related to the system (politics, policies and priorities), the organisation (planning, local alliances, models of care, policies and procedures), the community (service access, cohesiveness, socio-economic status, transport and environment) and characteristics of both the population and the health professional are core drivers of quality care (Burley & Greene 2007). In Australia, rural nurses work at many different levels, in multifaceted and diverse roles (Mills et al 2010). Some practise at advanced levels, combining education, research, management and consultancy (Mills et al 2010). Rural NPs are among those who conduct advanced-level, generalist practice, meeting the needs of a wide range of population groups in their community (Mills et al 2010).

Rural health care in New Zealand has traditionally been provided by a mix of GPs and PNs, district nurses and public health nurses. Although much rural health care is still provided in this way, a growing shortage of GPs and an increasing awareness of the positive impact of nursing has seen an increasing trend towards developing nursing models of care (New Zealand Institute of Rural Health 2008). These models include rural NPs, 'by Maori for Maori' nursing initiatives providing care to rural Maori populations, nurse-led clinics and nurse-led hospitals. Work is currently underway in New Zealand to develop a rural nursing workforce strategy. The strategy is aimed at enhancing rural nurses' abilities to contribute to population health in a variety of areas, which also requires an increase in the number of rural NPs (Kai Tiaki Nursing New Zealand 2009; New Zealand Institute of Rural Health 2008).

New Zealand rural NPs describe their role as including advanced health assessments, diagnostic reasoning, pharmacology for specialised prescribing and preparation for medical emergencies, which includes special primary response in medical emergencies (PRIME) training (O'Connor 2009a). All work within collaborative models of care, most having a set of standing orders for medications and diagnostic testing although some have achieved prescribing rights. Maloney-Moni (2006) describes the work she does as an NP with a rural Maori population using a kaupapa Maori model (Maori-centred model), demonstrating improving health outcomes for the families/whānau she is working alongside. Maloney-Moni's research and research by Litchfield (2004) have demonstrated how a rural nurse-led clinic has improved access to health care for those from lower socio-economic groups and Maori, by creating nurse–community

partnerships. It is vital that rural nurses in New Zealand extend this type of research to demonstrate that these nurse-led models are clearly linked to improvements in the health of the people with whom they are working. Like nurses and midwives in other countries, issues facing rural practitioners in New Zealand include funding constraints, variable employment structures, an ageing workforce, recruitment and retention issues, access to educational opportunities, and lack of a clear career pathway (Litchfield & Ross 2000; New Zealand Institute of Rural Health 2008; Goodyear-Smith & Janes 2008). These issues require further research. Research is also needed to illustrate the impact of collaborative practice on health care and health outcomes, as we discuss in the section to follow.

PARAMEDIC PRACTICE IN THE COMMUNITY

Paramedics play an important role in the provision of primary care in Australia and New Zealand. However, there is the potential for paramedics to utilise a more comprehensive PHC approach to practice, and, in New Zealand a paramedic practitioner role is being considered as a way of expanding the practice of paramedics in PHC. Paramedic practitioners are those with advanced skills who are able to deliver holistic care and treatment within a variety of PHC settings (Cooper & Grant 2009). The paramedic practitioner is able to assess the environment, consider the determinants of health, and determine the availability of family support prior to decision-making. The vision for New Zealand is to see the paramedic practitioner able to assess, treat and either discharge or refer a person on to further care. A review of the literature on paramedic practitioners and emergency care practitioners showed the value of paramedic practitioners in providing efficient care, as patients seen by paramedic practitioners were transported to hospital 25% less than patients seen by ordinary paramedics (Cooper & Grant 2009).

Point to ponder

Paramedics will have an increasing role in the provision of primary health care in rural and urban settings as new models of collaboration develop between health care providers.

Working as team members, paramedic practitioners have also been found to improve interprofessional collegiality, patient satisfaction and cost-effectiveness of services (Cooper & Grant 2009; Dixon et al 2008). Nurses must be aware of changes in paramedic practice and develop opportunities to work collaboratively with paramedics and paramedic practitioners to provide effective PHC in the community.

In Australia, Victorian RANs work collaboratively with paramedics in a partnership with Rural Ambulance Victoria, which helps both professions share knowledge and skills with a view towards more efficient and sustainable services (Burley & Greene 2007). In Queensland, a similar model has been adopted, where research conducted by the Queensland Ambulance Service indicated the need for an expanded scope of practice for rural paramedics (Reeve et al 2009). They now have the opportunity to attend a university-based National Population Health Education for Clinicians course, which has proven to be successful in encouraging a PHC focus to their practice. As well as improving emergency management, this education has encouraged better interdisciplinary teamwork and collaboration with rural and remote nurses for community health promotion and chronic disease management (Reeve et al 2009). Collaborative models involving paramedics are also a growing trend in other countries. One unique rural model of care is the NP-paramedic-family physician model implemented in a Canadian island community (Martin-Misener et al 2009). The model was developed with input from health professionals as well as community members, to capitalise on existing strengths and services, and identify their priorities for new programs. Evaluation has shown high ratings of acceptability and satisfaction from both residents of the community and the health professionals, whose model of care was based on successful collaborative teamwork. The collaboration has improved accessibility to care for the previously under-served population as well as proving cost-effective (Martin-Misener et al 2009). Other models of collaborative practice are proliferating in the UK and the US. Emergency nurses are working with paramedics in the UK to provide home visits 7 days a week as part of a national Transforming Community Services program (Nursing Standard 2009). In addition to emergency care, paramedics often work with community mental health nurses as part of mental health emergency response teams. However, the role of the community mental health nurse is rapidly expanding, as we discuss in the section to follow.

COMMUNITY MENTAL HEALTH NURSING PRACTICE

The role of community mental health nurses revolves around promoting mental health. Mental health is a state of wellbeing in which an individual realises his or her own abilities, can cope with the normal stresses of life, work productively and fruitfully, and is able to make a contribution to the community (Herman et al 2005). For community mental health nurses the health promotion role is particularly challenging, given that most policies and programs for mental health are focused on mental health services for those with a mental illness, rather than preventing mental ill health (Raphael 2009).

Point to ponder
Community mental health nursing is one of the most highly demanding types of community practice.

This is problematic, given that the research evidence indicates that the sources of mental health are embedded in the socially determined conditions within which people develop personal control over their lives, or where they are trying to cope with the effects of social deprivation, stress, degradation or experiences of stigma (Raphael 2009).

Community mental health nursing is one of the most highly demanding types of community practice. It requires a collaborative systems approach to ensure coordination and continuity of care (Proctor 2006). The trend towards deinstitutionalisation of those with a mental illness, population ageing and the complexity of client needs have created inordinate demands for community mental health nurses (CMHN) (Elsom et al 2009; Thompson et al 2008). The challenges of this specialised area of practice include work intensification caused by mental health nursing and psychiatrist shortages, increasing levels of unstable clients in the community for long periods of time prior to admission to psychiatric facilities, a large burden of administrative responsibilities, legal considerations in all cases they deal with and changing models of service provision (Henderson et al 2008). The emotional demands of the role creates inordinate stress, particularly where there is constant change in the models of care provided (Rose & Glass 2006). One challenge has been the shift to coordinating care for those with mental illnesses in general practice, rather than in specialist teams, which was the model used in the past. For the CMHN this often creates a blurring of roles and adds additional layers of administration and documentation on top of a heavy case load, as referrals are organised, liaison systems put in place, and competing ideologies are dealt with (Crawford et al 2007; Henderson et al 2008; Nolan et al 2004). The multidimensional role of CMHNs is constantly evolving with changes in health policies and personnel and the need to maintain multiple relationships and referral networks that often cross service boundaries, regulatory authorities and cultures, especially in Indigenous communities (Crawford et al 2007; Wilson & Crowe 2008).Together these factors create substantial work stress, yet the role attracts infrequent recognition (Burnard et al 2000; Crawford et al 2007; Funakoshi et al 2007; Henderson et al 2008).

Internationally, CMHNs have responded to the breadth of practice required in a PHC, social model of health, even though in the UK, they do not have legislative influence. This means that they practise under the power vested in medical officers and social workers (Hurley & Linsley 2007).

Point to ponder
Although community mental health nurses are challenged by the complexity of changing work environments, in many countries they are responding by embracing the principles of primary health care in their practice, and refocusing their goals on health and social equity.

In Australia and New Zealand, CMHNs have recognition in the respective acts, and are registered to act as responsible clinicians within their scope of practice (Hurley & Linsley 2007). In rural areas CMHNs are often the only mental health professional, and therefore they must act as a resource to others as well as carrying a case load that they cannot defer to someone without mental health skills (Henderson et al 2008). In both rural and urban areas their practice often involves home visits, in which the major role lies in monitoring changes and preventing

hospital admissions (Thompson et al 2008). Home care by CMHNs includes developing programs for rehabilitation and medication management, assisting people with parenting, personal relationships, adjustment reactions and activities of daily living, as well as supporting caregivers, especially those dealing with psychogeriatric conditions and their behavioural outcomes (Funakoshi et al 2007; Gaul & Farkas 2007; Moniz-Cook et al 2008; Thompson et al 2008).

Point to ponder
Many CMHNs are advanced practice nurses. Their practice involves medication management, ordering diagnostic tests, referrals, and recommendations for treatment.

Henderson et al (2008) report that nearly two-thirds of community mental health practice involves medication management. A study of their roles in 2009 indicated that the practice of as many as 70% of Australian CMHNs is focused on recommending new medications, changes to medications or adjustments in dosages (Elsom et al 2009). In the UK, a similar study found that 89% of CMHNs undertook this type of role (Nolan et al 2001). This level of responsibility for medication advice reflects an expanded role, and requires CMHNs to have extensive knowledge of psychotropic medications, which is often a fuller understanding of the indications, contraindications, interactions and side effects than the GPs who are coordinating their patients' care (Elsom et al 2009).

The CMHNs' level of clinical decision-making is clearly beyond the scope of practice of many other nurses working in the community. In addition to medication management it includes ordering diagnostic tests, referrals to specialists, recommendations for involuntary treatment and authorisation of sick certificates (Elsom et al 2009). Because of workforce shortages, suggestions have been made that support workers in mental health should be used to provide greater access to care for those with mental illnesses. However, this type of role requires a clear skill set and role demarcation for both the support workers and the CMHNs (McCrae et al 2008).

One of the major roles played by CMHNs involves work with those identified as having intellectual disabilities. In the UK a review of the practice of specialised 'community nurses for people with learning disabilities' (CNPLD) shows that their role is becoming more like CMHNs (Barr 2006). The role is expanding in response to the UK policy to promote social inclusion and health facilitation for those with intellectual disabilities. As a result, nurses are engaging more in health screening, monitoring, and coordinating care in the home and community, effectively addressing primary, secondary and tertiary care (Barr 2006). This inclusive approach is congruent with the PHC goal of empowerment, which is extremely important for those with intellectual disabilities, given the stigma and vulnerabilities they experience (Gaul & Farkas 2007). Caring for those with intellectual disabilities remains an under-developed aspect of the mental health nursing role, especially in Australia and New Zealand where the psychiatric model of care has continued to dominate treatment approaches (Taua & Farrow 2009). However, this is changing, with recent legislative steps to promote the rights of people with disabilities and their carers and the trend towards community-based treatment (Jorgensen et al 2009; Slevin & Sines 2005). This has led to a greater focus on social inclusion by addressing issues of poverty, communication skills, access to leisure opportunities, family relationships and education, all of which could help minimise the impact of vulnerability factors for those with intellectual disabilities (Devine & Taggart 2008). What remains is to ensure the new service initiatives and models of practice are informed by a body of nursing research evidence to guide future developments (Griffiths et al 2009).

Since implementation of the Primary Health Care Strategy (MOHNZ 2001) in New Zealand, ongoing work has focused on the needs of people with mild to moderate mental health issues in community settings. While it is recognised that most people with mild to moderate mental health issues can be effectively cared for in PHC settings, this care has frequently been dependent on their health provider's interest and expertise in the area of mental health (MOHNZ 2002). Funding to establish primary mental health initiatives across New Zealand has seen the development of a variety of models of care designed to meet the needs of these groups, including a model of shared care between GPs and mental health nurses. However, the business model of general practice is seen to be inadequate in allocating sufficient time to those with mental health needs (O'Brien et al 2006). With the inception of primary mental health coordinators (often

CMHNs) who have been appointed in many communities across New Zealand, a more collaborative approach has been achieved with greater potential for the future (O'Brien et al 2006). These specialised nurses provide needs assessment and service coordination for service users, mentoring of general practice staff, stronger links between primary and secondary services, advocacy for service users, case management and counselling services, and advice to general practice staff on referral options (Dowell et al 2009). Evaluation indicates that up to 80% of service users benefited from the variety of interventions offered in PHC settings (Dowell et al 2009).

> **Point to ponder**
> Specific funding has been allocated in New Zealand to develop primary mental health care initiatives. Primary mental health coordinators who are often CMHNs have been appointed in many New Zealand communities.

OCCUPATIONAL HEALTH NURSING

Occupational health nursing extends the goals of PHC to the workplace. It is a specialist area of community or public health nursing, where nurses provide workplace education, health promotion, clinical services, case management and other industry-specific innovations to keep the workplace and its workers safe and healthy (Guzik et al 2009; Marinescu 2007). Occupational health nurses (OHNs) practise in partnership with workers, worker groups and employers to plan health care that is accessible, empowering, and part of a comprehensive and continuing health conservation process. The uniqueness of OHN is manifest through a bilateral advocacy role, where the interests of both employee and employer are a priority in health planning. This is occasionally daunting, as it requires diplomacy, high-level communication skills, understanding of interpersonal and industrial relations, and familiarity with professional and government standards and legislation. Other factors influencing OHN practice include knowledge of environmental issues, the context and expectations of the employing organisation, employer and union philosophy and policies, budgetary restraints, and the nurse's scope of practice, professional supports and educational opportunities.

Contemporary trends in workplace health also have an impact of the OHN role. Population ageing and the global financial crisis of 2009 has seen more older persons continuing to work longer, and many of these older workers also suffer from chronic conditions. Changes to family life have created an increase in the number of women in the workplace. With increases in global migration, today's workplaces also have high proportions of workers from minority groups, and they are often in lower level jobs that require sensitivity to language and cultural issues (Marinescu 2007).

OHN practice has changed considerably since the 'industrial nurse' role was developed as a subset of the public health role early in the 20th century (Schwem 2009). At that time, where industries were localised to small communities, the objective of occupational health was often to ensure containment of illness in the workplace to prevent any infections spreading from there to the community (Schwem 2009). Since mid last century, rapid industrial expansion and globalisation with its multinational, highly competitive corporations, have created occupational health environments that are more systematic and focused on cost-containment, worker productivity and return on investments (Marinescu 2007). This has meant that the OHN role has shifted from a medical agenda for onsite diagnosis and treatment, to one where they must make a rational business case for health promotion programs on the basis of increased efficiency and evidence-based change management strategies (Marinescu 2007). To meet these obligations the nurse often combines the role of health professional with that of a business partner, which requires high-level management skills as well as advanced clinical knowledge (Marinescu 2007).

Managing health and productivity in many industries in the US is integrated within a health and productivity management (HPM) model (Marinescu 2007). This is a multidimensional approach to develop employee-centred occupational safety programs and activities aimed at improving workers' morale, reducing turnover, managing absences, and improving performance, productivity and work satisfaction (Marinescu 2007; Wallace 2009; Zinner 2006). The role is congruent with PHC in being focused on population health and the social determinants of health. Health planning is based on the premise that the worker requires not only a healthy workplace but a healthy community, family and society (Marinescu

2007). Numerous best-practice examples illustrate the state of the art in OHN, which include a number of trends as outlined in Box 4.2.

Point to ponder

Occupational health nurses provide workplace education, health promotion, clinical services, case management and other industry-specific innovations to keep the workplace and its workers safe and healthy.

Although safety remains a significant part of many OHN roles, often there is a safety officer employed in the workplace to provide first aid and develop injury surveillance and prevention programs. However, OHNs in many workplaces also undertake these roles, and must have sufficient

BOX 4.2 TRENDS IN OCCUPATIONAL HEALTH NURSING

Current practice	rather than	Historical practice
Evidence-based practice		tradition
Worker performance		absenteeism
Economic outcomes		health care costs
Employee prevention		treatment
Population		individual focus
Health focus		disease or illness
Multiple risk factors		single factors
Employee-centred interventions		program-centred
Creating a culture of workplace health and safety across the organisation		enforcements
Focus on communication, management, leadership skills		worker v management

(Marinescu 2007)

environmental knowledge to participate in primary, secondary and tertiary prevention (Rogers et al 2007). Primary prevention includes screening, surveillance and coordination of the role of team members in planning workplace health and safety and preventing illness or injury. This requires assessment skills and extensive knowledge of the workplace itself and its particular hazards. Ergonomic knowledge is helpful in this type of assessment, to understand the fit between the worker and their interface with the work environment. Ergonomic risks can include boredom, glare, repetitive motion, poor workstation–worker fit, lifting heavy loads or tasks that require the worker to assume an abnormal position. Physical hazards can include such things as extremes of temperature, noise, radiation or poor lighting. Biological hazards include exposures to chemical or various biological agents. Psychosocial hazards are those that produce inordinate stress, such as shiftwork, or negative interpersonal relationships on the job.

> **Point to ponder**
> Occupational health nurses are skilled in assessing the interface between the worker and their work environment; in particular, ergonomic assessment.

Stress is a major workplace hazard, particularly with company reorganisation and downsizing, often affecting management staff as well as those whose jobs are under threat (Wallace 2009). The OHN can help monitor worker stress, providing education, counselling, worksite stress reduction programs or referrals to specialist services (Olszewski et al 2007; Wallace 2009). Another aspect of primary prevention is ensuring sufficient information for planning and implementation of workplace initiatives. For example, a hazard survey may be conducted as part of the OHNs primary prevention activities. Where such a survey exists, it is usually up to the OHN to make it readily accessible to all members of the workforce. Most companies also have a disaster plan, which may have been developed with input from the OHN, who then takes a leading role in disseminating it to the workforce and assuming responsibility for intermittent updates. Disaster planning requires close collaboration with emergency services, other health professionals, and workplace health and safety personnel (Lobaton Cabrera & Beaton 2009).

> **Point to ponder**
> Occupational health nurses are integrally involved with primary, secondary and tertiary intervention planning to achieve optimal health outcomes for workers.

Secondary prevention requires knowledge of the workforce and any pre-existing conditions that may place their health or wellbeing in jeopardy. This information is often garnered during the pre-employment health examination and updated during periodic health assessments. To respond to any injuries or illness episodes in the workplace the OHN typically needs to be skilled in primary care such as first-aid procedures, crisis intervention and trauma management. Workplace violence is increasing in many places, including threats, physical or emotional abuse, stalking or sexual harassment (Olszewski et al 2007). The risk of violent incidents, and high levels of workplace stress creates the need for nurses to maintain counselling skills and an extensive referral network. The OHN may adopt a case management model, where (s)he works with employees with a chronic illness or disability to help them manage their condition and prevent acute episodes in the workplace (Aziz 2009). In this role the OHN is the care coordinator, providing the collaborative link between the employee, their GP, PN, specialists, social worker, physiotherapist or other health professional (Aziz 2009).

In many cases OHNs also become involved in helping workers with retirement planning (Zinner 2006). Today's workforce is comprised of an unprecedented number of workers who are planning on working well into their 60s, and many require modifications to the work environment. The OHN is often the main advocate for older workers, especially where the workplace has rigid shifts and common work styles and conditions (Zinner 2006). Older workers can make an important contribution to the workplace if their working life is flexible, and their needs for various ergonomic modifications are accommodated. Some require changes because of reduced eyesight or impairments from various illnesses (Wallace 2009). The OHN can help facilitate a smooth transition to flexible work for older persons by encouraging policies and practices amenable to their needs, helping the workers themselves develop a realistic concept of their future health, encouraging self-discovery of what they value, and helping them evaluate needs in their living environment as well as the workplace (Zinner 2006).

Tertiary prevention is aimed at minimising any compromises to health, or helping restore workers' health following any injury or illness. Included are strategies to help people in their transitions back to work after a workplace incident, or counselling to help people resolve any issues surrounding job restructuring or retraining. Recovery and rehabilitation following illness or injury often requires ongoing liaison with the worker's family physician and may also involve family members, depending on the circumstances. Many OHNs maintain a range of health intervention programs to engage workers while they are recovering from an illness episode or injury. These include employee assistance for those with substance abuse problems, corporate smoking cessation, and workplace health and fitness programs. Parallel with these in-house programs the OHN usually maintains a database of agencies that can help workers offsite. The information network required for all of these activities is extensive, and a major part of the OHN role. This extends to maintaining in-depth knowledge of government, health and safety agency, industry- and workplace-specific policies and procedures that have been developed to protect the workers and the workplace (Rogers et al 2007).

In countries such as Australia, Canada and the US, where OHN is highly developed, evidence-based practice is an expectation of the role. In some cases, this is linked to the extra education required for OHN practice. In some settings NPs undertake the occupational health role, and they have attracted high satisfaction ratings by workers (Guzik et al 2009). Studies conducted in Australia indicate that a variety of professionals and para-professionals such as physiotherapists and occupational therapists also undertake an occupational health and safety role (Mellor & St John 2009). Like their North American counterparts the role of Australian OHNs has shifted towards health promotion and injury prevention, which has been welcomed by OHN managers (Mellor & St John 2009). The areas where further development needs to take place is in advancing the knowledge base for practice through further research (Mellor & St John 2009).

The WHO Healthy Workplace movement that began in the 1980s has attracted an extensive network of healthy workplace initiatives (Online. Available: www.search.who.int/search?ie=utf8&; site=default_collection&client=WHO&proxysty [accessed 18 August 2009]). However, few have been established or managed by nurses working as OHNs. With few exceptions, many of these programs have also been developed on the basis of physical, psychological and behavioural life-style-related outcomes rather than organisational capacity building (Whitehead 2006b). A lack of evaluation studies has also delayed development of models to guide practice. Addressing this deficit in the research agenda requires a transformational approach that would see the research agenda move from the 'healthy lifestyle in the workplace' tradition to a more contextualised, participative model of developing capacity for sustainable workplace health. Whitehead (2006b) suggests that this would be better achieved using an organisational change action research cycle, where collaborative research into existing and potential workplace problems, structures and processes is intended to inform future developments for change.

COLLABORATIVE MODELS OF NURSING AND MIDWIFERY IN THE COMMUNITY

As we outlined under the different specialist roles above, the models of care within which Australian and New Zealand PHC nurses practise vary according to national, regional or state programs, the practice context and the degree of remoteness from services. Some are considered 'generalist specialists' who provide 'womb to tomb' primary, secondary and tertiary level care, as well as trauma and first line management (Mills et al 2009). However, the roles of nurses specialising in child health, school health, occupational health, practice nursing and a plethora of other roles are specialist roles, and typically designated as such.

Point to ponder
The growing demands on nurses working in community settings increases the imperative to develop collaborative models of nursing and midwifery care.

The dual challenges many face in being specialised as well as remote can include the pressure of enormous workloads. Because of the burden of care, some nurses have suggested facilitating a practice role where the second level nurse (enrolled nurse) undertakes advanced education for an enhanced scope of practice to ensure that community needs can be met (Nankervis et al 2008). Another alternative has been to organise care planning and coordination around a shared care model, where co-location of services can help improve the efficiency of services. Models of shared care have been shown to improve resource use in rural areas as long as the coordination of care is central to activities.

With the growing acceptance of PHC world-wide, numerous collaborative models of care have evolved. In the US a movement called 'consumer-driven health care' has spawned a rapidly growing industry of convenient care by NPs working with allied health professionals such as pharmacists and physiotherapists to offer accessible, quality care in shopping centres and retail outlets at lower cost than medical care (Miller 2009). These nurses work from standardised protocols sanctioned by a collaborating physician. This idea, which has forged new ground in the US, has also been adopted by Australian NPs who have established 'revive clinics' in shopping centres offering treatments and health promotion services 7 days a week (Online. Available: www.reviveclinic.com.au/ [accessed 17 August 2009]). In Western Australia the Revive Clinics and the Pharmacy Alliance Group have collaborated on planning one-stop-shop pharmacies that will employ NPs to assess and treat minor infections, colds and flu. These have been criticised by the Australian Medical Association as 'supermarket medicine', staffed by people (NPs) who do not understand holistic care (Online. Available: www.au.news.yahoo.com/thewest/a/-/national/5813445/nurse-clinics-are-supermarket [accessed 28 August 2009]). NPs working closely with the pharmacists on this expansion of services have been supported by the Health Ministry, which is working towards population health rather than medically dominated service provision.

Midwifery practice includes the 'shared care' model, in which midwives and medical practitioners (GPs and obstetricians) have a shared protocol for professional support for childbirth (Lombardo & Golding 2003; The North Staffordshire Changing Childbirth Research Team 2000). Another collaborative model is group antenatal care, where women attend antenatal care to build friendships and support networks as well as having access to expert midwives as facilitators (Teate et al 2009). The advantages of shared care include greater

continuity of care by at least one member of the shared care team, and a healthy evidence-based dialogue between health professionals to ensure access and equity to safe, high-quality care (Bai et al 2009). Another version of shared care is team midwifery, where a number of midwives share care for a designated number of women. This is in contrast to a case management model, where one midwife provides continuity of care by providing the care throughout pregnancy, birth and follow-up (The North Staffordshire Changing Childbirth Research Team 2000). New Zealand has this type of model called the Lead Maternity Carer (LMC) where the mother chooses the midwife, GP or obstetrician to lead her pregnancy care (Online. Available: www. kiwifamilies.co.nz/Topics/Pregnancy/Choosing+ an+LMC.html [accessed 19 August 2009]). The development of the LMC model has seen New Zealand midwives take on the majority of deliveries in that country. Consultation between midwives and the health sector has focused on improving the links between maternity care providers and those whose roles primarily focus on implementing the PHC strategy to improve population health and reduce inequalities (MOHNZ 2008).

> **Point to ponder**
> Midwives frequently use a shared care model to care for pregnant women. Shared care has been shown to improve use of scarce resources — particularly in remote areas.

The key to successful collaboration in a shared care model lies in having common aims and goals, clarity of communication and interaction with other team members, and shared decision-making (Teate et al 2009; Woodhouse 2009). The model of care needs to be tailored to the group's needs rather than based on historical funding decisions, role demarcations, or assessments of various population groups elsewhere (Allan et al 2007; Freeman et al 2004; Teate et al 2004). In midwifery care, the ideal model is an equal partnership between the mother and midwife or the team of midwives (Freeman et al 2004). It is underpinned by the philosophical standpoint that pregnancy and childbirth are normal events, and the midwife's role is to help the woman experience a normal pregnancy, labour, birth and postnatal period. Importantly, midwifery is always woman-centred and intended to provide the woman with continuity of caregiver throughout her childbearing experience (Freeman et al 2004). The role of the midwife in New Zealand is clearly entrenched within the PHC strategy. Midwives in Australia are working towards a greater PHC focus, and this has attracted support from the Commonwealth government which is advocating legislation to allow midwives to access the Medical Benefits Schedule (MBS) and the Pharmaceutical Benefits Scheme (PBS), and to be granted professional indemnity for their birthing practice.

Case study

Millie, Jim's mother, is diagnosed with diabetes mellitus and high blood pressure, much to the dismay of the rest of the family. However, her practice nurse, working through the PHO, enrols her in the 'Care Plus' program that has been running successfully throughout the district and the rest of New Zealand. Care Plus provides Millie with an individual care plan and access to increased nurse visits throughout the year as she learns to manage her conditions. One month into her management program her husband, Harold, was made redundant. Bored at home, Harold joined the local seniors' exercise program and met a friend who was involved with the local squash group. He decided to join, as in his younger years he was quite good at the game. However, he fractured his ankle in the second game. Fortunately, the Accident Compensation Corporation (ACC) covered Harold for the health care he required following his injury and paid for much of the physiotherapy he needed as he recovered.

Meanwhile in Australia, Jim and Maria are expecting a visit from Maria's cousin Massimo and his wife Anna, who live in Naples. They are bringing their three children (Rocco age 4, Julita age 8 and Giovanni age 11) over to Sydney for a month's holiday. Jim's job is going well, and he decided to get involved in the workplace health and safety committee. He is enjoying this and has some ideas for an employee health program that would include smoking cessation and nutrition counselling for those who wanted to take part. This idea came to him as Lily had brought a note home from school outlining a four-pronged program her school nurse was going to develop as part of healthy nutrition in the school.

Samantha's child care manager has contacted Maria to express her concern that Samantha may either be shy or slightly behind the other children developmentally. The behaviours causing her concern include Samantha tending to withdraw from any noisy play when all the children get together. She seems to prefer to sit on the side rather than join in and the child care manager is unsure as to whether she is just shy or might have a developmental problem.

REFLECTING ON THE BIG ISSUES

- Nurses and midwives undertake a variety of community roles with some common elements and some unique features.
- Many aspects of the roles of nurses and midwives are related to the practice setting and the regulatory environment that determines their scope of practice.
- Population ageing and increasing rates of chronic illnesses have a significant impact on the roles of many community nurses.
- Models of interdisciplinary collaboration can provide better health outcomes in communities.
- All nursing and midwifery specialties in the community suffer from a lack of research evidence that would advance the knowledge base and help provide role clarity.
- Nurses' professional activities could be enhanced by standardising titles and expectations, and developing evaluation studies of the impact of their practice.

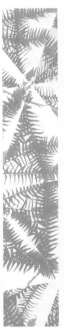

Reflective questions: how would I use this knowledge in practice?

1 What elements of PHC cut across the range of nursing, midwifery and paramedic practice areas?

2 As a practice nurse what would be your role in the Care Plus plan for managing Millie's diabetes?

3 What would be the implications of Millie and Harold living one and a half hours from the nearest hospital? Would this affect the way their care was coordinated?

4 What four major elements would Lily's school nurse be planning to include in her health nutrition plan for the school?

5 As the occupational health nurse how could you help Jim with his plan for smoking cessation and better nutrition in the workplace?

6 As the child health nurse, what would be your approach to assessing Samantha's behavioural issues at child care?

7 Draw an updated genogram of the Miller family that includes their visiting relatives.

Research-informed practice

Read the article by Allan, Ball and Alston (2007) 'Developing sustainable models of rural health care: a community development approach'.

These authors outline a community development approach to sustainable rural health services. Included in the article is the recommendation to conduct 'asset mapping' as a way of developing a systematic profile of the community.

• Explain how you would use this information to develop a 'think global, act local' community development plan.

• How would you encourage dissemination of this type of initiative?

• What research does this suggest for the future?

References

Allan J, Ball P, Alston M 2007 Developing sustainable models of rural health care: a community development approach. Rural and Remote Health 4(7):1–13

Armstrong F 2004 More than just bandaids: the emerging role of school nurses. Australian Nursing Journal 11(10):18–21

Association of State and Territorial Directors of Nursing (ASTDN) 2009 The public health nurse's role in achieving health equity: eliminating inequalities in health, Position Paper. ASTDN. Online. Available: www.astdn.org (accessed 10 August 2009)

Aston M, Meagher-Stewart D, Edwards N, Young L 2009 Public health nurses' primary health care practice: strategies for fostering citizen participation. Journal of Community Health Nursing 26:24–34

Australian General Practice Network (AGPN) 2007 National practice nurse workforce survey report. Australian General Practice Network, Canberra. Online. Available: www.generalpracticenursing.com.au/stie/content.cfm?page_id=32208&;current_category_code=4059 (accessed 16 August 2009)

Australian Nursing Federation (ANF) 2009 Primary Health Care in Australia. Primary Health Care Working Group. ISBN 978-0-909599-61-4. ANF, Canberra

Aziz B 2009 Making more of nurses. Occupational Health 61(5):22–3

Bai J, Gyaneshwar R, Bauman A 2009 Models of antenatal care and obstetric outcomes in Sydney South West. Australian and New Zealand Journal of Obstetrics and Gynaecology 48:454–61

Baid H, Bartlett C, Gilhooly S, Illingworth A, Winder S 2009 Advanced physical assessment: the role of the district nurse. Nursing Standard 23(35):41–6

Barnes M, Courtney M, Pratt J, Walsh A 2003 Contemporary child health nursing practice: Services provided and challenges faced in metropolitan and outer Brisbane areas. Collegian 10(4):14–19

—— 2004a School-based youth health nurses: roles, responsibilities, challenges, and rewards. Public Health Nursing 21(4):316–22

—— 2004b School based youth health nurses' role in assisting young people access health services in provincial, rural and remote areas of Queensland, Australia. Rural and Remote Health 4:279 Online. Available: www.rrh.deakin.edu.au/ (accessed 22 August 2009)

Barr O 2006 The evolving role of community nurses for people with learning disabilities: changes over an 11 year period. Journal of Clinical Nursing 15:72–82

Barry C, Gordon S, Lange B 2007 The usefulness of the community nursing practice model in grounding practice and research: narratives from the United States and Africa. Research and Theory for Nursing Practice: An International Journal 21(3):174–84

Benner P 1984 From Novice to Expert: Excellence and Power in Nursing Practice. Addison-Wesley, Menlo Park, California

Besner J 2004 Nurses' role in advancing primary health care: a call to action. Primary Health Care Research and Development 5:351–8

Bidmead C, Davis H, Day X 2002 Partnership working: What does it really mean? Community Practitioner 75(7): 256–9

Bonsall K, Cheater F 2007 What is the impact of advanced primary care nursing roles on patients, nurses and their colleagues? A literature review. International Journal of Nursing Studies 45:1090–02

Briggs C 2006–07 Nursing practice in community child health: developing the nurse–client relationship. Contemporary Nurse 23(2):303–11

Brooks F, Kendall S, Bunn F, Bindler R, Bruya M 2007a The school nurse as navigator of the school health journey: developing the theory and evidence for policy. Primary Health Care Research & Development 8:226–34

Brooks K, Davidson P, Daly J, Halcomb E 2007b Role theory: A framework to investigate the community nurse role in contemporary health care systems. Contemporary Nurse 25:146–55

Brooks K, Davidson P, Daly J, Hancock K 2004 Community health nursing in Australia: a critical literature review and implications for professional development. Contemporary Nurse 16(3):195–207

Buchan J, Calman L 2005 Skill-mix and policy changes in the health workforce: nurses in advanced roles. OECD Health Working Papers no. 17, Paris, OECD

Burley M, Greene P 2007 Core drivers of quality: a remote health example from Australia. Rural and Remote Health 7(611):1–12

Burnard P, Edwards D, Fothergill A, Hannigan B, Coyle D 2000 Community mental health nurses in Wales: self-reported stressors and coping strategies. Journal of Psychiatric and Mental Health Nursing 7:523–8

Bushy A 2000 Orientation to Nursing in the Rural Community. Sage, Thousand Oaks, Cal

Caffrey R 2005 The rural community care gerontologic nurse entrepreneur: role development strategies. Journal of Gerontological Nursing 31(10):11–16

Carolan M 2004–05 Maternal and child health nurses: a vital link to the community for primiparae over the age of 35. Contemporary Nurse 18(1–2):133–42

Catalano T, Kendall E, Vandenberg A, Hunter B 2009 The experiences of leaders of self-management courses in Queensland: exploring health professional and peer leaders' perceptions of working together. Health and Social Care in the Community 17(2):105–15

Chapman L, Smith A, Williams V, Oliver D 2009 Community matrons: primary care professionals' views and experiences. Journal of Advanced Nursing 65(8):1617–25

Chiarella M 2009 Australian Government National Health and Hospitals Reform Commission Discussion Paper. New and emerging nurse-led models of primary health care. UTS, Sydney

Child and Family Health Nurses Association (CAFHNA) 2000 Competency Standards for Child and Family Health Nurses (2nd edn). CAFHNA Standards & Practices subcommittee, NSW Inc., Sydney

Clendon J 2004–05 Demonstrating outcomes in a nurse-led clinic: how primary health care nurses make a difference to children and their families. Contemporary Nurse 18(1/2):164–76

—— 2009 Motherhood and the Plunket book: a social history. Unpublished doctoral thesis. New Zealand, Massey University, Wellington

College of Nurses Aotearoa 2010 Nurse Practitioners New Zealand. Online. Available: www.nurse.org.nz/nurse_practitioner/np_contact.htm (accessed 23 February 2010)

Comino E, Harris E 2003 Maternal and infant services: examination of access in a culturally diverse community. Journal of Paediatric Child Health 39:95–9

Commonwealth of Australia 2009 Capabilities for Supporting Prevention and Chronic Condition Self-management. DOHA and Flinders University, Canberra

Cooper S, Grant J 2009 New and emerging roles in out of hospital emergency care: a review of the international literature. International Emergency Nursing 17:90–8

Crawford P, Brown B, Majomi P 2007 Professional identity in community mental health nursing: a thematic analysis. International Journal of Nursing Studies 45:1055–63

Crooks V, Andrews G 2009 Community, equity, access: core geographic concepts in primary health care. Primary Health Care Research & Development 10:270–3

Currie L, Watterson L 2009 Investigating the role and impact of expert nurses. British Journal of Nursing 18(13):816–24

Daly W, Carnwell R 2003 Nursing roles and levels of practice: a framework for differentiating between elementary, specialist and advanced nursing practice. Journal of Clinical Nursing 12:158–67

DeBell D 2006 School nurse practice: a decade of change. Community Practitioner 79(10):324–7

Devine M, Taggart L 2008 Addressing the mental health needs of people with learning disabilities. Nursing Standard 22(45):40–9

DiCenso A, Auffrey L, Bryant-Lukosius D, Donald F, Martin-Misener R, Matthews S, Opsteen J 2007 Primary health care nurse practitioners in Canada. Contemporary Nurse 26(1):104–15

Dixon S, Mason S, Knowles E, Colwell B, Wardrope J, Snooks H, Gorringe R, Perrin J, Nicholl J 2008 Is it cost effective to introduce paramedic practitioners for older people to the ambulance service? Results of a cluster randomized controlled trial. Emergency Medicine Journal 26:446–51

Dowell A, Garrett S, Collings S, McBain L, McKinlay E, Stanley J 2009 Evaluation of the primary mental health initiatives: summary report 2008 University of Otago and Ministry of Health New Zealand, Wellington

Downes C, Pemberton J 2009 Developing a community matron service: a neighbourhood model. Nursing Standard 23(44):35–8

Downie J, Chapman R, Orb A, Juliff D 2002 The everyday realities of the multi-dimensional role of the high school community nurse. Australian Journal of Advanced Nursing 19(3):15–24

Duffield C, Gardner G, Chang A, Catling-Paull C 2009 Advanced nursing practice: a global perspective. Collegian 16:55–62

Edwards N, MacDonald J 2009 Building nurses' capacity in community health services. International Journal of Nursing Education Scholarship 6(1):1–18

Edwards N, MacLean Davison C 2008 Social justice and core competencies for public health. Canadian Journal of Public Health 99(2):130–2

Elsom S, Happell B, Manias E 2009 Informal role expansion in Australian mental health nursing. Perspectives in Psychiatric care 45(1):45–53

Expert Advisory Group on Primary Health Care Nursing 2003 Investing in health: Whakatohutia te Oranga Tangata A Framework for activating primary health care nursing in New Zealand. Ministry of Health New Zealand, Wellington

Falk-Rafael A 2006 Globalization and global health. Advances in Nursing Science 29(1):2–14

Finlayson M, Sheridan N, Cumming J 2009 Nursing developments in primary health care 2001–2007. Wellington, Victoria University of Wellington. Online. Available: www.vuw.ac.nz (accessed 10 August 2009)

Fisher Robertson J, Brandt Baldwin K 2007 Advanced practice role characteristics of the community/public health nurse specialist. Clinical Nurse Specialist 21(5):250–4

Forbes A, While A 2008 The nursing contribution to chronic disease management: a discussion paper. International Journal of Nursing Studies 46:120–31

Forbes A, While A, Ullman R, Murgatroyd B 2007 The contribution of nurses to child health and child health services: findings of a scoping exercise. Journal of Child Health Care 11(3):231–47

Freeman L, Timperley H, Adair V 2004 Partnership in midwifery care in New Zealand. Midwifery 20:2–14

Funakoshi A, Miyamoto Y, Kayama M 2007 Managerial support of community mental health nurses. Journal of Advanced Nursing 58(3):227–35

Gardner A, Hase S, Gardner G, Dunn S, Carryer J 2007 From competence to capability: a study of nurse practitioners in clinical practice. Journal of Clinical Nursing 17:250–8

Gardner G, Carryer J, Dunn S, Gardner G 2004 Nurse practitioner standards project. ANMC, Canberra

Gaul C, Farkas C 2007 Perspectives on psychiatric consultation liaison nursing. Public health and mental health: a model for success. Perspectives in Psychiatric Care 43(4):227–30

Goodyear-Smith F, Janes R 2008 New Zealand rural primary health care workforce in 2005: more than just a doctor shortage. Australian Journal of Rural Health 16:40–6

Green J, Lo Bianco J, Wyn J 2007 Discourses in interaction: the intersection of literacy and health research internationally. Literacy and Numeracy Studies 15:19–27

Green R, Reffel J 2009 Comparison of administrators' and school nurses' perceptions of the school nurse role. Journal of School Nursing 25(1):62–71

Greenhill J, Mildenhall D, Rosenthal D 2009 Ten ideas for building a strong Australian rural health system. Rural and Remote Health 9(1206):1–7

Griffiths P, Bennett J, Smith E 2009 The size, extent and nature of the learning disability nursing research base: a systematic scoping review. International Journal of Nursing Studies 46:490–507

Guzik A, Nivison Menzel N, Fitzpatrick J, McNulty R 2009 Patient satisfaction with nurse practitioner and physician services in the occupational health setting. American Association of Occupational Health Nurses Journal 57(5):191–7

Halcomb E, Davidson P, Daly J, Griffiths R, Yallop J, Tofler G 2005 Nursing in Australian general practice: directions and perspectives. Australian Health Review 29(2):156–66

Halcomb E, Hickman L 2010 Development of a clinician-led research agenda for general practice nurses. Australian Journal of Advanced Nursing 27(3):4–11

Harrison S, Lydon J 2008 Health visiting and community matrons: progress in partnership. Community Practitioner 81(2):20–2

Hayes L 2005 Public health and nurses … what is your role? Primary Health Care 15(5):22–5

Hegney D, McCarthy A, Pearson A 1999 Effects of size of health service on scope of rural nursing practice. Collegian 6:21–42

Henderson J, Willis E, Walter B, Toffoli L 2008 Community mental health nursing: keeping pace with care delivery? International Journal of Mental Health Nursing 17:162–70

Henwood T, Eley R, Parker D, Tuckett A, Hegney D 2009 Regional differences among employed nurses: a Queensland study. Australian Journal of Rural Health 17:201–7

Herman H, Sazena S, Moodie R (eds) 2005 Promoting Mental Health. WHO, Geneva

Hurley J, Linsley P 2007 Expanding roles within mental health legislation: an opportunity for professional growth or a missed opportunity? Journal of Psychiatric and Mental Health Nursing 14:535–41

Jorgensen D, Parsons M, Gundersen Reid M, Weidenbohm K, Parsons J, Jacobs S 2009 The providers' profile of the disability support workforce in New Zealand. Health and Social Care in the Community 17(4):396–405

Journal of School Nursing 2008 The American Academy of Pediatrics Policy Statement. The role of the school nurse in providing school health services. Journal of School Nursing 24(5):269–74

Kai Tiaki Nursing New Zealand 2009 Developing a rural nursing workforce strategy. Kai Tiaki Nursing New Zealand (15)3:8

Keleher H, Joyce C, Parker R, Piterman L 2007 Practice nurses in Australia: current issues and future directions. Medical Journal of Australia 187(2):108–66

Kilpatrick S, Cheers B, Gilles M, Taylor J 2009 Boundary crossers, communities, and health: exploring the role of rural health professionals. Health & Place 15:284–90

Kool B, Thomas D, Moore D, Anderson A, Bennetts P, Earp K, Dawson D, Treadwell N 2008 Innovation and effectiveness: changing the scope of school nurses in New Zealand secondary schools. Australian and New Zealand Journal of Public Health 32(2): 177–80

Kotter J 1995 Leading change: why transformation efforts fail. Harvard Business Review 73(2):59–67

Krothe J, Clendon J 2006 Perceptions of nurse-managed clinics: a cross-cultural study. Public Health Nursing 23(3): 242–9

Kruske S, Barclay L, Schmied V 2006 Primary health care, partnership and polemic: child and family health nursing support in early parenting. Australian Journal of Primary Health 12(2):57–65

Lange B 2006 Mutual moral caring actions: a framework for community nursing practice. Advances in Nursing Science 29(2):E45–E55

Lee G, Fitzgerald L 2008 A clinical internship model for the nurse practitioner program. Nurse Education in Practice 8:397–404

Lenthall S, Wakerman J, Opie T, Dollard M, Dunn S, Knight S, MacLeod M, Watson C 2009 What stresses remote area nurses? Current knowledge and future action. Australian Journal of Rural Health 17:208–13

Lewin K 1951 Field Theory in Social Science. Harper & Row, New York

Litchfield M 2004 Achieving Health in a Rural Community: A Case Study of Nurse–Community Partnership. Central Publishing Bureau, Hastings, New Zealand

Litchfield M, Ross J 2000 The Role of Rural Nurses: National Survey. Centre for Rural Health, Christchurch New Zealand

Lobaton Cabrera S, Beaton R 2009 The role of occupational health nurses in terrorist attacks employing radiological dispersal devices. American Association of Occupational Health Nurses Journal 57(3):112–19

Lombardo M, Golding G 2003 Shared antenatal care. Australian Family Physician 32(3):133–9

Long K, Weinert C 1989 Rural nursing: developing the theory base. In: Lee H, Winters C (eds) Rural Nursing: Concepts, Theory and Practice (2nd edn). Springer, New York, pp 3–16

MacLeod M, Kulig M, Stewart J, Pitblado N, Roger J, Knock M 2004 The nature of nursing practice in rural and remote Canada. The Canadian Nurse 100(6):27–35

Maloney-Moni J 2006 Kia mana: A Synergy of Well-being. Copy Press, Nelson, New Zealand

Marinescu L 2007 Integrated approach for managing health risks at work — the role of occupational health nurses. American Association of Occupational Health Nurses 55(2):75–87

Markham T, Carney M 2007 Public health nurses and the delivery of quality nursing care in the community. Journal of Clinical Nursing 17:1342–50

Martin-Misener R, Downe-Wamboldt B, Cain E, Girouard M 2009 Cost effectiveness and outcomes of a nurse practitioner-paramedic-family physician model of care: the Long and Brier Islands study. Primary Health Care Research & Development 10:14–25

May K, Phillips L, Ferketich S, Verran J 2003 Public health nursing: the generalist in a specialized environment. Public Health Nursing 20(4):252–9

McCoy C 2009 Professional development in rural nursing: challenges and opportunities. The Journal of Continuing Education in Nursing 40(3):128–31

McCrae N, Banerjee S, Murray J, Prior S, Silverman A 2008 An extra pair of hands? A case study of the introduction of support workers in community mental health teams for older adults. Journal of Nursing Management 16:734–43

McMurray R, Cheater F 2004 Vision, permission and action: a bottom up perspective on the management of public health nursing. Journal of Nursing Management 12:43–50

Mellor G, St John W 2009 Managers' perceptions of the current and future role of occupational health nurses in Australia. American Association of Occupational Health Nurses Journal 57(2):79–87

Miller K 2009 Consumer-driven health care: nurse practitioners making history. Nurse Practitioner Journal 5(1):31–4. Online. Available: www.npjournal.org (accessed 10 August 2009)

Mills J, Birks M, Francis K 2009 Research aims to improve remote area nursing in Queensland. Australian Nursing Journal 16(8):34–35

Mills J, Birks M, Hegney D 2010 The status of rural nursing in Australia: 12 years on. Collegian 17:30–7

Mills J, Fitzgerald M 2009 The changing role of practice nurses in Australia: an action research study. Australian Journal of Advanced Nursing 26(1):16–20

Ministry of Health New Zealand (MOHNZ) 1998 Report of the ministerial taskforce on nursing. MOHNZ, Wellington

—— 2001 The Primary Health Care Strategy. MOHNZ, Wellington

—— 2002 Primary Mental Health: a Review of the Opportunities. MOHNZ, Wellington

—— 2003 Primary Health Care and Community Nursing Workforce Survey — 2001. MOHNZ, Wellington

—— 2008 Maternity Action Plan 2008–2012: Draft for Consultation. MOHNZ, Wellington

Moniz-Cook E, Elston C, Gardiner E, Agar S, Silver M, Win T, Wang M 2008 Can training community mental health nurses to support family carers reduce behavioural problems in dementia? An exploratory pragmatic randomised controlled trial. International Journal of Geriatric Psychiatry 23:185–91

Moses K, Keneally J, Bibby H, Chiang F, Robards F, Bennett D 2008 Beyond bandaids: Understanding the role of school nurses in NSW — Project summary report. Online. Available: www.caah.chw.edu.au/projects/summary_report.pdf (accessed 24 August 2009)

Munns A, Downie J, Wynaden D, Hubble J 2004 Changing focus of practice for community health nurses: advancing the practice role. Contemporary Nurse 16(3):208–13

Nankervis K, Kenny A, Bish M 2008 Enhancing scope of practice for the second level nurse: a change of process to meet growing demand for rural health services. Contemporary Nurse 29(2):159–73

National Association of School Nursing (NASN) 2005 Roles of the school nurse. NASN Newsletter 20(6):9–13

New Zealand Institute of Rural Health 2008 Discussion Paper for Moving Forward in Rural Health. New Zealand Institute of Rural Health, Cambridge, New Zealand

New Zealand Nurses Organisation (NZNO) 2008 Advanced nursing practice — NZNO position statement. Online. Available: www.nzno.org.nz/Site/Professional/AN/ANP_Position_Statement.aspx (accessed 8 August 2009)

New Zealand Nurses Organisation & The College of Nurses Aotearoa (NZ) Inc 2007 Investing in Health 2007: an update to the recommendations of Investing in Health: A framework for activating primary health care nursing (2003, Ministry of Health). New Zealand Nurses Organisation & the College of Nurses Aotearoa (NZ) Inc, Wellington

Nolan P, Haque M, Badger F, Dyke R, Khan I 2001 Mental health nurses' perceptions of nurse prescribing. Journal of Advanced Nursing 36(4):527–34

Nolan P, Haque M, Bourke P, Dyke R 2004 A comparison of the work and values of community mental health nurses in two mental health NHS trusts. Journal of Psychiatric and Mental Health Nursing 11:525–33

Nursing Council of New Zealand 2008 Competencies for the Nurse Practitioner Scope of Practice. Nursing Council of New Zealand, Wellington. Online. Available http://www.nursingcouncil.org.nz/download/74/np-competencies-sept09.pdf (accessed 18 June 2010)

Nursing Standard 2009 Editorial Nurses help lead the transformation in delivery of community care services. Nursing Standard 23(43):12–13

O'Brien A, Hughes F, Kidd J 2006 Mental health nursing in New Zealand primary health care. Contemporary Nurse 21(1):142–52

O'Connor T 2009a The delights and dilemmas of rural nursing. Kai Tiaki Nursing New Zealand 15(3):16–17

—— 2009b Innovative approaches to extending the role of the rural practice nurse. Kai Tiaki Nursing New Zealand 15(3):20–3

Olszewski K, Parks C, Chikotas N 2007 Occupational safety and health objectives of Healthy People 2010: a systematic approach for occupational health nurses — part 11. American Association of Occupational Health Nurses Journal 55(3):115–23

O'Neill M, Cowman S 2008 Partners in care: investigating community nurses' understanding of an interdisciplinary team-based approach to primary care. Journal of Clinical Nursing 17:3004–11

Patterson E, McMurray A 2003 Collaborative practice between registered nurses and medical practitioners in Australian general practice: moving from rhetoric to reality. Australian Journal of Advanced Nursing 20(4):43–8

Pearce C, Marshman J 2008 A framework for specialist nurses. Nursing Management 15(3):18–21

Phillips C, Pearce C, Dwan K, Hall S, Porritt J, Yates R, Kljakovic M, Sibbald B 2008 'Charting new roles for Australian general practice nurses'. Abridged Report of the Australian General Practice Nurses Study. Australian Primary Health Care Institute, Canberra

Plunket Society 2008 Annual Report 2008, 'Today's children, Tomorrow's Future'. The Royal New Zealand Plunket Society, Wellington New Zealand

Por J 2008 A critical engagement with the concept of advancing nursing practice. Journal of Nursing Management 16:84–90

Porritt J 2007 Policy development to support nurses in general practice: an overview. Contemporary Nurse 26(1):56–64

Proctor N 2006 Mental health nursing for individual, community and organisational benefit. Preface, Contemporary Nurse 21(1):vii–ix

Raphael D 2009 Restructuring society in the service of mental health promotion: are we willing to address the social determinants of mental health? International Journal of Mental Health Promotion 11(3):18–31

Reeve C, Pashen D, Mumme H, De La Rue S, Cheffins T 2009 Expanding the role of paramedics in northern Queensland: an evaluation of population health training. Australian Journal of Rural Health 16:370–5

Roberts D 2009 What do school nurses really do? National Association of School Nurses Newsletter School Nurse doi 10.1177/1942602X09337518

Robinson F 2009 Practice nurse comes of age. Practice Nurse 37(10):11–12,14

Rogers B, Stiehl K, Borst J, Hess A, Hitchins S 2007 Heat-related illnesses the role of occupational and environmental health nurse. American Association of Occupational Health Nurses Journal 55(7):279–87

Rogers E 2003 Diffusion of Innovations (5th edn). The Free Press, New York

Rose J, Glass N 2006 Community mental health nurses speak out: the critical relationship between emotional wellbeing and satisfying professional practice. Collegian 13(4):27–32

Rowe J, Barnes M 2006 The role of child health nurses in enhancing mothering know-how. Collegian 13(4):22–6

—— 2008 Infants and their families. In: Barnes M, Rowe J (eds) Child, Youth and Family Health Strengthening Communities. Elsevier, Sydney pp 110–28

Ryan K 2008 Health promotion of faculty and staff: the school nurse's role. The Journal of School Nursing 24(4):183–90

Schneiderman J 2006 Innovative pediatric nursing role: public health nurses in child welfare. Pediatric Nursing 32(4):317–23

Schroyen B, George N, Hylton J, Scobie N 2005 Encouraging nurses' physical assessment skills. Kai Tiaki Nursing New Zealand 11(10):14–15

Schwem M 2009 Generalized public health and industrial nurses work together. Public Health Nursing 26(4):380–2

Searle J 2007 Nurse practitioner candidates: shifting professional boundaries. Australasian Emergency Nursing Journal 11:20–7

Sen A 2000 Development as Freedom. Knopf, New York

Senior E 2009 How general practice nurses view their expanding role. Australian Journal of Advanced Nursing 26(1):8–15

Sheehan R, Barclay L 1999 An audit of 24 hour parent help lines across Australia. Good Beginnings Project. Online. Available: www.goodbeginnings.net.au/main.php?page=library (accessed 23 November 2009)

Slevin E, Sines D 2005 The role of community nurses for people with learning disabilities: working with people who challenge. International Journal of Nursing Studies 42:415–27

Smith S, Firmin M 2009 School nurse perspectives of challenges and how they perceive success in their professional nursing roles. Journal of School Nursing 25(2):152–62

Spriggle M 2009 Developing a policy for delegation of nursing care in the school setting. Journal of School Nursing 25(98):125–7

St Leger L 1999 The opportunities and effectiveness of the health promoting primary school in improving child health — a review of the claims and evidence. Health Education Research 14(1):51–69

Swearingen C 2009 Using nursing perspectives to inform public health nursing workforce development. Public Health Nursing 26(1):79–87

Swiadek J 2009 The impact of health care issues on the future of the nursing profession: the resulting increased influence of community-based and public health nursing. Nursing Forum 33(1):19–24

Talbot L, Verrinder G 2010 Promoting Health: A Primary Health Care Approach (4th edn). Elsevier, Sydney

Taua C, Farrow T 2009 Negotiating complexities: an ethnographic study of intellectual disability and mental health nursing in New Zealand. International Journal of Mental Health Nursing 18:274–84

Teate A, Leap N, Schindler Rising S, Homer C 2009 Women's experiences of group antenatal care in Australia — the Centering Pregnancy Pilot Study. Midwifery doi:10.1016/j.midw.2009.03.001

The North Staffordshire Changing Childbirth Research Team 2000 A randomized study of midwifery caseload care and traditional 'shared care'. Midwifery 16:295–302

Thompson L 2008 The role of nursing in governmentality, biopower and population health: family health nursing. Health and Place 14:76–84

Thompson P, Lang L, Annells M 2008 A systematic review of the effectiveness of in-home community nurse led interventions for the mental health of older persons. Journal of Clinical Nursing 17:1419–27

Tkaczyk J, Edelson A 2009 School nurses a bridge to suicide prevention. National Association of School Nurses School Nurse doi 10.1177/1942602X09333894:125–7

Toofany S 2007 Do district nurses have a public health role? Primary Health Care 17(5):21–4

United Kingdom Department of Health 2004 The NHS improvement plan: putting people at the heart of public services. The Stationery Office UKDOH, London

Victorian Government 2004 An evaluation of the Victorian Secondary School Nursing Program. Executive Summary. Victorian Government Department of Human Services, Primary and Community Health Branch. Online. Available: www.eduweb.vic.gov.au/edulibrary/public/stuman/nursing/ssnpevaluation.pdf (accessed 24 August 2009)

Victorian School Nurses (ANF, Vic Branch) Special Interest Group 2010 School Nursing Professional Practice Standards. VSN, Melbourne

Wainwright P, Thomas J, Jones M 2000 Health promotion and the role of the school nurse: a systematic review. Journal of Advanced Nursing 32(5):1083–91

Wakerman J 2009 Innovative rural and remote primary health care models: what do we know and what are the research priorities? Australian Journal of Rural Health 17:21–6

Walker L 2010 Practice nursing. In: Walker L, Patterson E, Wong W, Young D General Practice Nursing. McGraw-Hill, Sydney, pp 2–23

Wallace M 2009 Occupational health nurses — the solution to absence management? American Association of Occupational Health Nurses Journal 57(3):122–7

Wallis K, Smith S 2008 Developmental screening in paediatric primary care: the role of nurses. Journal for Specialists in Paediatric Nursing 13(2):130–4

Weist M, Paternite C, Wheatley-Rowe D, Gall G 2009 From thought to action in school mental health promotion. International Journal of Mental Health Promotion (1193):32–41

Whitehead D 2006a The health-promoting school: what role for nursing? Journal of Clinical Nursing 15:264–71

—— 2006b Workplace health promotion: the role and responsibility of health care managers. Journal of Nursing Management 14:59–68

Wicklander M 2005 The United Kingdom National Healthy School Standard: a framework for strengthening the school nurse role. The Journal of School Nursing 21(3):132–8

Wilson B, Crowe M 2008 Maintaining equilibrium: a theory of job satisfaction for community mental health nurses. Journal of Psychiatric and Mental Health Nursing 15:816–22

Wilson S 2006 Health visitor or public health nurse? A Scottish study. Community Practitioner 79(9):289–92

Winters L, Gordon U, Atherton J, Scott-Samuel A 2007 Developing public health nursing: barriers perceived by community nurses. Public Health 121:623–33

Wong S, Regan S 2009 Patient perspectives on primary health care in rural communities: effects of geography on access, continuity and efficiency. Rural and Remote Health 9(1142):1–12

Woodhouse G 2009 Exploration of interaction and shared care arrangements of generalist community nurses and external nursing teams in a rural health setting. Australian Journal of Advanced Nursing 26(30):17–23

World Health Organization (WHO) 1996 Promoting Health Through Schools: The World Health Organization Global School Health Initiative. WHO, Geneva

—— 2005 Preparing a health care workforce for the 21st century. The challenge of chronic conditions. WHO Geneva

—— 2008 World Health Report 2008 Primary Health Care, Now More Than Ever. Online. Available: http://www.who.int/whr/2008/whr08_en.pdf (accessed 14 July 2009)

—— 2009 Health systems development nursing and midwifery. WHO. Online. Available: www.searo.who.nt/en/Section1243/Section 2167/Section 2168_14388.htm (accessed 31 March 2009)

Yarwood J 2008 Nurses' views of family nursing in community contexts: an exploratory study. Nursing Praxis in New Zealand 2(2):41–51

Zinner P 2006 Preparing the work force for retirement — the role of occupational health nurses. American Association of Occupational Health Nurses Journal 54(12):531–6

Zurmehly J 2007 A qualitative case study review of role transition in community nursing. Nursing Forum 42(4):162–70

Useful websites

http://www.ngala.com.au/ — early parenting support in Western Australia

http://www.tresillian.net/ — early parenting support in New South Wales

http://www.plunket.org.nz/ — Royal New Zealand Plunket Society

http://www.starship.org.nz/paediatric-update/ — New Zealand telemedicine programs

http://www.mindnet.org.nz — Vibe — mental health promotion and prevention newsletter

http://www.mentalhealth.org.nz — New Zealand mental health promotion

http://www.ncc-wch.org.uk/ — UK National Collaborating Centre for Women's and Children's Health

http://www.maternitycoalition.org.au/ — Australian national maternity action plan

http://www.goodbeginnings.net.au/ — Australian good beginnings program

http://www.aifs.gov.au — Australian Institute of Family Studies

http://www.msd.govt.nz/about-msd-and-our-work/publications-resources/research/nz-families-today/ — New Zealand Families Today

http://www.kidshealth.org.nz/ — New Zealand kidshealth

http://www.anu.edu.au/aphcri/ — Australian Primary Health Care Research Institute

http://www.ruralhealth.org.au/ — Australian National Rural Health Alliance

http://www.acphd.org/AXBYCZ/Admin/DataReports/07_step3_direction.pdf — Alameda County Public Health Department Community Assessment focusing on asset mapping

http://www.cyh.com/SubContent.aspx?p=102 — Australian Parent Helplines

http://www.reviveclinic.com.au/ — Australian 'Revive' Nurse Practitioner clinics

http://www.who.int/occupational_health/publications/healthy_workplaces_model_action.pdf — WHO Healthy
  Workplace Initiatives

http://www.aaohn.org — American Association of Occupational Health Nurses

http://www.cdc.gov/niosh — American National Institute for Occupational Safety and Health

http://www.schoolnursesnsw.asn.au/200.html — NSW School Nurses Association

http://www.australia.gov.au/topics/health-and-safety/occupational-health-and-safety — Australian Government
  sites for Occupational Health and Safety

http://www.nurse.org.nz — College of Nurses (Aotearoa) primary health care nurses network

http://www.moh.govt.nz/moh.nsf/indexmh/nursing-initiatives — Nursing initiatives in New Zealand

http://www.cph.co.nz/About-Us/Health-Promoting-Schools.asp — NZ Canterbury District Health Board site for
  health-promoting schools

http://www.chnwa.org.au — Community Health Nurses Western Australia website

http://www.nnnet.gov.au/ — National Nursing and Nursing Education Taskforce (N3ET) NP standards

http://www.nzno.org.nz/groups/colleges/college_of_practice_nurses/about_us — NZNO College of Practice
  Nurses website

http://www.nurse.org.nz — Nurse Practitioners of New Zealand website

http://www.nzno.org.nz/groups/colleges/college_of_primary_health_care_nurses — NZNO College of Primary
  Healthcare Nurses website

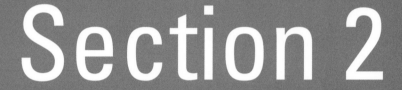

Section 2

Sustainable health for the family and the individual

Chapter 5 **Healthy families**

Chapter 6 **Healthy children**

Chapter 7 **Healthy adolescents**

Chapter 8 **Healthy adults**

Chapter 9 **Healthy ageing**

INTRODUCTION TO THE SECTION

This section reflects the importance of promoting health and wellness at each stage along the life course from birth to death. Chapter 5 focuses on the contemporary family, as the central element in the development and sustainability of individual and community health. Families are pre-eminent from conception through birth and throughout a child's life course. Their most significant role is evident in their ability to provide a healthy start to young people's lives. Along the developmental pathway family structures and processes are dynamic, changing with circumstances and events. These changes are also framed by the social determinants of health, which determine the extent to which families are able to provide early and sustained support for its members. This directs us to examine the many ways families are shaped by, and interact with, the social and cultural processes of the society that provides the context to their development.

In this 21st century, families are increasingly diverse, presenting a tapestry of different types and configurations, all of which influence and are influenced by factors outside the boundaries of family life. One of the most significant issues for families in this era is coping with the way the global economy has reshaped the work environment, and the effects of changes in workplace culture on dual earner families, their roles and relationships. Another global change flows from rapid communication systems and various technologies, which have also brought families from one community into contact with many others throughout the world. Sharing values and ideas with other cultures has caused provocative changes to family life. In today's society, young people's expectations and values are often more closely aligned to those of families in other parts of the world than to previous generations of their own family of origin. There is also greater diversity among populations due to cross-border migration for both voluntary reasons and because of civil conflicts. These migrations pose challenges for families, which we discuss in Chapter 5. In this chapter we also address some of the most pertinent issues for families in

the embrace of changing community and societal values, including the impact of family separation, divorce and the violence that can disrupt family stability. We also address the affect of community life on rural and caregiving families, and strategies for providing adequate and culturally appropriate support structures to help families and their communities live more vibrant, harmonious lives.

Child health is commonly understood as the most significant indicator of how families, neighbourhoods, communities and nations are able to provide health-enhancing conditions for daily living. Investing knowledge, resources, time and space to develop healthy, educated, well supported lives for infants and children shows the extent to which health is valued in the enabling community. Chapter 6 addresses health and potential, with the child at the centre of interest. The burgeoning body of research into biological embeddedness and the role of environmental stimuli are also addressed in this chapter. A long and trustworthy body of evidence now points conclusively to the critical and sensitive moments in a child's life when preset conditions interact with external stimuli to establish patterns for healthy adulthood. Each community has a unique capacity for nurturing young people, maximising their opportunities in the environmental, economic, social, political and cultural realms. Health professionals can be invaluable to this process by helping community members analyse their capacity to create optimal conditions for child health and development.

The health status of adolescents in any community provides a barometer of a community's progress in creating and supporting a healthy start to life, and creating a template for the future. At this crucial stage, a large segment of the population is launched from childhood to adulthood, from dependence to independence. How adolescents deal with the various challenges and negotiate the many transitions of a few delicate years often heralds how well they will cope with the transitions of adult life. The impact of peer pressure and social structures is among the most important determinants of adolescents' experiences and lifestyle choices. Chapter 7 explores the concept of the adolescent 'at promise' rather than 'at risk', in the expectation that there are some ways nurses and other health care professionals can bring the promise of adolescence to fruition. The chapter also focuses on adolescent resilience and some of the collaborative strategies communities and family members can use to help foster health literate adolescents and guide them toward competent and socially responsive adulthood. This is based on the knowledge that successes in adolescence are predictive of the extent to which young people will become healthy adults and create their own healthy families, neighbourhoods and communities.

Healthy adulthood reflects the culmination of socially and environmentally supported choices for health and wellness made by individuals at earlier stages of their development. Adulthood is also the time when many chronic diseases emerge and when the risks of ill health or injury are acute. For younger adults, particularly parents, social and occupational pressures loom large and the discussion extends to issues related to formal and informal work and family life that were introduced in Chapter 5. In the older adult population the outcomes of health service provision are also visible, as by the time most people reach adulthood, they have encountered the health care system on at least one occasion. These encounters may be aimed at redressing a clinical problem, providing an opportunity for illness prevention in the future, or both. In Chapter 8, the major risk factors and lifestyle determinants of healthy adulthood are discussed in a way that acknowledges the influence of the environment and social structures on personal choices for health. The chapter also reinforces the need for intergenerational consideration of health and illness. Longevity and longer working lives challenge our historical diminished expectations of people in later adulthood. We reconceptualise those years as a type of extended middle age, which has its own set of challenges for nurses, midwives and other health professionals. The chapter culminates in

an argument for 'third places', the kind of places where people go beyond work and home, to find social succour and respite from their busy lives.

Chapter 9 provides an examination of the features of healthy ageing. Managing chronic conditions is of major concern in this part of life's pathway, and we revisit some of the main strategies for helping people shape their lifestyles and their communities to promote healthy ageing. Like that of children, older people's health is punctuated by sensitive moments, the accumulation of stressors and strengthening incidents along the life course. To assist older people requires intergenerational sensitivity and a need to see older people as located along the critical pathway that begins in childhood. A social perspective of ageing is outlined, including the need to attend to older people's numerous transitions; those related to family members joining or leaving the family home, retirement, loss and the adjustments of widowhood. Our role in assisting older people to expect and then to achieve, health and wellness is paramount at this time of life, as older people rely more heavily than others on advice and guidance from those who they encounter in a range of health services. This includes measures to counter ageism and to strengthen older people's voices in the policy arena.

Throughout these chapters in Section 2, we use the Ottawa Charter for Health Promotion as a guide to working with each of the population groups. It is offered as a framework for situating practice within the goals of healthy public policy, creating supportive environments, strengthening community action, developing personal skills, and reorienting health services. The Millers also feature in each chapter, as the case study unfolds with a different focus for each, ranging from the family, to the children, adolescents, adults, and older persons. As you read through the chapters we encourage you again to think about the big issues, some of which we mention at the end of each chapter, and reflect on practice and its evidence base.

Chapter 5

Healthy families

INTRODUCTION

Few people would challenge the notion that the family is the most important influence on the health of a society. The family is where individuals are nurtured and guided to adopt and adapt beliefs, behaviours, values and attitudes that will help their members become healthy and competent citizens of wider worlds. As mentioned in Section 1, there are many influences on health and development that arise from the interactions between families and communities. Some of the most important of these are habits of mind and action that emerge from a child's early experience in the family. Daily interactions between family members create opportunities for inherent traits and predispositions to be shaped into positive or negative behaviours in relation to health and wellbeing. These become habitual and refined as they are reinforced and nurtured, and as family members interact with others external to the family. Families with children play an important role in nurturing their children along their developmental pathways. This has a reciprocal effect on parents or caregivers as each interaction provides not only an opportunity for parental dialogue, but also renewed consideration of the way adult family members are relating to one another. For families without children, regardless of their constitution, interactions are also major opportunities for mutual nurturing and the development of adult competence to deal with the world outside the family.

> **Point to ponder**
> Family is the most important influence on the health of a society.

Adult family members make lifestyle choices, and this can be crucial to a child's decision-making in relation to healthy lifestyles. Children's choices are cultivated by what is observed and modelled within the family, and how family health is entrenched in the social conditions and relationships beyond the family. In this respect, families play a significant gatekeeping role as the main link between individuals and their environments. Because families themselves are dynamic, their roles change in various ways and this has implications for family health and wellbeing. As individual family members change and develop in the encounters of daily life, the family as an entity also changes to adapt to the outside world, which affects its ability to provide a supportive environment for its members. Each opportunity to adapt and change can be used to share strengths and challenges, and to teach younger family members the skills to be self-regulating and competent, to create and sustain health and wellbeing as they negotiate the critical stages along the pathways to adulthood.

In a contemporary world where change is both rapid and constant, the way family members transact and adapt to the precariousness of their environments determines the extent to which the family can provide solace and refuge, comfort, succour and direction to each of its members. Families that are able to provide a firm grounding for their members to deal with outside stressors can vitalise the community in ways that cultivate understanding, tolerance and social cohesion. Alternatively, a lack of strong family bonds to shelter or protect family members from the outside world can have harmful effects on its members and cast a shadow over the community. As health professionals, it is essential that we understand the way families are changing and being changed by contemporary life. Towards that end, this chapter examines the family in the context of today's social changes and the role of nurses, midwives and other health professionals in helping them achieve health.

THE FAMILY, COMMUNITY AND SOCIETY

When we think of family, some of us think of the protective envelope that provides a refuge from the stresses and strains of contemporary society. Others

Objectives

By the end of this chapter you will be able to:

1 discuss the major changes affecting families in society
2 examine social trends related to demographic patterns, separation and divorce, parenting, family violence, the needs of rural families, migrants, refugees and family caregiving
3 develop professional strategies for meeting the needs of contemporary families in today's society
4 describe modifiable elements of social environments that could help promote non-violence and harmony in the family
5 identify community goals for sustaining family health
6 devise a set of research priorities that will help inform family change.

see family as a combat zone, a kind of repository for the collective problems of both the inside and outside world. Most people hold a view of family that lies somewhere between these two extremes. The family is the filter, or mediating structure that functions as a gatekeeper between individuals, their culture and the wider society. It is a conduit through which society transmits to individuals its social and cultural norms, roles and responsibilities. The family also acts as a communicative structure from within, providing a scaffold for interactions, with the goal of bonding individuals into a cohesive whole with shared attitudes, values and opinions. When this goal is achieved, the family is able to give voice to needs and preferences, which should, in turn, inform societal policies and processes that can vitalise the community.

Point to ponder

Family acts as a protective gatekeeper between individual family members and their culture, and the wider society.

Most communities situate the family at the centre of social life. From the seeds sown and nurtured in the family, members make decisions affecting access to health care and social services, prevention of illness, preservation of the natural and built environment, the cultivation of knowledge and good governance. These are the essential elements of a healthy society. However, family life can also exert a negative influence on these decisions, subduing or constraining individuals

and circumstances, precipitating illness, endangeringtheir environment or failing to protect its members from harm. Families are therefore the pivot point around which communities and societies revolve. As the foundational human institution the family has been described as:

> a cooperative economic and protective powerhouse delivering mutual care and goods and services to its members; a source of succour, nursing and welfare when needed; and a social organisation in miniature providing education, ethical instruction, recreation, entertainment, companionship, and love.
>
> (Maley 2009:1)

The 'fit' between the family and society is an indication of social cohesion and mutually beneficial goals and bonds of trust, which are the cornerstones of social capital (Hancock 2009; Putnam 2005). Thinking of the family in terms of social capital ultimately means that family members are part of the system of normative obligations created in the wider society. The norms and standards of the society are reinforced within kinship structures, and the institutions external to the family, such as schools and workplaces (Furstenberg 2005). This process is not imposed from outside the family, rather it occurs as an exchange of interests, sometimes as a symbolic exchange of affection, esteem, respect and cultural norms (Furstenberg 2005). In this era of globalisation and mass migration, the families of most societies, especially in the wealthy countries, are more culturally and linguistically diverse (CALD) than in the past. The challenge for health professionals is to explore ways of promoting and supporting family cohesion and the transmission of strengths, needs and preferences along developmental pathways. Promoting family health is complex, uncertain and fluctuating, determined by how a family is constituted, their previous experiences and their particular needs (Hartrick Doane 2005). This is, at times, a daunting challenge, given that it occurs in the face of constant change, but it also contains new understandings of the many contextual factors that influence family health, which is stimulating to all of us who are curious about the world and its people.

DEFINING THE FAMILY

Defining the family is important for several reasons. These include some of the most important social and structural determinants of health, such as the socio-legal family environment. Socio-legal arrangements dictate who is included in insurance policies, which members have access to children's school records, who can be a part of a joint tax return or bank account, and who is eligible for reproductive assistance, sick leave, death benefits, child support, superannuation or other means of income security. Some definitions of family are more traditional, for example, explaining the family on the basis of a common place of residence.

Point to ponder
Family has been defined in multiple ways. One of the more useful definitions tells us that family is 'whoever the family says it is'.

Another approach to defining the family is within the rubric of family systems theory, where the family is seen as an entity in itself, consisting of subsystems (of siblings, for example), which interact with the family as a whole and with its surrounding environment. The family system may be related by blood ties, marriage, legal adoption or residence, or by bonds of reciprocal affection and mutual responsibility (Wright & Leahey 2009). In addition to geographic, biological/genetic or cultural affiliation, the family may be defined according to constituent members, family structures, family relationships and/or lifestyle preferences. Within this type of perspective, individuals become families through personally constructed kinship, social and cultural networks informed by their ideologies and continuity of relationships (Crisp & Taylor 2009). Clearly, there is no typical

family form or common definition of the family. Wright and Leahey's (1987) explanation that the family is 'whoever the family says it is' may therefore be the most enduring and practical way of defining the family.

Contemporary notions of 'family' focus on the fact that families are constructed and transformed in the context of their members' interrelationships and interactions with one another. These are dynamic, changing over time depending on family type, structure and events in the family's history. For example, a nuclear family constituting two parents and a child may have fewer, but equally meaningful interactions than a separated family where the child is nurtured across two households. As the child grows the number and type of interactions (s)he experiences may depend on the degree to which each familial household experiences a stable structure or periods of relative stability.

Point to ponder
Families are constructed and transformed in the context of the interrelationships and interactions family members have with one another.

The event of additional children joining either or both families affects interactions between all members in both households, as do the various milestones in their development. In addition, a range of factors create changes affecting adult family members' relationships with one another, including economic, employment, environmental, social or health changes, and the adults' ages and stage in life. Intergenerational families, often described as extended families, may also have unique interactions to accommodate various members' stages in life. Changes tend to affect family members differentially, so individual experiences vary. However, in general, families are a microcosm of adaptive interactions that are determined by historical events, cultural mores, preferences for spiritual or lifestyle activities, and connections to their neighbourhood and community.

FAMILY FUNCTIONS

Although families experience considerable diversity in forms and functions, family roles tend to revolve around goal setting, conflict resolution, caregiving, nurturing and using internal and external resources for the advantage of family members (Friedman 1992). Duvall and Miller (1985) describe the family's general functions as the following:

- Affection — an affectionate family environment provides the conditions within which family members can learn to trust one another and those external to the family.
- Security and acceptance — having basic physical and emotional needs nurtured within the family instils a sense of safety and security that will promote the ability to be accepting of others.
- Identity and a sense of worth — reflecting on family interactions allows family members to develop a sense of who they are and how their unique characteristics are linked to those of others.
- Affiliation and companionship — throughout the life span the family creates a sense of belonging among members, which establishes a template for bonding together and with others.
- Socialisation — the family transmits a cultural and social identity that will embody the family's history and values and thus contribute to the community's collective identity, particularly in multicultural communities. This influences community cohesion.
- Controls — within the family all members come to recognise the rules and boundaries that provide realistic standards for public behaviour.

FAMILY DEVELOPMENTAL PATHWAYS

Developmental theorists suggest that families and their members go through various stages, each of which is quantitatively and qualitatively different from adjacent stages. These individual and family development trajectories are unique. They are generally based on personal experiences or particular ways family members have themselves been nurtured in the past, as well as their intentions for the future. Traditional family theorists contend that family stages, and their correspondent tasks are relatively consistent, designed to meet the family's biological requirements, cultural imperatives and shared aspirations and values. The stages are as described in Box 5.1.

BOX 5.1 STAGES OF FAMILY DEVELOPMENT

- The beginning stage of partnership or marriage, where the task is relating harmoniously to the kin network and planning the family.
- The stage of parenthood where the young family is established as a stable unit.
- The stage of raising preschool children where the need for protection and space, integration and socialisation predominates.
- The children-at-school stage where school achievement is promoted while the adults attempt to maintain a satisfying marital relationship.
- Families with teenagers, where the family attempts to integrate and communicate its values, lifestyles, moral and ethical standards.
- Launching centre families, where the children begin to leave home and the role of parents shifts to encouraging independence. As the older children marry, new adult family members are welcomed into the family.
- The post-parenting stage, where the parents attempt to maintain a sense of physical and psychological wellbeing through a healthy environment, sustaining satisfying relationships with children and ageing parents and re-strengthening the marital relationship.
- Retired families, where the partners attempt to maintain comfortable living arrangements, maintain intergenerational family ties and sometimes, learn to cope with the loss of a partner.

(Duvall 1977; Gottleib & Feeley 2000)

Although these developmental stages may apply to a nuclear family consisting of two parents and a child or children, the most common family form in today's society is a cohabiting couple. This challenges previous notions of what constitutes a family, and when family life actually begins. For cohabiting families marriage is not the starting point for family life. Instead, we live in an era where love and consent have replaced marriage as the condition permitting sex, cohabitation and childbearing (Thornton 2009). From this perspective, the beginning of family life may vary according to the couple's lifestyle choices. Cohabitation can be a normative stage where a couple lays the foundation for the future, including marriage and children (premarital cohabitation), or it may be an exploratory relationship between the partners to see whether or not they are sufficiently compatible to make a commitment to one another (Lichter & Qian 2008; Tach & Halpern-Meekin 2009). In some cases, adults may engage in serial cohabitation, either prior to or following marriage (Lichter & Qian 2008). This type of family does not conform to the nuclear family stages as outlined above. Nor do families who experience separation and/or reconstitution, through repartnering, remarriage or by changing their members' social orientation. Instead, many families live in transient groupings where the family straddles one or several stages at once and members have to learn quickly to adapt to the blending of two families and the intermittent involvement of non-resident members.

> ### Point to ponder
> Family form and structure have changed considerably over the past decades. Where once the nuclear family of mother, father and children was the norm, today, 'family' may take many different forms: from single or partnered adults, to families comprising multiple generations.

When family members are separated or divorced there are often many new transitions, such as establishing various boundaries, dealing with children's access to parents, consolidating new relationships, reconstituting the family unit and planning for step-parenting.

Family forms such as homosexual couples or intergenerational families also have non-standardised structures and their own unique challenges. Intergenerational families may be characterised by the presence of elders or by older children leaving home and returning, sometimes more than once. Single adults living together as a family of friends also experience unique stages in their development that are not dependent on children's developmental stages. So, although it is useful to consider various developmentally related family tasks and roles, a categorisation truer to today's families is simply single or married adults living as a couple, with or without children; married adults living with young, teenage or adult children; people living alone; and intergenerational families comprising any of the above.

CHANGING FAMILIES, CHANGING PARTNERS, CHANGING ROLES

As mentioned previously, family roles are usually dynamic, adapting to meet family goals and the ebb and flow of developmental and circumstantial events in family members' lives. A century ago when many families lived as an economic unit predominantly on properties, roles were relatively predictable. Nuclear families of husband, wife and several children were the norm. Few children were born to unmarried mothers, and cohabitation without marriage was rare and stigmatised by social norms (Maley 2009). The husband was considered the head of the family, the wife was its heart. Children and parents worked together towards the major goal of productivity and economic survival. Since the industrial revolution that followed World War II, family members have undertaken more diverse roles. One reason for this was the breadth of opportunities that came with industrial development, which opened up women's access to the world of work outside the home.

The women's movement of the 1970s was an important part of the socio-cultural revolution that followed industrialisation. The movement, called the 'women's movement' or the 'feminist movement', promoted the idea that women should have choices, rather than predetermined roles as wives and mothers. This was accompanied by a relaxation of sexual morality, reinforced by accessible contraception and a lack of social censure for marriage alternatives such as cohabitation (Maley 2009). By the end of the 1970s women's voices demanded release for women from traditional expectations of family life, and many began to separate their roles, choosing to work in the market economy as well as at home (Maley 2009). Abundant employment opportunities also inspired many women to undertake further education which they may have previously forgone to establish a family. These vast social changes have had profound effects in Western. One effect has been a decline in the birth rate. Another has been an increase in family separation and divorce. Yet another has been a dramatic increase in child care outside the family home.

> ### Point to ponder
> Industrialisation and the women's movement have had a profound impact on family roles and structures.

The information age of the 1980s and 1990s further expanded choices for both women and men, with opportunities in the information technology industry. Electronic media presented some people with the choice to work at home, while others chose to remain positioned in the workplace. Each option offered advantages and disadvantages. The workplace continued to provide greater opportunities for women to move up the career ladder, while home work allowed greater flexibility. Theoretically, the introduction of flexible work arrangements seemed to present an ideal opportunity to advance social change, including a greater sharing of household duties and parenting. However, four decades after the women's movement, the majority of women receive little assistance from partners in relation to the family's domestic responsibilities. In the workplace, they have yet to achieve parity with men in wages or executive opportunities. Women also experience greater job insecurity, partly because of family-related absences from the workplace (Schultheiss 2006). On the surface it seems that women have become emancipated from the predetermined roles of their mothers. Yet, for many, the new freedom created by the women's movement has meant additional, rather than substitute roles, because, contrary to expectations, changes in the workplace have not altered gendered norms of behaviour in the home (Ezzedeen & Ritchey 2008). As a result, many women continue to return home from work to complete a 'second shift' of child care and housework. This burden of dual roles often disrupts harmony in the home, creating a dual source of stress.

Globalisation has also had a major impact on the female workforce, with many women being relegated to lower-paid jobs at the end of large commodity chains. It has exacerbated job insecurity for women, many of whom work in low-wage service industries, which is a particular burden for immigrant women who are disadvantaged in numerous other ways. However, the increased competitiveness of globalised industries has also created work intensification for men. Like their female co-workers, they have had to adapt to rapidly changing employment environments without the job security of past decades, where rewards flowed from persistence and loyalty rather than rapid transitions to a series of new workplaces.

The challenges of the 21st century are multiplied many times over for migrant families. As we mentioned in Chapter 2, globalisation has precipitated

Point to ponder

Despite the promise of the women's movement and the expectation of flexible working hours engendered by the information age, women in most families remain in the dual role of primary caregiver and worker.

a mass migration of families across porous borders, and this has affected family, social and cultural life in their country of origin as well as in the host countries. Opening up national borders to migrants, and increasing the diversity and range of opportunities for women has provided greater financial and social independence for those previously excluded from these opportunities, and created the impression of a fairer society in countries of the West. However, expansion of opportunities has also been blamed for severe shortages of some predominantly female jobs, such as nursing and teaching.

From an equal opportunity perspective, presenting women with access to broader choices in the workplace can be seen as a successful outcome of the women's movement. Yet, the sweeping changes in society have irrevocably changed family life. The trend towards separation and divorce that began in the 1970s has continued, although at a slower rate now than at the turn of the century (Australian Bureau of Statistics [ABS] 2009; United Kingdom Office for National Statistics 2009). Since 1970 the Australian marriage rate has halved, while the divorce rate continues at a rate of approximately 12% after five years of marriage (Maley 2009). Similar figures exist in New Zealand with a 29% drop in marriages since 1971 and, as of 2006, a divorce rate of 11.9% (Families Commission 2008). Cohabiting couples have even higher rates of separation, with 40% of these relationships ending after five years (Maley 2009). These trends are a global phenomenon, representing the disappearance of social censure for cohabitation, declining religious sanctions and changes in family law systems, which have eliminated barriers to divorce (Byrd 2009; Maley 2009; Thornton 2009).

Point to ponder

Since 1970 in both Australia and New Zealand, the marriage rate has nearly halved, and the divorce rate after five years is now 12% and 11.9% respectively.

In 2006 57% of all adults aged over 16 years in New Zealand were partnered and living together (Families Commission 2008). In 2009, 65% of Australian adults lived in a couple relationship, most cohabiting or 'socially married' (ABS 2009; Maley 2009). Approximately 39% live together as a precursor to marriage, with the rest in a long-term partnership or cohabiting following divorce or separation (ABS 2009; Maley 2009). Of those who do marry, most wait until they are older than in the past to do so (ABS 2009; Commonwealth of Australia 2008; Families Commission 2008). When couples are uncertain of their future together or worried about losing their jobs, having children is often put on hold. This has led to increases in the proportion of couple-only families delaying childbirth, and older members of the population ageing (the 'empty nesters') (Commonwealth of Australia 2008). The number of one-parent families with dependent children has increased slowly over the past decade to 11% in Australia and 21% in New Zealand, with a slight increase in those headed by males (Commonwealth of Australia 2008; Families Commission 2008). The trend toward living alone has also increased, representing 23% of the Australian and New Zealand population (ABS 2007a; Statistics New Zealand 2006).

Over the past 2 decades, liberalisation of marital laws in some countries (Canada, the United Kingdom, South Africa and some states in the United States) has resulted in a trend toward greater acceptance of marriage between homosexual couples (Kluwer 2000; Le Bourdais & Lapierre-Adamcyk 2004). This is also a social trend in Australia and New Zealand. Civil union became legal for same sex couples in New Zealand in 2004 (Civil Union Act 2004. Online. Available: www.legislation.govt.nz/act/public/2004/0102/latest/whole.html [accessed 20 October 2009]), and in 2006 there were 430 civil unions (of which 80% were same sex unions).

> **Point to ponder**
> New Zealand introduced civil union for same sex couples in 2004. Australia continues to lobby for the same rights.

In Australia, groups lobbying for equal rights in marriage have attempted to secure similar legislation, and a Galaxy poll indicates that it would be widely supported by the public (Online. Available: www.australiamarriageequality.com/ [accessed 28 October 2009]). However, the legal issues are as yet unresolved. In 2008 same sex relationships were estimated to be around 1% of all couples in Australia (Commonwealth of Australia 2008). However, because many gay couples do not report their relationship in census data, there is uncertainty about the proportion of the population this represents (ABS 2009).

Among Australian and New Zealand families the majority (61% and 42% respectively) are raising children, most in 'intact' couple families (ABS 2007b). However, the number of children born to single women has increased dramatically, with one-third of all births born to unmarried or cohabiting women (Maley 2009). Despite a slowing of the divorce rate over the past decade, separation and divorce continue to leave many adults raising their children on a part-time basis (ABS 2009; Commonwealth of Australia 2008). Among families raising children, parents doing so without a partner represent 22% of Australian families and 18% of New Zealand families (ABS 2009; Statistics New Zealand 2006). Trends indicate a growing number of children (22%) living in blended families, and an increasing number (1% of families with children) being cared for by grandparents, although these proportions are higher for Indigenous people (ABS 2007a; Commonwealth of Australia 2008; Families Commission 2008).

Divorce is a major concern for contemporary families. Among de facto couples the rate of divorce is three times that of married couples (Commonwealth of Australia 2008).The highest rates of divorce are among blended families, which may be due to the complexity of remarrying after divorce (Crisp & Taylor 2009). The most significant outcome of this is that young adults in today's world are the first generation to experience marital instability and remarriage as a family norm (Sassler et al 2009). Many have lived with cohabiting parents and partners, dividing their time and emotional energy between stepfamilies and a variety of step siblings, and they are faced with the prospect that up to half of them may divorce themselves (Sassler et al 2009). These current patterns of union dissolution and remarriage may be intergenerational, as they have created a demographic momentum to reproduce divorce and family instability (Teachman 2002).

Point to ponder

Divorce is having a significant impact on contemporary family structure and function. Of greatest concern is the long-term impact of divorce on children.

In addition to the impact of divorce on society and its children, researchers from the Australian Institute of Family Studies (AIFS) report on the negative effects of instability in marriage and cohabitation as perceived by those experiencing divorce or separation. These indicate:

- dissatisfaction with their current life by both males and females following divorce
- men feel a lower sense of social support
- women experience poorer health
- divorced, single women have low satisfaction with life
- remarriage restores life satisfaction (DeVaus et al 2007).

Married people tend to live longer and be healthier than single people, and their children are less at risk for ill health or poor education outcomes (Maley 2009). Children raised by both biological parents score higher on measures of psychological adjustment, self-esteem and academic success (Sassler et al 2009). On the other hand, children of divorce have poorer health and educational outcomes, experience more behavioural and emotional problems, have a higher propensity to fall into delinquency and crime, are more often in danger of being abused and neglected, and experience more unstable and unsatisfying relationships themselves (Maley 2009; Sassler et al 2009).

FERTILITY, CHILD BEARING AND POPULATION TRENDS

The dramatic changes to family life since the social revolution of the 1960s and 1970s have had a pronounced effect on fertility, child bearing and projections for the future of the population. Marital instability and the decision of many women to delay child bearing until they have established their careers, have conspired against fertility rates, so there are fewer children being born, most to older (<30) first time parents (Commonwealth of Australia 2008; Maley 2009; Families Commission 2008). The birth rate in Australia has declined from 3.5 children in 1961 to 1.93 in 2007, and

in New Zealand from 4.3 in 1961 to 2.1 in 2007. These rates differ according to socio-economic advantage, with those from low socio-economic advantage (migrants, those with lower education, Indigenous women) having the most births. For example, the Indigenous fertility rate is 2.4 babies per mother in Australia, and 2.8 babies per mother for Maori in New Zealand (Commonwealth of Australia 2008; Families Commission 2008). A similar pattern of declining fertility rates is also evident across Europe and the US (UK Office for National Statistics 2009). Because infertility is a growing problem the rate of couples receiving assisted reproduction technologies has increased markedly over the past decade, to where children from in vitro fertilisation represent 3% of all babies being born to Australian mothers (Commonwealth of Australia 2008).

Point to ponder

Although fertility rates are declining in Australia and New Zealand, these rates differ according to socio-economic advantage. Those from low socio-economic advantage have the most births.

The implication of low fertility rates is that some countries, including Australia, have begun to rely on immigration to sustain the population (Commonwealth of Australia 2008). Although the fertility rate in New Zealand is currently at replacement level, this is predicted to decrease below replacement level by 2016 (Families Commission 2008). In this case, immigration will also become the most likely means of sustaining the New Zealand population. Although this is one solution, increasing the migrant population is only short term and does not provide the strong family systems that are a vital element in sustaining a vigorous and prosperous society (Maley 2009). Migrant families lend vibrancy to the community, especially when there are 'family reunion programs' that allow a migrant to bring other family members to the host country. However, it is also important for a society to replace itself to ensure sufficient young people to sustain the economy when older people retire and to care for them during ageing. This is a major concern for most countries, and we will discuss this further in relation to population policies in Chapter 13. What the trends suggest, is that by the year 2050, the Australian population over 65 is likely to rise to around 25% of the total population, while the proportion of younger people in the workforce who contribute to the economy will decline. The implication of this is that there will only be 2.7 people of working age to support each retiree, which is around half of the current workforce (Commonwealth of Australia 2008, 2010). Similarly, in New Zealand, the population aged over 65 is predicted to increase to 25% by 2051 (Dyson 2002) and although the workforce is predicted to grow overall, this growth rate will slow as the workforce ages (Statistics New Zealand 2008).

> ### Point to ponder
> By 2050–51 the respective populations over the age of 65 in Australia and New Zealand will have increased to 25% of the total population in each country. This will result in a large number of retirees with far fewer people working to support them.

Smaller family size is also a concern to demographers and child health specialists. One effect of small families is the number of children growing up without siblings, and the impact of this will likely not be fully realised until the children are adults. Another important consideration is the potential for families with young children to become the minority in the population. This could have implications for the way communities are developed or transformed if they become oriented towards meeting the needs of the older population rather than children. Although it is possible that in future, families will be caring for more adults than children, the impact of an adult-oriented community would be the lack of an influential voice for young families in the public arena. Already the built environment is showing the signs of demographic change, with some housing developments being tailored to older singles and child-free couples.

With children pushed to the margins of public consciousness it is difficult to imagine who will champion the causes of family-friendly environments, including schools, workplaces, leisure and health services, or the need for communities to be actively involved in children's development (Stanley et al 2005; Weston 2005).

Despite concerns about child health and development, society needs to maintain a parallel consideration of elders' needs as they age. The continuing decline in the number of younger adults in the working population may provide difficulties in terms of providing care and financial support for older people from the tax base generated by younger workers. Although migration may help even out the need for workers in the short term, in the longer term, it is not a viable solution, given that migrant populations are also ageing. It is an interesting dilemma, with many ethical issues, primarily in relation to the implications of selecting certain people for migration without exploitation. In addition, a lower tax base places those living alone with disabilities or the vulnerability of ageing at risk for a lower quality of life. This is of concern with nearly one-quarter of the population living alone (ABS 2009). If the trend towards living alone continues, it could also create a shortage of housing, and drive prices upward to where they are not affordable to many, whether these are young families or older people. More importantly, when individuals work long hours and live isolated lives there is a risk to family life and ultimately, community cohesion. However, there are a number of obstacles to increasing fertility rates. Despite government incentives such as child care subsidies, increasing the baby bonus or paid parental leave, there is a constellation of factors responsible for low birth rates that should be addressed. These include the need for equitable availability of child care centres, family and community support, gender relations at home and at work, family-friendly workplace policies, and parity of wages for women and men.

FAMILIES AND WORK

A major social trend of the past few decades that has had a profound effect on family life is the steady and dramatic transformation of the workforce (Palladino Schultheiss 2006). Across most countries the trend is towards large increases in dual-earner families and single parents in the workplace, and rapid transformation of the nature of work, all of which have had an unsettling effect on family life (Palladino Schultheiss 2006; Wierda-Boer et al 2009). Of course, unemployment has the most significant impact on the family, leaving family members without the resources for mutual support. For those employed, there has been a major trend towards casualisation of the workforce, which leaves many young families with little job security. Casualisation along with the trend towards working longer hours is thought to account for some couples delaying or forgoing children (Zubrick et al 2008).

Casualisation, part-time work and parental leave

Australia has a relatively large proportion of parents who work part-time (45% for women and 15% for men), which is higher than other Organisation for Economic Co-operation and Development (OECD) countries which serve as a benchmark (Commonwealth of Australia 2008). One reason for this may be the high cost and unevenness in access to formal child care. Most couples access flexible arrangements to share child care, with the most common employment pattern being a 'one and one-half earner' arrangement, where the father works full-time and the mother part-time (Commonwealth of Australia 2008). However, 35% of children up to age 4 and 14% of those aged 5–11 attend formal child care (Commonwealth of Australia 2008). Many Australian women, who comprise 58% of the workforce, return to work on a part-time basis in the first year after giving birth, which reflects family-friendly leave provisions, flexible working arrangements and the availability of affordable child care in their situation, but this is not standard across all workplaces. The Australian *Workplace Relations Act 1996* provides 52 weeks, unpaid leave following the birth of a baby, which can be shared between the parents (Commonwealth of Australia 2008). Some employers provide paid maternity leave for various lengths of time but this is left to their discretion, and just over half of Australian mothers are receiving paid parental leave (Commonwealth of Australia 2008).

Point to ponder

One of the most important trends to impact on family life over the past decades has been the rapid increase in the number of families in which both parents work.

In New Zealand, most adults in families with dependent children work at least some hours per week (Families Commission 2008). Over the past decade, there have been a range of family-friendly policies introduced to support them. These include 14 weeks, paid parental leave (under the *Parental Leave and Employment Protection (Paid Parental Leave) Act 2002* and its amendment in 2004), and 20 free hours of teacher-led care and education for 3- and 4-year-olds. Despite these policies, attaining the right mix of working hours and equitable distribution of work and child care responsibilities remains challenging for families (Colmar Brunton 2006). Over 29% of families with dependent children work 80 or more combined hours per week (Families Commission 2009a). Such long working hours bring multiple challenges for families and many call on extended-family members to assist with child care responsibilities. In particular, grandmothers frequently provide child care, often at great personal cost, given that many grandmothers today are engaged in part-time employment of their own, and many have carer responsibilities for an older family member. Child care therefore presents a major issue for social policy planners. For many mothers, difficult and stressful work, financial pressures and often an overlay of guilt from having to place their children in child care, may be acting as disincentives to having children at a time when there is a need for increased, rather than decreased birth rates.

Work and stress

The workplace of the 21st century generates considerable stress for workers. Globalisation has precipitated some of the changes, which include constant downsizing, outsourcing work and relocating industries to gain economies of scale. These changes are a result of the need for companies to respond quickly and competitively to global markets. As a result, Australian men work longer hours (43–45) than men in most other OECD countries (Commonwealth of Australia 2008; Zubrick et al 2008). Some workers caught in the competitive ethos have been forced to either seek alternative employment or relocate to other regions or other countries, which has implications for family life. In many workplaces the 'structure, pace and experience of work has intensified at a time when family structures have weakened in their ability to buffer workers from the stress of the economy' (Palladino Schultheiss 2006:334). In some cases, workers experience a sense of embeddedness or social connection with their work culture and workmates, which links them to a work-defined community. For others, work brings a sense of alienation and disconnection (Palladino Schultheiss 2006). Because both types of responses reflect the social worlds within which people interact, the boundaries between work and personal life are somewhat artificial and fluid.

Point to ponder

Growing demands in the workplace have seen both men and women work considerably longer hours than in the past. This can have profound implications on family life.

Stress in either the work or personal context can leak across the boundaries, creating difficulties, particularly where work is undertaken in highly competitive surroundings (Wierda-Boer et al 2009). This 'spillover' is more likely for those with inadequate coping skills, and it can erode a person's self-concept, making both their personal and work role difficult (Michel et al 2009; Palladino Schultheiss 2006; Wierda-Boer et al 2009). The challenges are more difficult for immigrant groups, especially if they experience stereotyping, restricted opportunities for advancement, bias or discrimination (Palladino Schultheiss 2006). For migrants from cultures that value traditional gender roles, work 'spillover', can be intense, particularly for men working in environments where gender roles are unfamiliar (Wierda-Boer et al 2009).

Conflicts in either work or family relationships can either stimulate or inhibit career progress, work-related tasks and family functioning. Both sides of the work–home boundary require clear navigation, and this begins with the opportunity to reflect on the goals of each (Palladino Schultheiss 2006). Palladino Schultheiss (2006) explains that the discourse of 'work–life' balance or 'work–family' balance may have created the misunderstanding that balance, in terms of time, involvement and satisfaction, is attainable.

Point to ponder

Achieving work–life balance is challenging for both men and women as careers become central to the identity of the individual.

For many people, successful work–family balance is often precarious. Like many men, women's careers are central to their identities. They have

high demands in the workplace, often having to outperform expectations, with their careers costing them more in their private lives than men's (Ezzedeen & Ritchey 2008). Some women find they must breach workplace standards that require masculine behaviours, but they also have a parallel problem in breaching social norms of caregiving, often having to relegate child care to outsiders (Ezzedeen & Ritchey 2008). However, researchers have found that support from co-workers and family members can provide a significant buffer for work–family conflict (Ezzedeen & Ritchey 2008; Michel et al 2009).

Those women with consistent, accessible and reliable support tend to be better equipped to weave the roles together than those without support (Palladino Schultheiss 2006). Ezzedeen and Ritchey's (2008) study of senior executive women found that while married women in high-level positions enjoyed concrete assistance with tasks from their spouses, what they most valued was their emotional support. This was particularly helpful when spouses could listen empathetically to their concerns and not try to fight their battles for them. They valued husbands' help with family members and their participation in household affairs, even when they were able to hire extra help. This type of assistance was seen as supporting their esteem, making a difference to their ability to cope with work pressures (Ezzedeen & Ritchey 2008). Support at home and in the workplace is extremely important for parents. However, not all parents receive this type of support. A large study of Australian parents indicated that approximately one in four felt they were receiving only low levels of support, which could be predictive of clinically significant psychological distress (Zubrick et al 2008). For those who did receive support, this was from family, parents, friends and a feeling of connection with their community (Zubrick et al 2008).

Gender issues and work

Conversations about the elusive (and some would say mythical) 'work–family balance' tend to focus on either single parents or dual-earner couples. However, gender issues are often hidden in workplace relationships. Lesbian, gay and bisexual families, unmarried partners with and without children also experience workplace difficulties, which can be exacerbated by stigma, isolation and invisibility (Palladino Schultheiss 2006).

The most evident issue is the gendered wage gap between male and female workers, but others include the disadvantage experienced by many women because of their responsibility for parenting-related absences. Other issues concern the language used in the workplace. for example, the 'working mother' term, which has no parallel 'working father' term. This maintains the stereotype that family responsibilities belong exclusively to mothers (Palladino Schultheiss 2006). Single employees without family responsibilities also have a unique set of issues, including the risk of having unequal access to benefits, a lack of respect for non-work life, occasional work expectations that exceed those with family responsibilities and social exclusion (Casper et al 2007). This set of discriminatory influences represents a backlash to the family-friendly workplace where more desirable assignments may be given to employees who are perceived to have greater needs because of parental responsibilities. Research indicates that this type of discrimination may be more problematic for those in low status, lower income jobs than those in a more privileged position (Casper et al 2007). Clearly, the goals of a family-friendly workplace should be inclusive and equitable working expectations and the provision of equal opportunities for all employees.

What's your opinion?

If a person in the workplace does not have family responsibilities, should they be expected to carry the load for a person in the workplace who does have family responsibilities and seeks to achieve a work–family balance?

A further workforce pressure in contemporary society lies in the growing number of older workers. Many older workers, especially older women, are seeking to delay retirement to respond to government policies that have reduced the affordability of living on a pension. Other changes affecting older workers flow from greater use of retrenchment and job redundancies for those unable to keep up with a highly competitive marketplace. On the other hand, some older workers stay in the workplace longer because of robust health, made possible by new medical technologies, or for other personal or professional reasons.

Fly-in fly-out families

Although each style of employment poses challenges to family life, the increase in the fly-in fly-out (FIFO) employment pattern in Australia has had a major impact on many families. Among other factors, the global economy and engineering technologies have contributed to an unprecedented resources boom in Australia that is expected to continue. The vast wealth of resources in regional and rural areas and a shortage of local workers have led companies to recruit large numbers of workers from urban areas with attractive remuneration. The workers fly to the exploration and mining or related infrastructure sites for several weeks at a time, then return home for a short break. While they are away, working hours are long with minimal time off. Leave can be unpredictable, as it is predominantly dictated by workplace need, with little room for negotiation by the worker. Another challenge lies in the worker's place of residence. Although there is an advantage to living in a place of their choosing (Guerin & Guerin 2009) if this is not a major city, there may be a further burden of travel for the worker. Many companies arrange to fly a worker in and out of the nearest capital city, which can be at a distance from workers living in regional or rural areas. In these cases, additional transportation costs to the capital city are self-funded.

Point to ponder

A fly-in fly-out family is one where the primary income earner spends several weeks working at a remote location away from the family, then returns for a short break at home before returning to work.

Despite substantial wages, the pervasiveness of the FIFO worker, or, in some cases, the drive-in drive-out (DIDO) worker (Guerin & Guerin 2009), has meant that some city suburbs and regional areas have large numbers of women raising their children without their partner for extended periods. Family life for those in the FIFO work pattern is somewhat similar to that of defence force families during periods of deployment, yet it is unique in that workers have numerous and frequent transitions in and out of the family environment. Unlike the military, where families have access to extensive training and counselling services, private FIFO employers provide little or no preparation for these transitions. Another issue surrounds the personal hardships associated with living in temporary accommodation with little or only intermittent health and social services (Guerin & Guerin 2009).

> **Point to ponder**
> A fly-in fly-out father has been likened to a non-residential father following divorce. Both parents and children have to constantly adjust to multiple entries and exits into family life.

For parents, the FIFO arrangement presents constraints to family life that are similar to those of separated families. The experience of the FIFO father can be similar to that of non-residential fathers following divorce, in that both parents and children have to make constant adjustments to the multiple entries and exits into family life. For these fathers, missing children's significant events or developmental milestones is a source of stress and anxiety. Moving from a partnered life to single men's accommodation also creates a plethora of stressors. These can include feelings of separation from family and support systems, exacerbated by a lack of telephone and internet access, and having little access to recreational facilities or time for relaxation. Some cope with the isolation in unhealthy ways, with alcohol or illicit substances. For the mothers left behind, anecdotal evidence indicates that some experience a sense of abandonment and isolation akin to being a sole parent. Mothers who have previously enjoyed the closeness of a partner relationship are forced to assume total responsibility for child care and the logistics of raising a family, as well as helping the children cope with their father's absences.

Although there is wide variation in the way individuals cope with these multiple transitions the accumulation of stress can lead to family disruption, depression and relationship breakdown. Some families adapt to this lifestyle by resettling in communities with a large number of FIFO families who provide an informal support system with a strong social network of families with a similar family situation.

> **Point to ponder**
> Support for the FIFO family remains scarce, with few agencies yet to provide appropriate services to meet the needs of this growing group of families. Nurses will have a growing role in supporting these families as the FIFO phenomenon becomes more common.

Research into the unique challenges encountered by FIFO families is slowly evolving. A small study of young men's views on the FIFO lifestyle indicated that having a positive attitude and effective coping mechanisms helps with psychological functioning and relationships while they are away, and adjustments when they make the transition to home (Carter & Kaczmarek 2009). A study by Taylor and Graetz Simmonds (2009) examined family qualities that enable FIFO families to function and enhance their satisfaction with family life. The families in this study, who completed a number of family assessment measures, were generally satisfied and had adapted to FIFO schedules by their commitment to flexibility and positive communication. Gallegos' (2006) in-depth interviews with FIFO family members also found communication crucial to their adjustment. She interviewed family members involved in the FIFO lifestyle to examine the transitions they experience. Participants in her study outlined the issues in relation to work and family roles, family identity issues, child development and attachment concerns, decision-making and communication challenges related to parenting, and dealing with emotional responses of all family members to the father's work schedule (Gallegos 2006). Suggestions from both workers and their partners included the need to improve the flow of information from support agencies about the realities of parenting in this type of lifestyle, and ensuring that information from the industry is clear on work schedules, travel requirements and entitlements (Gallegos 2006).

Communication from employers is particularly important, and the parents in Gallegos' (2006) study believed induction sessions should be provided for both parents. These could include a site visit where feasible, provision of safety information with emergency contact numbers, and information on policies related to family crises, fatigue management and company expectations. Parents also recommended support sessions for families on managing the stress of the emotional cycle associated with the FIFO employment and development of strategies for connecting parents, perhaps through industry websites. They also identified the need to implement an emergency home child care service or other practical supports that may be required when the father is absent (Gallegos 2006).

FIFO employment can add to the strain on marital relationships, or it can help build resilience. For cohabiting couples with a partner working in FIFO employment, there can also be difficulties in consolidating the partnership because of the intermittent nature of their relationships. In these cases, parenting and/or marriage is often delayed indefinitely until the couple can visualise a predictable future together. These couples spend the majority of their time as single adults, which can be socially awkward, leading to feelings of relationship insecurity. Like married couples, they transition frequently from the freedom of making their own decisions and organising their lifestyle according to personal needs to accommodating their part-time partner's needs when he/she arrives home. This can create a power imbalance in the couple relationship, and erode social relationships because of the tentativeness of their social life.

The Western Australian Government Department for Communities has developed a booklet for mothers to help them deal with parenting issues while their partner is away working (Support for Mum When Dad Works Away, Online. Available: www.community.wa.gov.au/DFC/Resources/ Parenting [accessed 23 April 2010]). However, support mechanisms for FIFO families are generally limited. Few counsellors are trained or have counselling experience in helping FIFO families. Extended-family members and friends often have limited understanding of their circumstances. This can lead to judgemental attitudes towards the worker and misunderstandings of why they are so often absent from the family home. There is also little understanding of the guilt experienced by the partners left behind when they develop other relationships and support systems outside the partnership. For nurses and other health professionals seeking to help these families or other families experiencing the strains of separation, non-judgemental interactions are paramount. The main objective of interventions with FIFO families is to help family members explore their feelings and ways of coping with the difficulties FIFO

employment presents for family relationships. In some cases, this is the role of the child and family nurse who encounters the parent in the context of child care visits. In other cases, the occupational health nurse onsite or employed by the company usually has an in-depth understanding of the issues and can help the worker explore his/her feelings and the implications of FIFO employment for family relationships. The issues surrounding FIFO employment illustrate the important role of nurses who work in a variety of community settings. In each case, they have to maintain a focus on the entire family and the particular circumstances within which they maintain health and wellbeing.

COUPLE RELATIONSHIPS

Although today's families assume various forms and styles, the intimate couple relationship remains central to family members' health and wellbeing. A strong, intimate couple relationship with warmth and open communication provides family members with a model for other relationships both within and external to the family. The importance of the couple relationship has been the subject of research studies demonstrating that parents' intimate relationship acts as a template for the quality and satisfaction of their children's subsequent relationships (Eldar-Avidan et al 2009; Ongaro & Mazzuco 2009; Sassler et al 2009). The type of partner an individual chooses to share her/his life depends on personal attitudes, values, norms of behaviour, identity and prior experience. All of these influences can be shaped either by their family of origin or events in their life (Ongaro & Mazzuco 2009). Becoming parents is a major event in the lives of many couples, one that

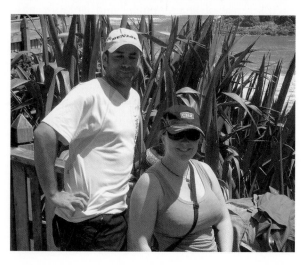

can cause difficulties in the couple relationship because of a decrease in their intimate or leisure time together (Claxton & Perry-Jenkins 2008). On the other hand, children can actually contribute to marital stability, acting as a deterrent to separation because of the financial, social and emotional costs of marital dissolution (Hewitt 2009).

Social influences on couple relationships

Societal changes also exert an influence on young adults' relationships. Couples are influenced by the general tolerance for divorce and cohabitation that exists in most societies, which was not tolerated in the past (Thornton 2009). In past times, traditional patterns of union formation saw many couples make companionate decisions about partnering, where a mate was chosen on the basis of compatibility. Today, there is a greater focus on individualised decisions, where a person seeks a partner who will support their personal development (Goldscheider et al 2009; Uecker & Stokes 2008). This does not negate the importance of the need for companionship, such as the need to spend leisure time together and share common interests (Claxton & Perry-Jenkins 2008). What is important is that couples understand each other's needs at the outset and throughout their relationship, and have a commitment to mutual self-development.

Social policies also affect couples' propensity to make decisions about marriage or cohabitation. In conservative areas such as exist in parts of the US, where marriage promotion schemes have been instituted to ensure young people's exposure to liberal family values, there is greater pressure on couples to marry (Heath 2009). Certain other social environments have a more laissez faire attitude, where young people are left to make up their own mind about partnering and marriage.

Parental marital history is another important influence on the choice of a partner and the style of partnership. Those who have been previously exposed to marital disruption tend to choose partners with similar experiences and often defer marriage until after a period of cohabitation (Goldscheider et al 2009). The timing of partnering or marriage also tends to be variable, sometimes influenced by socio-demographic factors. For example, rural women, those with a strong religious commitment, and those of low socio-economic status often marry earlier than others (Uecker & Stokes 2008).

Gender roles have always played a part in partner formation. Since the beginning of the feminist movement, women's preferences have changed, and women in the 21st century place less importance than in the past, on signs that a man is a good provider. Men, on the other hand, tend to place some importance on women's earning power, which has not historically been an influence in choosing a partner (Goldscheider et al 2009). Research also shows that for a woman, having children acts as a deterrent to finding a partner, unless a man has children of his own, especially for men with higher education levels (Goldscheider et al 2009). On the other hand, women with children are less likely to enter into a union with a man who has no marital or parental experience (Goldscheider et al 2009).

> **Point to ponder**
> Social policy and societal expectations can influence a couple's choices around marriage, cohabitation and the timing of children.

Relationship satisfaction

Because of the growing number of couple separations researchers have devoted an inordinate amount of time to studying partnership satisfaction (Claxton & Perry-Jenkins 2008). Most Australian married couples report that they are highly satisfied with their relationship, while those who are divorced, especially non-resident parents, report low levels of satisfaction (Commonwealth of Australia 2008). Research in the US indicates that cohabitors who marry often report lower marital quality and less satisfaction with their relationship than married couples (Lichter & Qian 2008). Research in the US indicates that co-habitors who subsequently marry often report lower marital quality and less satisfaction with their relationship than those whose initial union was marriage. This may be because committing to marriage in the first instance may be an indication of more realistic expectations than cohabitation. Reasons for this may be related to the tentativeness of living together, which feeds unrealistic expectations of their future as a couple. Cohabiting couples are less likely to pool resources and they must negotiate a number of decisions that may lead to conflict; for example, purchasing a home, having children, or dealing with relatives and friends. When a person has experienced multiple transitions from one union to another a stable relationship is less likely. This may be due to the fact that many serial cohabitors are from low socio-economic groups, some of whom have few resources for a successful marriage (Lichter & Qian 2008). However, it can also reflect an individual's lack of marriage commitment, their unconventionality, or it can be a function of the ease at which successive break-ups have been completed. For those cohabitors who do marry, the odds of divorce have been found to be double of those who have only ever lived with the one person they married (Lichter & Qian 2008). Research has also shown that marital quality tends to be poor among couples who have had a child during cohabitation, which may be explained partly by selection and partly by experience (Tach & Halpern-Meekin 2009). As a result, some individuals (low socio-economic groups, those who are depressed or mistrust their partner) may self-select to cohabit and have a child, a decision that might be daunting to others. The importance of commitment to marriage or partnership is widely recognised. Byrd (2009) explains three aspects of marital commitment in terms of social, interpersonal and legal elements. Personal reasons include an individual's preference to stay married, which may be an orientation towards sharing with a compatible other, the mutual benefit gained and personal fulfilment.

What's your opinion?
Couples who cohabitate report lower marital quality and less satisfaction with their relationship than married couples. What reasons do you think contribute to this finding?

Moral reasons for committing to another relate to feelings of obligation towards the marriage. Structural aspects reflect the constraints or barriers to not being married which can include children's disadvantage and financial considerations (Byrd 2009). Despite encountering difficulties such as financial strains, the arrival of children or challenging events, a strong relationship is multidimensional, the product of what is valued, shared goals, responses to experiences, and the potential of maintaining self-identity within the partnership.

Ideally, a couple relationship is one that:

> promotes the individual wellbeing of each partner and their offspring, assists each partner to adapt to life stresses, engenders a conjoint sense

of emotional and sexual intimacy and which promotes the long-term sustainment of a mutually satisfying relationship within the cultural context in which the partners live.

Halford (2000:14)

HEALTHY COUPLES, HEALTHY FAMILIES: COMMUNICATION AND RESILIENCE

A committed, well-functioning and stable relationship is associated with greater resilience to stressful events, better physical and mental health, greater work productivity and more effective parenting (Black & Lobo 2008; Guzzo & Lee 2008; Sanders, in Halford 2000; Waite & Gallagher 2000). Conversely, relationship problems are associated with increased potential for domestic violence, poor health, loss of productivity in the workplace and poor parenting (Halford 2000; Zubrick et al 2008). The risks for poor couple relationships are both static and dynamic. Static risk factors that predict breakdown include separation, divorce or violence in the family of origin, serial cohabitation, marrying young or having a history of depression or anxiety. Dynamic or changeable risk factors include poor communication and conflict management, unrealistic expectations of the relationship, inadequate mutual partner support, lack of balance between individual and shared activities, and inequitable division of household responsibilities (Halford 2000).

Point to ponder
A committed, well-functioning and stable relationship is associated with greater resilience to stressful events, better physical and mental health, greater work productivity and more effective parenting.

Relationship risks are also incurred at certain transitions in life: the critical moments in a family's development. These include the initial transition to marriage or cohabitation, the transition to parenting, subsequent re-partnering, times of family crisis, major illness and/or retirement (Halford 2000). The most significant transition is often the one that tests a couple's ability to manage personal attachment issues at the inception of their life as a family, as they learn to accommodate a highly dependent individual into their family

(Guzzo & Lee 2008). This transition has been described as 'relatively abrupt, adverse in nature, large in magnitude and likely to persist' (Lawrence et al 2008:41). Successful transition to parenting allows a couple to develop a secure base of emotional and social wellbeing. Most new parents experience a decline in their marital satisfaction, beginning in the latter stages of pregnancy and lasting throughout the first 12 months (Lawrence et al 2008). This effect is variable, depending on whether the pregnancy was expected, their level of satisfaction prior to the pregnancy and the ease of parenting (Lawrence et al 2008). Most parents return to a state of equilibrium in their relationship once they have adjusted to the normative decline in their couple relationship precipitated by parenthood (Claxton & Perry-Jenkins 2008).

The importance of family communication cannot be overstated. Family values, behaviours and relationships are encompassed in the way members communicate with one another and value one another's sense of self. Healthy communication patterns help each family member learn about others' needs and preferences and how to make personal choices in a supportive and trusting environment (Black & Lobo 2008). The main characteristics of successful family communication include clarity, open emotional expression, and collaborative problem-solving (Black & Lobo 2008). These help each member of the family develop personal self-esteem, self-regulation, trust and mutual respect (Cutrona 2004; Halford 2000).

> **Point to ponder**
> Effective communication strategies and shared power structures within families contribute to the creation of healthy families.

Family members need opportunities to express their feelings, thoughts and concerns; to receive active encouragement of spontaneity and authenticity; to have honest, constructive resolution of conflicts; and to receive clear, consistent and unambiguous messages that convey affection, support and acceptance (Friedman 1992).

Communication and power

A lack of clear communication can create confusion and misunderstanding, leading to mistrust and insecurity (Black & Lobo 2008). Where one family member dominates and controls communication and actions, others become disempowered. Healthy power structures in the family have a more egalitarian structure where there are flexible opportunities for sharing power, and for complementing, rather than subordinating one another. In a healthy family, individual members understand their respective roles in the family hierarchy and the extent to which they have authority over family decisions. This requires clear, predictable understanding of family role expectations and a commitment to sharing authority. Protracted problems with communication and power relations are destructive, often characterised by withdrawal and unresolved anger (Black & Lobo 2008). At their most serious, they can lead to family breakdown (Halford 2000). Communicating with compassion and understanding through conflicts is particularly important in developing individual comfort and security and helping children learn to work through problems in the future (Black & Lobo 2008). Ongoing dysfunctional communication and inter-parental discord can cause an accumulation of harmful effects for children. Parental depression may be a cause or consequence of family dysfunction, and this has a profound effect on child outcomes. Research has shown that the offspring of depressed parents are three times more likely to suffer from anxiety disorders, major depression or substance abuse in adulthood (Weissman et al 2006). Together, the co-existence of parental depression and marital conflict creates a multiplier effect, increasing children's risk for emotional insecurity (Kouros et al 2008).

Communication and change

Positive patterns of communication are significant during all periods of family change. Contemporary families have less predictability in their lifestyles than in previous times, more transitions and different configurations. Culture, experience, and personal and contextual factors conspire to create numerous permutations in the way family members adapt to change. Some families are able to accommodate variety and change without too many problems, allowing members their own pathways and styles of coping with change, while others hold fast to a level of protectiveness that may not be helpful to individual members. Most families interact along a continuum of responses, which change over time. To some extent, the family's responses to change depend on the degree to which their boundaries are more or less porous; the extent to which they tend to allow the external world in, and, in turn, open themselves to the outside world. This may also change as members adapt to different circumstances. For example, a tightly woven family with relatively closed boundaries may be temporarily helpful in times of grief and bereavement, which usually occur following a death in the family, or when family members depart the family home to begin their own lifestyle. However, if the family is overly protective in the event of this type of change, family members may not develop the skills they need to personally adapt to the situation or to other changing circumstances. If the family is able to maintain itself as a unit, to balance personal grief and individual needs while allowing compassion and help from others, there is a greater likelihood that family members will develop a more balanced and harmonious perspective. However, this also depends on the characteristics of individual members, some of who may find greater strength within, rather than outside the family.

Point to ponder

Positive patterns of communication are even more important in families during times of change.

Adaptation and resilience

The key to successful adaptation to change revolves around self-knowledge and being able to access the type and timing of support as it is needed, and being flexible and committed to others. These help build resilience in the face of change and tolerance for others' needs, strengths and patterns of adjustment. Family resilience is developed throughout the family lifecycle; the product of positive relationships that are enhanced and refined through problem-solving (Black & Lobo 2008). In this respect, resilient families demonstrate a potential for growth out of adversity, occurring through the exchange of a repertoire of positive coping behaviours and attributes. These include a positive outlook, spirituality, family member accord, flexibility, communication, financial management, time together, mutual recreational interests, routines and rituals, and social support (Black & Lobo 2008). Families who have a high level of resilience tend to survive the most difficult times, including the traumas of separation and divorce.

MARRIAGE, SEPARATION, DIVORCE AND PARENTING

Although researchers have been interested in studying marriage since the late 1800s, the past 30 years have seen heightened research and policy interest in marriage, separation and divorce and their effect on families (Walker 2004). A substantial body of research evidence has investigated the differential experiences of married and non-married couples to show the effect of marriage on personal health and wellbeing (Wright 2005). Many of these studies conclude that marriage has beneficial effects, but these are not experienced equally by men and women; nor are they consistent across time (Penman 2005). Women tend to be more satisfied with marriage in younger age groups, but become more dissatisfied as they get older, which may help explain the dramatic decline in marriages that endure over time, given that most separations are initiated by women (Halford 2000; Hewitt 2009; Penman 2005). The high rate of separation also illustrates a feminist, egalitarian perspective that traditional marriage serves patriarchal societies and it supports the suggestion that today's marriages should focus more on mutual affection and individual preferences than on maintaining societal standards (Amato 2004).

Point to ponder

Research demonstrates that marriage has beneficial effects but that these are not experienced equally by men and women, nor are they consistent across time.

Amato (2004) divides the scholarly debates on marriage into two camps: the marital decline perspective and the marital resilience perspective. The former group sees the retreat from marriage and the spread of single-parent households as a sign of individualistic norms that contribute to numerous social problems, including poverty, delinquency, violence, substance abuse, declining educational standards and the erosion of neighbourhoods and communities. In contrast, the latter group argues that separation and divorce provides a second chance for happiness and an escape from dysfunctional families. This side argues that poverty, unemployment, poorly funded schools, discrimination and the lack of health and other public services represent a more serious threat to the health of society than does the decline in married, heterosexual, two-parent families (Amato 2004). Most people believe that family separation and divorce present the greatest challenges in modern social life, given that most family members involved experience some kind of trauma, which remains for long periods after the marriage has ended. For some people, having experienced divorce in one's family is particularly detrimental to a healthy relationship. Divorce is a complex and long-lasting event which diverts a person's life course and requires new roles and relationship patterns as well as integration of events and emotions (Eldar-Avidan et al 2009). In terms of the family as a system, divorce affects the subsystems as well as the couple divorcing. This has effects on relatedness, closeness and differentiation among all family members, which influences their responses and reactions (Eldar-Avidan et al 2009).

Point to ponder

Separation and divorce have significant effects on the family. Successful coping and adaptation can be maximised if the divorce is harmonious and if stress is minimised.

For some family members, divorce creates new ways of coping and can be capacity building. Successful coping and adaptation can be maximised if the divorce is harmonious, if stress is minimised, and if the residential parent is able to sustain authoritative parenting and not inflict a parent role on the child (Hetherington 1999).

Divorce and parenting

The rate of divorce in society is a major challenge for parents. Numerous studies have shown that children raised by two happily and continuously married parents have the best chance of developing into competent and successful adults (Hetherington & Kelly 2002). Couples who maintain a satisfying relationship have been found to have skills, attitudes and behaviours that translate into higher levels of parental warmth towards their children (Zubrick et al 2008). A number of early studies on the effect of divorce on children

focused on studying children's resilience and the reasons why some children become resilient and well adjusted, while others experience negative and pervasive effects (Amato & Rivera 1999; Kouros et al 2008). Some of this research sought to allay the fears of separating parents that their actions would have adverse effects on their children by showing that it is better for the children when parents separate rather than remaining in a home with high marital conflict (Hetherington 1999; Louis & Zhao 2002; Wallerstein et al 2000). However, after 25 years of studying the effects of divorce on children, researchers have concluded that many of the children who showed resilience soon after divorce had difficulties with their own relationships when they became adults (Hetherington & Kelly 2002; Sassler et al 2009; Wallerstein et al 2000). Hetherington (1999) suggests that this may have been due to a lack of studies comparing children's adjustment in high-conflict divorced and non-divorced families. The more recent findings are also linked to increases in low-conflict divorces, which are less readily accepted by children, and a decline in their economic wellbeing (Eldar-Avidan et al 2009).

Although some children show resilient behaviours, more often than not, they experience distress, apprehension, confusion and anger in response to marital conflict and divorce (Amato 2004; Hetherington 1999; Kouros et al 2008; Wallerstein et al 2000). As adults, children of divorce also experience higher marital instability themselves and tend to have a reduced belief in marriage as a long-lasting institution (Ongaro & Mazzuco 2009; Teachman 2002). Many young women whose parents have divorced enter into cohabitation rather than marriage and delay parenthood (Ongaro & Mazzuco 2009). For most young people, especially adolescents, adjusting to the transitions that follow separation and divorce presents an enormous personal challenge. Young adolescents have the highest rates of difficulty adjusting to marital separation and step-family life (Russell & Bowman 2000). This appears to be related to a lack of consistency. Many children of divorce experience transient family groupings and a number of stressful challenges as the family establishes various boundaries, deals with children's access to parents, consolidates new relationships, reconstitutes the family unit and plans for step-parenting.

> **Point to ponder**
> The impact of divorce on children and adolescents is significant. Although some children demonstrate resilience, it is distress, apprehension, confusion and anger that are more common.

Divorce and the blended family

The blending of two families can be a difficult situation with many ups and downs as some or all of the members of both families become part of the core family for indeterminate lengths of time. Parental conflict, distress and the adjustments of divorce place children at risk for such negative outcomes as depression, withdrawal, conduct disorder, poor social competence, health problems and academic underachievement (Halford 2000). Children's emotional difficulties include a profound sense of loss when parents are too preoccupied with their own adjustment to adequately meet their emotional needs, and when the parent–child relationship deteriorates. Inadequate role modelling or a lack of support can create lasting difficulties for children in developing intimate relationships as adults (Eldar-Avidan et al 2009). On the other hand, when both parents are sensitive, responsive, nurturing and able to stimulate their children, there is a greater likelihood of favourable outcomes for children (Berlyn et al 2008).

The impact of divorce on parents

Parents are also at risk of poor outcomes from marital dissolution, with the most prevalent problem being financial difficulties, especially for residential parents, the majority of whom are mothers (Smyth 2004a). Women who become the head of a separated household tend to be affected most by economic difficulties, referred to as either the 'feminisation of poverty', or the 'pauperisation of motherhood'. The poverty of mothers raising children alone has been documented throughout the world and is not only an issue for the women themselves but, as many researchers have discovered, it is the most significant predictor of child outcomes (Keating & Hertzman 1999; Stanley et al 2005; United Nations Family Planning Association [UNFPA] 2000). Because women are most often the partner seeking dissolution of a marriage, they have attracted criticism for complaining about impoverishment, but this is a reality for many, given the difference in each partner's earning capacity. It is also an example of gender inequity in terms of what both men and women are entitled to, in life as well as the workplace. For single mothers, being the parent in the home has the advantage of being accessible to children at times of their greatest need, and being part of significant moments in their lives.

> **Point to ponder**
> Parents are also at risk following divorce. Women who go on to become head of a separated household are at particular risk of economic difficulties following marriage dissolution.

Non-resident parenting

Despite a growing proportion of single-father families, most men become non-resident parents following divorce (Goldscheider et al 2009). These fathers typically experience a deterioration of their lifestyle related to shrinking finances, but men tend to recover to a greater degree than their former wives. A more serious problem for non-resident fathers is their difficulty in maintaining a warm and enduring father–child relationship with their children (Eldar-Avidan et al 2009; Le Bourdais et al 2002; Swiss & Le Bourdais 2009). The reasons for this relationship difficulty are related to the father's pre-divorce parenting practices and relationships, financial resources, his satisfaction with access arrangements, his relationship with the children's mother in terms of parenting, the closeness of his residence to the children, and their age, stage and gender (Swiss & Le Bourdais 2009). The presence of another man acting as the social parent to his children may also affect a non-resident father's relationship with his children (Berger et al 2008). Studies of fathering comparing 'biological fathers' and 'social fathers' have shown mixed results, with some indications that social fathers engage in higher cooperative parenting styles and accept more shared responsibilities for parenting than married fathers. However, this may be due to the mother's selection of this type of husband, or because the new social father may be working to ensure quality and stability in the new relationship (Berger et al 2008).

> ### Point to ponder
> Men are more likely than women to become the non-residential parent following divorce. Although men experience deterioration in financial circumstances in these cases, the greatest impact on men is on their relationship with their children.

The importance of fathers remaining involved with their children is widely acknowledged, as fathering plays a significant role in children's health and wellbeing (Halle et al 2008). When both parents cooperatively plan to meet children's needs without conflict there is a greater likelihood of fathers' ongoing involvement with their children (Swiss & Le Bourdais 2009). The advantages of father involvement include economic, social and developmental benefits for children as well as higher satisfaction among fathers for their role as parents (Berlyn et al 2008; Gillies 2009; Swiss & Le Bourdais 2008). Where legal arrangements dictate access and child support, there may be lower levels of contact between fathers and their children, often because of financial difficulties. This has a reciprocal effect on both fathers and their children, as the father's emotional state can influence the quality of his parenting (Halle et al 2008). A large body of research has shown an association between the quantity and quality of father involvement and improved cognitive outcomes for their children (Amato & Rivera 1999), while the absence of a paternal figure has been linked to lower academic achievement and increased conduct disorder in children (Pfiffner et al 2001). A study in the UK on paternal interactions with infants under 1 year of age showed that the more hours fathers spent with their children the happier the child was (Lewis et al 2008). Clearly, when children have adequate access to their father, there are numerous gains for the children and a greater chance of fathers being satisfied with their parental role and remaining close to their children (Le Bourdais et al 2002; Lewis et al 2008).

Parenting and child support

Child support laws can also disadvantage low socio-economic fathers by requiring a greater proportion of their finances than wealthier men (Swiss & Le Bourdais 2009). Low-earning fathers may be further disadvantaged by having to work variable shifts or during weekends when their children are available to see them. Swiss and Le Bourdais (2009) suggest that these difficulties faced by fathers are not well understood in the legal justice system, and practical factors should therefore be taken into account by those determining father access. Their employment often dictates the extent to which they can be involved in their children's lives, yet without employment they are unable to provide for their family (Gillies 2009). In many cases, when financial barriers or the multiple responsibilities of two families arise, fathers tend to distance themselves, which reduces children's opportunities to have the advantage of both parents' support.

Although many people survive the emotional trauma of marital separation, it is often one of the most stressful events in a person's life. For men who become non-residential parents, the effects include poor health and wellbeing, which often lasts up to 10 years, especially if the relationship has ended against their wishes (O'Brien & Rich 2002). The risks to health are most evident in the period immediately following separation, particularly if initial interventions are 'legalistic, adversarial, distancing, or uncoordinated' (Moloney 2005:14). The separation of fathers from the family home can also lead to ongoing isolation of the father, which has been known to last into older age. Without the civilising influence of the family, many divorced fathers are at risk of being the population most in need of support during ageing (Gillies 2009; Lin 2008).

Divorce and the rights of the child

In many countries, new approaches to divorce laws have followed the lead set by the British *Family Law Act of 1992*, which mandated a parenting plan to be devised at the time of divorce. This ensures that the rights of children supersede the rights of either parent. Parenting plans represent one of the most important initiatives in helping families adjust to divorce. They are designed to document both parents' negotiated goals and intentions to ensure safety, physical and emotional care, education and legal responsibilities throughout their children's childhood. Parenting plans consist of detailed information on children's living arrangements and contact schedules, financial support, parents' decision-making responsibilities and dispute-resolution processes (Smyth 2004b).

Development of a parenting plan also helps to separate the processes of resolving money and property disputes from those involving the children. The plan is based on a humanising approach to providing for the children's wellbeing after parental separation to help to counter the effect of emotionally intense legal negotiations that often interfere with rational decision-making.

> ### Point to ponder
> Parenting plans document both parents' negotiated goals and intentions to ensure the safety of children during and following divorce. They are one of the most important initiatives available to assist families adjusting to divorce.

Attitudes towards divorce and parenting are changing, and this is having an effect on the language of the law as well as parenting. In the past, conflicts between separating parents often interfered with positive parenting. Many of these conflicts were related to custody of children. With an increasing body of research into post-divorce parenting, the child-rearing role of both parents is acknowledged, regardless of residence (Gillies 2009; Lewis et al 2008; Lin 2008; Swiss & Le Bourdais 2009). New legislation in many countries has seen the language of separation and divorce changed to reflect the fact that custody of children is no longer the most important issue. Instead, the emphasis is on allowing children access to parents, rather than the other way around. This elevates the role of the non-residential parent to a more equal status than previously, when the emphasis was on survival of the single-parent-headed household. Today, it is expected that both parents will create opportunities to contribute to their children's development not only financially, but emotionally and socially as well.

The focus of contemporary research into divorcing families is not so much on laying blame, as it is in emphasising the importance of parental support in ensuring love, security and support to achieve healthy social and cognitive development in children (Eldar-Avidan et al 2009; Kouros et al 2008; Swiss & Le Bourdais 2009; Wallerstein et al 2000). Widespread public debate about marriage, fertility, reproductive technologies and adoption have also drawn areas of discrimination into sharp focus. As a result, there is greater visibility of diverse family

forms and a family's rights to raise children, regardless of the family composition. However, when the subject of family diversity is aired publicly, it tends to attract heated criticism from those who believe that alternative family forms erode family values. The people on this side of the argument tend to favour the neoliberal, moral right wing of politics, which is often argued on the basis of a narrow religious view of what constitutes a legitimate family (Heath 2009).

>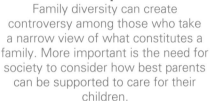
> ### Point to ponder
> Family diversity can create controversy among those who take a narrow view of what constitutes a family. More important is the need for society to consider how best parents can be supported to care for their children.

Coltrane (2001) argues that confining the debate to what constitutes a 'legitimate family' encourages rigid social mores such as premarital sexual abstinence, male family headship, females having to identify with the family, and resistance to feminism, homosexuality, cohabitation, abortion and related issues. Instead, the discourse of family issues should recognise the gendered and generational power dynamics that disadvantage both mothers and fathers when the children are not at the centre of policies and practices (Fletcher 2008; Gillies 2009). Clearly, there is a need in society for consideration of how parents can be supported in doing the best they can for their children. A good start would be to refrain from discriminating comments about parents who choose to remain at home to raise their children or who would like to take advantage of family-friendly child care policies, but cannot for reasons of maintaining employment (Gillies 2009). Polarised arguments to the right or the left side of politics do the family a disservice by focusing attention on morality and historical family structures, rather than jobs, poverty, equity, diversity, safe neighbourhoods, parenting, child care and health care; in other words, the social determinants of health that make families strong.

VIOLENCE IN THE FAMILY

One of the greatest risks to the health and wellbeing of families is violence among family members, the infliction of abuse by one family member against another. This can include child to parent violence, elder abuse, intra-familial abuse or intimate partner violence, the latter of which is the most frequent form of violence in the family (Schofield & Walker 2008; Stewart et al 2004–05; Thornton et al 2008). Abusive intimate relationships can be categorised in terms of legal, fear-based or injury-based definitions (Sheehan & Smyth 2000). The legal definition includes the occurrence, attempt or threat of violence. Fear-based violence includes any act or threat to a person, causing fear for their wellbeing and safety. Injury-based violence refers to the severity of the act, as one that requires clinical intervention (Sheehan & Smyth 2000).

In the 1990s a declaration by the United Nations (UN) identifying violence against women as a human rights violation attracted global attention and outrage (Campbell 2001). Also in the 1990s, the WHO declared domestic violence a public health problem, and in 1995 the World Conference for Women in Beijing incorporated women's right to live without violence into a set of recommendations to the 23rd special session of the UN General Assembly (UNFPA 2000). In 2002, in response to continuing rates of violence around the world, WHO commissioned a first World Report on Violence and Health (Heise & Garcia-Moreno 2002). These reports by the WHO and the UN drew international attention to what is now considered a major public health problem affecting families and communities.

Point to ponder

Family violence is one of the greatest risks to the health and wellbeing of families. Nurses have a significant role in screening for and supporting victims of family violence.

Intimate partner violence

The most common form of violence in the family, intimate partner violence (IPV) is linked to gendered power relations (Vincent & Eveline 2008). Regardless of the type of abuse, a major element in this type of violence is the power and control exerted over the woman by her partner, who may have exclusive access to family resources. Without personal resources many women tend to stay in abusive families to ensure their children have a home. However, this leaves the situation unchanged, and the woman typically becomes more disempowered over time, causing low self-esteem, self-worth and self-confidence (Wilson et al 2004–05). Women in this type of relationship become trapped within a cycle of daily disempowering conditions. This is because relationships between intimate partners are unlike any other social relationships in that they involve a wide range of contacts, eating, sleeping, co-parenting, playing, working, decision-making and sexual activity (Liang et al 2005). Liang et al (2005:75) explain that the 'fluid, liberal, and intimate nature of these interactions may make subtle violations and abuses difficult to detect and harder still to understand or define'. Over time many women suffer severe, complex and protracted physical and emotional ill health and a range of sequelae that include chronic ill health, depression, anxiety and stress-related syndromes from the abusive situation (Schofield & Walker 2008; Tower et al 2006).

Point to ponder

Intimate partner violence (IPV) is violence directed towards the intimate partner in a relationship. IPV is most often directed towards a woman by a man.

IPV is thought to affect somewhere between 20% and 40% of women, with a lack of certainty due to under-reporting. One-third of Australian women with a current or former partner report having experienced at least one form of violence, with 40% experiencing at least one incident of physical or sexual violence since age 15 (Murray & Powell 2009). A study in New Zealand showed that 34% of women in Auckland had experienced IPV at some time in their lives, with 5% of women reporting violence in the previous 12 months (Fanslow & Robinson 2004). The accuracy of figures on violence against Indigenous women is particularly unclear, given the propensity of many Indigenous families to protect family and kinship culture at their personal expense. Figures suggest that Indigenous women are thought to be up to 45 times more likely to be victims of IPV and 10 times more likely than non-Indigenous women to be murdered (Vincent & Eveline 2008). However, the experience of Indigenous women is complex and includes a combination of factors related to colonisation history, racism and marginalisation as well as their social and economic vulnerability (Cripps & McGlade 2008).

Societal factors also have an impact on violence in the home. IPV, like rape and other forms of sexual coercion occur in a microcosm of societal conditions fuelled by economic exclusion and patriarchal attitudes of entitlement (McMurray 2006; Moloney 2008). When this becomes entrenched in society, it sends a signal to women that they are not worthy of participating in certain aspects of social life. IPV is therefore a public health problem that compromises the capacity of women and children who are its victims to live safe, dignified, empowered lives (McMurray 2006). Victims of IPV are often subjected to multiple forms of abuse, with many women experiencing a combination of physically threatening acts, verbal abuse and sexual violence (Schofield & Walker 2008). The cost to society is substantial, both socially and economically (Murray & Powell 2009). The abuse of women is a violation of societal norms of behaviour in a civilised society. Yet the injustice continues without sanction from politicians or policy makers, especially for Indigenous women whose perpetrators are excused on the basis of alcohol and drug abuse, or 'problems' in their community (Vincent & Eveline 2008), which we discuss in Chapter 11.

IPV and the children

In some families, there is a co-occurrence of IPV and child abuse (Wilson et al 2004–05; Terrance et al 2008). In the US the overlap between woman and child abuse is estimated at 30–70% per year, with more than 3 million children witnessing their mothers being abused (Johnson & Sullivan 2008). Studies in Australia and New Zealand found that 23% and 17% respectively had witnessed violence in the home against their mother or step-mother in the previous year (Adolescent Health Research Group 2008; Indermaur 2001). Witnessing such violence was also associated with an increased likelihood of being both a victim of violence and of perpetrating it (Families Commission 2009b). Indermaur's (2001) study estimated that 14% of Australian children in two-parent families are exposed to family violence, but the prevalence grows exponentially to where it is estimated that 41% of children living with their mother and a new partner witness violence in the family. This is a serious threat to child health and wellbeing in that witnessing violence can cause children to experience the same psychological and behaviour problems as having been abused themselves (Johnson & Sullivan 2008).

Point to ponder
Studies in Australia and New Zealand have found that 23% and 17% of children respectively, had witnessed violence in the home against their mother or step-mother.

Observing and experiencing violence creates a 'cradle of violence' for antisocial adulthood (Strauss 2001:187). The signs that a child is becoming violent may be evident even before adolescence, when normal rebelliousness deteriorates into child-to-mother violence. Child-to-mother violence is often disguised as juvenile delinquency, rather than being disclosed as an intentional act perpetrated against a parent to intimidate, or cause physical, psychological or financial damage (Stewart et al 2004–05). Like other forms of violence, a child's aggressive behaviour is often covered up in the home because of parents' hesitancy to be judged incompetent, so the parents often end up assuming blame for their own victimisation (Stewart et al 2004–05). Social learning theory (Bandura 1977) suggests that when children are exposed to violence they may acquire aggressive behaviour patterns based on what they observe in the home, developing the perception that violence and aggression are normal and acceptable (Proctor 2006). This can be exacerbated if they live in a violent neighbourhood or community, where children and adolescents may experience a wide range of negative outcomes, including internalised distress and symptoms of post-traumatic stress disorder (Proctor 2006). Exposure to community violence has been linked to aggressive, antisocial, disruptive behaviours, physiological markers of stress, social maladjustment in the peer group, diminished academic achievement and early onset of substance abuse (Proctor 2006).

For separating parents, the rates of violence are difficult to estimate, as many couples experience unprecedented levels of conflict during and for some time after separation and divorce. For those cases that reach the family court, no separate statistics on family violence are kept as distinct from undifferentiated parenting disputes (Shea Hart & Bagshaw 2008). A woman's decision to end her marriage is often a precipitating factor for violence and this may be exacerbated by the injustice felt by male partners in an era of heightened awareness of men's roles in parenting. Heightened awareness of issues around fathering and the protracted grief experienced by many men often precipitates violence, even among men who have not previously been violent or where violent behaviours have not been part of their lives. Separation may also be a trigger to violence in migrant men, particularly those from cultures where violence is more readily tolerated than in their host country. Other factors may be related to the major changes in power relations when couples migrate to a country where women have greater authority and status than in their country of origin, when migrant women first enter the workplace, and in families without extended family support (Naeem et al 2008).

MIGRANT FAMILIES AND HEALTH

The transition to a new country is complex for all family members and affects family interrelationships in both subtle and overt ways. Some families experience a conflict of competing cultures, as young family members straddle old and new ways of thinking about such things as child care, being working parents, separation and divorce, and the need for space and solitude in their frenetic lives. These situations can evoke intense emotion from those who prefer to see the family as a source of stability rather than change. In contrast, some families embrace changes, especially if it means improvement in the family's lifestyle or health, wellbeing or opportunities for prosperity.

> **Point to ponder**
> Migration to a new country can create new opportunities for families but can also be one of the most stressful periods in a family's life course.

Most immigrant families migrate to countries with better opportunities than they have previously experienced because of poverty, dangerous or destructive living conditions, political or individual freedom, or to provide better opportunities for their children (Chuang & Gielen 2009). Leaving their homes, friends and relatives is stressful, as is the need to make adjustments to completely new lifestyles, social, education and employment systems. This can be extremely challenging if they also encounter discrimination, prejudice and feelings of isolation (Chuang & Gielen 2009). Once migrant families do make the transition, their culturally bounded view of parenting may be challenged by their children's assimilation into the new culture, transforming family dynamics and values across the generations (Chuang & Gielen 2009). This can be difficult for parents, especially if they have been used to extended family support in their country of origin.

Migration and family life

Migration from poor to wealthy countries creates tensions for all concerned, but the emphasis in public opinion seems to be placed on the strain on the host country's resources from waves of migration. At the same time, there is widespread debate over how to meet skills shortages. Obviously, the two issues are being discussed in the same arena, but there remains a need for stronger discussion as to how migrant people can be educated and employed in the areas of greatest need without disempowering them, or denigrating their lifestyles. The timing of migration is also important to family life and can be disruptive to family stages (Clark et al 2009). In many cases, young families make the transition to both parenthood and a new country at the same time, which increases their level of transitional stress. A lack of support at this time has a potential negative effect on subsequent patterns of family development and the family's ability to connect with the wider community. Sometimes the transition of migration is made easier by resettlement in a place where there is an enclave of people sharing the same ethnic identity, but this is not always possible, especially if employment dictates otherwise. Searching for adequate employment after resettlement can place multiple strains on family members, especially if they experience multiple moves to be close to their workplaces. Additional family disruptions may occur when adolescent children attempt to adjust to their new surroundings, and are made responsible for siblings at the same time as they are transitioning to school or the new environment (Hafford 2009).

Migrants, refugees, stress and coping

Economic deprivation or traumatic pre-migration experiences can also have profound effects on the family's adaptation to the new environment. Some families endure long periods of adjustment when family members have experienced torture and trauma, changing roles, separation or death of family members, language difficulties or cultural behaviours that conflict with their country of origin (Lewig et al 2009). These difficulties can be eased if support systems are provided by health and social service professionals who have a good understanding of their unique experiences and expectations (Lewig et al 2009). Lewig et al's (2009) research into refugee families' parenting challenges in South Australia found that the major challenges were linked to tensions between Australian laws and cultural norms and traditional cultural parenting beliefs and practices. Disciplining children was a particular area of difference in parenting. Refugee families found the inappropriateness of physical discipline in Australia challenging, as they had been used to stronger control over children's behaviour (Lewig et al 2009). Parents also believed that child care should be undertaken in the family, often by older siblings. They were also concerned about the lack of structured activities in the community where mothers could meet one another and share parenting skills, as well as activities for adolescents after school to encourage their engagement with the community (Lewig et al 2009).

Point to ponder

Refugee families face particular challenges when arriving in a new country. Many refugees have been subject to or witnessed torture, trauma, separation or death of family members.

Other research into the migrant experience shows that it is an extended process rather than a discrete event that affects family life for many years after physical relocation (Lassetter & Callister 2009). Even for voluntary migrants the processes of adaptation create health effects linked to the 'stress of the move, climate differences, racism, separation from family members and modifications in their physical environment, lifestyle and cultural milieu' (Lassetter & Callister 2009:94). These effects are linked to the interplay of structural and cultural factors (Clark et al 2009). Some factors may interfere with acculturation or cause deteriorating health, including disease exposure, risky behaviours such as alcohol and tobacco consumption, lifestyle exposure to non-nutritious foods and inaccessible culturally appropriate ingredients, unhealthy habits, a lack of holistic health care and experiences with racism (Lassetter & Callister 2009).

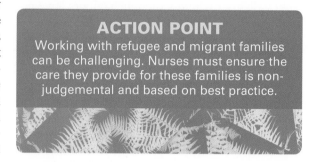

ACTION POINT

Working with refugee and migrant families can be challenging. Nurses must ensure the care they provide for these families is non-judgemental and based on best practice.

Adjustment to a new country can also be confronting if norms in the host country are incompatible in terms of religious or moral values (Clark et al 2009; Lassetter & Callister 2009). However, protective factors, such as marital stability, or serial migration, where family reunion programs have brought more than one generation of the family to the same area, can help families adjust to their new environment (Clark et al 2009). The post-migration environment is also important in establishing a pattern for the future, as well as helping families work through their adjustment. Essential elements in this process include the presence of cultural and religious supports, accessible education and health care resources, social support services and a political environment in their resettlement country that is amenable to peace and stability. (see Box 5.2)

FAMILIES DEALING WITH ILLNESS

Many families provide informal family care for illness for one or more of their members. In many cases, illnesses in children are transient and although they present logistical difficulties associated with employment schedules, they are not a source of major stress. However, other families have protracted caring responsibilities for someone with chronic illness or disability, or during the period of palliative care for someone at the end of life. Although families have always had to deal with illness, injury and death, in today's society, with so many people either living alone, or where both adults in a household work full-time, there is a declining pool of family members available to provide caregiving. Consequently, those who are available experience a larger burden of care than they would in the past, when large families were able to share caregiving arrangements among various family members.

The New Zealand government has one of the most open refugee policies in the Western world, being one of only 10 UN member states who accept refugee quotas over and above those arriving spontaneously at their borders. New Zealand is a party to both the 1951 Convention and the 1967 Protocol Relating to the Status of Refugees. Annually, the New Zealand government accepts a refugee 'quota' of 750 places mandated by the office of the United Nations High Commissioner for Refugees (UNHCR). These refugees arrive in groups of 125 six times each year. The New Zealand government gives preference to refugees who fall under the categories of 'women at risk', those needing 'protection', and those with a 'medical condition or disability'. An additional 1800 asylum seekers arrive in New Zealand annually and apply for asylum on arrival. Once in New Zealand, 'quota' refugees spend six weeks at a refugee resettlement centre where they undergo medical assessment, receive English language lessons and gain information on life in New Zealand. After the initial six-week period, the refugees travel to their new homes in a variety of locations throughout New Zealand. An attempt is made to co-locate refugees from similar cultures to assist in the transition to life in New Zealand (Online. Available: www.refugeehealth. govt.nz [accessed 26 February 2010]). The New Zealand government also accepts 300 sponsored family members to reunite with refugees who have already resettled in New Zealand. Research into the resettlement process in New Zealand found that the process of resettlement is ongoing and that some refugees may never fully participate in life in New Zealand to the same extent as other residents. Refugees however did report feeling safe in New Zealand and that for the most part people and organisations were friendly and helpful (New Zealand Immigration Service 2004).

Point to ponder
Families who provide care to a family member experiencing disability contribute the equivalent of around $30.5 billion worth of care to the Australian economy, with little in the way of reciprocal support.

Family caregiving provides a major contribution to the 20% of Australians and 17% of New Zealanders who live with some type of disability (Australian Institute of Health and Welfare [AIHW] 2008; Bascand 2006). This has been estimated to represent around $30.5 billion worth of caregiving services per year in Australia (Commonwealth of Australia 2008). Indigenous Australians experience even higher rates of disability (36%) than non-Indigenous Australians, and these represent a larger proportion of severe, chronic and long-term core activity limitations, placing an inordinate burden on caregiving families (AIHW 2008). Maori have higher rates of disability compared to all other ethnic groups in New Zealand. Of particular note is the burden of disability for Maori appears at a significantly younger age — 80% of Maori experiencing disability were aged under 45 years compared with 54% of the European New Zealand population (Bascand 2006).

Family caregiving issues

Adults, predominantly women aged 35–39 experience the greatest burden of care, as many are 'sandwich carers', acting as the primary caregiver for children as well as older persons with disabilities or ageing parents. Most carers live with those needing their assistance, spending 20 hours or more a week, with some taking on full-time caring responsibilities of 40 hours or more a week (Commonwealth of Australia 2008). Older carers often have chronic illnesses of their own, and this can create considerable personal stress, especially for those who live in the same home as the person requiring assistance. Many pay a high price financially, as they are unable to maintain paid employment at the same time as they fulfil their caring responsibilities.

Point to ponder
Family caregiving places considerable stress on those providing the care — most often women aged 35–39 who are likely to be trying to simultaneously care for children and elderly parents, and hold down a job.

Additional financial pressures arise from the need to purchase special equipment, health services or respite care (Commonwealth of Australia 2008). Because of the financial disadvantage researchers have found a strong link between disability and poverty (Fremstad 2009). With population ageing the future burden of caregiving in the family will be significant, as many older people require some form of assistance, ranging from help with hearing devices to the constant help needed for those with dementia (Commonwealth of Australia 2008). Deinstitutionalisation of the mentally ill and policies that have eliminated many disability and aged care services have also placed increased burden of care on family caregiving. Other pressures on informal caregivers are related to increased rates of family breakdown, leaving even fewer family members available for caregiving, especially for their elders. The economic difficulties experienced by many families reflect parallel problems in the health care industry, which is increasingly required to do more with less. We live in an era of 'drive-through' health care, where the cost of caring for people in hospital has proven prohibitive for all but the most critically ill. This has resulted in shorter stays in hospital and more people being discharged home 'quicker and sicker', with highly complex needs. These people usually have access to some home care, but the amount and acuity of their care that is absorbed by family members is significantly greater than in the past. It also places a burden on hospital staff, who find that developing health literacy in patients and family members within a 24-hour hospital stay is almost impossible. The ongoing challenge for all concerned with home and community care is to ensure there are opportunities for patients and carers to develop the knowledge and skills required for self-management, and this requires ongoing attention to the adequacy of community-based services.

Caring for children with disabilities

One of the most difficult caring challenges is in caring for a child with intellectual disability. These family caregivers typically provide care over long periods of time, which can create serious family strain (Tsai & Wang 2009). Caring for a chronically disabled child can also lead to feelings of guilt, separation from society, depression, marital problems and anxiety about their child's future (Tsai & Wang 2009). The imperative to care for a chronically disabled child often continues into adulthood, presenting further challenges for the family. Unlike families whose children do not have disabilities, their adult children are unable to achieve independence and leave the family home. Unable to seek their identity outside the family unit during this phase of life, those with disabilities must continue to define themselves within the home, which deprives them of a normal transition to adult life (Todd & Jones 2005).

Point to ponder
One of the most challenging family caregiving roles is caring for a child with an intellectual impairment.

As with all family members dealing with a chronic illness, caregivers for those with a disability suffer from fatigue and emotional irritability, particularly where there is a lack of social support (Tsai & Wang 2009). This can create emotional overload, leading to stress, burnout and constant worry (Jeon et al 2005). For caregivers of family members with severe mental illness such as schizophrenia, carer concerns revolve around the occurrence of a crisis. The intermittent, episodic nature of acute crises requires constant vigilance, similar to caring for a family member with epilepsy, diabetes, asthma or a cardiac condition. When the problem is mental illness finding appropriate sources of respite is difficult due to the unpredictable nature of acute episodes and the need for highly skilled staff and resources (Jeon et al 2005).

Caregiver stress

Although health professionals attempt to provide sufficient information and support to family caregivers, research studies have revealed that they often overestimate family members' health-related knowledge, underestimate the ill person's functional status, have poor understanding of the family's cultural needs and are sometimes insensitive to the family's intergenerational needs (Donelan et al 2001; Kinrade et al 2009; Teel & Carson 2003). As a result, family members may be left to deal with medical crises, symptom management and other maintenance issues with less than adequate professional backup, relying primarily on their own judgement, wisdom and resourcefulness. This is a stressful undertaking and it may cause or exacerbate physical or emotional illness in the caregivers, or cause burnout, where they are no longer able to provide care sensitively (Knafl & Gilliss 2002). Over time, family carers may experience gradually diminishing levels of support from others whose intentions may have been to provide long-term support, but who simply become victims to ongoing stress themselves (Stewart 2000). Caregivers are also disadvantaged by having to forgo predictability and long-term planning for their own lives as they become trapped in a situation where they are unable to make career changes, relocate, or implement retirement plans (Donelan et al 2001). After long periods of time, some caregivers find that the burden of care precipitates a much faster deterioration in their physical and mental health than they had anticipated and they may withdraw from social interactions and be at risk of developing clinical depression.

Point to ponder
Family caregivers experience significant stress, often having to forgo their own life aspirations in order to care for others.

The sense of social isolation experienced by caregivers can be severe. In some cases, the family becomes isolated either by the desire of the ill person to remain out of public view, or by the altruistic desire to manage the situation as well as possible (Sanders 1995; Tsai & Wang 2009). Often, the caregiver gets caught up in a cycle of caring without respite, becoming exhausted to the point of emotional breakdown. Whether this occurs because of a lack of available resources, a situation that prevents accessing help, or an unwillingness to seek assistance, it is a dysfunctional state for both the caregiver and the rest of the family. All families need cooperation and support from others, mutual caring and a sense of control, especially those who are called upon to assist with such an important task as managing another's illness. The challenge for health advocates is to recognise the bi-directional impact of family caregiving and to help families in this situation become empowered to develop the resources and support mechanisms required for the health of all members (Teel & Carson 2003; Tsai & Wang 2009).

RURAL FAMILIES

The burden of family caregiving is often pronounced for families living in rural areas, where resources for family support are extremely scarce. Because of this, rural families have been forced to become resourceful in finding ways to rely on family members, friends and religious and voluntary agencies for support, rather than the health care system (Hunsucker et al 1999). The problem becomes magnified many times over for Indigenous and migrant families living in rural or remote areas, who often have few culturally sensitive resources to assist them.

Point to ponder
32% of the Australian population and 15% of the New Zealand population live in rural and remote areas.

The proportion of people living in Australian rural and remote areas is approximately 32% of the population, dispersed throughout nearly three-quarters of the land (AIHW 2008). In New Zealand, approximately 15% of the population live rurally, however comparisons are difficult as standard definitions of rural versus urban do not exist. For example, New Zealand defines a main urban area as having 30 000 or more people (Statistics New Zealand 2004), while the Australian definition lists a population centre of 100 000 or more people as a main urban area. Compared with families in urban environments, rural families have higher rates of illness, disability and mortality, all of which are exacerbated by poor access to care and caregivers (AIHW 2008; Ward et al 2005). Their disproportionate health status increases with the distance from metropolitan health services, and it is not clear how much of the difference is a result of biological factors, structural determinants of health or the rural lifestyle (Bourke et al 2009). What is known is that the rural and remote population has lower socio-economic status and lower levels of education compared with families living in urban environments (AIHW 2008). The other aspect of this population group that makes differentiation difficult is that rural communities also contain disproportionately large numbers of Indigenous people, whose health is compromised by factors other than geography (ABS 2005). Rural life may be a protective factor for some Indigenous people, providing them with a closer sense of 'country', and we'll discuss this further in Chapter 11. However, like other rural families, they may be disadvantaged by the lack of access to services and support systems.

Social determinants of the health of rural families

In the current climate, rural and remote area dwellers have less financial security than in past times, especially when they have experienced years of drought and more competitive markets for their goods due to the global economy. This has eroded the health status of many families, which is often compromised by exposure to harsh environments, occupational hazards associated with rural work and long working hours. Some rural dwellers, especially those who have fallen on hard times, have used risk-taking behaviours, such as smoking and heavy use of alcohol as a way of coping (Dade Smith 2004). Cultural influences on behaviour can also interact with the social isolation of living in rural and remote areas to influence family health or ill health, especially where there are cross-cultural tensions (Payet et al 2005).

Point to ponder

Globalisation and the resultant competitive international market have decreased the financial security of many rural and remote families leading to increasing socio-economic disadvantage for many families.

Other lifestyle pressures exist in the more remote settlements, which are disadvantaged by unreliable and expensive communications, continually rising fuel costs and a lack of access to fresh food, safe housing, adequate education and health services. As a result, young children and their families in remote and rural communities lack the advantages of having access to the internet and other educational tools for developing health literacy and skills for a changing workplace. Because of the lack of educational opportunities many adolescents leave home early to study in cities. When the family business is farming, their departure can create additional work pressures for those left behind. It can also be difficult for parents, especially for farming families who often spend more time with their children than urban families. For young people, the isolation and loneliness of being separated from the family can cause stress and difficulties associated with dislocation at a time when they most need family support.

Point to ponder

Rurality impacts on people's access to health services. Few options for accessing care limit rural families' choice of health care provider, in some cases, meaning a family does not seek care and does their best to 'manage'.

Another difference between urban and rural people lies in the way rural people use health services. Most people make greater use of hospital emergency departments for primary care (AIHW 2008). This can be a problem for family members seeking the personalised care and privacy of a general practitioner, as there are few alternatives for care. Interventions for mental illness, family conflicts or other issues may rely heavily on friendship networks rather than professionals, which can pose difficulties in a small community. Rural women in particular, who experience violence may have unique needs that are not acknowledged by either police or health care professionals, and geographic isolation can amplify their perpetrator's control over them and their subsequent loneliness and isolation. In some cases, the prominence of firearms in a traditional, patriarchal rural home can heighten women's vulnerability by creating fear and intimidation (Wendt 2009). Some rural women in this situation become trapped in violent relationships through 'financial insecurity, dependency, and stress; a perceived lack of confidentiality and anonymity; and stigma attached to the public disclosure of violence' (Wendt 2009:175). A study of rural women's experiences of violence indicates that they would like to have opportunities to disclose the reality of their situation, not be stereotyped in terms of societal expectations of rural life and norms of behaviour (Wendt 2009).

FAMILY LIFE IN THE 21ST CENTURY

Regardless of location, the family unit is today diverse and dynamic in its composition, perceptions and performance. What it means to belong to a family is defined in many ways, depending on the meanings held by family members and the ways they are bound together. The family itself is a metaphor for belonging and this should have a positive connotation for quality of life and life satisfaction. But despite the strength in connectedness, the family is also the most fragile of all human institutions; the place where we hold our deepest tensions, fears and hatreds, and sometimes violence, madness and despair (Curthoys 1999). For some families, having a wider range of choices has enhanced the quality of members' lives, while in others, the result has been dissatisfaction and disharmony. In the wealthy nations, the escalation of industrialisation into a highly competitive global marketplace has played havoc with family expectations. In the developing world, death, disease and civil strife are re shaping the family. In all countries, politicians dictate family structures and processes, through policies that either enhance or mitigate against various notions of 'family' and the capacity of families to evolve in their preferred direction. The only certainty is change. In the face of unremitting change, families will need the support of societal structures and policies and the commitment and guidance of health professionals to ensure sustainability throughout the precariousness of this century.

Goals for healthy families

The goals for healthy families are aimed at creating societies that will provide:

- physical, emotional and cultural support for all families
- access to a family-friendly means for economic sustainability
- a common bond from which to relate to the outside world
- opportunities for self-development for each of its members
- a connection to other families
- a sense of place, heritage and continuity.

To achieve these goals, strategies for assisting families must be linked to the wider social and cultural context of their lives.

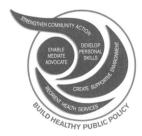

BUILDING HEALTHY PUBLIC POLICY

The term 'family-friendly policy' has become increasingly distorted with political usage. A family-friendly policy is designed in collaboration with families who will be not only recipients, but co-creators of strategies that enhance health and wellbeing. Yet, often, governments devise family-friendly policies on the basis of economic gains and without genuine collaboration with those who would enrich policies with practical wisdom. For example, parents should be involved in planning child care policies and other policies to deal with education, child health services, transportation, women and men's health and a range of other areas that affect family life.

> **Point to ponder**
> The family is one of the most important structures in society, yet also one of the most vulnerable. The development of family-friendly policies is imperative for the long-term sustainability of the family.

Family-friendly policies must be inclusive, which means they gather input from people in a variety of cultures and lifestyles. Such policies need to be based on in-depth knowledge of the various permutations of family life and the actual experiences of families. This means, for example, that policy-makers should take into account the obstacles to access that exist when parents cannot leave their employment to access child care entitlements, especially where unpaid leave is financially difficult (Gillies 2009). With parental input, family policies will be better able to avoid discriminatory language, such as describing separated fathers as 'deadbeat dads'. Likewise, they should be balanced and fair when describing mothers who make a conscious choice to stay home and raise their children. These comments disparage all parents trying to do their best in the circumstances and changes to family life (Gillies 2009).

Marriage policies

Some important gains have been made in the policy arena for Australian and New Zealand families. In New Zealand the policy allowing civil unions, mentioned previously has created a more equitable situation for non-traditional, same-sex unions. In Australia, the policy that led to increasing the family allowance has had a modest effect on the fertility rate. Following the lead of industry, where 50.8% of all large organisations are now paying maternity leave to employees, the Australian Commonwealth government is considering a policy for paid maternity leave (Online. Available: www.tanyaplibersek.fahcsi.gov.au/internet/tanyaplibersek.nsf/content/bus_fem [accessed 28 August 2009]).

Greater flexibility in workplace policies is another family-friendly policy goal. However, in some cases, flexible work schedules are too difficult for parents, so these should be developed with an understanding of the difficulty parents have in accessing them (Gillies 2009). Family-friendly policies also need to be cognisant of the need to integrate fathers' needs into policy targets and activities, especially when fathers have problems with flexible working hours (Berlyn et al 2008; Gillies 2009). Father involvement can be promoted by greater intersectoral collaboration, including cross-service discussions of how workplace policies affect social service policies and child access as determined by legal orders. Closer collaboration would provide an opportunity to solve some of the challenges faced by both men and women who have intermittent or variable work patterns affecting family life, such as occurs with FIFO families or those who must travel for work.

Another policy area requiring attention revolves around ensuring that the legal system supports parenting and families. Family law is a major concern for family advocates because current Australian and New Zealand law, like that of other countries, allows unilateral divorce, which can be imposed upon an unwilling and possibly exploited spouse with legal impunity. This creates a disincentive to work towards partnership stability and responsibility (Maley 2009). However, in cases of violence, such laws help promote safety, usually for the woman. Maley (2009) suggests that the current trend towards unilateral decision-making in child custody arrangements are not helpful. A fairer system would be to require all applications for divorce to be consensual, and include agreed terms of settlement. Where this is too difficult the application should be contingent on a court hearing from both parties to discuss all issues surrounding the application, including the wellbeing of the children. He believes that if there was an incentive to negotiate the terms of the settlement, the outcomes may be more reasonable than at present where the partner who may not have wished the divorce ends up living their lives in anger (Maley 2009).

Parental and children's rights policies

Policies governing children's access to parents are highly debatable. They require ongoing discussion by legal authorities as well as those who advocate for family health and wellbeing, particularly in the light of shared parenting agreements. The Australian *Shared Parental Responsibility Act of 2006* (Sweet & Power 2009) has been an attractive policy initiative for some families, but for others, it has had the untoward effect of depriving a child of basic needs. The extreme example of this is the mandate for shared parenting in very young infants who are breastfeeding. Regular interruptions to breastfeeding have had a detrimental effect on both the child and the breastfeeding mother, which illustrates the lack of practical decision-making in some family law judgements (Sweet & Power 2009). The other side of this policy argument is based on the notion that the move towards shared parenting has given more children access to their fathers than they would have previously had.

Policies protecting human rights and non-violence

Violence in the home and community has become a more visible policy issue since the activism of the feminist movement in the 1970s (Murray & Powell 2009). A positive step in developing government policies to address the true nature of violence against women has been to reframe 'family violence' within a human rights discourse (Murray & Powell 2009). This means that each of us has a right to be safe and to have equality of opportunity. For women, unequal status in many areas compromises their human rights. Indigenous women, for example, are marginalised by gender, culture, economic and historical factors such as colonisation. This 'intersection' of factors impinges on their human rights. Yet policies are developed on the basis of 'family violence', a term that tends to overlook the gendered issues of economic and social inequality inherent in violence against women. Therefore, situating responses to domestic violence within women's right to have control over their lives is a more appropriate foundation for policy development (Murray & Powell 2009). It is the approach advocated by the United Nations Declaration on the Elimination of Violence Against Women (UN 1993).

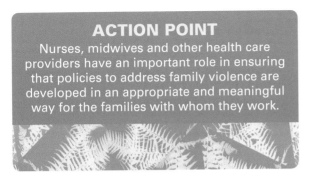

There also remains a need for appropriate discussion of Indigenous women's violence, to include 'the combined effects of racism, colonisation, and the socio-economic disadvantages of unemployment, poverty and social isolation' (Murray & Powell 2009:542). Such an inclusive, culturally embedded policy response to the issue of violence against Indigenous women would be more appropriate in drawing attention to the social and structural determinants of their health and wellbeing.

Policies designed to reduce community violence should be developed to respond to young people's need for a peaceful community in which to successfully negotiate their psychosocial development (Proctor 2006). In addition to legal and policing issues to promote safety, policies should also cover emergency accommodation for those made vulnerable by violence, especially for women and their children having to leave their home. Many report lengthy and fragmented bureaucratic processes in obtaining safe, secure and affordable housing, and in ensuring continuity of their relationship with their children (Johnson & Sullivan 2008; NSW Women's Refuge Movement & UWS Urban Research Centre 2009). In some cases, women's lack of housing creates an untenable situation, where their children are at risk of being taken into care by child protection workers because of their homelessness (NSW Women's Refuge Movement & UWS Urban Research Centre 2009). Policies that take into account the services required in the short and longer term can be more helpful than a single emergency response.

Inclusive policies

Public policies represent the shared values of society, which can reflect a moment in time or a vision for the future (Murray & Powell 2009). Implementation of policies is likely to be more equitable when they are developed from a deep understanding of the people affected by them. Inclusiveness should therefore be a major concern for all family policies. The way a family is defined sets boundaries for inclusion and exclusion when funding allocations are made. Government policies should therefore be developed in consultation with the community and the families who reside there, rather than be instigated above the grassroots level. For example, government agencies that fund programs for ageing families on the basis of such criteria as age and frailty, fail to recognise that in doing so, they may sever a vital relationship between ageing couples or siblings who may need to remain together as a first priority. Older families with caregiving needs, and families with children suffering disabling conditions can find the maze of social service policies difficult to understand or access, particularly when they change with each new government. This brings the role of advocating for families in clearer focus, and provides the impetus for all nurses, midwives and health professionals to have a working knowledge of policies and how they affect various families.

Policies for vulnerable families

The special needs of rural and migrant families, those with extended family households, Indigenous people and those whose family of definition is based on sexual preference need to also be addressed within a family-friendly context. The status of refugees is a classic case where families are being imperilled by unhealthy policies. Detaining those who have sought asylum from global conflict, for example, without preserving family integrity, contradicts the human rights principles of actively engaging with people to encourage participation in decision-making and self-help. As Lewig et al (2009) have found it is important that the receiving culture learn as much as possible about the needs of migrant and refugee families, particularly in terms of parenting. From this base of information policies can be developed that are both responsive to their needs and culturally appropriate.

In many of our large cities, we are surrounded by open, public debate on how to create cohesive, vibrant, trusting, family-friendly environments. Every town, city and community seems to aspire to a model of improving its image as a repository of social capital. At the local council level, interdisciplinary teams are developing policies for clean air, water conservation, more green spaces for recreation and better opportunities for education. This acknowledges the important role of communities in health and acceptance of the social determinants of health. In Australia, the state of Victoria now mandates city-council-level health and wellbeing policies, with many other states following its lead. This is one of the most important policy developments of recent times, as it entrenches the notion that it takes a whole community to raise a family. Numerous policies have also been developed around safety and quality of life. These include food security policies, public awareness of nutrition and food safety, new standards of food packaging, labelling and marketing, pricing sanctions and elimination of junk food advertising to deter families from overconsumption of high cholesterol and fatty foods, alcohol and tobacco.

Policies protecting the community

At the global level, we have seen the policies of the most powerful governments move further away from social programs by severely limiting budget allocations to programs that would ensure health and safety for families raising children. This is ironic at a time of declining rates of childbirth and widespread knowledge of the inequities between rich and poor. At the national level, government policies protect markets abroad, yet there is no policy support to ensure local markets are able to compete with their goods, or that local community services are available for those most in need of them. New Zealand, which has the advantage of national policy development, has been better able to facilitate policies for families across both Islands. With the fragmentation of policies in Australian states this has not yet been achievable. Policies for rural communities are virtually non-existent, despite the need to revitalise rural areas in order to leave a safe, cohesive and vibrant environment for the next generation. Bushy (2005) suggests that an integrated approach needs to be taken to address both personal and population health needs in rural communities to address the skills shortages that are leaving many people without health professionals and to invest in infrastructure to maintain ongoing health and independence of those citizens who have endured severe hardship in the country areas. One of the most vocal advocates for rectifying rural disadvantage is Australia's National Rural Health Alliance (NRHA), which is also connected to rural organisations in other countries, such as Canada. The NRHA maintains an ongoing commitment to keep rural issues on the policy agenda, lobbying for the retention of commercial and social services, health professionals, culturally safe Indigenous health services, education and infrastructure to support rural families.

CREATING SUPPORTIVE ENVIRONMENTS

In the rush of today's busy lifestyles, the need for community and societal support has never been greater. Supportive communities can develop ways of providing safety for families where abuse or other types of trauma are interfering with their health and wellbeing. Caregiving families, rural families, Indigenous families and those suffering family disruption need sensitive, resourceful health professionals to understand their needs. Those dealing with domestic abuse need equally sensitive treatment, and when they present to hospitals, and other health and community services, professionals working in these environments should be aware of the signs indicating that the person is living under threat. One of the most important elements of helping families is to convey a sense of non-judgemental support. Often the language we use to describe single mothers or divorcees or those who have chosen single parenthood is less than supportive. In some cases, our expressions are actually discriminatory as we refer to 'single-parent families', where the family actually consists of two parents, but is headed by one adult residing in the home. In this case, the terms 'separated family', or 'one-parent household' may be more appropriate and less dismissive of the parent who lives outside the family home.

Parent groups

First time mothers gain enormous benefit from parent groups. Some groups are organised informally, from neighbourhoods or churches, but where these are not available, health professionals have an important role to play in bringing new and experienced mothers together, or in helping to connect several first time mothers. The benefit of these types of groups is well documented. Hanna et al (2002) report on a Cochrane Review of 23 studies showing that such parenting programs can make a significant contribution to the short-term psychosocial health of mothers. Similarly, fathers need support and reinforcement to become involved in parenting, especially in accessing resources and receiving guidance on the needs of their children (Berlyn et al 2008; Halle et al 2008).

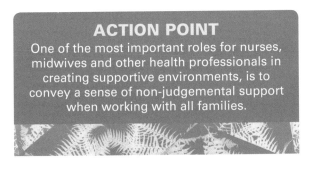

ACTION POINT
One of the most important roles for nurses, midwives and other health professionals in creating supportive environments, is to convey a sense of non-judgemental support when working with all families.

The needs of mothers heading family households alone are well documented and there is no argument against them needing support for themselves and their children. However, fathers' needs are often overlooked and many have begun to respond to supportive environments such as men's outreach services, father and son camps, or father-friendly places where they can pick up and drop off their children if necessary. Man-friendly services, with materials written in male-oriented language, are especially important for migrant and/or Indigenous men, and those living in rural areas who may be isolated from others (O'Brien & Rich 2002). Similarly, our language needs to reflect various forms of families, including gay and lesbian couples with or without children.

Culturally inclusive support

Non-judgemental support is also required in the way we respond to people's need to balance the conventions of their culture with the circumstances of their lives. For example, it is unacceptable in some communities to be divorced, yet violence against women and children is tolerated because it is embedded in people's culture and social mores. We can all assist families by becoming knowledgeable about other cultures and developing mutually supportive systems for cultural safety. This means shifting our own values to acknowledge different families' sense of history, heritage and rituals (Campbell 2001) and developing strategies for incorporating this knowledge into our plans for assisting them.

Formal agencies established to help women victims of violence can provide crucial help at the time a woman and her children leave home (Liang et al 2005). However, to be effective there must be inter-agency collaboration and information sharing, which is difficult in a situation where confidentiality is a primary concern and mandatory reporting of child abuse may see a woman lose her children (Malik et al 2008). Agencies and institutions need to understand the significant role of informal social support and the extent to which friendship networks can act as a protective factor when a woman has experienced traumatic events (Liang et al 2005). Women's shelters or refuges can be invaluable in providing ongoing nurturing and support for women who have experienced violence. These can act as a one-stop-shop for a continuum of services that include safety planning, support groups, children's services, advocacy and transitional accommodation (Liang et al 2005; NSW Women's Refuge Movement & UWS Urban Research Centre 2009). These support networks can often provide a vital source of security and hope for the future (NSW Women's Refuge Movement & UWS Urban Research Centre 2009).

Understanding women who have been victims of violence is the first step in providing support. This requires us as nurses to facilitate a woman's transformative journey, to allow her the time and space, and to encourage her to relate her story in her way in a caring, supportive environment (Davis & Taylor 2006). It is important to know that a woman's experience of violence, her coping style, her circumstances and her help-seeking are not universal (Liang et al 2005). Each of these can be multi-layered and unique. Yet, as we discussed in relation to women in the workplace, women who have fled violent homes are often judged according to maternal stereotypes. These include the 'all-sacrificing mother, the all-knowing mother, and the nurturing mother/breadwinning father' (Johnson & Sullivan 2008:243). This type of stereotypical thinking holds mothers to a higher standard of caregiving responsibility than their male partners. Social and institutional failures to hold the perpetrators responsible for their actions create a situation of entrapment, where women and often their children cannot escape a violent home because of economic reasons and fears for their safety (Johnson & Sullivan 2008). A further level of disadvantage can occur when the legal system becomes involved, with mothers becoming subjugated to the unequal power dynamics of the courts, often because of a lack of familiarity with the processes involved (Malik et al 2008).

STRENGTHENING COMMUNITY ACTION

The key to strengthening community action is family empowerment, which can be achieved by acknowledging family competence and preferences. One of the most important elements in helping families negotiate health is to support the many nested contextual influences that either constrain or support a family's health and development capacity (Pinderhughes et al 2001). These influences may include culture, neighbourhood, family members' behaviours and the variety of strategies and networks used to achieve 'connectedness' with the outside world (Pinderhughes et al 2001). This requires attention to family members' perceptions, to ascertain how they view the many aspects of family life. An ecomap, illustrating family members' different connections and networks can help identify family strengths and environmental influences as illustrated in Appendix H.

Supporting family decision-making

As nurses and midwives working with families, our role is to allow family members to 'own' their own problems, rather than telling them what to do. As an effective family practitioner, we provide the information and guidance that will assist them with self-management and making informed choices. Guidance therefore includes social action, to ensure that families are aware of the influences in society which affect their functioning and development. For example, in rural areas, stereotypical notions of rural culture may interfere with accurate assessment of health issues (Wendt 2009). Family assessment can ascertain how rurality is experienced by family members. Families should also be involved in the type of early education opportunities their children are able to access, and this requires intersectoral planning between educators, health professionals and others involved in the health and social development of children. A family-inclusive approach in the settings of people's lives also recognises the plethora of influences in a family's environment, thereby incorporating an ecological, relational approach to decision-making.

Family support in the workplace

In the workplace, one target for social action is in lobbying for changes in organisational culture (Russell & Bowman 2000; Smyth 2004b). Companies need to recognise that worker loyalty will be multiplied many times over by systems of work that allow people to fulfil the obligations of both family and work. There are advantages for the whole of society from

> **ACTION POINT**
> Assist workplaces to develop a culture of support for families.

workplaces where family values are recognised, where family stress and conflict is dealt with openly, and where career options are not precluded because of family responsibilities. Good managers recognise the value added to their productivity from supporting family members with greater flexibility and attention to their emotional needs. This means that managers become involved in helping people understand the importance of developing emotional intelligence, developing self-awareness, self-management, social awareness and social skills, to anticipate and handle emotional challenges and to interact with co-workers in healthy, non-bullying ways in the workplace (Goleman 2000). Providing a supportive work environment benefits the whole family, as parents who are fulfilled at work come home to their families without the sense of exhaustion that stifles parent–child relationships. At work, as in other settings of their lives, family members should have access to health-related information, and someone to help them filter what is useful to their quest for health. In this respect, the workplace can be a source of health literacy, providing a foundation for people to make decisions on how to approach certain problems or issues in their lives. It is a more family-sensitive, empowering approach than trying to engineer families' strategies for change or critical decisions. This is particularly important in our information age, when the sheer volume of information people access on the internet can be bewildering.

> **ACTION POINT**
> Using family assessment tools such as ecomaps can help identify family strengths and the contextual issues that influence family development.

Family advocacy

Social action is also necessary to bring about widespread change to the allocation of health resources to support families in all their geographic, cultural, social and developmental configurations. This is a highly political undertaking, and family members often seek professional assistance in identifying the time and place for contributing their views. A PHC approach, where families are considered as partners in planning, dictates the need for ongoing communication. The communications media has awakened us to the large number of hidden facets of family issues and sparked a debate over the public versus private nature of the family, including issues of collective morality. As health professionals, it is important that we stay involved in community dialogue, to provide the opportunities for family members to weigh in to debates that affect their health and wellbeing, and to transmit helpful information to them. To be of real assistance to families, we must keep issues of concern to them at the centre of public focus.

> ## ACTION POINT
> Get involved with what is happening in your community.

DEVELOPING PERSONAL SKILLS
We hear much today about skills shortages, and, as mentioned above, policies should be developed carefully and inclusively, to create employment for successive generations of young people. This is particularly important with declining fertility and an ageing society that will require care and economic support for many years to come. A generation unemployed can develop neither the skills nor experience to provide infrastructure for an ageing society unless there is access to education and training programs and ongoing support for those undertaking skills development courses. In countries with low unemployment, it is easy to overlook the need for building both personal and community skills, but it is important to have both. People are affected by work, whether they experience a lack of work or work stress. This component of their lives is substantial, and many people require strategies for building resilience that can transfer across the work-to-home boundaries. These strategies can be discussed during health encounters in the context of promoting an ecological perspective where people work towards harmony in all of the settings of their lives. This is

a capacity development approach, wherein the relational aspects of family life can be explored and validated as major steps on the pathway to community cohesion, trust and capacity for change.

Supporting civic participation
The rise of the voluntary sector over the past decade has shown the improved sense of wellbeing that occurs in communities where volunteering and participation in community life has become the norm. This makes a significant contribution to social capital. The contribution of volunteers should be recognised, and their needs considered, especially those caring for family members with illness. Volunteers need ongoing communication as a safety net to assist them in making caregiving decisions and help with skill development. As we outlined in Chapter 4, telephone helplines are invaluable for parenting support and advice as well as guidance when an ill family member's condition changes or moves to a different level of need. Parents' groups and self-help groups can also provide opportunities to begin a dialogue on personal development that will help all family members prepare for the future. These volunteer groups should also attract ongoing recognition as their activities can make the difference between confident parenting and caregiving or feelings of social isolation.

Supporting family relationship skills

Although family life is coloured by the normal ups and downs of daily life, satisfaction is both the entry and end-point of the couple relationship. It is an ideal to which most young people aspire and a source of consternation among those who either find it elusive, do not understand it when they find it, or have found it and lost it. Lorraine Wright (2005), a family nursing scholar, contends that the greatest challenge and opportunity in family nursing is marriage. She argues that we have paid too little attention to marriage in our practice, education and research agenda, particularly as it has such a powerful effect on health and illness. Compared with people who are unmarried, married couples tend to have higher incomes, greater emotional support and better health. To some extent this is because they generally have better nutrition, 'take better care of themselves, and live a more stable, secure and scheduled lifestyle' (Wright 2005:346).

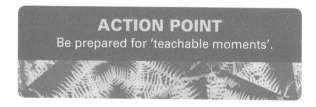

ACTION POINT
Be prepared for 'teachable moments'.

One of the most important things we, as health professionals can do to assist families is to understand at least the foundation of family relationship skills, so that our guidance and referrals are appropriate. For example, Halford (2000) describes the basic couple interactions for relationship success including intimate and self-disclosing communication, effective conflict management, partner mutual support, positive day-to-day interactions and shared positive activities. Couples often need guidance from health professionals at the 'teachable moment', such as child health visits or school health encounters. In some cases these include aspects of their intimate relationship, such as resuming sexual activity following childbirth to try to promote closeness at this time (Williamson et al 2008). In addition, becoming informed about parenting plans can help ease the strain on separated parents. As family health practitioners, if we can help family members develop self-esteem by feeling competent as parents and as partners, they have a better opportunity to build healthy communities. A further service to parents lies in helping them teach their children effective ways of coping with family stress, not only in the short term, but as a long-term strategy for living (Kouros et al 2008). This is crucial in so many families who are undergoing marital disruption, particularly with the prospect of long-term effects on the children. This involves ensuring that intervention programs for children of divorce are both proactive and reactive (Eldar-Avidan et al 2009). This approach would provide guidance to parents on responding according to children's ages and developmental stage, as well as including culturally appropriate support for the family unit and sibling subsystems (Eldar-Avidan et al 2009).

REORIENTING HEALTH SERVICES

A family-sensitive, family-focused approach to helping means that the family and its issues lie at the centre of models of care. All health professionals need ongoing education and skills updates in relation to contemporary issues, such as family violence, the sequelae to marital breakdown, the stress of working families and the needs of caregivers.

Communication, empathy and empowerment are the most important goals, especially where there is a need to encourage disclosure of sensitive issues such as family violence (Wong et al 2008). Some health professionals shy away from dealing with difficult issues such as IPV because of a fear of opening 'Pandora's box' and being unsure of what to do to help. In some cases, failure to ask questions that might have clarified the level of risk to a mother and her children has had dire consequences (Wilson et al 2004–05). This reinforces the importance of accurate assessment as a basis for health service planning.

Assessment and screening

Women seeking help for violence in the home have reported that they want health professionals, including their doctors to ask about this type of situation, responding positively to an empathic approach (Wendt 2009; Wong et al 2008). Hegarty

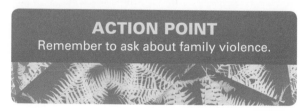

ACTION POINT
Remember to ask about family violence.

et al (2008) suggest a general practice program that combines screening for violence, health professional training, and a counselling intervention, to help women develop self-awareness and self-worth. Screening has also been the focus of large-scale initiatives among Australian and New Zealand emergency departments, with some Australian state governments supporting screening, and the New Zealand government committing to screening as part of its national health policy (De Vries et al 1996; Koziol-McLain et al 2008; Ritchie et al 2009; Schimanski & Hedgecock 2009). Following the development of the New Zealand Family Violence Intervention Guidelines in 2002, several hospitals have adopted regular screening for all women over the age of 16 attending emergency departments for injuries (Ritchie et al 2009; Schimanski & Hedgecock 2009). Child health nurses in New Zealand (Plunket and Tamariki Ora/Well Child nurses) have also incorporated screening for family violence as part of their everyday practice. Screening involves three safety questions, followed by a 20-minute assessment tool and referral for those women disclosing violence (Schimanski & Hedgecock 2009). This is an admirable step in helping alleviate the problem, even though it is not consistently applied in other settings. Screening for violence often depends on nurses' knowledge and understanding, their level of comfort in dealing with violence, time and support from others (Ritchie et al 2009). However, despite these barriers, it is important that this type of program should continue as a basis for education and other interventions as well as maintaining women's safety (Schimanski & Hedgecock 2009).

Family-centred care

Many of the roles discussed in the previous chapter have a major focus on families, whether this is in the child health clinic, the school, home, community or the workplace. Family-centred nursing in a wide range of dimensions is a crucial part of contemporary nursing practice (Yarwood 2008). Adopting a family-centred approach allows nurses to help empower family members, such as victims of violence, by identifying, then working towards a more enabling, strengths-based approach to the victim's future (Wilson et al 2004–05). Yarwood's (2008) interviews with a range of New Zealand nurses also revealed how family nurses work within families' 'relational web' of dynamic and complex family issues, according to Hartrick Doane and Varcoe's (2005) model of relational practice. Guided by the model, they are able to ensure a multidimensional approach embedded in family needs and contexts (Yarwood 2008). A similar approach is also advocated by the WHO. In Europe, the WHO has commissioned a multinational study of the role of family nurses in integrating the goals of PHC into general practice (Hennessy & Gladin 2009). Like their counterparts in Australia and New Zealand, these nurses were found to be working within interdisciplinary teams, adopting an extended health promotion and advocacy role to ensure family health (Hennessy & Gladin 2009).

Health professionals

Health services in most urban environments are characterised by an over-reliance on medical practitioners. In rural areas, the shortages of practitioners are acute and health promotion services sparse. The success of health professionals in rural areas relies on their ability to develop effective partnerships with families and the community (Francis et al 2008). We have a responsibility to connect the needs of families in the community with best practice in the cities, the rural areas and the wider

global agenda. Developing collective social consciousness and viewing the community as full partners in care can help with the equitable rationalisation of resources. Community members also have strong insights into the major economic and demographic changes affecting their communities from fertility rates, ageing, migration and wars, to employment and development patterns. Regional needs can often be identified from intersectoral, community collaboration and these should become part of the local as well as larger health agenda. In implementing PHC, it is important that links be made between the policy arena and people's access to health services. This involves making sure that links between policy and practice address not only health status and demographic information, but education, social protection, child care, housing, land use, the preservation of cultural and societal values, and adequate investment in health professionals. The latter includes the distribution of personnel across rural and urban areas, as well as permeable services that promote access for vulnerable people to move in and out of the system with ease (Beckfield & Krieger 2009; Peiris et al 2008).

Evidence-based practice

In working with families, new combinations of skills and services need to be developed from a base of research evidence to inform accessible, adequate and appropriate care. The evidence base for family nursing begins with a quest for understanding families, rather than searching for certainty, then examining ways of working with them from practice-derived knowledge (Hartrick Doane 2005). To date, there is a serious shortage of studies on the separating or divorcing family, and a dearth of investigations on appropriate ways of assisting couples undergoing marital separation. We need to redress these deficiencies and also reorient our research strategies from focusing on problems to case studies of what works, to provide exemplars of good and best practice in family care. To this body of evidence we should add our practice-based arguments for preventative care, which is visionary, culturally and regionally relevant, and inventive. Caring, as the fundamental essence of professional practice, mandates our involvement in social and political processes. This guides us towards extending our role into society in order to work intersectorally at optimal capacity as community partners to secure access, equity and empowerment for better health and wellbeing.

Case study

Maria's sister Deirdre immigrated to Australia shortly after Maria and is married to Taine. They live close to Maria and Jim in Sydney. Taine is of Maori descent and has a large extended family in New Zealand but came to Sydney for work in the early 1990s where he met Deirdre. Taine works as a truck driver and is frequently away from home for long periods of time. Deirdre has a full-time role at home caring for their five children. The oldest of their children is Tama who is 17 and in his final year of high school. Tama intends to go to university next year and study biology, eventually hoping to get into forensic science. Deirdre and Taine are full of expectation with the idea of having a son at university. His next sister, Susie, is 15 and attends the same high school as Tama. She has a boyfriend Joseph. The other siblings are Mark, aged 13, Aroha, aged 5, and Ella, aged 3. The family seems happy to outsiders but there has been a history of intimate partner violence, leaving each family member to cope in their own way.

REFLECTING ON THE BIG ISSUES

- Family life is multidimensional and consists of not only the family system but sibling subsystems.
- One of the primary goals for empowering young people is ensuring they have access to education.
- Family violence takes many forms, and interventions must be culturally appropriate, maintaining safety for all family members.
- Family health and wellbeing is a product of individual and family interactions and the way family members interact with the external world, including the immediate community and society.
- The role of nurses, midwives and other health professionals in fostering family health involves engaging as partners with family members to help them build resilience.
- Nursing interventions should be based on research evidence as well as careful assessment of the family and the circumstances and events surrounding them.

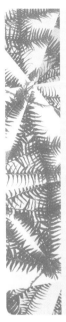

Reflective questions: how would I use this knowledge in practice?

1 Draw a genogram of Maria's family that includes Deirdre and Taine's family members.

2 What are the implications of family violence for the members of Deirdre and Taine's family?

3 What family goals would you establish to ensure health and wellbeing for all family members?

4 How would you approach family assessment if you were conducting a home visit?

5 Would you alert the school nurse of any problems with the family? Why or why not?

6 What communication strategies would you use to ensure all members of the family were moving towards resolving any ongoing conflicts?

7 What resources would you use to ensure you had access to current research evidence for your actions?

Research-informed practice

Read the article by Black and Lobo 2008 'A conceptual review of family resilience factors'. Using their recovery factor characteristics (Table 1) develop a plan for working with Deirdre and Taine and their family.

References

Adolescent Health Research Group 2008 Youth'07: the health and wellbeing of secondary school students in New Zealand. Initial findings. The University of Auckland, New Zealand

Amato P 2004 Tension between institutional and individual views of marriage. Journal of Marriage and the Family 66(4):959–65

Amato P, Rivera F 1999 Paternal involvement and children's behavior problems. Journal of Marriage and the Family 61:375–84

Australian Bureau of Statistics (ABS) 2005 The Health and Welfare of Australia's Aboriginal and Torres Strait Islander Peoples. Cat No. 4704.0, ABS, Canberra

—— 2007a Australian Social Trends. Cat No. 2102.0, Canberra. Online. Available: www.abs.gov.au (accessed 8 August 2009)

—— 2007b Divorces, Australia 2007. Online. Available: www.abs.gov.au/AUSSTATS/abs@.nsf /mf/3307.0.55.001 (accessed 25 August 2009)

—— 2009 Couples in Australia, Australian Social Trends. Online. Available: www.abs.gov.au/ AUSSTATS/abs@.nsf/Lookup/4102.0Main+ Features20March%202 (accessed 25 August 2009)

Australian Institute of Health and Welfare (AIHW) 2008 Australia's Health 2008. AIHW, Canberra

Bandura A 1977 Social Learning Theory. Prentice-Hall, Englewood Cliffs, NJ

Bascand G 2006 Disability Survey: 2006. Statistics New Zealand, Wellington

Beckfield J, Krieger N 2009 Epi + demos + cracy: Linking political systems and priorities to the magnitude of health inequities — evidence, gaps and a research agenda. Epidemiologic Reviews Advance

Access www.DOI 10.1093/epirev/mxp002 (accessed 12 June 2009)

Berger L, Carlson M, Bzostek S, Osborne C 2008 Parenting practices of resident fathers: the role of marital and biological ties. Journal of Marriage and Family 70:625–39

Berlyn C, Wise S, Soriano G 2008 Engaging fathers in child and family services. Occasional Paper No. 22, Australian Government Department of Families, Housing, Community Services and Indigenous Affairs, Canberra

Black K, Lobo M 2008 A conceptual review of family resilience factors. Journal of Family Nursing 14(1):33–55

Bourke L, Humphreys J, Lukaitis F 2009 Health behaviours of young, rural residents: a case study. Australian Journal of Rural Health 17:86–91

Bushy A 2005 Needed: quality improvement in rural health care. Guest Editorial, Australian Journal of Rural Health 13:261–2

Byrd S 2009 The social construction of marital commitment. Journal of Marriage and Family 71:318–36

Campbell J 2001 Global perspectives on wife beating and health care. In: Martinez M (ed.) Prevention and Control of Aggression and the Impact on Its Victims. Kluwer Academic/Plenum Publishers, New York, pp 215–27

Carter T, Kaczmarek E 2009 An exploration of generation Y's experience of offshore fly-in/fly-out employment. The Australian Community Psychologist 21(2):52–66

Casper W, Weltman D, Kwesiga E 2007 Beyond family-friendly: the construct and measurement of singles-friendly work culture. Journal of Vocational Behavior 70:478–501

Chuang S, Gielen U 2009 Understanding immigrant families from around the world: introduction to the special issue. Journal of Family Psychology 23(3):273–8

Clark R, Glick J, Bures R 2009 Immigrant families over the life course. Journal of Family Issues 30(6):852–72

Claxton A, Perry-Jenkins M 2008 No fun anymore: leisure and marital quality across the transition to parenthood. Journal of Marriage and Family 70:28–43

Colmar Brunton 2006 Work, family and parenting study: research findings. Ministry of Social Development, New Zealand, Wellington

Coltrane S 2001 Marketing the marriage 'solution': misplaced simplicity in the politics of fatherhood. Sociological Perspectives 44(4):387–418

Commonwealth of Australia 2008 Families in Australia: 2008. Department of the Prime Minister and Cabinet, Canberra

—— 2010 The Intergenerational Report 2010. Online. Available: www.treasury.gov.au/gr/gr2010/report/pdf/01 (accessed 12 February 2010)

Cripps K, McGlade H 2008 Indigenous family violence and sexual abuse: considering pathways forward. Journal of Family Studies 14(2–3):240–53

Crisp J, Taylor C 2009 Caring for families. In: Crisp J, Taylor C (eds) Fundamentals of Nursing. Elsevier, Sydney, pp 129–57

Curthoys A 1999 Family fortress: chronicles of the future. The Australian, 13 November, Sydney

Cutrona C 2004 A psychological perspective: marriage and the social provisions of relationships. Journal of Marriage and Family 66(4):992–9

Dade Smith J 2004 Australia's Rural and Remote Health: a Social Justice Perspective. Tertiary Press, Croydon, Melbourne

Davis K, Taylor B 2006 Stories of resistance and healing in the process of leaving abusive relationships. Contemporary Nurse 21:199–208

De Vries R, March L, Vinen J, Horner D, Roberts G 1996 Prevalence of domestic violence among patients attending a hospital emergency department. Australian and New Zealand Journal of Public Health 20:364–8

DeVaus D, Gray M, Qu L, Stanton D 2007 Divorce and Personal Wellbeing of Older Australians. Paper presented to Australian Social Policy Conference, University of New South Wales, Sydney

Donelan K, Falik M, DesRoches C 2001 Caregiving: challenges and implications for women's health. Women's Health Issues 11(3):185–200

Duvall E 1977 Marriage and Family Relationships (5th edn). Lippincott, Philadelphia

Duvall E, Miller B 1985 Marriage and Family Development (6th edn). Harper & Row, New York

Dyson R 2002 Health of Older People Strategy: Health Sector Action to 2010 to Support Positive Ageing. Ministry of Health New Zealand, Wellington

Eldar-Avidan D, Haj-Yahia M, Greenbaum C 2009 Divorce is a part of my life … resilience, survival, and vulnerability: Young adults' perception of the implications of parental divorce. Journal of Marital and Family Therapy 24(10):30–46

Ezzedeen S, Ritchey K 2008 The man behind the woman. A qualitative study of the spousal support received and valued by executive women. Journal of Family Issues 29(9):1107–35

Families Commission 2008 The Kiwi nest: 60 years of change in New Zealand families. Families Commission, Wellington New Zealand. Online. Available: www.familiescommission.govt.nz/research/the-kiwi-nest (accessed 26 February 2010)

—— 2009a Finding time: parents' long working hours and time impact on family life. Families Commission, Wellington New Zealand. Online. Available: www.familiescommission.govt.nz/research/work-life-balance/finding-time (accessed 26 February 2010)

—— 2009b Family violence statistics report. Families Commission, Wellington, New Zealand. Online. Available: www.familiescommission.govt.nz/research/family-violence/family-violence-statistics-report (accessed 26 February 2010)

Fanslow J, Robinson R 2004 Violence against women in New Zealand: prevalence and health consequences. New Zealand Medical Journal 117(1206):1173–85

Fletcher R 2008 Father-inclusive practice and associated professional competencies. Australian Family Relationships Clearinghouse Briefing 9:1–10

Francis K, Chapman Y, Hoare K, Mills J 2008 Australia & New Zealand Community as Partner. Wolters Kluwer Lippincott Williams & Wilkins, Philadelphia

Fremstad S 2009 Half in ten: why taking disability into account is essential to reducing income poverty and expanding economic inclusion. Center for Economic and Policy Research, Washington. Online. Available: www.cepr.net (accessed 6 October 2009)

Friedman M 1992 Family Nursing: Theory and Assessment (3rd edn). Appleton Century-Crofts, New York

Furstenberg F 2005 Banking on families: how families generate and distribute social capital. Journal of Marriage and Family 67:809–21

Gallegos D 2006 Fly-in fly-out Employment: Managing the Parenting Transitions. Centre for Social and Community Research, Murdoch University, Perth

Gillies V 2009 Understandings and experiences of involved fathering in the United Kingdom: exploring classed dimensions. Annals of the American Academy of Pediatric Social Services 624 doi 10.1177/0002716209334295

Goldscheider F, Hofferth S, Spearin C, Curtin S 2009 Fatherhood across two generations. Factors affecting early family roles. Journal of Family Issues 30(5):586–604

Goleman D 2000 Emotional Intelligence. Bantam Books, New York

Gottleib L, Feeley N 2000 Nursing intervention studies: issues related to change and timing. In: Stewart M (ed.) Community Nursing: Promoting Canadians' Health (2nd edn). WB Saunders, Toronto, pp 523–41

Guerin P, Guerin B 2009 Social effects of fly-in-fly-out and drive-in-drive-out services for remote Indigenous communities. The Australian Community Psychologist 21(2):7–22

Guzzo K, Lee H 2008 Couple relationship status and patterns of early parenting practices. Journal of Marriage and Family 70:44–61

Hafford C 2009 Sibling caretaking in immigrant families: understanding cultural practices to inform child welfare practice and evaluation. Evaluation and Program Planning doi:10.1016/j.evalprogplan.2009.05.003

Halford K 2000 Australian Couples in Millennium Three. Commonwealth of Australia, Canberra

Halle C, Fowler C, Dowd T, Rissel K, Hennessy K, MacNevin R, Nelson M 2008 Supporting fathers in the transition to parenthood. Contemporary Nurse 31:57–70

Hancock T 2009 Act Locally: Community-based population health. Report for The Senate Sub-Committee on Population Health, Victoria BC, Canada. Online. Available: www.parl.gc.ca/40/2/parlbus/commbus/senate/com-e/popu-e/rep-e/appendixBjun09-e.pdf (accessed 17 July 2009)

Hanna B, Edgecombe G, Jackson C, Newman S 2002 The importance of first-time parent groups for new parents. Nursing & Health Sciences 4:209–14

Hartrick Doane G 2005 Family nursing: challenges and opportunities: the challenge and opportunity of complex uncertainty. Journal of Family Nursing 11(4):350–3

Hartrick Doane G, Varcoe C 2005 Family nursing as relational inquiry: developing health-promoting practice. Lippincott Williams & Wilkins, Philadelphia

Heath M 2009 State of our unions. Marriage promotion and the contested power of heterosexuality. Gender & Society 23(1):27–48

Hegarty K, O'Doherty L, Gunn J, Pierce D, Taft A 2008 A brief counseling intervention by health professionals utilising the 'readiness to change' concept for women experiencing intimate partner abuse: The *weave* project. Journal of Family Studies 14(2–3):376–88

Heise L, Garcia-Moreno C (eds) 2002 World Report on Violence and Health. WHO, Geneva

Hennessy D, Gladin L 2009 Report on the evaluation of the WHO multi-country family health nurse pilot study. Online. Available: www.euro.who.int/document/E88841.pdf (accessed 23 August 2009)

Hetherington E 1999 Should we stay together for the sake of the children? In: Hetherington E (ed.) Coping With Divorce, Single Parenting, and Remarriage. Lawrence Erlbaum Associates, New York, pp 93–116

Hetherington E, Kelly J 2002 For Better or For Worse: Divorce Reconsidered. Norton, New York

Hewitt B 2009 Which spouse initiates marital separation when there are children involved? Journal of Marriage and Family 71:362–72

Hunsucker S, Frank D, Flannery J 1999 Meeting the needs of rural families during critical illness: the APN's role. Dimensions of Critical Care Nursing 18(3):24–33

Indermaur D 2001 Young Australians and Domestic Violence. Australian Institute of Criminology, Canberra

Jeon Y, Brodady H, Chesterton J 2005 Respite care for caregivers and people with severe mental illness: literature review. Journal of Advanced Nursing 49(3):297–306

Johnson S, Sullivan C 2008 How child protection workers support or further victimize battered mothers. Journal of Women and Social Work 23(3):242–58

Keating D, Hertzman C 1999 Developmental Health and the Wealth of Nations. The Guilford Press, New York

Kinrade T, Jackson A, Tomnay J 2009 The psychosocial needs of families during critical illness: comparison of nurses' and family members' perspectives. Australian Journal of Advanced Nursing 27(20):82–8

Kluwer E 2000 Marital quality. In: Milardo R, Duck S (eds.) 2000 Families as Relationships. John Wiley, Chichester, pp 59–78

Knafl K, Gilliss C 2002 Families and chronic illness: a synthesis of current research. Journal of Family Nursing 8(3):178–98

Kouros C, Merrilees C, Cummings E 2008 Marital conflict and children's emotional security in the context of parental depression. Journal of Marriage and Family 70:684–97

Koziol-McLain J, Giddings L, Rameka M, Fyfe E 2008 Intimate partner violence screening and brief intervention: Experiences of women in two New Zealand health care settings. Journal of Midwifery Women's Health 53:504–10

Lassetter J, Callister L 2009 The impact of migration on the health of voluntary migrants in Western societies. Journal of Transcultural Nursing 20(1):93–104

Lawrence E, Cobb R, Rothman A, Rothman M, Bradbury T 2008 Marital satisfaction across the transition to parenthood. Journal of Family Psychology 22(10):41–50

Le Bourdais C, Juby H, Marcil-Gratton N 2002 Keeping in touch with children after separation: the point of view of fathers. Canadian Journal of Community Mental Health 4:109–30

Le Bourdais C, Lapierre-Adamcyk E 2004 Changes in conjugal life in Canada: is cohabitation progressively replacing marriage? Journal of Marriage and Family 66(4):929–42

Lewig K, Arney F, Salveron M 2009 Challenges of parenting in a new culture: implications for child and family welfare. Evaluation and Program Planning doi:10.1016/j.evalprogplan.2009.05.002

Lewis S, West A, Stein A, Malmberg L, Bethell K, Barnes J, Sylva K, Leach P 2008 The families, children and child care project team. A comparison of father-infant interaction between primary and non-primary care giving fathers. Child Care Health and Development doi 10.1111/j.1365-2213.2008.00913.x

Liang B, Goodman L, Tummala-Narra P, Weintraub S 2005 A theoretical framework for understanding help-seeking processes among survivors of intimate partner violence. American Journal of Community Psychology 36(1/2):71–84

Lichter D, Qian Z 2008 Serial cohabitation and the marital life course. Journal of Marriage and Family 70:861–70

Lin I 2008 Consequences of parental divorce for adult children's support of their frail parents. Journal of Marriage and Family 70:113–28

Louis V, Zhao S 2002 Effects of family structure, family SES, and adulthood experiences on life satisfaction. Journal of Family Issues 23(8):986–1005

Maley B 2009 Family on the Edge: Stability and Fertility in Prosperity and Recession. CIS Policy Monograph 101, Centre for Independent Study, Sydney

Malik N, Ward K, Janczewski C 2008 Coordinated community response to family violence: the role of domestic violence service organizations. Journal of Interpersonal Violence 2(7):933–55

McMurray A 2006 Peace, love and equality: nurses, interpersonal violence and social justice. Preface, Contemporary Nurse 21:vii–x

Michel J, Mitchelson J, Pichler S, Cullen K 2009 Clarifying relationships among work and family social support, stressors, and work–family conflict. Journal of Vocational Behavior doi:10.1016/j.jvb.2009.05.007

Moloney L 2005 Government's response to the family law maze: the family relationship centres proposal. Journal of Family Studies 11(1):11–35

Moloney L 2008 Violence allegations in parenting disputes: reflections on court-based decision-making before and after the 2006 Australian law reforms. Journal of Family Studies 14(2–3):254–70

Murray S, Powell A 2009 What's the problem? Australian public policy constructions of domestic and family violence. Violence Against Women 15(5):532–52

Naeem F, Irfan M, Zaidi Q, Ayub M 2008 Angry wives, abusive husbands: relationship between domestic violence and psychosocial variables. Women's Health Issues 18:453–62

New South Wales Women's Refuge Movement and the UWS Urban Research Centre 2009 The impact of housing on the lives of women and children post-domestic violence crisis accommodation. NSW Women's Refuge Movement Resource Centre, Sydney

New Zealand Immigration Service 2004 Refugee voices: a journey towards resettlement. New Zealand Immigration Service, Wellington

O'Brien C, Rich K 2002 Evaluation of the Men and Family Relationships Initiative. Commonwealth Department of Family and Community Services, Canberra

Ongaro F, Mazzuco S 2009 Parental separation and family formation in early adulthood: evidence from Italy. Advances in Life Course Research doi.10.1016/j.alcr.2009.06.002

Palladino Schultheiss D 2006 The interface of work and family life. Professional Psychology: Research and Practice 37(4):334–41

Payet J, Gilles M, Howat P 2005 Gascoyne growers market: a sustainable health promotion activity developed in partnership with the community. Australian Journal of Rural Health 13:309–314

Peiris D, Brown A, Cass A 2008 Addressing inequities in access to quality health care for indigenous people. Canadian Medical Association Journal 179(10):985–6

Penman R 2005 Current approaches to marriage and relationship research in the United States and Australia. Family Matters 70:26–45

Pfiffner L, McBurnett K, Rathouz P 2001 Father absence and familial antisocial characteristics. Journal of Abnormal Child Psychology 29:357–67

Pinderhughes E, Nix R, Foster M, Jones D 2001 Parenting in context: impact of neighborhood poverty, residential stability, public services, social networks, and danger on parental behaviors. Journal of Marriage & Family 63(4):941–53

Proctor L 2006 Children growing up in a violent community: the role of the family. Aggression and Violent Behavior 11:558–76

Putnam R 2005 Civic Renewal and Social Capital. Round Table Discussion. Alcoa Research Centre for Stronger Communities, Curtin University, Perth

Ritchie M, Nelson K, Wills R 2009 Family violence intervention within an emergency department: achieving change requires multifaceted processes to maximize safety. Journal of Emergency Nursing 35(2):97–104

Russell G, Bowman L 2000 Work and Family Current Thinking, Research and Practice. Commonwealth of Australia, Canberra

Sanders M (ed.) 1995 Healthy Families, Healthy Nation. Australian Academic Press, Brisbane

Sassler S, Cunningham A, Lichter D 2009 Intergenerational patterns of union formation and relationship quality. Journal of Family Issues 30(6):757–86

Schimanski K, Hedgecock B 2009 Factors to consider for family violence screening implementation in New Zealand emergency departments. Australasian Emergency Nursing Journal 12:50–4

Schofield M, Walker R 2008 Innovative approaches to family violence. Editorial, Journal of Family Studies 14(2–3):160–6

Schultheiss D 2006 The interface of work and family life. Professional Psychology: Research and Practice 37(4):334–41

Shea Hart A, Bagshaw D 2008 The idealized post-separation family in Australian family law: a dangerous paradigm for children in cases of domestic violence. Journal of Family Studies 14(2–3):291–309

Sheehan G, Smyth B 2000 Spousal violence and post-separation financial outcomes. Australian Journal of Family Law 14(2):102–12

Smyth B 2004a Post-separation fathering: what does Australian research tell us? Journal of Family Studies 10(1):20–49

—— 2004b Parent-child Contact and Post-separation Parenting Arrangements. Australian Institute of Family Studies, Report No. 9, AIFS, Melbourne

Stanley F, Richardson S, Prior M 2005 Children of the Lucky Country. Pan Macmillan, Sydney

Statistics New Zealand 2004 New Zealand: a rural/urban profile. Statistics New Zealand, Wellington

—— 2006 Census data. Online. Available: www.stats.govt.nz/Census/2006CensusHomePage/QuickStats/quickstats-about-a-subject/national-highlights/households.aspx (accessed 26 February 2010)

—— 2008 National Labour Force Projections: 2006 (base) — 2061. Online. Available: www.stats.govt. nz/browse_for_stats/work_income_and_spending/ Employment/NationalLabourForceProjections_ HOTP06-61.aspx (accessed 26 February 2010)

Stewart M 2000 Social support, coping, and self-care as public participation mechanisms. In: Stewart M (ed.) Community Nursing: Promoting Canadians' Health (2nd edn). WB Saunders, Toronto, pp 83–104

Stewart M, Jackson D, Mannix J, Wilkes L, Lines K 2004–05 Current state of knowledge on child-to-mother violence. Contemporary Nurse 18(1–2):199–210

Strauss M 2001 Physical aggression in the family. In: Martinez M (ed.) Prevention and Control of Aggression and the Impact on its Victims. Kluwer Academic/ Plenum Publishers, New York, pp 181–200

Sweet L, Power C 2009 Family law as a determinant of child health and welfare: shared parenting, breast-feeding and the best interests of the child. Health Sociology Review 18(1):108–18

Swiss L, Le Bourdais C 2009 Father–child contact after separation. The influence of living arrangements. Journal of Family Issues 30(5):623–52

Tach L, Halpern-Meekin S 2009 How does premarital cohabitation affect trajectories of marital quality? Journal of Marriage and Family 71:298–317

Taylor J, Graetz Simmonds J 2009 Family stress and coping in the fly-in fly-out workforce. The Australian Community Psychologist 21(20):23–36

Teachman J 2002 Childhood living arrangements and the intergenerational transmission of divorce. Journal of Marriage and Family 64:717–29

Teel C, Carson P 2003 Family experiences in the journey through dementia diagnosis and care. Journal of Family Nursing 9(1):38–58

Terrance C, Plumm K, Little B 2008 Maternal blame. Battered women and abused children. Violence Against Women 14(8):870–85

Thornton A 2009 Framework for interpreting long-term trends in values and beliefs concerning single-parent families. Journal of Marriage and Family 71:230–4

Thornton J, Stevens G, Grant J, Indermaur D, Chamarette C, Halse A 2008 Intrafamilial adolescent sex offenders: family functioning and treatment. Journal of Family Studies 14(2–3):362–75

Todd S, Jones S 2005 Looking at the future and seeing the past: the challenge of the middle years of parenting a child with intellectual disabilities. Journal of Intellectual Disability Research 49:389–404

Tower M, McMurray A, Rowe J, Wallis M 2006 Domestic violence, health and health care. Women's accounts of their experiences. Contemporary Nurse 21:186–98

Tsai S, Wang H 2009 The relationship between caregiver's strain and social support among mothers with intellectually disabled children. Journal of Clinical Nursing 18:539–48

Uecker J, Stokes C 2008 Early marriage in the United States. Journal of Marriage and Family 70:835–46

United Kingdom Office for National Statistics 2009 Divorces. Online. Available: www.statistics.gov.uk/ cci/nugget_print.asp?ID=170 (accessed 20 September 2009)

—— 2009 European Context. Online. Available: www. statistics.gov.uk/CCI/nugget.asp?ID=1314&Pos=4&C olRank=2&Rank=160 (accessed 20 September 2009)

—— 2009 Living Arrangements. Online. Available www.statistics.gov.uk/cci/nugget_print.asp?ID=1652 (accessed 20 September 2009)

United Nations 1993 Declaration on the Elimination of Violence Against Women. Online. Available: www. un.org/documents/ga/res/48/a48r104.htm (accessed 9 October 2009

United Nations Family Planning Association 2000 The State of World Population 2000. United Nations, New York

Vincent K, Eveline J 2008 The invisibility of gendered power relations in domestic violence policy. Journal of Family Studies 14:322–33

Waite L, Gallagher M 2000 The Case for Marriage. Broadway Books, New York

Walker A 2004 A symposium on marriage and its future. Journal of Marriage & Family 66(4):843–7

Wallerstein J, Lewis J, Blakeslee S 2000 The Unexpected Legacy of Divorce: A 25 Year Landmark Study. Hyperion, New York

Ward B, Anderson K, Sheldon M 2005 Patterns of home and community care service delivery to culturally and linguistically diverse residents of rural Victoria. Australian Journal of Rural Health 13:348–52

Weissman M, Wickramaratne P, Nomura Y, Warner V, Pilowsky D, Verdeli H 2006 Offspring of depressed parents: 20 years later. The American Journal of Psychiatry163:1001–8

Wendt S 2009 Constructions of local culture and impacts on domestic violence in an Australian rural community. Journal of Rural Studies 25:175–84

Weston R 2005 Having children or not. Overview, Australian Institute of Family Studies. Family Matters 69:1–8

Wierda-Boer H, Gerris J, Vermulst A 2009 Managing multiple roles. Personality, stress and work–family interference in dual-earner couples. Journal of Individual Differences 30(1):6–19

Williamson M, McVeigh C, Baafi M 2008 An Australian perspective of fatherhood and sexuality. Midwifery 24:99–107

Wilson D, McBride-Henry K, Huntington A 2004–5 Family violence: Walking the tight rope between maternal alienation and child safety. Contemporary Nurse 18(1–2):85–96

Wong S, Wester F, Mol S, Romkens R, Hezemans D, Lagro-Janssen T 2008 Talking matters: abused women's views on disclosure of partner abuse to the family doctor and its role in handling the abuse situation. Patient Education and Counseling 70:386–94

World Health Organization 2002 World Report on Violence and Health. WHO, Geneva

Wright L 2005 Family nursing: challenges and opportunities. Marriage: it matters in sickness and in health. Journal of Family Nursing 11(94):344–9

Wright L, Leahey M 1987 Nurses and Families: a Guide to Family Assessment and Intervention (2nd edn). FA Davis, Philadelphia

—— 2000 Nurses and Families: a Guide to Family Assessment and Intervention (3rd edn). FA Davis, Philadelphia

—— 2009 Nurses and Families: a Guide to Family Assessment and Intervention (5th edn). FA Davis, Philadelphia

Yarwood J 2008 Nurses' views of family nursing in community contexts: an exploratory study. Nursing Praxis in New Zealand 24(2):41–51

Zubrick S, Smith G, Nicholson J, Sanson A, Jackiewicz T, The LSAC Consortium 2008 Parenting and families in Australia, Social Policy Research Paper No 34, Department of Families, Housing, Community Services and Indigenous Affairs, Australian Government, Canberra

Useful websites

http://www.aifs.gov.au/ — Australian Institute for Family Studies

http://www.aracy.org.au — Australian Research Alliance for Children and Youth

http://www.communities.wa.gov.au/childrenandfamilies/parentingwa/Pages/default.aspx — Parenting tips

http://www/families.gov.au — Australian Department of Families, Children and Parenting

http://www.familycourt.gov.au/ — Family court matters

http://www.pfsc.uq.edu.au — The University of Queensland Parenting and Family Support Centre

http://www.relationships.com.au/ — Information on relationships, family, love and life

http://www.ruralhealth.org.au — National Rural Health Alliance

http://www.SDOH@YorkU.ca — Social Determinants of Health

http://www.snaicc.asn.au — Secretariat of National Aboriginal and Islander Child Care

http://www.stats.govt.nz/analytical-reports/nz-family — New Zealand child and family information

http://www.nswccl.org.au/issues/glbt.php — NSW Council for Civil Liberties

http://www.australianmarriageequality.com — Australian Marriage Equality

http://www.familiescommission.govt.nz — New Zealand Families Commission — research and publications to support the family

http://www.communities.wa.gov.au/childrenandfamilies/Pages/default.aspx — Resource for FIFO families

Chapter 6

Healthy children

INTRODUCTION

One of the greatest indicators of health and wellness in a community is the extent to which it invests in and nurtures its children. As we outline in this chapter, the research on child health is growing at a rapid rate, and there is widespread understanding that the most important avenue to good health in any community is supporting a healthy start to life. This includes support for parents from the time they begin to plan a family, through conception, childbirth and parenting. Community life is crucial to good parenting, and it requires commitment at all levels of society to develop community structures and processes that will be helpful to parents and others who interact with children.

The governments of most Western nations have declared their commitment to the health and wellbeing of their communities by promoting and supporting child health initiatives. Australia and New Zealand share this commitment. Compared with children in other Organisation for Economic Co-operation and Development (OECD) countries, children in this part of the world are doing relatively well, but there are still areas for improvement. The past several years have seen declining rates of mortality related to injuries, and declining hospitalisations for asthma. There have been improved survival rates for children with leukaemia, greater immunisation coverage, and increases in the number of children meeting national physical activity guidelines and reading and numeracy standards (Australian Institute of Health and Welfare [AIHW] 2009a).

Point to ponder

One of the greatest indicators of health and wellness in a community is the extent to which it invests in and nurtures its children.

However, other benchmarks require attention, including rising rates of severe disability, diabetes and tooth decay. This indicates a need to keep up the momentum towards better health for children, promoting safety and oral health. Another challenge lies in trying to reduce the time children spend in front of a television or computer screen, and increasing their physical activity. In addition, there is a need to support parents in promoting healthy lifestyles, harmony in the home, and sustaining sufficient resources to circumvent risks to family life. As nurses and midwives, we must also remain vigilant to ensure that families at risk of injury, low socio-economic status (SES), a lack of access to services or with relationship difficulties are brought to the attention of those agencies that can help them. This also includes drawing attention to the education system and those who allocate resources to promote equity of access for rural, remote and Indigenous children.

Disadvantage among Indigenous children and their families is by far the most urgent issue for all health professionals. We have a major role to play in helping communities achieve equitable health outcomes by drawing attention to the disparities, and framing solutions in terms of primary health care (PHC). This is a major priority of government health strategies in both Australia and New Zealand (AIHW 2009a; Ministry of Health New Zealand [MOHNZ] 2001, 2002a). It will be important for current and future generations of Indigenous children to work towards an evidence base for health policy and planning. Nursing and midwifery research can add value to this by gathering important data from our communities, showing not only the importance of an early, healthy start to life, but the local contextual strengths and constraints that impact on healthy childhoods.

At the community level, there are enormous challenges for parenting and child health from

Point to ponder
One of the most pressing issues in both Australia and New Zealand is the inequitable disadvantage experienced by Indigenous children in both countries.

some of the societal changes mentioned in the previous chapter. These include increasing population diversity, the need for work and family harmony, financial constraints and the need for accessible, affordable child care. Understanding these as global, as well as local issues can help us connect knowledge of child health and wellbeing in our communities with that being generated elsewhere. This will help us understand how we are all similar, rather than different, and how we can learn from one another how to make things better for children. Guided by the principles of PHC we seek common ground as a basis for promoting a socially just world. In the process, we have to ensure that our work continues to create a thirst for the kind of wisdom that will help provide a safe, healthy, equitable, accessible and culturally appropriate pathway from before birth to the end of life. Then, we can use this knowledge as the impetus for change that will sustain our children well into their future.

THE HEALTHY CHILD

Healthy children can be defined on the basis of a wide variety of indicators. Being born healthy gives a child a head start, whereas coming into the world with a disability or some form of abnormality compromises a child's chance of good health.

After birth, health also depends on the family, and having opportunities to lead a healthy, nurtured and well-nourished lifestyle with a minimum of stress. Children's health is a product of receiving warm and consistent parenting, a good educationand health services when these are required; and having more protective factors in their environment than risk factors. These determinants of healthy childhood are underpinned by several theories of child health and development.

Point to ponder
A healthy child is one that experiences warm and consistent parenting, a good education, receives health services when needed, and has access to more protective and fewer risk factors in their environment.

For example, Bronfenbrenner's (1979) theory of social ecology or 'bioecology' focuses on interactions between the child, parental care and features of the family's environment. The resources a family brings to these interactions include income, time, and human, psychological and social capital (Brooks-Gunn et al 1995; Zubrick et al 2000). In combination, these resources help parents build the capacity to support child health and development in the context of their community and society (Li et al 2008).

Another theory, self-efficacy theory, explains how parents make decisions about their behaviour (Bandura 1977). This perspective argues that individuals choose behaviours they believe will lead to certain outcomes, which they usually believe

Objectives

By the end of this chapter you will be able to:

1 identify the most important influences on child health in contemporary society
2 describe the major risk and protective factors that influence child health
3 develop a set of community level strategies for promoting good parenting
4 explain how you would assess the resource base in any given community for supporting child health
5 describe how you would use the principles of primary health care to create a model for child health promotion in the community
6 identify the nursing roles that provide a common base of expertise for child health and parenting across a range of settings (school, clinic, home visiting, play groups).

they can carry out. Bandura's self-efficacy theory suggests that when parents are provided with both information and trust in their own judgement, they will be more likely to make decisions that promote better health for their children. A third theory, Bowlby's (1969) theory of human attachment, posits that newborn infants are predisposed to seek attachment to their caregivers in times of stress, illness or fatigue. Attachment is also important for parents. When parents have had secure attachments in their lives they will be sensitive, responsive, engaged caregivers for their own children (Olds 2002).

BIOLOGICAL EMBEDDING AND CHILDHOOD STRESS

Children begin life with a set of predispositions, biologically embedded to respond to what lies within the sphere of their life. This 'biological embeddedness' provides a template for interactions between children and the array of social and environmental circumstances of their lives, as they develop. Children's interactions with the world around them at 'critical moments' (times of heightened sensitivity) along their developmental pathway determine their endocrine, neurological, cardiovascular and immunological development, and how they learn to modify incoming stressors (Hertzman 2001a, 2001b; Mustard 1996, 1999). Critical pathway interactions are therefore instrumental to children's development. They provide opportunities for children to embed health enhancing behaviours in the early stages of their lives, which literally helps 'sculpt' their developing brains to build their coping capacity for later life (Mustard 2007).

Point to ponder
Children's interactions with the world around them at 'critical moments' in their development help them embed healthy behaviours in the early stages of their lives.

In some cases, children's cultural, spiritual and physical environments allow them to use their biological strengths to greater advantage. In other cases, children fail to reach their potential because of socio-cultural determinants. These can include cycles of intractable poverty, or a lack of healthy

policies for child support, or a lack of high-quality day care, adequate parental support or environmental protection. Instead of enhancing their coping capacity, certain combinations of these social factors may conspire to stifle a child's ability to be nurtured in the community (Shonkoff et al 2009). This can create inequalities for children that persist into adult life in two ways. The first is by accumulating damaging adversities during sensitive developmental periods. So, for example, traumatic exposure to psychologically and physically stressful experiences during a very early sensitive period of life could establish effects that become permanently incorporated into the child's regulatory physiological processes.

Current research has found that these physiological mechanisms can lead to coronary artery disease, cancers, alcoholism, depression and substance abuse, as well as being linked to obesity, physical inactivity and smoking (Shonkoff et al 2009). For this reason, interventions to deal with these diseases in adulthood are nowhere near as effective as ensuring a healthy childhood relatively free from stress. An alternative explanation to why childhood stress leads to adult diseases is called 'weathering' of the body, which occurs under persistent adversity (Shonkoff et al 2009). In this situation, the increased wear and tear induced by too many stressful experiences deregulate and overuse the pathways that were originally designed for an individual's adaptation to stress. This accelerates the ageing processes. Cumulative exposure to stress creates an 'allostatic load' which activates stress management systems in the brain to the extent that they become pathogenic instead of adaptive (Shonkoff et al 2009).

Point to ponder
Exposure to psychologically and physically stressful experiences in childhood can impact on health as an adult.

SOCIO-ECONOMIC FACTORS AND CHILDHOOD STRESS

Pathogenic effects can be created when children live in impoverished families, where they can be exposed to numerous stressors. These stressors include such things as maltreatment, traumatic fear, family conflict and/or chaos, inadequate nutrition, recurrent infections, having mentally unstable or absent parents, punitive parental behaviour, neighbourhood violence and dysfunctional schools (Shonkoff et al 2009; Waldegrave & Waldegrave 2009). Research shows that these social stressors affect many children from lower SES backgrounds through heightened activation of their stress-responsive systems (Shonkoff et al 2009; Waldegrave & Waldegrave 2009). Because of this burden of stress it may be impossible to completely reverse the neurobiological and health consequences of growing up poor. On the other hand, an emerging body of research is showing that positive parent–child interactions, exposure to a new vocabulary and stability of parental responsiveness can actually alter a child's physiological responses (Hackman & Farah 2009). Parental social support, especially from family members, and having the support of services and schools can help moderate the impact of adverse circumstances for children (Zubrick et al 2008). Stress in children can therefore be buffered by stable and supportive relationships at the family, community and societal levels (Shonkoff et al 2009; Zubrick et al 2008). This is cause for optimism in promoting child and family health.

As mentioned in the previous chapter, the quality of the parental relationship is a significant influence that can lead to either sensitive parenting or disruptive relationships between parents and their children (Finger et al 2009). This reflects the importance of focusing on intergenerational health. Where the community and society provide supportive environments for families, there is a greater likelihood that parents will make healthy choices for parenting practices, and personally, modify any risky behaviours that leave them vulnerable to ill health. This, in turn, affects the likelihood of their children leading healthy lifestyles.

> **Point to ponder**
> The quality of the parental relationship has a significant influence on the relationship between parents and their children.

Clearly, investing in children and their parents should be the major priority for ensuring good health across the life course and across the population (Shonkoff et al 2009). This is illustrated in Figure 6.1.

GLOBAL CHILD HEALTH, DISADVANTAGE AND POVERTY

The health of the world's children is of concern to everyone who claims global citizenship. Most children in the world are cared for and loved, but other children suffer from violence, exploitation and abuse. Approximately 200 million children globally are not achieving their full development potential (Commission on the Social Determinants of Health [CSDH] 2008). Every day, more than 2000 die from an injury (World Health Organization [WHO] 2008b). In some regions, children are sexually abused or forced into child marriages,

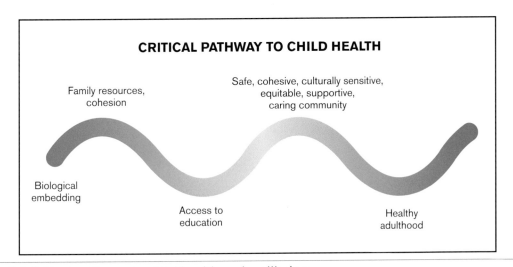

Figure 6.1 Critical pathway to child health and wellbeing

while others may be trafficked into exploitative conditions of work. Just over one billion children under the age of 5 live in the midst of armed conflict (United Nations Childrens Fund [UNICEF] 2009). Infant mortality is improving in some countries, but in the African countries, rates have either stagnated or lost ground, primarily due to poor access to health care (WHO 2008a). Although there have been some improvements in countries where there has been greater access to water, sanitation, drugs and antenatal care, globally, there are still nearly 10 million child deaths per year (WHO 2008a).

Point to ponder

While most children in the world are cared for and loved, more than 2000 children a day die in the world as the result of an injury, and over 1 billion children under the age of 5 live in the midst of armed conflict.

In addition to these poor morbidity and mortality rates, global and national inequities are not being resolved, especially in developing nations. Approximately 51 million children are not registered at birth, leaving them without the protection they should have from social institutions (UNICEF 2009). In 33 countries, less than half of all births are attended by health professionals (WHO 2008a). More than one-third of young women in developing countries were married as children (UNICEF 2009). More than 70 million girls have undergone female genital mutilation, and 150 million children aged 5–14 are engaged in child labour. Others are trafficked into prostitution or other forms of exploitation (UNICEF 2009). Child poverty is also persistent. Despite worldwide attention to child poverty throughout the past 100 years, about 600 million children continue to live in absolute poverty, trying to survive on less than $US1 per day (UNICEF 2007). The main problem in many of these countries is an actual expansion of disparities between the wealthy and the poor, which leaves many poor children with little hope for the future (WHO 2008a).

In the countries of the West, *relative* child poverty continues to be a major problem. Relative poverty refers to those children living in homes receiving less than 50% of the median national income, and this affects approximately 15% of children in Australia and New Zealand

BOX 6.1 IMPACT OF IMPOVERISHMENT IN CHILDHOOD

High infant mortality

High unintentional injury rates

Low birth weight

Poor overall child wellbeing

Low immunisation rates

Juvenile homicide

Low educational attainment

Non-participation in higher education

Dropping out of school

Aspiring to low-skilled work

Poor peer relations

Bullying at school

Teenage pregnancy

Physical inactivity and childhood obesity

Not having breakfast

Mental health problems, including loneliness

(Emerson 2009)

(Emerson 2009). The effects of living in relative poverty have been demonstrated in a wide-ranging body of research (Emerson 2009), summarised in Box 6.1.

An interesting analysis of young people's perspectives on poverty was conducted in the United kingdom (UK) to see how the children themselves experienced disadvantage (Redmond 2008). A review of nine studies where children's views were sought found that children living in relative poverty were not as concerned about the lack of resources as they were about family relationships and being excluded from activities that their peers can access (Redmond 2008). Social exclusion therefore had the most profound impact on their lives as a result of relative poverty. This was experienced in not being able to access the tools of virtual communication (phones, computers) to connect with their peers. The children coped with this type of social exclusion by relying heavily on family life to help them cope. For children who live in rural and remote areas, these effects are even more intense. Some children adapt to these difficulties with resourcefulness and optimism, while others experience anxiety, pessimism and reduced aspirations for the future (Redmond 2008).

CHILDREN AND HOMELESSNESS

At the extreme end of poverty, a growing number of children are rendered homeless, even in the wealthiest countries. Homelessness is a source of grave concern in the United States, where in a CNN poll found that 1 in 50 American children faced homelessness in 2005–06 (Online. Available: www.cnn.com/2009/US/03/10/homeless.children [accessed 14 October 2009]). In Australia during the financial crisis of 2008–09, homeless families with children accounted for one-quarter of the homeless population of nearly 79 000 (AIHW 2009b). In New Zealand, homelessness is a largely invisible problem, with some imprecision in the number of homeless. Although Statistics New Zealand released a formal definition of homelessness in 2009 (Statistics New Zealand 2009), there are also cases of 'concealed homelessness', a situation where people have no other option but to share someone else's accommodation. This is a growing concern.

Point to ponder

While few children in Australia and New Zealand live in absolute poverty, relative poverty is a significant issue for children in both countries.

In addition to having a lack of housing, there has been a growing trend towards women and children using women's refuge services as temporary safe housing (National Collective of Women's Refuges 2007). The negative health and social impact of this situation is an immediate problem, as these children are prone to injury, violence and behavioural problems. It is a social tragedy in wealthy countries. Although some cases of homelessness are a result of families becoming victims of changing socio-economic circumstances, other cases of child homelessness reflect parental neglect or abuse. Children who have been neglected or abused have the same types of negative developmental outcomes as mentioned opposite in Box 6.1, particularly lower social competence, poor school performance and impaired language ability (AIHW 2009a; Waldegrave & Waldegrave 2009). In addition, child victims of maltreatment or abuse do not acquire the skills to be self-regulating, which interferes with their ability to control emotions and behaviour. This impedes the development of independence and self-sufficiency later in life

(Schatz et al 2008). A longitudinal study of New Zealand children found that children with severely disturbed childhood behaviours have a number of risks in later life, including the risk of committing violent offences, attempting suicide and becoming teenage parents (Fergusson et al, in WHO 2009a). As others have found, the residual effects of child abuse often last throughout the child's life, especially among those who have been sexually abused, and those who do not disclose the abuse (Ming Foynes et al 2009; Pereda et al 2009). As we mentioned in Chapter 5, some victims of abuse grow up to become perpetrators of abuse themselves (AIHW 2008).

INDICATORS OF CHILD HEALTH IN AUSTRALIA AND NEW ZEALAND

A comprehensive report on child health in Australia in 2009, indicates where progress has been made in reducing risk and increasing protective factors, and identifies health issues that continue to be problematic (AIHW 2009a). No similar barometer of child health has been reported for New Zealand children, although a monitoring framework provides the basis for key indicators of child health (Craig et al 2007). What we do know from recent comparative data is that New Zealand lags behind Australia in a number of international child health indicators, including infant mortality rates, immunisation, deaths from accidents and injury, relative income poverty of children and material wellbeing of children (UNICEF 2007).

Point to ponder

New Zealand lags behind Australia in a number of key child health indicators, including infant mortality, immunisation and relative income poverty of children.

The main health issues for children in Australia are mental disorders, chronic respiratory conditions such as asthma, and neonatal conditions. As in other Western nations, injuries are the leading cause of death in children aged 1–14, with 10–14-year-old boys having 2.5 times the rate of injuries for girls in this age group. For all Australian children the leading causes of injuries are falls, land transport accidents, accidental poisoning, burns, scalds and assault. The other most prevalent conditions causing childhood deaths are cancers and diseases of the nervous system (AIHW 2009a). Injury deaths have been reduced over the past decade because of fewer land transport accidents, accidental drowning and submersions. Infants have the highest rates of injury death of all children's age groups, although infant mortality can be due to factors related to pregnancy. The mortality rate among infants and young children have steadily declined as a result of adequate neonatal intensive care units, increased community awareness of risk factors for sudden infant death syndrome (SIDS) and the rate of childhood immunisation, which covers 93% of Australian 2-year-olds. The rate of Australian infant mortality and childhood deaths compares favourably with other OECD countries in ranking, just above the median level, but only for non-Indigenous children.

New Zealand children are most likely to be acutely hospitalised for injuries/poisoning, gastro-enteritis and asthma. Arranged admissions to hospital are most often for cancer/chemotherapy and dental conditions, with the most common reason for children's hospital admissions in 2004 being insertion of grommets (Craig et al 2007). In the same year, SIDS (now often referred to in New Zealand as sudden unexpected death in infancy or SUDI), was the most common cause of mortality for children aged under 1 year, with injuries the most common cause for children over the age of one. As is the case for Australian children, the leading causes of injury among children were motor vehicle accidents and falls. Drowning also figured highly among causes of death among New Zealand children (Craig et al 2007).

HEALTH INDICATORS FOR INDIGENOUS CHILDREN

Although infant mortality has halved in the years 1986–1998 in Australia, since 2006 it has been comparatively stable in Indigenous children (AIHW 2009a). Aboriginal and Torres Strait Islander (ATSI) children experience a significantly higher rate of under 5 mortality than non-Indigenous children, including three times higher infant mortality, and three times as many childhood injuries. Half of all Indigenous infant deaths are due to perinatal problems; low birth weight and complications of pregnancy, with congenital conditions and diseases like SIDS being responsible for the remainder. Indigenous children are nearly five times

more likely to die of SIDS. They are also eight times more likely than non-Indigenous children to be the subject of child protection orders for child abuse, neglect and maltreatment. Injury deaths are also more than four times greater in remote areas, where many Indigenous children live.

Point to ponder

Indigenous children in Australia and New Zealand are at greater risk of poor health outcomes than non-Indigenous children in both countries.

New Zealand's Indigenous children are also at greater risk of poor health outcomes than non-Indigenous children. When Maori children in New Zealand are born, they are more likely than European children to have a low birth weight, die in infancy, enter primary school with poorer hearing, have oral health problems, have experienced respiratory issues, and be at greater risk of unintentional injuries (Dyall 2007). Maori children are also more likely to be exposed to domestic, sexual and criminal violence in the home (Dyall 2007).

CHRONIC ILLNESSES IN CHILDHOOD

The chronic conditions of asthma, diabetes and cancer are increasing in Australian children, with 40% experiencing at least one condition of 6 months or more duration, and boys suffering disproportionately (55%). Indigenous children have a greater prevalence of chronic conditions and hospitalisation rates than non-Indigenous children as well as a 30% greater prevalence of disabilities (AIHW 2009a). Among all Australian children, there has been a significant increase in type 2 diabetes over the past decade, more so for girls. The incidence of cancers among children has remained relatively stable over this time, with improved survival because of advanced treatments, and a decline in mortality. Cancer prevalence is greater in boys than girls (55%). The proportion of Australian children having allergies and asthma is equal highest (with Costa Rica) among OECD countries, whereas the prevalence of other chronic conditions is relatively similar to the other countries.

Children in New Zealand experience similar chronic conditions to Australian children. New Zealand has one of the highest reported occurrences of asthma in the world, with 25% of children reporting asthma symptoms (Howden-Chapman et al 2008). Although overall hospital admissions for asthma have declined over the past decade, ethnic disparities persist with higher rates for Maori and Pacific children than for European children (Craig et al 2007). While it is acknowledged that childhood obesity and associated type 2 diabetes are increasing in prevalence among New Zealand children, figures are not readily available. However, it is known that, like other conditions, Maori and Pacific children are over-represented in obesity and diabetes statistics (Kedgley 2007).

Point to ponder

The chronic conditions of asthma, diabetes and cancer are increasing among Australian and New Zealand children.

Cancer is relatively rare among New Zealand children, with leukaemia accounting for approximately one-third of all cases (Craig et al 2007). Cancer prevalence is, however, increasing across all types, but with a corresponding decrease in mortality, which is expected to continue into the foreseeable future (Craig et al 2007).

Approximately 8% of Australian children and 11% of New Zealand children have disabilities that interrupt their interactions and effective participation in society, with physical disabilities more common in girls, and intellectual disabilities more common in boys. Disabling conditions among children range from moderate impairments for home and school life to those that severely limit core activities of development and require lifelong support (AIHW 2009a; Craig et al 2007).

Point to ponder

Approximately 8% of Australian children and 11% of New Zealand children experience some type of disability that interrupts their ability to participate in society.

Other indicators of child health and wellbeing include having good dental health, physical activity and nutrition, and being breastfed from birth (AIHW 2009a). Internationally, dental health is improving due to better public health programs,

water fluoridation, and improved oral hygiene and disease management (AIHW 2009a). Figures on the oral health of Australian children are not current, but it appears that they are above the OECD standard on the number of tooth decays. In New Zealand, however, the figures are concerning, with no improvement in the rate of dental caries since the early 1990s. Only 50.7% of 5-year-olds in New Zealand live in communities with fluoridated water supplies (Craig et al 2007).

NUTRITION, PHYSICAL ACTIVITY AND THE SOCIAL DETERMINANTS OF CHILD HEALTH

In terms of nutrition and physical activity, most Australian and New Zealand children meet the national guidelines of 60 minutes of activity every day, but very few meet the nutrition standard for fruit and vegetable consumption (AIHW 2009a; Craig et al 2007). In addition, only one-third report that they conform to the 'screen guidelines', which recommend no more than 2 hours of non-educational screen time (computers, video, TV) per day. These guidelines are based on the fact that children who engage in more than 2 hours of screen time per day are more likely to be overweight; be less physically active; drink more sugary drinks; snack on foods high in sugar, salt and fat; and have fewer social interactions (Commonwealth Scientific and Industrial Research Organisation [CSIRO] 2009).

Although most Australian and New Zealand children are within a normal weight range, approximately one-fifth of Australian children and one-tenth of New Zealand children are overweight or obese (AIHW 2009a; MOHNZ 2008a). Those who are disadvantaged socially, economically and geographically are at increased risk of becoming overweight due to a lack of available, accessible and affordable fresh fruit and vegetables and opportunities for exercise. Pacific children in New Zealand are 2.5 times, and Maori children are 1.5 times more likely to be obese than other children (MOHNZ 2008a). The majority of children are also active, meeting the standard of 60 minutes a day of some kind of physical activity, but nearly one-quarter do not meet this benchmark (AIHW 2009a). Children's nutrition and physical activity patterns have attracted worldwide attention because of the 'obesity epidemic' in many nations. The obesity epidemic has attracted widespread attention because it is commonly understood that the most prevalent cause of morbidity and mortality in adults in the 21st century are non-communicable cardiovascular and metabolic diseases (WHO 2008a). The most useful way to analyse these disease patterns and their causes in the population should begin with an examination of children's health, and the critical events that occur along the pathway to adulthood that instigate and perpetuate these diseases in epidemic proportion. A significant element of this type of analysis lies in analysing the social determinants of poor eating behaviours and inactivity patterns and the way these may be contributing to the obesity epidemic.

Point to ponder

Most Australian and New Zealand children meet recommendations for daily exercise, but few meet the standards for fruit and vegetable consumption.

Many researchers into obesity have focused on genetics, physiology, race/ethnicity, personal responsibility and freedom of choice, effectively creating the impression that inappropriate diets are either destiny or unwise choices (Drewnowski 2009). However, increased attention has been drawn to obesogenic food environments and the importance of economic factors as social determinants of poor eating habits (Drewnowski 2009). For example, low-income neighbourhoods tend to have many fast-food outlets and convenience stores, which encourages consumption of inexpensive foods with refined grains and high sugar and fat content. On the other hand, people living in affluent neighbourhoods have the wealth and access to healthy, low-fat foods. This difference in access illustrates the role of social inequality in dietary behaviour (Drewnowski 2009). Other studies take a more socio-cultural approach, arguing that poor dietary habits are environmental and intergenerational, the result of how the family environment socialises and controls a child's eating habits (Kime 2008). This perspective contends that the lack of structure in contemporary family life creates a more haphazard and less ordered way of eating that is sometimes chaotic, and can lead to less nutritious patterns of food consumption (Kime 2008). The other critical issue relevant to good nutrition is breastfeeding.

Breastfeeding

The research evidence supporting the health benefits of breastfeeding is unequivocal (AIHW 2009a). Compelling evidence suggests that breast-feeding protects infants against infectious diseases, including gastrointestinal illness, respiratory tract infections and middle ear infections (WHO 2005). Other possible benefits include a reduced risk of SIDS, type 1 diabetes and some childhood cancers, although the link between breastfeeding, asthma and childhood allergies is less certain (AIHW 2009a; Bryanton et al 2009; Kramer et al 2007). Having been breastfed may also reduce the incidence of high cholesterol, high blood pressure, obesity and diabetes later in life, and improve cognitive development (Horta et al 2007). More exclusive and longer periods of breastfeeding show the strongest associations between breast-feeding, lower rates of infant illnesses and better cognitive development (AIHW 2009a).

Point to ponder

The benefits of breastfeeding for both infant and mother are extensive. Nurses and midwives have an important role in supporting breastfeeding mothers and normalising the breastfeeding process.

Benefits of breastfeeding also extend to the mother, improving recovery after childbirth, reducing the risk of ovarian cancer and possible reduced risk of breast cancer, post-menopausal hip fractures, osteoporosis and maternal depression (Ip et al 2007; Productivity Commission 2009). Breastfeeding is also thought to improve mother–infant bonding and secure attachment (Allen & Hector 2005; Bryanton et al 2009). For these reasons, the WHO (2009b) guidelines recommend exclusive breastfeeding to 6 months of age.

No national studies on breastfeeding among Australian mothers have been conducted to date, so figures vary according to the state of residence. However, data collected for the Longitudinal Study of Australian Children (LSAC) on 5000 families show that 91% were breastfed at birth, and 46% continued to 4 months, with 14% continuing to the 6-month period as recommended by the WHO (2009b). New Zealand figures indicate that 70% of infants are exclusively breastfed at 6 weeks of age, at 3 months just over 50% of infants are exclusively breastfed, and by 6 months this has dropped to approximately 7.5% (MOHNZ 2008a). Of the latter, most were women who did not have to return to the workplace during that period of time (Zubrick et al 2008). The link between breastfeeding and work schedules confirms the complexity of breastfeeding behaviour in relation to the combination of individual and environmental factors (Commonwealth of Australia 2009). As revealed in the Australian National Review of Maternity Services, these include the health and risk status of mothers and infants, their SES, education, knowledge and skills, and support in the hospital, workplace, community, and policy environments (Commonwealth of Australia 2009). The review also cites a study in New South Wales, which found that mothers who returned to work fewer than 10 hours per week or who were self-employed had the highest rates of breastfeeding (Hector et al 2005).

Point to ponder
The UNICEF Baby-Friendly Hospital Initiative has been a significant factor in increasing breastfeeding rates globally.

A Queensland study of the influence of psychological factors on breastfeeding duration also identified factors that predict breastfeeding (O'Brien et al 2008). These include the mother's anxiety level, whether or not she had an optimistic disposition towards breastfeeding, self-efficacy, faith in breast milk for her baby, expectations and planned duration of breastfeeding prior to the birth, and the timing of making the decision to breastfeed (O'Brien et al 2008).

This body of research contributes important insights into the issues that may help encourage mothers to breastfeed. At the global level, the most significant factor in encouraging higher rates of breastfeeding in recent years has been the UNICEF Baby-Friendly Hospital Initiative, which began in 1992 (Online. Available: http://unicef.org.au/GetInvolved-Subs.asp?GetInvolvedID=99 [accessed 23 October 2009]). This is a structured method of encouraging breastfeeding, which has been adopted by a number of hospitals throughout the world as a consistent method of encouraging breastfeeding. However, women's busy lives outside the home and an early return to work after childbirth can run counter to successful breastfeeding, especially where workplace practices constrain a woman's ability to breastfeed her child. Clearly, family-friendly workplace strategies could go a long way to extending the rates of breastfeeding to meet the WHO guidelines. Community and peer support have also been identified as important to persevering with breastfeeding, and these will be incorporated into a future National Breastfeeding Strategy for Australian mothers to be developed in 2010 (Australian Health Ministers 2009). The development of a breastfeeding helpline (1800 MUM 2 MUM) is also expected to demonstrate a favourable impact on breastfeeding rates once national data are collected from users of this service (Commonwealth of Australia 2009).

Healthy pregnancy

The fruits of a healthy pregnancy are celebrated daily, throughout the world. For some mothers, though, a healthy pregnancy is a conquest of the human spirit over dire social circumstances, made worse by a lack of care and support. In developing countries, the rate of accessing antenatal care steadily increased throughout the 1990s, notably in countries like Indonesia and other parts of South-East Asia. However, in some areas, lack of access to care can place both mother and child in a perilous situation, especially if there are other co-morbid conditions, such as malaria or HIV/AIDS (WHO 2005). In response to this situation, the Commission on the Social Determinants of Health (CSDH) recommends a global comprehensive strategy to provide mothers and children with a continuum of care from pre-pregnancy through pregnancy and childbirth to the early years of a child's life (CSDH 2008). Their recommendations also include support for exclusive breastfeeding initiation within the first hour of life and for the first 6 months, skin to skin contact immediately after birth, extended breastfeeding to age 2, and educational support for children and their mothers. If these recommendations were adopted worldwide, it would have an intergenerational effect, shaping lifelong trajectories and opportunities for health as well as promoting mothers' educational attainment as a way of countering gender and other inequities (CSDH 2008).

Point to ponder
A healthy pregnancy is one of the key determinants for achieving a healthy childhood.

Other risks to healthy pregnancy lie in the workplace. Many pregnant women maintain full-or part-time employment, exposing them to workplace hazards. Others may be exposed to dangerous conditions in their home, neighbourhood or community. In any of these settings, the availability of sufficient nutritious food is an important influence on healthy pregnancy. A nutritional diet in pregnancy should have a high intake of fruits, plant foods and calcium and low intake of fat, salt, sugar and alcohol. Research also indicates that folic acid, one of the B vitamins, should be taken by pregnant women to help prevent spina bifida and other neural tube defects (AIHW 2008). Another important goal of pregnancy is to ensure that both parents are in good health and free from infections, harmful drugs or other substances that can interfere with the construction of a healthy child. It is important for expectant parents to understand the multiplier effects of all factors, to gain a clear understanding of how lifestyle factors can interact with biological or genetic factors and environmental circumstances to either enhance or override a child's healthy development.

Antenatal care

Antenatal care by a health professional from the earliest stages of pregnancy can help pregnant women and their partners identify the need for any dietary or lifestyle changes and ways of sustaining those changes throughout the pregnancy and beyond the birth of the child. It also provides an opportunity to help parents create the emotional foundations for the child's life; one of the most important elements of early parenting.

Point to ponder

Effective antenatal care provides an opportunity for parents to create the emotional foundations for a child's life.

Ultrasound examinations and population studies show that from about 10 weeks, an infant moves spontaneously, and by 15 weeks, movements may be felt as a reaction to the mother's laugh or cough, suggesting a response of self-protection or self-assertion (Shonkoff & Phillips 2000). During this stage, a high level of stress in the mother can affect the function of the fetal–placental unit, compromising fetal growth and causing a risk of pre-term birth or low birth weight (Hobel et al 2008).

Knowledge of this early neurological development of the fetus, along with our understanding of the effects of stress on neural development during the critical periods, underlines the importance of early and ongoing antenatal care (Hobel et al 2008; Shonkoff et al 2009).

An additional goal of antenatal preparation is to establish a birth plan, one that empowers parents to make decisions on the place of birth, and the choice of birth attendant or birth companion. Yet another important opportunity afforded by antenatal visits is the chance to discuss the diagnostic approach to the pregnancy, including the choice of vaginal or caesarean birth and whether or not an induction will be indicated. Antenatal preparation also provides an opportunity for parents to talk through their emotional needs in relation to parenting, which is especially important for pregnant adolescents and first time parents. The antenatal visits can therefore act as a platform for planning and empowerment as a parent. They provide an opportunity to establish a trusting relationship with a health professional and open up channels of communication that will help women develop the skills for lifelong decision-making (WHO 2005). Birth preparation includes gathering information about breastfeeding and how to access help with infant problems such as feeding, crying and sleep disruptions, which are typically the most problematic for parents, especially for their first child. Parents often use the antenatal visit to seek guidance on conditions such as Sudden Infant Death Syndrome (SIDS). The prevalence of SIDS has shown a dramatic, worldwide reduction, which, to some extent, is directly related to antenatal guidance, and campaigns urging parents to place their infants in a supine, or back-lying position while sleeping (AIHW 2008; Child and Youth Mortality Review Committee 2008).

Childbirth

For Indigenous mothers, the antenatal period and birth hold unique challenges, especially for those who live in rural and remote areas. Compared with non-Indigenous mothers, ATSI mothers have more births (2.4 in their lifetime) than non-Indigenous Australian mothers (Commonwealth of Australia 2009). Many are younger when they give birth and, if they attend antenatal classes, it is usually at a later stage of pregnancy and less frequently than non-Indigenous women. Teenage pregnancy is also more prevalent in Indigenous women (19%), compared with non-Indigenous mothers (4%). Indigenous neonatal deaths occur more frequently, and Indigenous babies are twice as likely to be low birth-weight, especially if they have not attended antenatal care (Commonwealth of Australia 2009). Maternal deaths are also much higher for Indigenous women, and many encounter a lack of culturally appropriate birth practices in the Australian health care system. The cultural preference of many Indigenous women is to have 'birth on country', which is a cultural rite of passage at childbirth, where women's identity and connections with the land and country are transferred, shared and celebrated (Commonwealth of Australia 2009). A number of culturally appropriate models of this type of birthing exist throughout Australia, mostly run by women in the local community, but these are limited to certain geographical areas.

Point to ponder

The cultural elements of birth are significant to many Indigenous women, providing important links to culture and the land.

For most mothers and their partners, childbirth is a joyous occasion, but there are also risks to health. These can include injuries to the vaginal canal, temporary anaemia due to blood loss and, for some mothers, dramatic changes in their emotional state. Another issue is the risk of infection from a surgical birth. This is a growing problem, with the rates of caesarean section increasing worldwide. The WHO (2005) guideline recommends a maximum proportion of 15% for caesarean sections compared with vaginal births, however the rate of caesarean births in many countries exceeds this proportion (Althabe & Belizan 2006; Anderson 2004; Moore 2005). In Australia the national rate is around 30%, and states such as Western Australia have recorded a rate of 33.9%, which has been rising annually (Gee et al 2007). In New Zealand the rate is 23.7% (MOHNZ 2008b). The rate of inductions at birth has also increased worldwide to 25–30% of births (MacKenzie 2006). This creates a set of other risks related to epidural analgesia, and morbidity such as birth injury and lengthened hospital stay (MacKenzie 2006).

Postnatal depression

One of the most serious challenges for many women at the time of childbirth is related to the emotional aspects of the experience. Postnatally, many women experience being a bit down for various lengths of time, and this may reflect a depressed mood or tiredness that can begin prior to the birth (Figueiredo et al 2009; Seimyr et al 2009). For some mothers, their emotional state evolves into the more serious problem of postnatal depression. Postnatal depression is reported to occur at a rate close to the rate of other types of depression in the population, in approximately 13% of mothers (Dennis et al 2009; Hewitt & Gilbody 2009). O'Brien et al (2008) found in their study of women birthing in two Australian hospitals, an unexpected rate of 44% of postnatal distress. Postnatal distress and depression have been linked to feelings of social isolation and lacking an intimate confidant or friend after the birth (Dennis et al 2009). Postnatal depression tends to develop in the first few months after the baby is born, with a peak in incidence at around 4–6 weeks (Hewitt & Gilbody 2009). Some of the factors contributing to postnatal depression are listed in Box 6.2.

BOX 6.2 FACTORS CONTRIBUTING TO POSTNATAL DEPRESSION

- Unwanted or stressful pregnancy.
- Poor relationship with the child's father or other family members.
- Criticism or lack of social support, either from family members or peers.
- Poverty and the social conditions it precipitates, such as crowding, substandard housing or unemployment.
- Being a migrant mother without a support network.
- Prior psychiatric problems or a history of depression.
- Stressful life events.
- Sleep deprivation or anxiety.
- Having an infant born with a medical problem or not surviving the birth.
- Poor physical health or coincidental adverse life events, such as the loss of a partner.
- Being depressed prior to birth.
- Having a depressed partner.

(Dennis et al 2009; Figueiredo et al 2009; WHO 2005)

Given widespread recognition of the significance of postnatal depression, the past decade has seen a burgeoning body of research into the condition. Studies have shown that it is the most common form of maternal morbidity after delivery, with health consequences for the infant and the woman's partner as well as herself (Dennis et al 2009). Infants and children are particularly vulnerable because of the impairment to maternal–infant interactions, which can cause attachment insecurity, developmental delay, and social and interaction difficulties. Researchers have found that less than 50% of postnatal depression cases are detected by health care professionals, which indicates the need to screen all new mothers for the condition (Hewitt & Gilbody 2009). Treating the condition with antidepressants is not always appropriate, particularly for breastfeeding mothers (Morrell et al 2009). Several studies, including a Cochrane systematic review, have shown that postnatal depression can be treated effectively with psychosocial and psychological techniques (Dennis et al 2009).

Point to ponder

Postnatal depression is a significant challenge for many women in Australia and New Zealand. It can have profound implications for the health of both mother and child.

Another study, that trialled a telephone-based peer support program by volunteer mothers over 12 weeks' postpartum, showed that this type of support reduced the incidence by half among those at risk of postpartum depression (Dennis et al 2009). The researchers concluded that telephone support is ideal for this purpose, given that it is flexible, private and non-stigmatising, and it overcomes the problems of accessibility to services, especially for mothers of low SES. Another trial of social support by health visitors in the UK that provided weekly one-hour sessions with new mothers for up to 8 weeks, also demonstrated dramatic reductions in the incidence of postpartum depression (Morrell et al 2009).

Men may also experience the effects of depression in the postnatal period. This depression is closely associated with maternal depressive symptoms and previous paternal depression (Ramchandani et al 2008) and has been demonstrated to place children at increased risk of emotional and behavioural problems (Schumacher et al 2008; Ramchandani et al 2008). Nurses and midwives must be aware of the signs and symptoms of depression among men in the early postpartum period and consider screening men for depression where indicated — particularly where the mother is experiencing depression (Schumacher et al 2008; Ramchandani et al 2008). There is some evidence that including fathers in antenatal preparation results in an increased awareness of the maternal experience and it has been suggested that father-specific sessions may be helpful in preparing men for the transition to fatherhood (Schumacher et al 2008).

CHILDREN'S PSYCHOSOCIAL WELLBEING

Measurements of mental health and wellbeing among Australian children are imprecise because of a lack of national data. However, it is likely that the rate of mental illness is likely to be similar to other OECD countries, with a prevalence of around 20% of children. In New Zealand, it is estimated that 17.6% of children under the age of 11 have some type of mental health problem with up to 5% suffering from conduct disorder (WHO 2009a; Craig et al 2007). In the US, it is estimated that one in 10 children suffers from an emotional disturbance severe enough to cause impairment (Herman et al 2009). Data from general practice have recorded rates of mental illness in children that include behaviour symptom/complaint (27%), ADHD (18%), sleep disturbance (14%) and depression/anxiety disorder (13%) (AIHW 2009a). Children with these complaints are disadvantaged not only from the disease, but also socially, in terms of stigma, discrimination, functional impairment and the risk of premature death (AIHW 2009a). Childhood depression is thought to be a significant issue for many children, overlooked, untreated and, in many cases, debilitating (Herman et al 2009). The mental health of immigrant children is a particular concern, especially those who are refugees and/or are living in detention centres awaiting status decisions. This affects approximately 1% of Australian children, who are refugees from war-torn countries. Most arrived through the government's Humanitarian Program and many live in relative socio-economic disadvantage (AIHW 2009a).

Mental ill health

Although mental illness may arise from birth it is also a product of social determinants within the family and the child's psychosocial world. Having a parent with mental illness can predispose a child to mental illness such as schizophrenia, bipolar disorder or depression, however these conditions may not develop without the interaction of non-genetic risk factors. Other precipitating factors include slow academic achievement, physical or psychological trauma, abuse and/or neglect, loss of family, or community and cultural factors, such as having low SES or being discriminated against (AIHW 2009a). Having a child with a mental illness is also traumatic for parents, who may suffer high levels of distress and depression that can lead to a vicious circle of stress and emotional ill health for all family members (Scharer et al 2009). For children from economically deprived families the presence of mental ill health may be both a cause and consequence, as economically deprived children have a high risk of behavioural or emotional problems that can manifest in childhood and persist into adult life.

Learning readiness and social development

Economic disadvantage in childhood is also linked to learning readiness, and this is an area that is attracting considerable research attention. Early learning enhances a child's functioning, including language development, literacy acquisition, cognitive processes, emotional development, self-regulation and problem-solving skills (Zubrick et al 2008). As a child makes the all-important transition to school, academic competence is important to him/her developing the ability to process feedback from the family, school and peer environment. Support through this transition can help children gain both cognitive and social competence. However, if the child encounters criticism or a harsh learning environment this may be more difficult, especially if the child has some emotional disadvantage on entry to school (Herman et al 2009; Zubrick et al 2008).

The preschool experience is critical to children developing the skills for lifelong learning, particularly in learning to read, as studies have found a link between reading problems in children and depressive illness (Herman et al 2009). With a large proportion of parents working outside the home, the quality of child care plays an important role in helping children develop a sense of belonging and the competence, independence and the community connectedness they require to grow into successful adults. Preschool and child care can help young children develop cognitive and social skills that prepare them for the transition to school, which can be a significant asset for children from low socio-economic environments (AIHW 2009a). This is achieved through positive adult–child interactions and regular opportunities for guided play with other children, which focus on early sensory and language development as well as a child's socialisation skills.

All of these factors have been found to lead to better language and social and emotional outcomes for children (McCain & Mustard 2002; Shonkoff & Phillips 2000; Mitchell et al 2008). High-quality child care organisations maintain basic health and safety measures, including standards aimed at preventing communicable diseases, especially for infants. These organisations have sufficient staff to child ratios to give each child attention that is appropriate to their age level. They also have qualified staff, and maintain relatively small groups to enable children to form caring relationships with one another, all of which contributes to learning readiness (AIHW 2009a).

The number of children attending early childhood education in New Zealand is increasing.

The introduction of 20 hours of free early childhood education for all 3-and 4-year-olds in New Zealand in 2007 was an acknowledgement of the importance of early childhood education to child health and wellbeing, particularly for children from lower socio-economic groups and for those with English as a second language (Mitchell et al 2008). The policy has had an impact on increasing children's participation in childhood education (Froese & Jenkins 2008).

There is some evidence that attending poor-quality early childhood education prior to 1–2 years of age can result in antisocial or worried behaviour among children both at the time and at entry to school, although this can be tempered by the subsequent provision of high-quality education (Mitchell et al 2008). Studies have also shown that young children attending poor-quality early childhood centres display an increased cortisol level, which is an indicator of stress. This can leave them more prone to infection (Mitchell et al 2008). With increasing numbers of children under the age of 3 years attending early childhood centres in New Zealand and Australia these issues are of concern. Clearly, high-quality standards, and regular monitoring in early childhood centres are required to ensure optimal outcomes for children.

The LSAC mentioned previously, is the first comprehensive national Australian study to examine learning readiness, gathering data on children's lives at regular intervals across infancy and middle childhood (Zubrick et al 2008). Among other factors relevant to child health and wellbeing, the researchers have explored the link between financial disadvantage and school readiness, finding that children at 4 and 5 years of age from low-income families had lower indicators of school readiness, particularly in language development (Zubrick et al 2008). At age 6 and 7, more children from low-income families have been found to experience literacy and numeracy difficulties than children from middle-income families (Smart et al 2008). Duncan and Brooks-Gunn (2000) explain that these effects occur through a convergence of factors from the quality of the children's home environment, the quality of parent–child interactions, early learning and child care outside the home, parental health and community conditions. School relationships are particularly important, which is being recognised worldwide because of increased attention to anti-bullying programs.

Point to ponder

Children from low-income families have lower indicators of school readiness prior to starting school and experience more literacy and numeracy issues once started at school than children from middle-income families.

Bullying is prevalent in most schools today, including those in Australia where 20% of boys and 15% of girls have been identified as victims of weekly bullying (AIHW 2009a). In New Zealand, 19.2% of calls to the 0800WHATSUP child and youth telephone counselling service in 2006 were for bullying, which was an increase from 14.9% of calls in 2003 (Craig et al 2007). A healthy school environment can counter bullying by working towards eliminating the power imbalance that can leave some students with physical, social or emotional harm, oppressed and isolated from the school community. All children need peer support at school, and this has implications for health and development. Without the support of peers many children can become discouraged and often fail to develop their learning potential (AIHW 2009a).

The LSAC data also revealed that around 58% of Australian 2–3-year-olds are being read to daily, which bodes well for their future literacy, as reading aloud to young children is considered the best way to instigate literacy acquisition. In 2009 benchmarks for learning development will be established through national administration of the Australian Early Development Index (AEDI). The AEDI will measure the five developmental domains of physical health and wellbeing; social competence; emotional maturity; language and cognitive skills; and communication skills and general knowledge. This will provide clearer data to guide programs for the future, aimed at ensuring that every child has an equal chance of making a successful transition to school, and subsequently having the literacy and numeracy skills to develop personal capacity and resilience (AIHW 2009a).

RESILIENCE

Whether children are born to traumatic conditions or to a more gentle life, their development capacity depends on their resilience, which is the key to personal and social competence. Resilience is a concept that captures how some children seem to have the ability to do well in life, regardless of the hardships imposed on them (Armstrong et al 2005; Stanley et al 2005). Resilient children survive the challenges of daily life through self-esteem and good problem-solving abilities (Silburn 2003).

Education, child care, parenting and other sectors that determine a child's environmental features all have major parts to play in helping develop resilience, and therefore their ability to cope with the future. A child's innate characteristics also seem to have an effect on resilience. Those who begin life with a positive temperament will often show resilience early, and demonstrate persistence and emotional regulation to adapt to life as they develop (Stanley et al 2005). Girls seem to be more resilient than boys, and this may be related to girls being more inclined to reach out and use social networks (Silburn 2003; Stanley et al 2005). Resilient individuals are also thought to have protective factors that tend to modify, ameliorate or change their responses to stressors. These protective factors include having an active approach to problem solving, an ability from infancy to get positive attention from others, being alert and autonomous, having a tendency to seek out novel experiences and to maintain an optimistic view, even in the face of distressing experiences (Armstrong et al 2005). With an enabling family, community and society their resilience will help them adapt throughout childhood and into adult life (Armstrong et al 2005) (see Figure 6.2).

Point to ponder

Resilience describes the ability of some children to do well in life despite having experienced significant hardships.

PARENTING PATTERNS AND CHILDREN'S HEALTH OUTCOMES

Parental health and wellbeing, especially family conflict and the mother's physical and mental health, play a significant role in children's health outcomes (Khanam et al 2008; Kiernan & Huerta 2008; Sanders 2002). Both maternal depression and family conflict have been identified as increasing a child's risk of developing behavioural or emotional problems, including substance misuse, antisocial behaviour or delinquency (Kiernan & Huerta 2008). The risk is greatest where there is protracted conflict and/or clinical depression extending beyond the normal circumstances of having a child. For most couples, marital quality declines once a first child is born, primarily because of sleep deprivation and, for mothers, overwork from housework and parenting responsibilities (Ahlborg et al 2009). However, with support, mutual tolerance and encouragement in their parental roles, most couples find the resilience to provide a harmonious home environment and positive parenting (Widmer et al 2009). Where there is

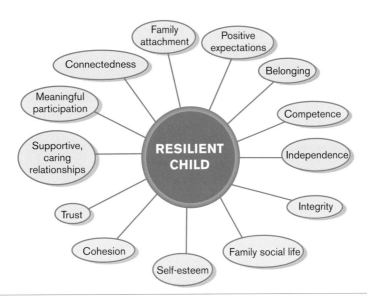

Figure 6.2 Universal needs for developing resilience in children

an absence of support for parenting or a lack of mutual support between the couple, children may be at risk of poor mental health outcomes.

> **Point to ponder**
> Parental health and wellbeing play a significant role in children's health outcomes.

Parenting style is an important determinant of children's health outcomes. Research in the 1960s and 1970s identified the three main styles of parenting as *authoritative, authoritarian* and *permissive*. Authoritative, characterised by high warmth and responsiveness, was seen as the most desirable (Baumrind 1966, 1971). Other researchers since that time have conceptualised parenting styles on the two broad dimensions of warmth and control (Chaudhuri et al 2009). Children of parents who are warm and emotionally available, yet encourage the child's development have been found to foster self-esteem, social skills and academic achievement (Chaudhuri et al 2009). This begins in infancy, with parental behaviours that maintain physical and emotional closeness, responding with quick, calming, soothing responses that provide control and security (Bryanton et al 2009). Dependable and predictable care is also important, managing a child's behaviour with consistency. Warmth and consistency are the opposite of hostile parenting reactions (McCain & Mustard 2002; AIHW 2009a). Hostile parenting is akin to Baumrind's (1966) authoritarian style of parenting, where parents use angry or coercive patterns of parenting with criticism, negativity and emotional reactivity. This is the type of harsh discipline that flows from family conflict or depression, which typically leads to poorer cognitive and social development in children (Kiernan & Huerta 2008; Whiteside-Mansell et al 2008; Zubrick et al 2008).

Parental warmth is expressed in affectionate behaviours, high positive regard, expressing enjoyment in the child's company, taking an interest and being involved in the child's activities, being responsive to his or her moods and feelings, and giving positive expression of approval and support (Zubrick et al 2008). Consistent parents are firm, structured, yet sensitive in their interactions with children. They set clear, developmentally appropriate boundaries and expectations for their chid's behaviours, following through with intentions and giving the child a sense of direction and competence (Zubrick et al 2008). This does not negate the fact that there is a reciprocal response in parenting, where parents respond differently to children with different temperaments, but in general, warmth, consistency and emotional availability lead to the most positive outcomes for children (Chaudhuri et al 2009; Zubrick et al 2008). They help foster the development of trust, security, self-worth and readiness to learn in the child, as well as a sense of self-efficacy in the parents, wherein they feel confident in their parenting capacity (Zubrick et al 2008).

> **Point to ponder**
> Parenting style has an impact on child health outcomes. Authoritative, authoritarian and permissive parenting are three types of parenting style. Authoritative parenting is characterised by warmth and responsiveness, and is the most effective parenting style of the three.

Some parenting behaviours create risk factors for children's health. These include teenage pregnancy, smoking and alcohol consumption during pregnancy, and consuming a non-nutritious diet with inadequate fruit and vegetables (AIHW 2009a; Khanam et al 2008). A poor diet before and during pregnancy and lactation can leave a mother deficient in vitamins and minerals that are essential to an infant's health. Teenage motherhood and fetal exposure to tobacco and alcohol can contribute to low birth-weight and poorer outcomes for the child. Adolescent mothers are also at risk of dysfunctional parenting because they are at an early stage of their own development and struggling with adjustment issues (Schatz et al 2008). Many have little understanding of the importance of refraining from alcohol and tobacco smoking during pregnancy, which is a major problem for Indigenous mothers, who have high teenage birth rates (four to five times that of non-Indigenous mothers) and high rates of smoking (AIHW 2009a; Craig et al 2007).

FAMILY LIFESTYLE PRACTICES

Family lifestyle practices are another important aspect of healthy childhood, especially in relation to smoking, diet and activity patterns.

This is significant, given that an entire generation of children in Western nations lives in the shadow of chronic lifestyle diseases and mental health problems that are often co-morbid with physical disease (AIHW 2008). Smoking is declining worldwide, and this is having a positive effect on children (AIHW 2008). However, research into obesity and lifestyle shows that many families continue to have less than optimal eating and activity patterns, both of which have harmful consequences for both physical and mental health (AIHW 2008). Obesity among members of Indigenous families is an even greater problem, as many are already at higher risk of cardiovascular disease and type 2 diabetes in adulthood (AIHW 2008).

Point to ponder

Family lifestyle practices such as smoking, diet and activity patterns are another important aspect of healthy childhood.

Obesogenic environments

Various explanations have been given for the 'overweight or obesity epidemic'. It is tempting to blame parents for the problems, but there is actually a web of social and environmental factors that have created this situation, many of which affect both parents and children. Solutions therefore have to be aimed at the broader circumstances that create unhealthy lifestyles for the entire family. First, there is a proliferation of food choices available to busy families these days and the foods marketed to them are often refined and calorie-dense. Many busy families tend to buy foods for convenience and price rather than nutrient value, adding to children's incentives to eat large quantities of fast, easily prepared foods. The trend towards more meals consumed outside the home, and a shift to larger portion sizes also play a part (Harnack et al 2000). Because fast foods are less filling than fresh fruits or vegetables and pleasurable to eat, children tend to eat larger quantities of them. Fresh fruits and vegetables are also more expensive than fast foods, but not as aggressively marketed (AIHW 2008). Marketing strategies also play a part. Promoting healthy alternatives by some fast-food outlets creates confusion as to what is in fact, 'healthy', and what may be laden with empty calories.

The education system also contributes to the epidemic. Public schools have reduced the physical education component of their curricula. With shrinking education budgets and a virtual explosion of curriculum content, physical education is easy to dispense with, especially where educational managers are not strong advocates of healthy lifestyles. Government regulatory agencies and various education authorities have been moving towards standardised curricula, and their plans often fail to include strong voices for physical education. Like other government agencies today, schools are required to manage risk in a way that reduces the threat of accidents and injuries, and these typically occur during sports and physical activities, making the reduction of sport and activity easy to justify. After-school programs have also changed. Because of the increase in working mothers, a large proportion of children attend after-school care, and these relatively low funded programs are easier to manage indoors. Where children do attend formal activities after school, the major focus of these is often oriented towards preparing them to compete in the intellectual, rather than lifestyle domain.

From the parents' perspective, it is more convenient to pick children up from school rather than have them ride their bikes. Concerns for children's safety also leave many students taking passive, rather than active transport to and from school. Together with a reduction in physical education classes at school, these factors mitigate against adequate activity at a time when children are becoming more obese (Salmon et al 2005). Children also seem to be involved in more sedentary home activities, with extended screen time now considered a health hazard. These factors are only part of the web of causation for the childhood obesity epidemic, and many individual and situational factors also have a role to play, including the workplace stressors that cause parents to be too exhausted to exercise with their children, and for some, a propensity to seek solace in non-nutritious foods. The solutions to the current obesity epidemic thus lie in a combination of healthier family lifestyles, and eliminating obesogenic environments. Lifestyle modification programs can risk blaming the victims. Because stress plays an important role in the metabolic syndrome that often leads to diabetes, it is important to be sensitive to the environmental influences that contribute to their behaviours. In the final analysis, responsibility for childhood obesity should be everyone's concern, especially given the knowledge that, if the trend continues, the current generation of children will be the first in the history of the world to have lower life expectancy than their parents (Stanley et al 2005).

KEEPING CHILDREN SAFE

Each day, 2000 children around the world die of unintentional injury, half of whom could be saved (WHO 2008b). In addition to 830 000 child injury deaths, millions more are left with lifelong disabilities. The most prevalent childhood injuries are from road traumas, drowning, burns, falls and poisoning. The highest rate (95%) of these injuries occurs in developing countries, especially African nations, where children die at 10 times the rate of Australian and New Zealand children, primarily from road traumas (WHO 2008b). Besides being the greatest cause of child mortality, childhood injuries also place an extraordinary burden on health care systems. For those children who survive accidental injuries, many are seriously disabled, creating a lifelong caregiving burden for families. When the child has been injured in the home, there is an often unrelenting emotional toll on family members. This is a major problem, as the most common injuries occur in or around the home.

ACTION POINT
Childhood injuries have a significant impact on nations throughout the world. Advocating for the creation of safe environments for children is one of the most important things a health professional can do to promote child health.

One of the things health professionals can do to promote child safety from injury is to lobby for healthy and protective environments within which young children grow, to ensure that the onus is on all of society to help keep children safe from harm. This approach has been effective in advocating for bike helmet use, safer roadways and bicycle paths, and seatbelts on school buses. Child and family health nurses also have a major role to play in fostering parental health literacy. Strategies include providing parents

with information on their child's capacity at each developmental stage, so they will be alert to the precautions needed to ensure their child is safe, or directing parents to the sources of parental advice on child safety, either in print form or on the internet. Family-friendly websites provide a wealth of encouragement for safety prevention, such as the practices maintained by UNICEF (www.unicef.org). The UNICEF site has a list of key messages for both the family and community, including those listed in Box 6.3.

Many childhood injuries are not caused by children's behaviour, but by the family's social circumstances. Factors related to the social environment include living in substandard housing, being in a one-parent household, low maternal education, large family size and parental drug or alcohol abuse (AIHW 2009a). The risk for Indigenous children is also greater, as many live in substandard housing and have poor general health. For some older children, the risks are multiplied by engaging in risky behaviours such as glue sniffing or other self-harming behaviours (AIHW 2008). Compared with non-Indigenous Australian children, Indigenous Australian children living in remote areas have additional risks for accidents and injuries from attending school in run-down

BOX 6.3 HELPING PARENTS KEEP CHILDREN SAFE

- Ensure that children are watched and kept in a safe environment.
- Keep children away from fires, cooking stoves, lamps, matches and electrical appliances.
- Take precautions to secure stairs, balconies, rooves, windows and play areas.
- Keep sharp objects such as knives, scissors and glass away from children.
- Keep small objects out of the reach of young children.
- Never store poisons, medicines, bleach, acid and liquid fuels in drinking bottles and keep away from children's sight and reach.
- Do not leave children alone when they are in or around water.
- Always accompany children under age 5 near roadways and teach safe road behaviour as soon as they can walk.

(UNICEF online. Available: http://unicef.org.au/GetInvolved-Subs.asp?GetInvolvedID=53 [accessed 23 October 2009]) buildings, often without working smoke alarms or other safety features. When the circumstances of Indigenous education fail to provide learning environments conducive to successful study, and the only physical and social spaces available to children are dangerous, their chances of a just, socially inclusive, healthy adulthood are greatly diminished. We elaborate further on these risks in Chapter 11.

> **Point to ponder**
>
> Strong family bonds help children make appropriate decisions about the various paths they will take towards independence.

To develop independence and empowerment in a positive and not isolating way, a child needs close attachments to family. From strong family attachments, young people are able to make decisions about the various paths they will take towards independence. These attachments also provide a blueprint for forming subsequent social relationships and a sense of social connectedness. Helping children acquire and refine skills at progressively higher and broader levels, sets the stage for later developmental tasks. Refining skills to the level of mastery helps children move from reaching and grasping, to walking, riding a tricycle, playing sport, and developing friendships and intimacies.

In mastering lower level skills, children learn confidence, self-esteem and a sense of control over their environment. This attracts recognition from others, a sense of pride, wellbeing and life satisfaction (Stanley et al 2005). Engaging with the wider community provides opportunities for children to make the most of their own capacities in the context of developing respect for those around them, a sense of integrity and 'civic friendship' (Stanley et al 2005:25). As a child grows to adulthood, civic friendship and civic participation can then grow into increasingly wider circles of trust, which helps foster community cohesion and social capital (Putnam 2005) (see Figure 6.3).

CRITICAL PATHWAYS TO CHILD HEALTH

From all the research into early parenting and development, we know that the health of children reflects the world into which they are born; the national policy environment that encourages or discourages the expression of their culture; their genetic make-up, and that of their parents; their ability to access education and early preparation for employment; the family's SES, including their place of residence; their access to, and preferences for health services; family harmony, the extent to which healthy behaviours are modelled in the family and community; and features of the physical environment.

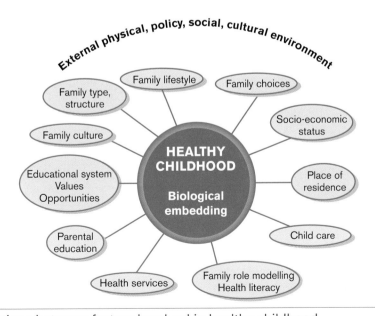

Figure 6.3 Interactions between factors involved in healthy childhood

The first critical step on the pathway to healthy children, as WHO (2005) advocates, is to focus on the health and wellbeing of women and this begins with educating women throughout the world. The pre-eminence of maternal education is validated in numerous studies demonstrating its significance to child survival (WHO 1999), in developing competence for life long coping (Mustard 2007) and in breaking the cycle of poverty (UNFPA 2000). It is commonly understood that children can reduce a woman's financial potential by interrupting employment during the years of peak growth in earnings. When mothers with low earning potential become separated or divorced, they and their children often become economically disadvantaged.

Point to ponder
The first critical step toward healthy children is the health and wellbeing of women.

Distress from the combined economic and interpersonal crisis often interferes with the mothers' work performance and the children's school performance. The quality of their lives is compromised by social stress, poor social networks, low self-esteem, high rates of depression, anxiety, insecurity and the loss of a sense of control (Wilkinson 1996). The longer the period of disruption and distress, the greater the probability that the mother and her children will fail to advance, for adequate mother and child attachment is difficult in the struggle to survive. As a result, both mother and child may have residual problems with relationships, precipitating an intergenerational tendency toward family breakup. Combined with higher fertility among less educated women, these break-ups drive a growing rate of cyclical poverty among women and children (WHO 2005; Wilkinson 1996). Research revealing the intricacies of this cycle demonstrates unequivocally that the pathway to health and wellbeing extends from pre-conception advice on diet, smoking, exercise and self-esteem, to political decisions aimed at enhancing structural support for families at all stages from birth through maturation to death (McCain & Mustard 2002).

A second critical pathway overlaps the first, in that health promotion activities should address the links between individual cognitive development and competence, and the aspects of society and the environment that either provide social

buffering, social risk or social enhancement. A socio-ecological view of child health includes both proximal and distal factors, some of which may be found in neighbourhoods, religious groups and nationalities, but most particularly in early childhood education (McCain & Mustard 2002; Zubrick et al 2008). This includes a need to better understand the residential composition of communities, including the larger societal forces that act to stratify groups by race, ethnicity and social class (CSDH 2008). Our interventions must also seek to address the constellation of factors such as quality of housing, child care facilities, schools, parks and recreational areas, businesses and transportation networks that allow us to appreciate children as agents in their daily activities and local habitats (Earls & Carlson 2001).

Point to ponder
The second critical step toward healthy children is that health promotion activities should focus on the link between individual development of the child and those aspects of society and the environment that enhance health.

Compelling data from child development research supports the contention that healthy children are more likely to develop from an environment of good early parental care which is supported by social and environmental factors (Zubrick et al 2008). Children also need to be seen from very early in life as learners, right from earliest child care to high school and beyond (Hertzman 2001b; Mustard 2007). When they are encouraged to develop the aptitudes they have, this will pull along learning in weaker areas, provided that, by age 4 or 5, they feel the impact of the community (Hertzman 2001a, 2001b). If not, they run the risk of carrying forward a developmental drag that could affect their mental and physical health, coping abilities and competence throughout their lives (McCain & Mustard 2002).

Goals for child health
The major health issues for children's health in today's society include adequate societal investment in the early years, supportive communities that protect and enable child and family health, health literacy for parents and their children, and continuing evolution of the evidence base for child and family health. The most optimal circumstance for a healthy

child is to be born into a child-friendly, healthy and safe family and community. To support parents in this endeavour nurses and midwives need to address key family practices, as outlined in Box 6.4.

To achieve child health in any community, all known risk factors and factors that develop children's resilience and capacity to cope with their environments must be acknowledged and incorporated into a community's goals and target for prevention, protection and health promotion. An intersectoral approach is essential, which is best argued within the strategies of the Ottawa Charter for Health Promotion (WHO, Health and Welfare Canada & CPHA 1986).

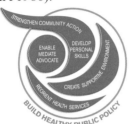

BUILDING HEALTHY PUBLIC POLICY

The greatest investment any society can make for the health of its people is one that facilitates the health of children. Health policies should therefore be developed on the basis of a commitment to child and family health. This is embedded in health and intersectoral strategies at the global, national and local levels. The United Nations Convention on the Rights of the Child, developed as a legally binding international instrument to guide the care and protection of children illustrates the global commitment (Online. Available: www.unicef.org/crc [accessed 21 October 2009]). The Millennium Declaration of 2000 addresses the explicit need to protect children from conflict, violence, abuse and exploitation (UNICEF 2009). Each of the Millennium Development Goals outlined in Chapter 1 are linked to the needs of children, from poverty reduction to educating children, eliminating gender inequality and reducing child mortality

---

BOX 6.4 NURSING AND MIDWIFERY GOALS FOR SUPPORTING PARENTS

- Maintaining culturally appropriate birthing and social support.

Some resources for ATSI women's birthing services include Congress Alukura in Alice Springs; Nganampa Health Council; Ngua Gundi Mother Child Project, Woorabinda, Queensland; Aboriginal Maternal and Infant Health Strategy (AMIHS) NSW; Strong Women, Strong Babies, Strong Culture, NT. For migrant women information can be accessed at: www.migrationinformation. org/Feature/display.cfm?ID=108).

- Breastfeeding exclusively for 6 months and continuing until the child is aged 2 or more.

Resources for breastfeeding are listed at the end of this chapter and include: www.breastfeeding. asn.au; www.babyfriendly.org.nz; telephone helpline 1800 686 2 686 (Australia) 0800 611 116 (New Zealand).

- Promoting physical growth and mental and social development, including interactions with others in the household.

- Recognising the need for assistance if required for infant settling or feeding. Resources are listed at the end of this chapter, including: www.plunket.org.nz; www.cs.nsw.gov.au/tresillian/default.cfm; www.ngala.com.au.

- Preventing child abuse and neglect.

- Accessing health services when required by maintaining sufficient health.

- Literacy to recognise needs and seek timely and appropriate care. Resources include www. healthinfonet.com.au; www.moh.govt.nz.

- Providing access to high-quality child care when required.

- Ensuring the home is peaceful and free from stress, conflict or violence.

- Mental/emotional health promotion with the aim of meeting the universal needs of belonging, competence, independence, learning readiness and connectedness to the broader environment.

- Keeping children safe from the harm of alcohol, tobacco or other toxic substances.

- Immunising children according to the national schedules (www.immunise.health.gov.au; www. moh.govt.nz).

- Preventing injuries and accidents (accessing helplines, local poison hotline).

- Maintaining food security in all neighbourhoods, promoting safe cooking with good ventilation.

- Maintaining health literacy through knowledge of resources for child health (AIHW 2009a; WHO 2005).

(UNICEF 2009). At the heart of all of these global policies is the need for equity at the start of life, to eliminate disparities and inequitable conditions, and provide a strong foundation for children along their life course (CSDH 2008). This requires policy coherence, commitment and leadership, as well as the integration of health in all government policies (CSDH 2008; WHO 2008a).

In New Zealand, the 2001 Primary Health Care Strategy set in motion a national set of policies to reduce social inequities with a focus on child, family and community health (MOHNZ 2001). In 2009, Australia developed its first national Primary Health Care Strategy with a similar intention (Online. Available: www.yourhealth.gov.au/internet/yourhealth/publishing.nsf/Content/nphcs [accessed 20 October 2009]). A national commitment to children has also been declared in the Australian National Agenda on Human Capital of the Council of Australian Governments (COAG) and the Stronger Families and Communities Strategy (2004–2009), both of which also address the social inclusion agenda of closing the gap on Indigenous disadvantage (AIHW 2009a). At the state level, similar principles are included in policy documents such as the Western Australian Aboriginal Maternal and Child Health Action Plan (Department of Health Western Australia [DOHWA] 2008).

ACTION POINT

The most valuable action a government can take to promote the health of children is to develop health policies that demonstrate a commitment to child and family health. As health professionals, our role is to contribute to policy-making at all levels, to ensure this commitment is realised.

The most important policy decision governments must make acknowledges the importance of antenatal care in providing and sustaining a good start for improving the health of the entire population. This is encompassed in the recommendations of the Australian Review of Maternity Services, which focus the country's service commitment on access and equity for parents and children (Commonwealth of Australia 2009. Online. Available: www.health.gov.au/maternityservicesreview [accessed 20 October 2009]). Policies governing antenatal and birth care, immunisation, support for breastfeeding both at home and in the workplace, and early childhood education can be argued on the basis of research into the link between good health and adequate support during pregnancy, the influence of early parenting, and the importance of the nested influences of neighbourhoods and communities in child health. Antenatal care and breastfeeding, in particular, have the capacity to increase life span, enhance quality of life and reduce the cost of illness care for the population, making them the most important policy focus in public health.

In 2002 the Ministry of Health New Zealand established national breastfeeding targets and a corresponding action plan (MOHNZ 2002b). It is expected that similar national initiatives will flow from adoption of the Australian Primary Health Care Strategy and the Australian Review of Maternity Services (Commonwealth of Australia 2009). A further policy initiative was launched in 2009 by the Australian Research Alliance for Children & Youth (ARACY), which created a Declaration and Call to Action to transform Australia for the future of its children (ARACY 2009). The declaration provides inspiration to galvanise researchers, policy-makers and child health advocates to value, nurture and respect children and young people so that they can thrive and reach their potential (see Appendix F).

Collaborative policy development

Healthy public policy for children involves ensuring that policies governing illness and injury surveillance, health and fitness promotion, family support systems and sustainable environments are all developed coherently, so that all influences on health are acknowledged by all sectors of society. This type of intersectoral collaboration is advocated in the Australian National Preventative Health Strategy which sets targets for reducing chronic illnesses through shared partnerships and acting early and throughout life (Preventative Health Taskforce. Online. Available: www.preventativehealth.org.au/internet/preventativehealth/publishing.nsf/Conte [accessed 15 October 2009]). The intention of this set of policy developments is to adopt a multidimensional approach to health and illness. This reflects the global initiative of embedding health in all policies (WHO 2008a).

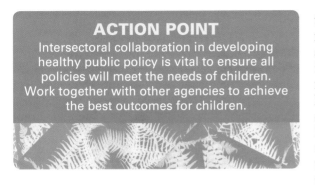

ACTION POINT

Intersectoral collaboration in developing healthy public policy is vital to ensure all policies will meet the needs of children. Work together with other agencies to achieve the best outcomes for children.

To date, the intersectoral approach has been more widely accepted in New Zealand than in Australia, primarily because of fewer layers of bureaucracy and a stronger commitment to working across sectors (Jacobs 2009). However, the Australian Preventative Health Strategy and PHC initiatives foreshadow a stronger government commitment to health in all policies, and intersectoral collaboration for the future. It is expected that in time, early child development (ECD) and parenting programs will be included in public policy structures that embrace all sectors relating to human health and development (AIHW 2009a; CSDH 2008; McCain & Mustard 2002). Despite the inclination toward intersectoral collaboration in New Zealand, there remains much to be done in relation to child health policy development. Although the Paediatric Society of New Zealand has developed a set of child health indicators from which to benchmark child health in New Zealand, there has been no government-led child health policy or action plan since 1998 (MOHNZ 1998). Although child health is embedded in various policy documents as outlined above, strategic direction in this area has been lacking over recent years, and there is a need for cohesive policies that provide a way forward for nurses, midwives, and other health professionals working in child and family health.

Policy collaboration is essential. This includes developing and monitoring manufacturing safety standards, housing standards and advertising codes of conduct, particularly in promoting tobacco products and junk food to children. Collaborative legislation such as that governing seat belts, bicycle helmets and child care workers is also intended to guide safe behaviour and environments. Laws mandating the licensing of child care workers, accreditation of child care providers and working with children's legislation are a visible signal of society's commitment to protect its most vulnerable citizens. There remains a need for national child care strategies and parental leave policies. A national inquiry into paid parental leave has made a number of recommendations for Australian parents, which have yet to be incorporated into legislation (Productivity Commission 2009). As mentioned earlier, New Zealand already has in place 14 weeks of paid parental leave. Leaving child care solutions to parents causes many families to suffer prolonged reductions in income, and a lack of opportunity for promotion once they revert to part-time work.

The Scandinavian countries of Denmark, Finland, Iceland, Norway and Sweden have the most generous entitlements to parental leave for both parents, which is expected to encourage fathers to become more involved in child rearing. Yet, in highly competitive workplaces, many fathers relinquish their right to this leave, particularly with persistent disparities between male and female salaries. This is one area where industrial policies would make a difference to both parental attitudes and child rearing. Initiatives to help parents maintain a balance between work and parenting are important, as conflicts between the two have been identified as a major contributor to mental health problems (Hertzman 2001b). Father-sensitive policies and services would also help reframe fathers' roles with their children as more inclusive in their emotional development rather than simply as the source of family finances (Fletcher 2008). See Box 6.5 regarding healthy food policy.

As a general rule, policies to promote better health among children should respond to children's holistic needs for balance and potential. This means that school boards and education authorities should become aware of the need to accommodate physical education programs as integral to children's development. Schools can also be effective in promoting child health by cultivating health literacy. One example of this is the focus on good nutrition, which is done well by many early child care providers as well as primary schools by eliminating high fat content from school canteens and promoting better nutritional standards. This is an attempt to balance healthy eating policies during the early primary school years with modifications to the environment within which children and their families make healthy choices.

> ### BOX 6.5 FOOD POLICY FROM THE SCHOOL TO FAMILY AND COMMUNITY
>
> In 1989 the School Food Program (SFP) was developed by the National Heart Foundation of New Zealand and introduced into both primary and secondary schools. The aim of the health promotion program was to support schools to make positive changes to their nutrition environments (Craig 2009). The program is now called the Healthy Heart Award for Schools: Tohu Manawa Ora — Kura. It has expanded its focus to include healthy lifestyles as well as nutrition, and is funded by the Ministry of Health. The program is based on four key areas of action: food and nutrition education as part of the curriculum; promotion of healthy food to the whole school community (including parents, teachers and children); community health promotion; and the development of healthy food policies. By taking a whole-school approach to nutrition and lifestyle, the program encourages schools to work towards bronze, silver or gold awards in recognition of their achievements. Evaluation of the program over time has seen the Heart Foundation respond to various criticisms and adapt the program accordingly. Research shows that addressing childhood nutrition in schools alone will have a limited impact on child health outcomes, but working within schools to develop broader, collaborative improvements to food policy is effective and appropriate (Craig, in Signal et al 2009).

CREATING SUPPORTIVE ENVIRONMENTS

Supportive environments for child health should begin with those conducive to healthy pregnancy. Ideally, services that provide health surveillance and monitoring for pregnant women would be readily available to all and accessible through workplace-based resources. With the current shortage of health care professionals, arrangements should be made to provide new parents with access to alternative sources of information and support to develop adequate levels of health literacy for parenting. This can be accomplished by ensuring appropriate online resources, or distributing information and resources in schools, child care centres or designated family support centres, allowing parents a choice in how and where they access information. Acting on the research evidence indicating the importance of a healthy start and the difficulties faced by separated families, parenting resource centres have been established in Australia and Canada. A website for family members, including children has been established by the Australian government to help provide guidance on children and parents' emotional needs, resources for family violence, financial and legal support (Online. Available: www.familyseparation.humanservices.gov.au [accessed 21 October 2009]).

> ### ACTION POINT
> Where health professionals are low in numbers, use other resources to create supportive environments for families with children. For example, the internet, schools and family centres are ideal locations for health promotion activities.

McCain and Mustard (2002) advocate for better use of school facilities for parenting resources, especially in evenings and on weekends, as well as during the day, to encourage community participation in early child development. Schools are also an ideal setting to provide dietary advice at opportune times for young families and this approach is particularly helpful to urban and rural families without other services, as they are often able to provide information that is both culturally appropriate and family-friendly. This sends a message to families that educational settings are places where young children can not only learn, but thrive, and that the family is as valued as the child. It also places the school squarely at the heart of the community, helping not only children, but their families as well.

As outlined in Chapter 4, the move towards having local councils more involved in health and wellbeing is a positive step in promoting supportive environments for health, and a sense of belonging, especially at the neighbourhood level. This also helps build trusting, cohesive environments through intersectoral commitments to children's education in the family, home and school. The potential for this type of collaboration lies in providing a base of support that can help children overcome the seeming hopelessness of a low socio-economic beginning.

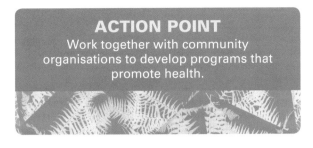

ACTION POINT
Work together with community
organisations to develop programs that
promote health.

In 2003, the UNICEF Innocenti Research Centre in Florence, Italy, advocated intersectoral, community support by creating the International Secretariat for Child Friendly Cities, whose aim is to shift responsibility for child health, education and protection to municipal councils. This is expected to provide a PHC approach in communities, where healthy, safe childhood becomes integral to community development (Online. Available: http://unicef.org.au/GetInvolved-Subs.asp?GetInvolvedID=53 [accessed 23 October 2009]). This global statement from UNICEF underlines the importance of the structural supports for child health and wellbeing; the macro forces within a child's environment that predict the extent to which children will do well. These include the global and national political environments and institutions that can create social injustice and health inequality, or responsive community care (Li et al 2009).

One example of a collaborative innovation between a group of child health researchers and the local council is the Swimming Pool Study, which was conducted in three remote Indigenous communities in Western Australia. The research team attracted funding from two government departments and worked with the local councils to build a swimming pool in each community, to respond to high rates of ear infections and skin sores, as well as high truancy and low activity rates, the latter related to the lack of facilities. In discussing the problems with local parents it was agreed to establish a 'no school no pool' policy to encourage attendance at school and provide an activity that would be fun and that could bring the community together to plan for the local children's health and wellbeing. Once the program was conceived, the pools were built and swimming lessons arranged. A swimming carnival has also been held in one community at the end of the five-year period, to motivate the local children and as an event to bring the community together. Evaluations conducted over a five-year period have shown marked reductions in the infections, dramatic improvements in school attendance and

a greater degree of cohesion among community residents who are making plans to sustain the use of the pools with local managers and the Royal Lifesaving Society (Lehmann et al 2006).

Point to ponder
Community strategies must
be inclusive of all members of
the community at all stages of
development, from implementation
to evaluation.

Similar collaborative ventures have seen New Zealand initiatives between Health, Sport and Recreation and local community health, social development and education groups (Jacobs 2009). One example is the iMove Nekeneke Hi! program in the mid-central region of the lower North Island. The iMove program encourages school students to choose between walking or riding a bicycle to school on a given day for a month. Students get a trip card which they get signed off and go into a draw to win on-the-spot prizes. The iMove program started as a pilot in two schools in 2006 and by 2008 over 30 schools were involved. While initially, the project was established by the Roadsafe Central coordinator, the success of the program has been dependent on the collaborative efforts of the police, the Palmerston North City Council, public health services, non-government organisations, local Maori health providers, primary health organisations (PHOs), the media and local sporting organisations (Ferry 2009).

Comprehensive strategies to address children's issues also take into account the increasing levels of immigrant, refugee, and culturally and linguistically diverse (CALD) families in the neighbourhood. Bringing CALD needs to the multi-sectoral agendas will help build tolerance in a community across politicians, health and education services, transport, the business community, the community council, consumer organisations, the police, juvenile justice authorities and any service clubs within the community. This type of collaborative approach focuses on ensuring safety and protection for all young people from a multidimensional perspective. Child-friendly neighbourhoods acknowledge the important effect of family and community environments on children's psycho-social, educational and criminal outcomes and entrench child safety and protection as every-one's concern (AIHW 2009a; Shonkoff & Phillips 2000).

STRENGTHENING COMMUNITY ACTION

It takes a community to create an empowering environment within which children's capacity can be developed. Ideally, this would be consti-tuted by a careful blend of voluntary, professional, business, faith-based and family organisations, to nurture children across the spectrum of childhood, irrespective of their abilities or level of disadvan-tage. Community partnership strategies can be helpful in building resilience in children, if they shift from a risk orientation to building children's competence. This approach places children at the centre of a community, and mobilises resources around them to transform the environments in which their lives are embedded (Vimpani 2000). Children's individual interactions with their social world should help them develop personal capac-ity within a safe, supportive, empowering learning environment (AIHW 2009a). To foster this kind of development at the school, neighbourhood and community level, parents, grandparents, teachers and others need to be made aware of their commu-nity's strengths and resources as well as the areas of particular risk to young children. Clear and vis-ible partnerships, with the child at the centre of the community, send a signal to children that their health and wellbeing are central to the way the community sees itself, and it gives them a sense of validation as they move through the various stages of childhood, learning to cope with life's chal-lenges and develop self-confidence and mastery at each stage.

> ### ACTION POINT
> Programs such as Family Start and Early Years, focus on strengthening community action for healthy childhoods. Be aware of the programs in your community and support families to access them.

Parent-to-parent programs and ECD programs like the United States Head Start program, the United Kingdom Home Start, the New Zealand Family Start, and Canadian and Aus-tralian Early Years strategies, have in common a focus on strengthening community action for healthy childhoods (CSDH 2008; DOHWA 2008; Downie et al 2004–05; McCain & Mustard 2002). Programs that use existing networks of volunteers, including grandparents, and health, welfare and education professionals, provide an outlet for new parents to express concerns and to share resources and strategies for parenting (Downie et al 2004–05). Like informal parent-ing groups, they can also provide an opportunity to socialise with others in similar situations, and thus guard against the ill effects of the isolation that new parenting often brings. This also helps strengthen community connectedness, which is particularly important for vulnerable first time families and those who may be at risk for adverse parenting approaches (Hanna et al 2002; Kelle-her & Johnson 2004).

Researchers have found that the most success-ful early intervention programs are those aimed at socially disadvantaged families, which use combined strategies for improving both child and parent outcomes (Watson & Tully 2008). Community programs to help these families are more effective when they begin before the child attends primary school, when they can help develop skills for learning and cognitive develop-ment, as well as good health (Brooks-Gunn 2003). Early intervention programs are also a vital element in improving the health of first time Indigenous mothers and their children and this is acknowledged in programs such as the Strong Mothers, Strong Babies, Strong Culture, which has been successful in the Northern Territory of Australia (Commonwealth of Australia 2009). A strengths-based approach has been used in a variety of child and parenting programs, focusing on empowering the family by identifying fam-ily members' strengths and capacity to do things for themselves (Green et al 2004). This approach has also been found to help build family relation-ships and cultural competence as well as health literacy and a connection to the wider community network of resources (Green et al 2004). Nursing and midwifery roles in community groups such as those mentioned above, are facilitative, bring-ing people together to strengthen their combined resources, and helping them compile a base of resources for any additional services required. Sometimes it is a matter of timing, being there to help draw attention to various issues of child health. At other times, it is an active involvement in building cohesion by bringing people together who need one another.

DEVELOPING PERSONAL SKILLS

It is up to health, education and community welfare groups to ensure that the community has appropriate educational opportunities for skills development for health carers, teachers and the children themselves. This is fundamental to developing community child-oriented capacity. Mandatory regulatory practices and compulsory in-service sessions for early child care and teaching personnel are designed to protect children, but many programs require only a minimum level of personal development. Community-based programs that help child workers remain connected to one another and maintain currency in their practice are a step further. In an era of evidence-based practice, it is also important that all professionals dealing with children have opportunities to share in the most recent research findings that guide their practices. Universities and colleges can be helpful in this respect, bringing people together as community residents, and providing courses that help them enhance their own capacity by building skills and strengths to cope with the challenges of their work. Personal development courses can also help reduce attrition among child care workers, which is a major problem today, given a rapidly growing need for child care, and a critical shortage of skilled health and welfare workers.

> **ACTION POINT**
> Facilitate connections between those involved in promoting the health of children by providing and encouraging participation in professional development programs.

One of the difficulties of parenting in contemporary society lies in managing child and family roles with formal work patterns. Many parents find themselves returning to work quickly after childbirth with little knowledge of developmental stages or children's needs, and a lack of extended family support. For some of these parents, the opportunity to access group-based positive parenting support programs is a lifeline to the wider community. Parenting programs have been found effective in helping reduce maternal depression and anxiety/stress, and in improving confidence, self-esteem and partner relationships, as well as improving child health outcomes (Fielden & Gallagher 2008). In Australia, nurses and other health professionals working in the community have successfully delivered the Triple P Parenting classes, which have had an important impact on early parenting skills (Zubrick et al 2005). Organisations such as Tresillian in New South Wales and Queensland, N'Gala in Western Australia and the Plunket Society in New Zealand emphasise the importance of building parenting capacity to ensure children's health and wellbeing. Evaluation of the New Zealand Plunket Parenting Education Program (PPEP) demonstrated that connecting parents to strong family and community networks can help build social capital that provides a foundation for children's social, emotional and educational needs (Fielden & Gallagher 2008). These programs are particularly effective when used in conjunction with individual interventions to support young families in their transition to parenthood.

REORIENTING HEALTH SERVICES

In the past, public health services included a relatively equitable distribution of family and public health nurses and child health specialists throughout the community, to support and assist parents in maintaining the health of their children. In Australia and New Zealand, the rationalisation of services has created inequities in service provision, with some families enjoying accessible neighbourhood centres for monitoring and guidance. Others, particularly those who live in rural areas or in the outer suburbs of large cities, have to rely on central hospital-based services and their local GP. It is interesting to hear of the reduction in child and family support programs in the same political context as the rhetoric about the 'family-friendly society', and then to ponder the effect of worldwide shortages of physicians, midwives, nurses and other health professionals. This is particularly concerning, given research findings that home-visiting interventions in Australia, the US and the UK from as early as 6 weeks of age have a positive impact on maternal, infant, family and home environment (Armstrong et al 1999, 2000; Barlow et al 2007; Olds 2002; Wilson et al 2008).

The most definitive evidence of the impact of nursing on children's health comes from a growing body of research into nurse-led models of care.

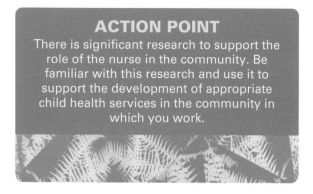

ACTION POINT

There is significant research to support the role of the nurse in the community. Be familiar with this research and use it to support the development of appropriate child health services in the community in which you work.

Analysis of a 25-year program of research into home visiting for low SES mothers in the US has shown that nurse home visiting improved parental care, reduced childhood injuries, improved maternal health and workforce participation, and reduced the number of pregnancies and the need for public assistance (Olds 2002). The results of similar studies in the UK have shown improvements in mother–child interactions, better health attitudes and behaviour, improvements to infant health and reduced risk of neglect or abuse (Barlow et al 2007). Studies in Australia and New Zealand have also shown that nurses play a key role in mandated child abuse and neglect cases (Fraser et al 2009; Rodriguez 2002). Because they are present in the community and home environments, nurses often have opportunities to observe childhood injuries and provide ongoing monitoring of children's health (Fraser et al 2009). This wide-ranging body of evidence cannot be overstated. Guidance and parenting support for new mothers has the potential to affect the health and development of children, enhance the parental life course for mothers, improve father involvement, and reduce the risks to children. Nursing and midwifery assessments of infant and family strengths and needs early in the postpartum period can reduce parenting stress, which can have a flow-on effect in reducing antisocial and detrimental behaviours such as smoking and substance abuse.

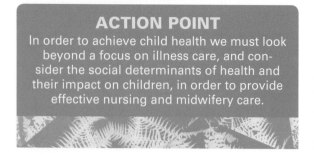

ACTION POINT

In order to achieve child health we must look beyond a focus on illness care, and consider the social determinants of health and their impact on children, in order to provide effective nursing and midwifery care.

With shrinking budgets and fewer personnel to meet family needs, our communities may become increasingly imperilled at the very time as we have determined the most appropriate way to help children. The evidence base indicates that the future of society rests in having all young children equipped emotionally and cognitively for their place in society. This should provoke us to look outside our professional boundaries at the social determinants and conditions that will help children become mentally and socially fit and able to cope with their lives. Health professionals who continue focusing only on illness care, and social workers who only focus on crisis events may be doing a disservice to families. Instead, the focus should be on interventions aimed at the whole of the population. This requires comprehensive PHC, with the addition of selective PHC to meet the needs of children with disabilities or special needs, such as mental illness (Scharer et al 2009; Woodcock & Tregaskis 2008). As mentioned in the previous chapters, this type of care reframes our health care systems towards equity, access, empowerment, cultural sensitivity and intersectoral collaboration.

Nurses are well prepared to work with others, and the partnerships between school nurses and teachers attest to the effectiveness of this (see Chapter 4). Collaboratively, the nurse–teacher team can align learning and health resources to make a significant contribution to health in the schools. They could also work with police and the judicial system that have in the past, focused their efforts on punishing and incarcerating, to develop programs to prevent children's antisocial behaviours. Nurses also play an important role in advocating for quality and monitoring of standards in child care organisations. This can be a part of their community level interventions, or by greater involvement with parents in their guidance of child care.

The issue for all involved in child health is to recognise that the organisation of health services continues to value illness care, even though the rhetoric proclaims a commitment towards prevention. In the interest of access and equity, all health professionals should work more closely together to ensure that families do not fall through the cracks of service provision. This involves greater teamwork and careful evaluation of services and health outcomes. It also requires examination of the best way to use existing resources, given the large number of health professionals about to retire with insufficient replacements. This is an important component of the ongoing agenda in health services research. Although there is a significant need to investigate specific health issues related to healthy child development, the need for safe care provision for all is a priority and it is a current and future challenge for researchers. Valuing children is valuing the future of society (CSDH 2008). There remains a need to demonstrate how valuing children can be translated into better outcomes for them, their families and communities.

Case study

Maria and Jim had been trying for a third child for some time and after an uneventful pregnancy, Maria has just given birth to a healthy baby boy (Luke). Maria had successfully established breastfeeding while in the hospital, but on her return home she has been struggling to settle Luke. Her nipples have become sore and swollen and Luke is fretful. She is visited by the child health nurse, then a lactation consultant. Luke is due for his first immunisations, and Samantha who is 3 is also due for immunisation, so Maria has made an appointment for both to be immunised. At the same time, both Jim and Maria have noticed Lily coughing at night and becoming breathless when she is exercising. After visiting the GP, Lily is diagnosed with asthma and, in conjunction with the GP and practice nurse, an action plan is developed to manage this.

REFLECTING ON THE BIG ISSUES
- The most important investment governments can make is in supporting child and family health.
- One of the most significant threats to child health is poverty.
- Healthy pregnancy and antenatal care establishes a platform for good health in childhood.
- Breastfeeding is the ideal for nourishing infants.
- The health of children in Australia and New Zealand is at a high standard relative to other countries of the West.
- Family lifestyle and parenting practices have a profound impact on child health.
- Nurse home visiting is one of the most important interventions to provide parenting support and guidance for child health.

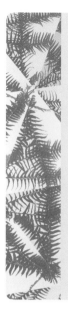

Reflective questions: how would I use this knowledge in practice?

1 What are the main priorities you would identify in a first home visit with Maria?

2 How would you assess the Millers' household environment for risks and protective factors for their children?

3 How would your knowledge of Jim's employment and Maria's volunteer work change your approach to assessing their needs?

4 Which support services in Maria and Jim's community would be most likely to provide support for their needs and that of their family?

5 Explain how you would ensure the Millers had sufficient health literacy for their parenting responsibilities.

6 Describe three aspects of their school or recreational setting that would be crucial to providing family support. For each, explain the importance of the setting in promoting child health and its link to PHC principles.

Research-informed practice

Read O'Brien et al's (2008) study on 'The influence of psychological factors on breast-feeding duration'.

• Do you think there is a 'psychological profile' that fits certain mothers and makes them more favourably disposed towards breastfeeding?

• What do you think are the most important determinants of breastfeeding?

• How would you use local services and professionals to provide breastfeeding support to immigrant mothers in your community?

• What elements would you include in a plan to support rural women in breastfeeding to the WHO standard?

References

Ahlborg T, Misvaer N, Moller A 2009 Perception of marital quality by parents with small children: a follow-up study when the firstborn is 4 years old. Journal of Family Nursing 15(2):237–63

Allen J, Hector D 2005 Benefits of breastfeeding. NSW Public Health Bulletin 16(3–4):42–6

Althabe F, Belizan JU 2006 Caesarean section: the paradox. The Lancet 368:1472–3

Anderson G 2004 Making sense of rising caesarean section rates. British Medical Journal 329:696–7

Armstrong K, Fraser J, Dadds M, Morris J 1999 A randomized, controlled trial of nurse home visiting to vulnerable families with newborns. Journal of Paediatrics and Child Health 35:237–44

—— 2000 Promoting secure attachment, maternal mood and child health in a vulnerable population: a randomized controlled trial. Journal of Paediatrics and Child Health 36:555–62

Armstrong M, Birnie-Lefcovitch S, Ungar M 2005 Pathways between social support, family well-being, quality of parenting, and child resilience: what we know. Journal of Child & Family Studies 14(2):269–81

Australian Health Ministers' Conference communiqué, November 13, 2009 National Breastfeeding Strategy endorsed. Media Release, Honourable Nicola Roxon, Canberra

Australian Institute of Health and Welfare (AIHW) 2008 Australia's Health 2008. AIHW, Canberra

—— 2009a A Picture of Australia's Children 2009. Cat No. PHE 112. AIHW, Canberra

—— 2009b Council of Homeless People. Online. Available: www.chp.org.au (accessed 14 October 2009)

Australian Research Alliance for Children and Youth (ARACY) 2009 Transforming Australia for our children's future. ARACY National Conference, 4 September, Melbourne

Bandura A 1977 Self-efficacy: toward a unifying theory of behavioral change. Psychological Review 84:191–215

Barlow J, Davis H, McIntosh E, Jarrett P, Mockford C, Stewart-Brown S 2007 Role of home visiting in improving parenting and health in families at risk of abuse and neglect: results of a multicentre randomised controlled trial and economic evaluation. Archives of Diseases of Childhood 92:229–33

Baumrind D 1966 Effects of authoritative control on child behavior. Child Development 37(4):887–907

—— 1971 Current patterns of parental authority. Developmental Psychology 4(1) Part 2:1–103

Bowlby J 1969 Attachment and Loss: Vol. 1, Attachment. Basic Books, New York

Bronfenbrenner U 1979 The Ecology of Human Development: Experiments by Nature and Design. Harvard University Press, Cambridge

Brooks-Gunn J 2003 Do you believe in magic? What can we expect from early childhood intervention programs? Social Policy Report 17(1):3–14

Brooks-Gunn J, Brown B, Duncan G, Anderson Moore K 1995 Child development in the context of family and community resources: an agenda for national data collections. The National Academy of Sciences, Washington

Bryanton J, Gagnon A, Hatem M, Johnston C 2009 Does perception of the childbirth experience predict women's early parenting behaviors? Research in Nursing & Health 32:191–203

Chaudhuri J, Easterbrooks A, Davis C 2009 The relation between emotional availability and parenting style: cultural and economic factors in a diverse sample of young mothers. Parenting Science and Practice 9:277–99

Child and Youth Mortality Review Committee, Te Rōpū Arotake Auau Mate o te Hunga Tamariki, Taiohi 2008 Fourth Report to the Minister of Health: Reporting mortality 2002–2005. Child and Youth Mortality Review Committee, Wellington

Commission on the Social Determinants of Health (CSDH) 2008 Closing the gap in a generation: health equity through action on the social determinants of health. Final Report of the Commission on Social Determinants of Health. World Health Organization, Geneva

Commonwealth of Australia 2009 Report of the maternity services review. Online. Available: www.health.gov.au/maternityservicesreview (accessed 19 October 2009)

Craig E, Jackson C, Han DY, NZCYES Steering Committee 2007 Monitoring the Health of New Zealand Children and Young People: Indicator Handbook. Paediatric Society of New Zealand, New Zealand Child and Youth Epidemiology Service, Auckland

Craig K 2009 The National Heart Foundation School Food Programme: a critique. In: Signal L, Egan R Cook L (eds) Reviews of Health Promotion Practice in Aotearoa New Zealand 2007–2008. Health Promotion Forum of New Zealand and Health Promotion and Policy Research Unit, University of Otago, Auckland, pp 24–31

Commonwealth Scientific and Industrial Research Organisation (CSIRO) 2009 Fact sheet: Recreational screen time. CSIRO, Canberra. Online. Available: www.csiro.au/resources/10-steps-for-healthy-families-ScreenTime.html (accessed 14 October 2009)

Dennis C, Hodnett E, Reisman H, Kenton L, Weston J, Zupancic J, Stewart D, Love L, Kiss A 2009 Effect of peer support on prevention of postnatal depression among high risk women: multisite randomised controlled trial. British Medical Journal 338a:3064-doi:10.1136/bmj.a3064

Department of Health Western Australia (DOHWA) 2008 Aboriginal maternal and child health action plan priorities for closing the gap. Government of Western Australia, Perth

Downie J, Clark K, Clementson K 2004–05 Volunteerism: community mothers in action. Contemporary Nurse 18(1–2):188–98

Drewnowski A 2009 Obesity, diets, and social inequalities. Nutrition Reviews 67 Suppl (1):S36–S39

Duncan G, Brooks-Gunn J 2000 Family poverty, welfare reform, and child development. Child Development 71(1):188–96

Dyall L 2007 Guest editorial: the impact of historical factors on Māori child health and potential ways forward in the future. In: Craig E, Jackson C, Han DY, NZCYES Steering Committee 2007 Monitoring the Health of New Zealand Children and Young People: Indicator Handbook. Paediatric Society of New Zealand, New Zealand Child and Youth Epidemiology Service, Auckland, pp 43–8

Earls F, Carlson M 2001 The social ecology of child health and wellbeing. Annual Review of Public Health 22:143–66

Emerson E 2009 Relative child poverty, income inequality, wealth, and health. Commentary, Journal of the American Medical Association 301(4):425–6

Ferry B 2009 iMove Nekeke Hi! In Signal L, Egan R Cook L (eds) Reviews of Health Promotion Practice in Aotearoa New Zealand 2007–2008. Health Promotion Forum of New Zealand and Health Promotion and Policy Research Unit, University of Otago, Auckland, pp 69–77

Fielden J, Gallagher L 2008 Building social capital in first-time parents through a group-parenting program: a questionnaire survey. International Journal of Nursing Studies 45:406–17

Figueiredo B, Costa R, Pacheco A, Pais A 2009 Mother-to-infant emotional involvement at birth. Maternal and Child Health Journal 13(4):539–50

Finger B, Hans S, Bernstein V, Cox S 2009 Parent relationship quality and infant–mother attachment. Attachment & Human Development 11(3):285–306

Fletcher R 2008 Father-inclusive practice and associated professional competencies. Australian Family Relationships Clearinghouse Briefing 9:1–10

Fraser J, Mathews B, Walsh K, Chen L, Dunne M 2009 Factors influencing child abuse and neglect recognition and reporting by nurses: a multivariate analysis. International Journal of Nursing Studies doi 10.1016666/j.ijnurstu.2009.05.015

Froese N, Jenkins M 2008 Early effects of free early childhood education: report to the Ministry of Education. Ministry of Education, Wellington

Gee V, Hu Q, Ernstzen A 2007 Perinatal statistics in Western Australia 2005. Department of Health Western Australia, Perth

Green B, McAllister C, Tarte J 2004 The strengths-based practices inventory: a tool for measuring strengths-based service delivery in early childhood and family support programs. Families in Society 85(3)3:326–34

Hackman D, Farah M 2009 Socio-economic status and the developing brain. Trends in Cognitive Science 13(2):65–73

Hanna B, Edgecombe G, Jackson C, Newman S 2002 The importance of first-time parent groups for new parents. Nursing & Health Sciences 4:209–14

Harnack L, Jeffery R, Boutelle K 2000 Temporal trends in energy intake in the United States: an ecologic perspective. American Journal of Clinical Nutrition 71(6):1478–84

Hector D, King L, Webb K, Heywood P 2005 Factors affecting breastfeeding practices: applying a conceptual framework. NSW Public Health Bulletin 16(3–4):52–5

Herman K, Reinke W, Parkin J, Traylor K, Agarwal G 2009 Childhood depression: rethinking the role of the school. Psychology in the Schools 46(5):433–46

Hertzman C 2001a Health and human society. American Scientist 89(6):538–44

—— 2001b Determinants of Health. Presentation to the Commission for Children and Young People (CCYP), Queensland Health. 21 November, Royal Children's Hospital, Brisbane

Hewitt C, Gilbody S 2009 Is it clinically and cost effective to screen for postnatal depression: a systematic review of controlled clinical trials and economic evidence. British Journal of Obstetrics and Gynae-cology doi:10.1111/j.1471-0528.2009.02148.x

Hobel C, Goldstein A, Barrett E 2008 Psychosocial stress and pregnancy outcome. Clinical Obstetrics and Gynecology 51(2):233–348

Horta B, Bahl R, Martines J, Victora C 2007 Evidence on the long-term effects of breastfeeding: systematic review and meta analyses. WHO, Geneva

Howden-Chapman P, Pierse N, Nicholls S, Gillespie-Bennett J, Viggers H, Cunningham M, Phipps R, Boulic M, Fjallstrom P, Free S, Chapman R, Lloyd B, Wickens K, Shields D, Baker M, Cunningham C, Woodward A, Bullen C, Crane J 2008 Effects of improved home heating on asthma in community dwelling children: randomised controlled trial. British Medical Journal 337: a1411

Ip S, Chung M, Raman G, Chew P, Magula N, DeVine D 2007 Breastfeeding and maternal and infant health outcomes in developed countries. Evidence Report/Technology Assessment, no. 153 Agency for Healthcare Research and Quality, Rockville, MD

Jacobs M 2009 New Zealand approaches to prevention. Public Health Bulletin SA 6(1):27–9

Kedgley S 2007 Inquiry into obesity and type 2 diabetes in New Zealand: report of the health committee. House of Representatives, Wellington

Kelleher L, Johnson M 2004 An evaluation of a volunteer-support program for families at risk. Public Health Nursing 21(4):297–305

Khanam R, Nghiem H, Connelly L 2008 Child health and the income gradient: Evidence from Australia. Australian Centre for Economic Research on Health, The University of Queensland, ACERH Working Paper No. 3, Brisbane

Kiernan K, Huerta C 2008 Economic deprivation, maternal depression, parenting and children's cognitive and emotional development in early child-hood. The British Journal of Sociology 59(40):doi:10.1111/j.1468-4446.2008.00219.x

Kime N 2008 How children eat may contribute to rising levels of obesity. Children's eating behaviours: an inter-generational study of family influences. International Journal of Health Promotion & Education 47(1):4–11

Kramer M, Matush L, Vanilovich I, Platt R, Bogdanovich N, Sevkovskaya Z 2007 Effect of pro-longed and exclusive breast feeding on risk of allergy and asthma: cluster randomised trial. British Medical Journal 335(7624):815

Lehmann D, Silva D, Tennant M, Wright H, McAullay D, Lannigan F 2006 The Swimming Pool Study 2000–2006. Telethon Institute for Child Health Research, Perth

Li J, Mattes E, Stanley F, McMurray A, Hertzman C 2009 Social determinants of child health and well-being. Health Sociology Review 18(1):3–11

Li J, McMurray A, Stanley F 2008 Modernity's paradox and the structural determinants of child health and wellbeing. Health Sociology Review 17(1):64–77

MacKenzie I 2006 Induction of labour at the start of the new millennium. The Journal of Reproduction and Fertility 131:989–98

McCain M, Mustard F 2002 The Early Years Study Three Years Later. Canadian Institute for Advanced Research, Toronto

Ming Foynes M, Freyd J, DePrince A 2009 Child abuse: betrayal and disclosure. Child Abuse & Neglect 33:209–17

Ministry of Education New Zealand 1996 Te whāriki: he whāriki mātauranga mō ngā mokopuna o Aotea-roa: Early Childhood Curriculum. Learning Media, Wellington

Ministry of Health New Zealand (MOHNZ) 1998 Child Health Strategy. MOHNZ, Wellington

—— 2001 The Primary Health Care Strategy. MOHNZ, Wellington

—— 2002a He Korowai Oranga Maori Health Strat-egy. MOHNZ, Wellington

—— 2002b Breastfeeding: A Guide to Action. MOHNZ, Wellington

—— 2008a A Portrait of Health. Key results of the 2006–07 New Zealand health survey. MOHNZ, Wellington

—— 2008b Maternity Action Plan 2008–2012: Draft for Consultation. MOHNZ, Wellington

Mitchell L, Wylie, C, Carr M 2008 Outcomes of early childhood education: literature review. Report to the Ministry of Education. Ministry of Education, Wellington

Moore M 2005 Increasing cesarean birth rates: A clash of cultures? Journal of Perinatal Education 14(4):5–8

Morrell C, Slade P, Warner R, Paley G, Dixon S, Walters S, Brugha T, Barkham M, Parry G, Nich-oll J 2009 Clinical effectiveness of health visitor training in psychologically informed approaches for depression in postnatal women: pragmatic cluster randomised trial in primary care. British Medical Journal 338:a3045 doi:10.1136bmj.a3045

Mustard J 1996 Health and social capital. In: Blane D, Brunner E, Wilkinson R (eds) Health and Social Organization: Towards a Health Policy for the Twenty-First Century. Routledge, London, pp 303–13

—— 1999 Social Determinants of Health, Presentation to University of Queensland Centre for Primary Health Care, 5 August, Brisbane

—— 2007 Experience-based brain development: scientific underpinnings of the importance of early child development in a global world. In: Young M, Richardson L (eds) Early Child Development: From Measurement to Action. World Bank, Washington, pp 43–71

National Collective of Women's Refuges 2007 Statistics July 2007. Online. Available: www.womensrefuge. org.nz (accessed 31 October 2009)

O'Brien M, Buikstra E, Hegney D 2008 The influence of psychological factors on breastfeeding duration. Journal of Advanced Nursing 63(4):397–408

Olds D 2002 Prenatal and infancy home visiting by nurses: from randomized trials to community replication. Prevention Science 3(3):153–72

Pereda N, Guilera G, Forns M, Benito J 2009 The international epidemiology of child sexual abuse: a continuation of Finkelhor (1994) 2009 Child Abuse and Neglect 33:331–42

Productivity Commission 2009 Paid parental leave: support for parents with newborn children. Productivity Commission inquiry report. Productivity Commission, Canberra. Online. Available: www.pc.gov.au/projects/inquiry/parentalsupport/report.pdf (accessed 19 October 2009)

Putnam R 2005 Civic Renewal and Social Capital Round Table Discussion. Alcoa Research Centre for Stronger Communities, Curtin University, Perth

Ramchandani P, O'Connor T, Heron J, Murray L, Evans J 2008 Depression in men in the postnatal period and later child psychopathology: a population cohort study. Journal of the American Academy of Child Adolescen & Psychiatry 47(4):390–8

Redmond G 2008 Children's perspectives on economic adversity: A review of the literature. Innocenti Discussion Paper No.IDP 2008-01UNICEF Innocenti Research Centre, Florence, Italy

Rodriguez C 2002 Professionals' attitudes and accuracy on child abuse reporting decisions in New Zealand. Journal of Interpersonal Violence 17(3):320–42

Salmon J, Timperio A, Cleland V, Venn A 2005 Trends in children's physical activity and weight status in high and low socio-economic status areas of Melbourne, Victoria, 1985–2001. Australian & New Zealand Journal of Public Health 29(4):337–42

Sanders M 2002 Parenting interventions and the prevention of serious mental health problems in children. Medical Journal of Australia 77 Suppl (7):87–92

Scharer K, Colon E, Moneyham L, Hussey J, Tavakoli A, Shugart M 2009 A comparison of two types of social support for mothers of mentally ill children. Journal of Child and Adolescent Psychiatric Nursing 22(2):86–98

Schatz J, Smith L, Borkowski J, Whitman T, Keogh D 2008 Maltreatment risk, self-regulation, and maladjustment in at-risk children. Child Abuse & Neglect 32:972–82

Schumacher M, Zubaran C, White G 2008 Bringing birth-related paternal depression to the fore. Women and Birth 21:65–70

Seimyr L, Sjogren B, Welles-Nystrom B, Nissen E 2009 Antenatal maternal depressive mood and parental-fetal attachment at the end of pregnancy. Abstract, Archives of Women's Mental Health 12(5):269

Shonkoff J, Boyce W, McEwen B 2009 Neuroscience, molecular biology, and the childhood roots of health disparities. Journal of the American Medical Association 301(21):2252–9

Shonkoff J, Phillips D 2000 From Neurons to Neighbourhoods: The Science of Early Childhood Development. National Academy Press, Washington

Signal L, Thomson G, Walton M 2009 Policy interventions to support primary schools in promoting healthy nutrition. Online. Available: www.wnmeds.ac.nz/academic/dph/research/heppru/research/childhood.html (accessed 7 November 2009)

Silburn S 2003 Pathways to Resilience. Telethon Institute for Child Health Research, Perth

Smart D, Sanson A, Baxter J, Edwards B, Hayes A 2008 Home to School Transitions for Financially Disadvantaged Children: Final Report. The Smith Family and the Australian Institute of Family Studies, Sydney

Stanley F, Richardson S, Prior M 2005 Children of the Lucky Country. Pan Macmillan, Sydney

Statistics New Zealand 2009 New Zealand definition of homelessness. Statistics New Zealand, Wellington

UNICEF 2007 Child poverty in perspective: An overview of child wellbeing in rich countries. UNICEF Innocenti Research Centre, Florence, Italy

—— 2009 Progress for children. A report card on child protection (no. 8). UNICEF Innocenti Research Centre, Florence, Italy

United Nations 2006 Convention on the Rights of Persons with Disabilities. UN, Geneva

United Nations Family Planning Association (UNFPA) 2000 The State of World Population 2000. United Nations, New York

Vimpani G 2000 Editorial: home visiting for vulnerable infants in Australia. Journal of Paediatrics and Child Health 36:537–9

Waldegrave C, Waldegrave K 2009 Healthy Families, Young Minds and Developing Brains: Enabling All Children to Reach Their Potential. Families Commission, Wellington

Watson J, Tully L 2008 Prevention and Early Intervention Update — Trends in Recent Research. NSW Department of Community Services Centre for Parenting Research, Sydney

Whiteside-Mansell L, Bradley R, McKelvey L, Fussell J 2008 Parenting: linking impacts of interpartner conflict to preschool children's social behaviour. Journal of Pediatric Nursing 2:1–12

Widmer E, Giudici F, Le Goff J, Pollien A 2009 From support to control: a configurational perspective on conjugal quality. Journal of Marriage and Family 71:437–48

Wilkinson R 1996 Unhealthy Societies: the Afflictions of Inequality. Routledge, London

Wilson P, Barbour R, Graham C, Currie M, Puckering C, Minnis H 2008 Health visitors' assessments of parent–child relationships: a focus group study. International Journal of Nursing Studies 45:1137–47

Woodcock C, Tregaskis C 2008 Understanding structural and communication barriers to ordinary family life for families with disabled children: a combined social work and social model of disability analysis. British Journal of Social Work 38:55–71

World Health Organization (WHO) 1999 The World Health Report 1999: Making a Difference. WHO, Geneva

—— 2005 Make Every Mother and Child Count. The World Health Report 2005. WHO, Geneva

—— 2008a World Health Report 2008: Primary Health Care, Now More Than Ever. WHO, Geneva

—— 2008b The World Report on Child Injury Prevention. Online. Available: www.who.int/violence_injury_prevention/child/injury/world_report/en (accessed 20 October 2009)

—— 2009a Mental Health, Resilience and Inequalities. WHO regional office for Europe, Copenhagen

—— 2009b Breastfeeding guideline. Online. Available: www.who.int/topics/breastfeeding/en (accessed 21 October 2009)

World Health Organization, Health and Welfare Canada & CPHA 1986 Ottawa Charter for Health Promotion. Canadian Journal of Public Health 77(12):425–30

Zubrick S, Smith G, Nicholson J, Sanson A, Jackiewicz, T, The LSAC Consortium 2008 Parenting and families in Australia, Social Policy Research Paper No. 34, Department of Families, Housing, Community Services and Indigenous Affairs, Australian Government, Canberra

Zubrick S, Ward K, Silburn S, Lawrence D, Williams A, Blair E, Robertson D, Sanders M 2005 Prevention of child behavior problems through universal implementation of a group behavioral family intervention. Prevention Science 6(4):287–304

Zubrick S, Williams A, Silburn S, Vimpani G 2000 Indicators of social and family functioning. Commonwealth Department of Family and Community Services, Canberra

Useful websites and helplines

http://www.who.int/topics/breastfeeding/en/

http://www.bfhi.org.au

http://www.babyfriendly.org.nz

http://www.lalecheleague.org.nz

http://www.aaca.com.au — Australian Children's Foundation

http://www.acsso.org.au — Australian Council of State School Associations

http://www.earlychildhoodaustralia.org.au — Early Childhood Australia, Inc

http://www.aifs.gov.au/ — Australian Institute for Family Studies

http://www.aracy.org.au — Australian Research Alliance for Children and Youth

http://www.austparents.edu.au — Early Childhood Learning Resources

http://www.beyondblue.org.au — Clinical depression

http://www.breastfeeding.asn.au — Australian Breastfeeding Association

http://www.cihi.ca/CIHI-ext-portal/internet/EN/Home/home/cihi000001 — Canadian Institute for Health Information

http://www.communities.wa.gov.au/childrenandfamilies/parentingwa/Pages/default.aspx — Parenting tips

http://www.curriculum.edu.au/elearning — Early Childhood Learning Resources — National Agenda for Early Childhood http://www.ehsnrc.org/— Early Head Start program

http://www.familycourt.gov.au/ — Family Court matters

http://www.healthinsite.gov.au/topics/Exercise_for_Children — Children's exercise programs

http://www.ichr.uwa.edu.au — Western Australian Institute for Child Health Research

http://www.media-awareness.ca/english/parents/ — Media Awareness Network for Parents

http://www.napcan.org.au — National Association for the Prevention of Child Abuse and Neglect

http://www.netdoctor.co.uk/health_advice/facts/depressionpostnatal.htm — Postnatal depression

http://www.nhmrc.gov.au/publications/synopses/wh29syn.htm — NHMRC Postnatal depression

http://www.nutritionaustralia.org — Nutrition Australia — Nutrition for Children

http://www.pfsc.uq.edu.au — The University of Queensland Parenting and Family Support Centre

http://portal.unesco.org/education/en/ev.php-URL_ID=17529&URL_DO=DO_TOPIC&URL_SECTION=201.
  html — UNESCO International Clearing House for Children and Violence on the Screen

http://www.refugeecouncil.org.au — Refugee Council of Australia

http://www.relationships.com.au/ — Information on relationships, family, love and life

http://www.snaicc.asn.au — Secretariat of National Aboriginal and Islander Child Care

http://www.childtrends.org/lifecourse/programs/infanthealthdev.htm — Infant Health and Development program

http://www.chp.org.au — Australian Council to Homeless People

http://www.plunket.org.nz — Largest provider of well child services in New Zealand

http://www.immunise.health.gov.au — www.ncirs.usyd.edu.au/facts/resources_patient-parent%20concern%20abo
  ut%20immunisation.pdf

http://www.health.govt.nz/ — www.dhs.vic.gov.au/earlychood

http://www.paediatrics.org.nz/— Paediatric Society of New Zealand

http://www.kidshealth.org.nz — Information on child health in New Zealand

http://www.aifs.gov.au/

http://www.healthinfonet.ecu.edu.au/ — Government website for health information

http://www.sidsandkids.org/

http://www.kidshelp.com.au — Kids helpline

1800 MUM 2 MUM (1800 686 2 686) — Australian breastfeeding helpline

http://www.moh.govt.nz/moh.nsf/indexmh/breastfeeding — Information on breastfeeding for mothers and health
  providers in New Zealand

Chapter 7

Healthy adolescents

INTRODUCTION

Adolescents are a vital part of community life, contributing energy and vibrancy to the population through the spirit of youth and a promise for the future. In most cases, their health and wellbeing is focused on school and the developmental tasks of adolescence. Compared to young children and adults, they are under-represented in health services, with health care often seen as incidental to their lives. Instead, the social sphere within which they interact is predominant. It is the pivot around which their lives and their identity revolves. Understanding the social lives of adolescents is fundamental to helping young people bridge their transitions safely within the protective umbrella of family, community and society. The challenges inherent in these transitions change daily.

Point to ponder

Adolescents are predominantly physically healthy. It is the social aspects of life as an adolescent that present the greatest challenge for achieving health and wellbeing.

The adolescent journey is sometimes described as fraught with confusion, conflict and risk. However, an alternative view sees adolescents 'at promise' instead of 'at risk'. When the family, school, neighbourhood and community lend timely, sensitive and appropriate support for their lives, they can indeed be at promise of creating a healthy future. On the other hand, if the social determinants embedded in the family, school, neighbourhood and community fail to provide a web of support for their transitions, there is a greater risk that they will begin their adult lives at a disadvantage. As a result, they may be confronted with compromised health status, failure to thrive, less than optimal resilience and fewer opportunities to add value to each step of the journey.

Adolescence is the most critical, the most interesting and the most tortuous stage on the journey to adulthood. In the early years of adolescent life, and later, in a stage of pre-adulthood, significant habits of mind and action are formed. These thoughts, attitudes and behaviours can mean the difference between health and ill health, confidence or low self-esteem, joy or depression, social competence and vitality, or isolation in later life. Many researchers of adolescent behaviours and attitudes write about risk and risk factors. But a strengths-based approach to analysing adolescent life would see each transition along the pathway to adulthood in terms of potential and possibilities. From this perspective, each challenge offers an opportunity to develop inner resourcefulness. This can be accomplished with the support of family, school and the social environment, each of which plays a critical role in connecting the various elements of adolescent life with one another.

As health professionals we are particularly interested in the journey as well as the outcome. Some of the main issues we'll address in this chapter include questioning what distinguishes the adolescent who progresses through the tortuous path to healthy adulthood from others who fall victim to high-risk behaviours. What sustains behaviours such as smoking, overeating, abusing alcohol or other harmful substances, unsafe sexual activities and self-inflicted injury beyond the stage of experimentation? Why are some young people better able to change the course of their life midstream and redirect their efforts towards a healthier future? How have some adolescents been successful, while others with seemingly similar backgrounds have slipped backwards into the abyss of unhealthy lifestyles? How are some young people able to face adversity and bounce back stronger for the challenge, while others become depressed and anxious? This chapter unpacks some of the evolving knowledge base underpinning adolescent life,

Objectives

By the end of this chapter you will be able to:

1 identify the factors influencing healthy adolescence

2 explain the social ecology of adolescent life

3 analyse the research evidence related to the role of family support in influencing adolescent health and wellbeing

4 identify goals for supporting and sustaining adolescents at promise

5 explain how a primary health care framework can be used in planning strategies for adolescent health

6 identify strengths and gaps in the research evidence base for working with adolescents.

examining the determinants of risk and potential, and the pathway to personal resilience, civic engagement and the skills for a promising future. The chapter concludes in an exploration of the ways nurses and other health professionals can provide assistance and ongoing support along the way.

THE DEVELOPMENT OF SOCIAL COMPETENCE

Adolescence is a period of rapid cognitive, psychological, social, emotional and physical changes in a person's life (Halpern-Felsher 2009). During adolescence young people establish caring, meaningful relationships. They also seek acceptance and belonging in social groups, and this helps them develop a capacity for interpersonal intimacy (Whitlock et al 2006). These social connections are developmental and they contribute to the important tasks of identity formation and the development of autonomy and independent thinking. Sculpting out an adult identity takes precedence over any other issue, as young people 'try on' a range of identities to establish a sense of themselves in relation to the world and various groups of people (Erikson 1963). Identity formation is a significant step in developing critical thinking ability. Some young people find this difficult, particularly when they are balancing personal changes and aspirations with the influence of family and friends. Peers and other social groups provide a mirror within which adolescents view themselves, which can be embarrassing or empowering in their struggle for self-identity and the formation of unique ideas (Price 2009).

Point to ponder

Identity formation is a key milestone for young people.

Without ongoing support from peer groups, families, schools and others within their social and cultural environments, some adolescents are easily led into patterns of behaviour that leave them feeling isolated, abandoned and without positive role models for successful development (Bronfenbrenner 1986). This illustrates the importance of a social ecological perspective of adolescent life. Everything is connected to everything else in their social world. Family, school, peers and the many contexts in which they interact all have an effect on one another. This includes their virtual social lives on the internet and other electronic media as well as the face-to-face interactions that frame the development of social competence. Positive role models in the home and school environment can help guide adolescents towards behaviours that help them navigate through the changes with a sense of comfort in their identity and relationships.

Family structure has an important influence on adolescent development. Many years ago young people had clear rites of passage from childhood to adult, spouse, parent and worker. In the 21st century, adolescents experience variable transitions in the public eye, which take place over an extended period of time. As we reported in Chapter 5, family structures have changed. Gone are the family norms where a father transferred to his son the means to a livelihood, and a mother passed her skills on to her daughter for a predetermined role as wife or mother. Today, many young people who grow up in families without two biological parents tend to see themselves as adults at a younger stage than those from intact families (Benson & Kirkpatrick Johnson 2009). This often results from having assumed a variety of roles in different family structures, households and family groupings. Family processes are also instrumental in influencing adolescent identity formation. These influences arise from the style of parenting (authoritarian, authoritative or permissive), and the extent to which parents exert social control and monitoring, warmth and closeness, a sense of responsibility and a clear sense of the adolescent's place in the hierarchy of family relations (Benson & Kirkpatrick Johnson 2009).

Point to ponder
Positive role models support young people as they develop social competence.

SOCIAL DETERMINANTS OF ADOLESCENT HEALTH, RISK AND POTENTIAL

The social ecology of adolescent development can be seen as a matrix of inter-related factors that influence adolescents' health and wellbeing. As with other population groups, the social determinants of their lives present strengths, weaknesses, threats and opportunities. The main strength of adolescents is that most tend to be physically well. The weaknesses or risks inherent in adolescent life generally revolve around the fact that, because they are in the formative stages of development, most adolescents are not yet able to take control of their lives or health-related decisions. However, good physical health is not always accompanied by good mental health. Identity formation and other psychosocial challenges place inordinate pressures on adolescents, which can pose threats to mental health. So although health status indicators may suggest that adolescents are among the healthiest groups in the population, their greatest threat to health lies in emotional, social and behavioural conditions of their lives that affect mental health (Australian Institute of Health and Welfare [AIHW] 2008; Ministry of Health New Zealand [MOHNZ] 2002).

The most conspicuous mental health issues for adolescents include the risk of depression, behavioural problems such as aggression or self-harm, adolescent pregnancy, substance misuse, sexually transmitted infections, eating disorders and obesity (AIHW 2008; MOHNZ 2002; World Health Organization [WHO] 2009). Many of these are inter-related. Approximately 10% of Australian adolescents suffer from a long-term mental or behavioural problem (AIHW 2008). In New Zealand, it is estimated that 22% of 15-year-olds and 36.6% of 18-year-olds have a mental health problem (Craig et al 2007). The most serious of these, requiring hospitalisation, are substance use and schizophrenia for adolescent males, and depressive episodes, eating disorders and self-harm for adolescent girls.

Adolescent deaths are primarily caused by injuries, many of which are also related to behaviours, with a strong link between alcohol consumption, substance abuse, attempted suicide and motor vehicle accidents. Adolescents are also at risk of conditions such as asthma, cancers such as leukaemia and skin cancer (melanoma). However, these are overshadowed by the problems created by binge drinking and illicit drug use, which can also be linked to unsafe sexual behaviours and the possibility of sexually transmitted infections (STIs) and adolescent pregnancy (AIHW 2008; Craig et al 2007). The most important social determinants affecting successful navigation through these conditions are family, school and social support.

Point to ponder
Common health issues for young people include depression, pregnancy, substance abuse, STIs and obesity.

Identity and body image: weight management and eating disorders

The quality of family life has been shown to be the most powerful influence on adolescent health, particularly in relation to nutrition and weight management, which continues to be a problem for adolescents. Around 20–22% of Australian and New Zealand adolescents are overweight, with 7–9% being classified as obese (AIHW 2008;

MOHNZ 2006). These problems are much greater for Indigenous adolescents in both countries (AIHW 2008; MOHNZ 2006). This creates risks for cardiovascular disease, diabetes and cancer in adult life, particularly when the risk is compounded by physical inactivity. Only a third of females and 46% of males participate in physical activity to the level recommended in Australian national guidelines (AIHW 2008). In New Zealand, young men aged 15–24 years are 1.5 times more likely to participate in physical activity five or more times per week than young women of the same age (MOHNZ 2008). Because overweight adolescents tend to become overweight adults, there is a strong belief that late childhood is the time to address unhealthy eating behaviours and optimal patterns of eating and activity. This is an important and complex challenge for health promotion interventions, given the known links between overweight, low self-esteem, stress, a lack of social support and the ultimate risk of depressive illness (Martyn-Nemeth et al 2009).

What's your opinion?
What socio-ecological factors influence the discrepancy between young men and young women's participation in physical activity?

There is a strong link between eating behaviours, stress and coping. Adolescents' coping strategies evolve throughout the period of adolescence, as puberty poses its own set of stressors. These include physical and hormonal changes which do not always follow a predictable path. Coinciding with the increase in the number and type of stressors, physical activity levels often decline throughout this period, especially for girls (Thunfors et al 2009). In many cases, parental work schedules reduce adults' control over mealtimes, and this can lead to poor eating habits among their children (Jui-Han & Miller 2009). In urban areas, adolescents also tend to gravitate to fast-food outlets as a place for socialising, and often substitute high salt, high sugar content foods for healthy meals at home with the family. Using food as a coping mechanism or developing fast-food habits can lead to overeating as a long-term pattern, especially if there is a lack of family and social support to buffer the effects of stress. This, in turn, can lead to lower self-esteem and depressive mood, which

creates a cycle of overeating and weight problems (Martyn-Nemeth et al 2009). Although rural youth do not have the same access to fast-food outlets, many eat because they are bored, feeling emotional or depressed, or because their friends are eating (Bourke et al 2009). The need to feel connected with peers can be a potent force in eating behaviours, and a way of feeling included in group activities.

Equally as difficult is the challenge of supporting adolescents with eating disorders. For some young people, disordered eating patterns may be due to individual and cultural factors that lead to a distortion of body image (DeLeel et al 2009). To some extent, the media contributes to the prevalence of eating disorders, by reinforcing unrealistic images of what constitutes an ideal body. Images of ultra-thin models and pop stars surround adolescent life, making them difficult to ignore. In the absence of positive role models, young people may adopt a view of their ideal self based on what they see in magazines and the media instead of what is feasible.

Point to ponder
The desire to 'fit in' with the group can lead to poor eating behaviours among adolescents.

The most common eating disorders are anorexia nervosa, bulimia and binge eating. Those with anorexia are thought to be obsessed with three forms of control: over their eating, their body weight and their food. This causes them to self-induce starvation out of fear of gaining weight (Ramjan 2004). Control issues may also lie at the core of bulimia and binge-eating disorders. In all three types of disorders, the young person may have an obsession with beauty or physical attractiveness, competitiveness and a desire to punish themselves as well as control their weight (Fairburn & Harrison 2003). Eating disorders are often accompanied by symptoms of depression and anxiety, irritability, mood swings, impaired concentration and a loss of sexual appetite, all of which begins a cycle of social withdrawal and isolation (Fairburn & Harrison 2003). In addition, they suffer from poor physical health, especially oral health and gastrointestinal disorders, which are related to inadequate nutritional status and/or purging after meals.

Eating disorders and family life

Although there may be many different factors involved, researchers have linked conditions such as anorexia nervosa and bulimia with family conflicts and parenting styles. The risks of these conditions are heightened when parents are too controlling, where their relationships with their adolescents are lacking in intimacy, and when they communicate inconsistent and irrational messages in relation to weight control (May et al 2006). Links have also been found between bulimia and low levels of maternal nurturance or responsiveness from family members (May et al 2006). Family meals have also been shown to have a profound effect on young people's eating patterns. Families who place high importance on regular family meals tend to have children with less disordered eating (Fulkerson et al 2006). This seems to be related to two factors: role-modelling healthy eating and promoting family cohesion (Rodgers & Chabrol 2009). Positive role modelling establishes good nutritional habits that tend to endure throughout adult life. On the other hand, teasing, parental dieting, restricting food or commenting on the beauty standards of media personalities can lead children to disordered eating. This is a particular problem among young girls who are often susceptible to parental body image attitudes, and are made vulnerable because of their own anxieties (Rodgers & Chabrol 2009).

Point to ponder

Family attitudes and behaviour towards eating can have a profound influence on young people's eating habits.

Family mealtimes can promote family cohesion through meaningful communication (Franko et al 2008). Because family meals have become victim to the hurried lifestyles of many dual-earner families, researchers have turned their attention to mealtime as a vehicle for family harmony. Research linking regular family meals with a cluster of risky adolescent behaviours has found that girls reporting more frequent family meals showed reduced substance use, higher school marks, fewer depressive symptoms, decreased risk of suicide attempts and less extreme weight control behaviours (Franko et al 2008). This is thought to arise from the closeness and enjoyment of regular meals

(Franko et al 2008). Parental conversations can also provide important lessons on how they solve everyday problems and deal with social pressures. Family mealtime conversations also provide opportunities for parental monitoring of adolescents' views and behaviours (Franko et al 2008). In addition, parents' use of alcohol at mealtimes can also have a major influence on alcohol consumption among adolescents. The combination of role modelling and family connectedness can be a vehicle for ensuring the lines of communication between parents and their adolescent children remain open. This helps establish a pattern for open and ongoing discussion of expectations and family standards (Haegerich & Tolan 2008; Velleman & Templeton 2007).

Risky sexual behaviours

Sexual risk-taking is one of a number of behaviours that underline the importance of decision-making in an adolescent's social development (Atkins & Hart 2008; Halpern-Felsher 2009). Unprotected sexual activity creates a risk for unwanted pregnancy and STIs such as *Chlamydia*, gonorrhoea, syphilis, genital warts (HPV) and HIV, as well as cervical and anal cancers (AIHW 2008). The risk of these outcomes increases with sex at an early age and the number of sexual partners (AIHW 2008; Craig et al 2007; Denny-Smith et al 2006). In Australia, the median age of first sexual intercourse has been estimated at 16, but it is decreasing (Williams & Davidson 2004). This is cause for alarm, as younger sexual debut creates a higher risk of unintentional pregnancy as well as STIs. A New Zealand survey of high-school students found that 15% of sexually active students either don't use or only sometimes use condoms and/or other forms of contraception (Adolescent Health Research Group 2008).

The problem of STIs is a particularly serious public health issue, and these infections have been increasing in Australia and New Zealand over the past decade. The incidence of HIV/AIDS is not increasing as rapidly as in the past, but many more people are now living with HIV/AIDS in the community (Nakhaee et al 2009). The personal impact on health from STIs can be severe, particularly if the infection is not detected immediately. For example, *Chlamydia* can be asymptomatic for a long period of time, and also increase the risk of HIV, which is a significant risk for older adolescents (Major-Wilson et al 2008). Many *Chlamydial* infections also progress to pelvic inflammatory disease (PID), which can lead to infertility (AIHW 2008). New Zealand has the dubious distinction of being named the '*Chlamydia* capital of the world' with regional laboratory rates consistently higher than in Australia, the United Kingdom (UK) and the United States (US) (Braun 2008).

Adolescent pregnancy is an ongoing concern in Australia and New Zealand, where, even though rates are declining, there remain high rates of adolescent conception compared to other OECD countries (AIHW 2009; Pinkleton et al 2008; Williams & Davidson 2004).

Point to ponder
Rates of STIs among young people remain high, with reports of variable condom usage.

In Australia, adolescent pregnancy occurs across the socio-economic spectrum and across all cultural groups, with the highest rates among Indigenous adolescents (Williams & Davidson 2004). In some Indigenous groups, this may be linked to traditional perspectives, where pregnancy and fertility are perceived as valued in their culture (DeVries et al 2009). In New Zealand, adolescent pregnancy is highest among young Maori and Pacific women and those living in the most economically deprived areas (Craig et al 2007).

The level of adolescents' knowledge about pregnancy and STIs is a cause for concern. One study of 500 adolescents in the US found that a large majority believed that birth control pills were a form of protection against STIs. More than two-thirds thought douching protected them from STIs, and 84% believed they were having safe sex if they confined their activities to one partner (Denny-Smith et al 2006). Even nursing students have been found to have misconceptions about sexual behaviour, leading researchers to conclude that risk factor screening for pregnancy and STIs is a vital aspect of health promotion (Denny-Smith et al 2006). Clearly, a lack of knowledge about the impact of unsafe sexual behaviour is a major concern. So too, is the fact that adolescent mothers have a higher level of risk for other behaviours such as alcohol and substance abuse, impoverishment, depression and other forms of social disadvantage. These conditions can compromise the young woman's health and wellbeing and create a greater likelihood of impediments to her future potential.

As we mentioned in Chapter 6, there are also negative outcomes for the child of an adolescent mother, as these mothers often fail to seek antenatal care. Adolescent mothers are disproportionately at risk of miscarriage, pre-term delivery, low birth-weight babies and many other complications of pregnancy that can affect their children (AIHW 2009). Children born to an adolescent mother who smokes tobacco or is involved in alcohol or substance abuse carry a higher risk of infection than the children of older parents. They are also more likely to be trapped in an intergenerational cycle of disadvantage themselves, be deprived of strong supportive networks or educational attainment, and girls often become adolescent mothers themselves (AIHW 2009; Haldre et al 2009).

Point to ponder
Adolescent mothers are at disproportionate risk of miscarriage, pre-term delivery and low birth-weight infants.

So why are younger adolescents having sex? Some believe it may be linked to cultural traditions, poor parent–child relationships, use of alcohol or marijuana, or a lack of personal skills at negotiating sexual behaviour (DeVries et al 2009). For some time, public speculation has also suggested a link between the highly sexualised images in the media and early sexual activities. Research studies have now confirmed this, demonstrating that sexual content in television programs is in fact, a precipitating factor in risky sexual behaviours. One study of adolescent pregnancy in the US found that those with high levels of exposure to sexual media content were twice as likely as others to experience pregnancy in the next three years (Chandra et al 2008). The influence of media images also reflects the importance of peer group norms. An Australian study of adolescents' perceptions of peer sexual attitudes and behaviours revealed that they overestimated the extent to which their peers were sexually active (Lim et al 2009). The researchers concluded that this could induce young people to alter their behaviours in ways that could promote early onset of sexual activity or increase the risks of unsafe sexual practices, especially related to condom use (Lim et al 2009).

Point to ponder
High levels of sexual content in the media is a precipitating factor for risky sexual behaviour among young people.

A number of researchers have focused on the reasons adolescents shy away from using contraception to prevent STIs and pregnancy. Sheeder et al (2009:302) contend that most adolescents 'are not cognitively and psychosocially mature enough to form intimate, mutually respectful, long-term interpersonal relationships'. Their sexual decisions are made in the moment, intuitively, based on romantic circumstances rather than rational thought. They have no prior experience of what it is like to bear a child, and rarely see the barriers or negative aspects of conception. Many also have a lack of knowledge or misperceptions about the risk of pregnancy or how it will impinge on their future goals (Haldre et al 2009; Sheeder et al 2009). This also affects her decisions about the pregnancy.

Choosing between persevering with or terminating a pregnancy is one of the most difficult issues that confront any woman, especially young adolescents. The adolescent mother's developmental stage, her level of self-esteem and her resources have profound effects on the outcomes of pregnancy. The social and political context in which reproductive choices are made also have a major influence on choices and their outcomes. Social mores and competing views on what is morally right or wrong can conspire against her reproductive choices, creating highly inflamed debates and polarised opinions. Sometimes this is too difficult an environment for a young person to deal with in such an emotionally charged situation. Social and cultural messages that convey resilience will support young women to make appropriate choices regarding pregnancy (Sparrow 2009).

Compounding risk: alcohol, drug use and tobacco smoking

A large number of adolescents who develop STIs or have unplanned pregnancies have experienced these because of decisions that were made while they were affected by either alcohol or illicit drugs. This is concerning, because even in small amounts and infrequent episodes, overuse of these substances can be dangerous and have far-reaching effects. Although the proportion of young people drinking alcohol has declined slightly in recent times, the proportion of those who are drinking at hazardous levels and engaging in binge drinking remains high (AIHW 2008; Australian Research Alliance for Children & Youth [ARACY] 2009; Velleman & Templeton 2007). This is a global phenomenon, raising concerns because it is a compromise to community life. It is estimated that 24% of young Australians drink at risky levels (ARACY 2009). In New Zealand 50% of young men and one in three young women aged 18–24 years are considered to have hazardous drinking patterns (MOHNZ 2008). In rural communities this is even higher, especially for Indigenous young people, with 70% of rural Australian adolescents more likely to die from risky drinking than those in urban areas (ARACY 2009). In rural areas, adolescents consume alcohol as a way of being socially included, as alternative social activities are often unavailable (Bourke et al 2009). Ingesting excessive amounts of alcohol or other substances can be considered a form of self-harming behaviour. Chronic excessive alcohol misuse is strongly correlated with other risks to health, including unsafe sexual activity, antisocial and criminal behaviours, injuries from motor vehicle accidents, and mental health problems (Velleman & Templeton 2007). Overuse of alcohol can also cause or exacerbate diabetes, heart disease, liver disease and a range of other threats to physical health.

Point to ponder
Hazardous drinking patterns are common among young people, and are strongly correlated with other risks to health, such as unsafe sexual activity, criminal behaviour and motor vehicle accidents.

The most recent Australian data show that, even though consumption of alcohol has been gradually decreasing over the past 30 years, more than 60% of Australian boys aged 16–17 and 52% of girls of this age ingest alcohol weekly. This is higher than the prevalence among New Zealand adolescents, where it is estimated that close to one-third of those aged 14–17 drink alcohol weekly, 30% of whom are heavy drinkers by this time (AIHW 2008). A small proportion of Australian adolescents use 'hard drugs' such as methamphetamine, cocaine, ecstasy, cannabis or other illicit substances, but the prevalence of drug use is declining (AIHW 2008). This is similar to the global situation, except that cannabis smoking remains high among adolescents in some other countries, while hard drug use is declining.

Although tobacco use has been declining over the past several decades, it is an ongoing problem for many adolescents in Australia and New Zealand (AIHW 2009). Some adolescents see smoking as a way of relaxing, dealing with boredom or stress, gaining independence or controlling weight (Bourke et al 2009). Tobacco is also known to be a 'gateway' drug, which may lead to ingestion of alcohol, cannabis or other harmful substances. Alarmingly, one UK study found that half of those who reported ever using drugs began smoking cannabis at age 10–15 (Velleman & Templeton 2007). Young people who try their first cigarette at the time of adolescence are at the highest risk of becoming daily smokers and they are the least likely to quit smoking (Sherman & Primack 2009). In addition, the longer-term effects of passive smoking of tobacco products are not only potentially fatal to the smoker, but compromise the health of others, including infants and young children (Hamilton 2003). For this reason, tobacco smoking is seen as the leading preventable cause of death and disease (Sherman & Primack 2009).

Point to ponder

Young people who try their first cigarette during adolescence are at high risk of becoming daily smokers.

Adolescent risk-taking in areas such as unsafe sexual behaviour or alcohol and substance misuse, has been described as a syndrome of behaviours, wherein engaging in one type of risk makes a person prone to engage in others (Leather 2009). Some risk-taking is thrill-seeking, often aimed at participating in peer group social life. Other risky behaviours are a form of rebellious, reckless or antisocial acts (Leather 2009). Some see adolescent risk-taking as a natural part of development, a type of adolescent play, while others link risky behaviours to the notion of invulnerability, a feeling among adolescents that they are invincible (Leather 2009). Despite these perspectives, it is not always helpful to stereotype reasons for

risk-taking given individual differences (Holland & Klaczynski 2009). What all researchers and scholars of adolescent life agree on is that for some clusters of risky behaviours, there are serious and enduring psychological and social repercussions. These can include threats to mental health, which are manifest in depression, suicide ideation, low self-esteem, poor body image, low social connectedness, a lack of academic performance at school and a poor quality of family life (Holland & Klaczynski 2009).

Depression, self-harm and suicide

The psychosocial conditions of adolescents' lives and their behavioural decisions can lead to depression, self-harm and in some cases, suicide. They can also result in some adolescents being subjected to violence, bullying at school and adopting a lifestyle that is detrimental to health. In the 21st century, depression is considered the leading cause of disability throughout the world, affecting 15–20% of adolescents (Herman et al 2009). The prevalence of depression varies with age and gender, with a higher incidence among girls (AIHW 2008). The social determinants of depression include family factors, such as having a parent who is mentally ill (Hayman 2009). Other factors include the interactive relationship between parent and child, and a variety of stressors that lie within a young person's physical, social and cultural context. For adolescents, these are usually their school and peer relationships, however parental work schedules that prevent family closeness have also been linked to the development of adolescent depression (Jui-Han & Miller 2009).

Depression has an impact on every aspect of an adolescent's life and can have dire consequences, including suicide, which is the leading cause of death among adolescents (Herman et al 2009). Major depressive disorder (MDD), or clinical depression, is a state of mental ill health where the emotional lows, often described as sadness, become pervasive (Herman et al 2009). Besides genetic factors, depression can be the result of an accumulation of stressful life events involving threat, loss, humiliation or personal defeat (Commonwealth of Australia 2008). Clinical depression is often confused with the wide-ranging mood swings and intense emotional highs and lows young people often experience during their adolescent years. These mood swings are a normal part of learning to respond to events and other people. However, some events and inter-actions with others can cause dramatic shifts in emotions that aren't quickly resolved. If these negative responses continue for a long period of time, it may be a sign that the person is slipping into a depressed state. Instead of bouncing back from a reaction or negative mood, the person may continue on a downward slide, often isolat-ing him/herself from others. Depression can be experienced differently by different individuals. It can make a person feel miserable or irritable most of the time. Some feel restless or agitated, while others feel down and tired all the time. Concen-tration may be difficult, and they can lose interest in their usual activities, overlook school or work responsibilities, and experience changes in their relationships with family members. They may be overcome by feelings of guilt or worthlessness and ultimately decide life is not worth living (Online. Available: www.youthbeyondblue.com [accessed 4 November 2009]).

ACTION POINT

Depression affects 15–20% of adolescents worldwide. Health professionals must undertake comprehensive health assessments when in contact with young people in order to detect signs and symptoms of depression.

One outcome of a depressed state can be self-harming behaviours. Self-harm or deliberate self-injury is often a repetitive act of cutting, carving or burning various parts of the body, pulling out clumps of hair or overdosing on over-the-counter drugs, the latter of which is not typically a suicide attempt (Gardner 2008). In a recent New Zealand survey, 25% of female high-school students and 16% of males reported self-harm (Adolescent Health Research Group 2008). Some self-harming adolescents report that they do so to escape deep distress, hopelessness and misery, to deal with anger and frustration, or to gain relief from inner tension and conflict, or punish others or themselves. Others report that it is a way of gain-ing control or feeling alive (Gardner 2008). Self-harm can also be the response of someone with a

psychiatric disorder or intellectual disability who is not able to express emotions verbally (Com-monwealth of Australia 2008).

Self-harm is rapidly increasing among adoles-cents and some researchers have questioned whether this is because it is so visible in the mass media. Like substance misuse and other negative aspects of youth culture, publicity about the condition on the internet and in the press may be providing an available emotional outlet for those who are predis-posed to self-harm (Velleman & Templeton 2007; Whitlock et al 2006). The presence of self-harming behaviours is understandably perplexing to parents (Rissanen et al 2009). Many feel guilt and shame, searching for meaning and understanding in their own lives to make sense of the behaviour. An Aus-tralian study of mothers of self-harming adoles-cents reported that they felt overwhelmed by their child's behaviour, and inadequate in their parent-ing skills (McDonald et al 2007). This made them feel isolated, ashamed and embarrassed, wonder-ing what circumstances in their own lives led their child to self-harm (McDonald et al 2007).

The relationship between self-harm and sui-cide is complex. Unfortunately, some self-harm behaviours result in unintentional suicide before the young person has been able to receive assis-tance for the underlying cause of their distress (Norman 2009). The risk for suicide is up to three times greater among those who turn to alcohol, particularly binge drinking, which has been identi-fied as the key differentiating factor in planned and unplanned suicide attempts (Schilling et al 2009). In some cases a self-harming adolescent will prog-ress to suicide because they have resisted disclos-ing their feelings for fear of becoming stigmatised (Norman 2009). This makes assessment of the problem difficult for everyone in the young person's web of influence. For parents, teachers, school nurses and other health professionals, the challenge lies in the fact that each person's experi-ence of stress is highly individual. The causes and extent of the self-harm are variable, and it is extremely difficult to judge which self-harming individuals will progress to the stage where sui-cide is attempted or completed. Some of the poten-tial causes of self-harm are listed in Box 7.1.

Recognising the risk of suicide

The treatment for depression typically involves drug therapy and psychological interventions, such as counselling and behavioural therapies.

BOX 7.1 POTENTIAL CAUSES OF SELF-HARM

- Mental illness such as depression or border-line personality disorder.
- Being the victim or perpetrator of bullying at school.
- Problems with parents.
- Stress surrounding academic performance.
- Hypersensitivity, loneliness.
- Alcohol or substance abuse.
- Family separation and divorce.
- Bereavement.
- Unwanted pregnancy.
- Experiences of abuse.
- Problems related to sexuality.
- Problems linked to race, culture or religion.
- Low self-esteem.
- Fears of being rejected.

(Mental Health Foundation 2006; Rissanen 2009)

Group programs that provide mutual support and focus on developing life skills can also be effective (Hayman 2009). However, for some, an unknown combination of factors conspires against recovery and there is a danger of lapsing into hopelessness. An attempt at suicide can be the result of a long history of mental illness or distress, or an impulsive or irrational act (Commonwealth of Australia 2008).

Point to ponder

The risk of suicide among young people experiencing depression is high. It is important to recognise the warning signs of an impending suicide attempt.

Over the past three decades the rates of suicide have declined, with some attributing this to the increased use of antidepressant medications, such as selective serotonin reuptake inhibitors (SSRIs), among adolescents (Bursztein & Apter 2008). For those who do attempt suicide there are usually some warning signs that signal their intention. These can include comments about suicide or death, expressions of hopelessness, rage, anger, revenge, or comments that they feel there's no way

out of the present state. The person may also begin withdrawing from friends or family, or experience abnormal anxiety, agitation or sleep disturbances, either not sleeping or sleeping all the time. They may begin consuming alcohol or other drugs. In some cases, they may begin to give away possessions, say goodbye to people close to them, or make actual threats that they are planning to commit suicide (Commonwealth of Australia 2008).

The 'tipping point' in deciding to commit suicide can be an argument with someone close, a relationship breakdown, a suicide by a family member, friend or associate, hearing a media report of a suicide, recurrence of an illness, an unexpected change in life circumstances or a traumatic event such as bullying, abuse or violence (Commonwealth of Australia 2008). In preparation for a suicide attempt, some adolescents will begin accessing suicide sites on the internet (Bursztein & Apter 2008). The most significant preventative measure for parents, teachers and health professionals is a strong understanding of the adolescent's experiences. To activate protective factors it is important to remain close enough to read the risk factors and warning signs, and to know when it may be time to call for specialised assistance. Precipitating factors or typical triggers are outlined in Figure 7.1.

ADOLESCENT LIFE IN THE COMMUNITY CONTEXT

To understand adolescent behaviour, Eckersley (2004) suggests it is necessary to disentangle the binary notions that characterise adult perspectives of adolescent life. In his view, we think of young people in terms of differences: between ill and well, marginalised and mainstream, the disadvantaged and the privileged, males and females. Instead, we should be studying young people's ideas, preferences and their notions of wellbeing and potential. Researchers tend to over-generalise adolescents' status and behaviours in population approaches that references them to too broad a group (Eckersley 2004). Scientifically measuring adolescents' collective behaviour may not be as helpful as seeing them in the ecological context, which includes the social and environmental determinants of their individual lives. Another flaw in some existing perspectives of adolescence lies in adopting too objective a gaze, trying to understand adolescents and their health risks and potential on the basis of problem behaviours rather than strengths.

Triggers and precipitating events

Risk factors	Warning signs	Tipping point	Imminent risk
• mental health problems • gender – male • family discord, violence or abuse • family history of suicide • alcohol or other substance abuse • social or geographical isolation • financial stress • bereavement • prior suicide attempt	• hopelessness • feeling trapped – like there's no way out • increasing alcohol or drug use • withdrawing from friends, family or society • no reason for living, no sense of purpose in life • uncharacteristic or impaired judgement or behaviour	• relationship ending • loss of status or respect • debilitating physical illness or accident • death or suicide of relative or friend • suicide of someone famous or member of peer group • argument at home • being abused or bullied • media report on suicide or suicide methods	• expressed intent to die • has plan in mind • has access to lethal means • impulsive, aggressive or anti-social behaviour

Figure 7.1 Typical triggers or precipitating events to suicide (Commonwealth of Australia 2008, LIFE p 23 with permission)

The major threats and opportunities of adolescent health are those embedded in the adolescent social culture, where interactions within their peer group can exert multiple pressures on their behaviours. As mentioned above, these behaviours can be positive or negative, helping the adolescent develop a strong sense of self or leading to certain clusters of problem behaviours (Haegerich & Tolan 2008). The social culture of young people in this century is markedly different from that of their parents. They are connected to the external world through a variety of electronic media. Their access to virtual peer groups creates a closer bond to like-minded individuals and to some whose lives are substantially different from theirs. These virtual networks are often used as benchmarks for adolescents' lives and behaviours. As a result, young people today have enormous decision-making challenges. The implication for parents, nurses and other health professionals is to seek understanding of the social influences on adolescents by assessing their perspective on these experiences.

An ideal assessment tool to help identify young people's needs is the HEADSSS assessment tool (Goldenring & Cohen 1988; see Appendix G). The assessment gathers information on the most common influences on an adolescent's life at home, school and in other social environments. The tool can help nurses gain a multidimensional, yet individual perspective of adolescent life. The assessment data can be used to foster closer engagement with their world, and ultimately, strategies to help

protect and nurture them through uncharted pathways. Assessment can also be collaborative, aimed at helping inform a whole-of-community approach. Teachers, administrators, parents, community members and others can encourage constructive opportunities and validate the adolescent's ability for decision-making. This approach is most likely to help the young person develop a positive sense of self (Borders 2009; Faulkner et al 2009; Waters et al 2009).

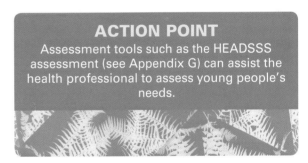

ACTION POINT
Assessment tools such as the HEADSSS assessment (see Appendix G) can assist the health professional to assess young people's needs.

Activities in the neighbourhood and community play an important role in a person's sense of self. Where these are supportive they can help foster civic engagement, trust and other aspects of social capital that help young people develop the competence and character to contribute to society (Duke et al 2009). Strong connections to the broader culture through volunteer work or various forms of community involvement also help provide a strong grounding for adult life (Duke et al 2009). The combination of civic engagement, strong family relationships and a caring school environment can help young people believe they are the agents of their own destiny. Developing academic, social and physical competence in the context of supportive family, school and social environments can ultimately lead to empowerment and the self-confidence for successful adulthood.

Point to ponder

Encouraging young people to become involved in school and community activities can help provide a strong grounding for adult life.

Adolescent life in the school context

The school plays a privileged and strategic role in adolescent development (Herman et al 2009). School offers the opportunity for peer socialisation, which can be the determining factor in adolescents' choices of healthy behaviours (Thunfors et al 2009). The school culture can also be a training ground for empathy, which is a protective factor for antisocial and aggressive behaviours (Estevez Lopez et al 2008). Empathy, where a person can understand and imaginatively enter into another's feelings, is also a core skill for developing appropriate friendship networks and partnerships. This helps young people develop mutually respectful relationships and reject those that are aggressive, especially when choosing a romantic partner. Teachers play a significant role in helping adolescents develop this level of social competence. Teachers who instil empathy, respect, courtesy, shared responsibility and a sense of community create a culture of reciprocal valuing, which helps prepare adolescents for adult life as workers and citizens (Estevez Lopez et al 2008). At school, bonding to others who share the goals of becoming academically competent, respectful and self-motivated reduces the likelihood of young people becoming drawn into substance abuse, smoking or other antisocial behaviours (Haegerich & Tolan 2008; Herman et al 2009). School connectedness is also a predictor of later mental health, acting as a protective factor against mental illness (Herman et al 2009; Shochet et al 2006).

Point to ponder

School can be the centre point of a young person's life. Positive school experiences may shape how a young person copes with peer group behaviours.

Many aspects of adolescent social life are centralised around school and peer group behaviours. Peer group norms and values can validate a young person's identity or sanction certain behaviours through criticism or ostracism (Hamilton et al 2009). For example, ownership of material possessions ('name-brand consumerism') can convey physical attractiveness, athletic prowess and social skills to others in the peer group (Hamilton et al 2009:1528). Like adults, some students wear or carry name-brand merchandise like a badge of honour. This can define them as part of an in-group culture, or it can be difficult for those whose socio-economic status (SES) does not provide the means to access the same consumer goods. Unequal financial status and perceptions of inequality can also widen the gap between the in-groups and out-groups. In most cases, the tensions between these groups are manifest in the school context and linked to their virtual world of social networking.

SCHOOL, HOME AND SOCIAL NETWORKING

Another aspect of adolescent life that influences emotional wellbeing is called peer contagion. As social learning theory suggests, a person's emotions, behaviours and moods are strongly influenced by the activities, interactions, thoughts and observations in their social group (Bandura 1977). Where peers are overly critical and unsupportive, young people can develop social anxieties that unchecked, can ultimately lead to depression. Teachers who try to nurture academic competence and self-determined behaviours, and who try to prevent social comparisons can help protect adolescents from such negative outcomes (Herman et al 2009). But this is increasingly difficult for the digital generation, whose interactions take place in the elusive environment of the internet and in mobile phone technology. In the electronic venue of cyberspace, their language and their messages can become transformed. The internet provides a greater opportunity for deception where 'identities can be protected, personalities can be changed, and young people have limitless liberties to interact and role-play' (Cassidy et al 2009:384). This capacity of anonymity has led to the rise of cyber-bullying using internet and mobile phone technologies, which today is one of the most challenging issues for teachers and parents.

Most adolescents are involved daily in social networking as a form of instant messaging, on sites such as MySpace, FaceBook, Twitter and Flickr. For some, these sites provide a virtual community, providing a vital connection to their peers. Many use the sites daily, communicating with each other about personal behaviours or concerns (Moreno et al 2009). But these technologies have also changed the rules of mockery, insults and harm, and they can be used as media for abuse. Abuses include posting defamatory messages on social networking sites; sending a hurtful message to someone by text, instant messaging or email; spreading rumours; stalking; threats; harassment; impersonation; humiliation by editing a picture to distort someone's image or excluding them from an online group (Cassidy et al 2009; Feinberg & Robey 2009). The rise of this type of abuse has grown over the past two decades since chat rooms first became popular.

Point to ponder
The internet and mobile phone technology has widened young people's social experiences, creating both risks and opportunities.

It is estimated that one-quarter of Australian and New Zealand young people have been cyber-bullied at some time, with 14–17-year-olds the most likely victims (Online. Available: www.today. ninemsn.com.au/article.aspx?id=840251 [accessed 2 November 2009] and www.nzherald.co.nz/youth /news/article.cfm?c_id=107&;objectid=10601177 [accessed 18 November 2009]). This is only marginally less of a problem than in the UK, the US and Canada where one-third of young people have been reportedly victimised in this way (Cassidy et al 2009; Feinberg & Robey 2009; Henshaw 2009). Although the abuse may technically occur away from school, it can undermine the school climate, interfering with the victim's school performance and placing them at risk for mental health problems. The victims are often the unpopular students, those who have poor coping skills and poor relationships, or who are dealing with an emotional episode such as a romantic break-up. Some become hyper-vigilant, feeling they cannot relax anywhere in the school environment. They are often made more vulnerable to manipulation by those with greater technological skill and a desire to remain online, which keeps them from reporting the problem to parents and teachers (Feinberg & Robey 2009).

Point to ponder
Cyber-bullying is a form of bullying that uses technology as a medium of harassment. Cyber-bullying can be pervasive in a young person's life and can be very difficult for a health professional to detect.

Students with a body image or weight problem are a particular target group for cyber-bullying. Like other forms of bullying, cyber-bullying often attacks the most sensitive students, many of whom are preoccupied with body image and social attractiveness. The adolescent years are a time when self-esteem tends to decline, especially in girls who are subjected to diverse and contradictory messages about their role and place in society. Young women are often exposed to gender stereotyping that suggests they are not good at some things (e.g. science), at the same time as they are challenged to succeed in these areas. Some of these stereotypical pressures set girls up for dissatisfaction with their bodies, which is difficult at a time when their growth defies the idealised body portrayed in the media (May et al 2006; Rodgers & Chabrol 2009). This has implications for body image and weight management. It also occurs when metabolic changes associated with puberty can cause girls to gain weight and cause boys to shed body mass, both of which can erode self-esteem. In some cases, eating disorders can actually be exacerbated by well-intentioned health educators urging adolescents to exercise and eat healthier foods, whether these messages are conveyed in person or in the media (Price 2009).

Concerns with weight control have also been linked to depression in adolescents. Boys may express concerns about being too small, while girls have been reported as worrying about thinness at as young as 5 years of age (May et al 2006).

Point to ponder

Adolescence is a time where challenges to self-esteem are high. Peers, media images and bullying can all place greater pressure on a young person to attempt to conform to often unattainable standards.

For most young people, these concerns arise around the time they become adolescents and decline somewhere around age 16 (May et al 2006). The way body image is handled in the school community can have a marked effect on the outcome. Recognising the importance of the problem has led many schools to develop programs designed to create awareness of the need for an ethic of care surrounding those at risk of all forms of bullying, especially in victimising those with weight problems. These programs also include websites that have been developed for easy access by students. In Australia, these include information from the Australian National Centre Against Bullying (NCAB) (Online. Available: www.ncab.org.au/ about/ [accessed 4 November 2009]), and advice on dealing with bullying from the Beyond Blue website (Online. Available: www.youthbeyondblue.com [accessed 4 November 2009]). In New Zealand, netsafe (www.netsafe.org.nz) has some useful resources on coping with cyber-bullying for young people, parents and teachers. A collaborative website between the New Zealand Police and Telecom (www.nobully.org.nz) also provides a range of resources on bullying.

RISK, RESILIENCE AND DECISION-MAKING

Adolescents whose parents remain closely connected with them throughout adolescence have a greater chance of becoming a resilient adult. Parents who negotiate control in a warm and loving environment, and praise their children for the development of competencies nurture the young person's internalisation of parental standards (Heaven & Ciarrochi 2008). Families who over-monitor their children can inhibit the development of adult identity, while low levels of family monitoring can accelerate identity formation (Benson & Kirkpatrick Johnson 2009). This has been reported in studies of early sexual debut, where under-controlled children were found to be more likely to respond to peer encouragement to engage in health damaging behaviours and situations that led to sexual risk-taking (Atkins & Hart 2008).

Point to ponder

Positive feedback nurtures independence and resilience in young people.

A large proportion of adolescent decisions revolve around friendships, academic studies, extra-curricular activities, lifestyle and consumer choices. These are all important in developing good judgement. Decision-making tends to follow a process of exploring all possible options, weighing these up in relation to desirability and possible consequences, assessing the probability that a given consequence will occur, and then deciding on the best course of action (Halpern-Felsher 2009). These are deliberate, rational, analytical processes that can be critical to developing as a socially competent, independent person. They are also important steps in learning to cope with stress, which helps build resilience. Even poor decisions can help build resilience if the consequences help them develop perseverance and strategies for moving on constructively from mistakes. Resilient people develop this type of strategic thinking as a way of coping with stress. This helps them when confronted with progressively complex challenges in the future (Beale Spence & Tinsley 2008). With the support of adults, their positive risk-taking behaviours (academic pursuits, taking on new challenges) are reinforced. Positive feedback from others nurtures independence and leads to the development of a repertoire of protective factors rather than risky behaviours. Armed with confidence and a sense that they are making their own decisions, young people have a better chance of achieving important goals in life.

HOPE AND SELF-ESTEEM

Two important elements along this developmental pathway are hope and self-esteem, both of which help adolescents adjust to adversity (Heaven & Ciarrochi 2008). High self-esteem refers to feelings of wellbeing positive peer group approval, active coping strategies and the expectation of success in life. Hope is a positive motivational state that comes from setting goals that are seen as achievable, even when they experience temporary setbacks (Heaven & Ciarrochi 2008). Hope

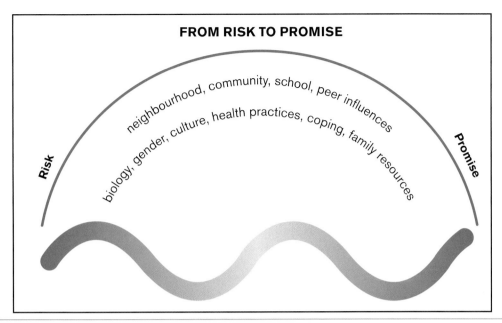

Figure 7.2 Pathway from risk to promise

and self-esteem can give a young person a 'future orientation'; that is, aspirations beyond the immediate moment (Haegerich & Tolan 2008). This is linked to impulse control. Theoretically, if adolescents believe they can get pregnant from having unprotected sex, develop lung cancer from smoking, or have a traffic accident from drink driving, they may be more likely to avoid those behaviours (Halpern-Felsher 2009). Although this is a logical expectation, many adolescents engage in risky behaviours because of a lack of experience in decision-making. In these cases, their perspective of future consequences is overridden by impulsive actions (Beale Spence & Tinsley 2008).

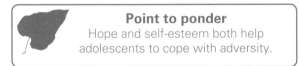

Point to ponder
Hope and self-esteem both help adolescents to cope with adversity.

Adolescent decisions to take risks often take place in emotionally laden and fast-paced situations, where they rely on intuitive, rather than rational, decision-making (Holland & Klaczynski 2009). Choices may be based on a decision that the perceived benefits (peer approval) are more immediately gratifying than the perceived costs (STIs, lung cancer). This has major implications for health promotion, in that even when they have knowledge and understanding of the consequences

of a certain decision, many adolescents will act on situational cues, emotions, stereotypes, memories and automatic responses (Holland & Klaczynski 2009). This explains why numerous programs focusing on behaviour, such as condom use, have had little effect. The good news is that once adolescents reach adulthood, impulsivity and emotional reactivity decline and most young people develop the cognitive ability for impulse control and better planning (Holland & Klaczynski 2009). The challenge is in supporting adolescents to reach adulthood safely!

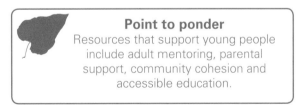

Point to ponder
Resources that support young people include adult mentoring, parental support, community cohesion and accessible education.

Developing social competence for life and resilience in the face of adversity focuses on strengths rather than deficits. The pathway for both implies the presence of both risks and promotive factors that either lead to a positive outcome, or reduce or avoid a negative one (see Figure 7.2). Promotive factors can be either assets or resources. Assets refer to the individual strengths of competence, coping skills and self-efficacy. Resources are supportive elements surrounding the adolescent, such as parental support, adult mentoring, community cohesion and other social environmental influences on adolescent health and development (Fergus & Zimmerman 2005). Resources in the adolescent's home and community environment may be seen as compensatory, such as gaining an education that helps overcome vulnerability or disadvantage, or they may be protective, such as having a highly supportive family.

COUNTERING RISK: HEALTHY ADOLESCENCE

The major objective for promoting health among today's adolescents should be to create healthy pathways to adulthood that overcome risk and promote resilience. A socio-ecological approach addresses the many dimensions and interrelationships among risk factors and guides best practice in risk reduction, prevention of ill health and promotion of health and wellness. In this respect, any planning strategies to counter risk should be comprehensive and mindful of how one type of behaviour or environmental situation affects all others. Strategies should also be developed on the basis of a sequential or life span approach, based on an understanding of adjacent stages of development. The settings of adolescent life should also be woven into any strategies, to reflect the environmental influences on behaviours and development and how these vary according to the home, neighbourhood, school, group, physical and broader socio-cultural environments. The objective of programs for improving and maintaining adolescent health and wellbeing is that they should harmonise the needs and aspirations of adolescents within an ecology of youth, one that is empowering and sustainable to develop lifelong habits and habitats of body and mind.

Goals for adolescent health

The major health issues impacting on adolescents include the following:
- mental and emotional health and maturity
- physical health and wellbeing
- minimisation of conditions that create risks to health and wellbeing
- sustainable lifestyle habits
- healthy environments
- adolescent-appropriate nursing and health services
- empowering structures and processes for successive generations.

Adolescent health begins with the community and society to create supportive infrastructures for health and wellness. Once again, the strategies of the Ottawa Charter for Health Promotion provide a framework for addressing the most salient issues for adolescent health.

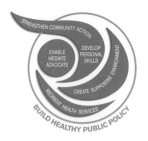

BUILDING HEALTHY PUBLIC POLICY

Healthy adolescence begins with healthy public policies. These include legislation to control alcohol, tobacco products, cannabis and illicit substances, as well as those that promote healthy nutrition guidelines, mental health and environments conducive to healthy lifestyles. Healthy public policies also include those aimed at reducing health disparities among young people living in disadvantaged or vulnerable circumstances. Policy development is tied to economic conditions, and with shrinking resources in many parts of the world, certain policies that would support adolescent health have been discarded. These include funding decisions for school health education, child health services, counselling and community support services. When these services decline there is a greater likelihood of poor school attendance and risky behaviours, all of which impinge on healthy adolescent development (Anderson Moore 2009).

Among the most important policies are those related to alcohol. Although adolescents consume alcohol for a variety of reasons, especially in response to peer pressure, perceived availability and opportunities to obtain alcohol make it seem more socially acceptable (Kuntsche et al 2008). Policies prohibiting certain types of alcohol or reducing availability have gained some support from policy-makers. The tax on 'alcopops' or premixed drinks, was a 2008 policy decision instituted by the Australian government, but there exists no evidence that it has been effective in changing the social acceptability of alcohol or drinking behaviours. This may be because other forms of alcohol are omnipresent in Australia and New Zealand, and adolescents have no difficulty accessing alternatives. Drinking behaviours are embedded in the culture, while the power of the alcohol industry remains strong. This makes it important to take a wide-ranging view of the problem of adolescent drinking, including advertising policies, restrictions on availability and price, police enforcement and a whole-of-society approach to promoting safe drinking behaviours (ARACY 2009).

> ## ACTION POINT
> Harm minimisation approaches have been effective in containing the spread of HIV, and may be useful in supporting adolescents to cope with other risky behaviours.

Policies governing what is portrayed on television and other media also have an effect on adolescent behaviour. The 'just say no' messages of conservative American governments have driven sexual behaviours below the radar, partly because of the mixed messages adolescents receive from the media. On the one hand, they are bombarded with highly sexualised messages, and on the other, they are cautioned to exercise abstinence. A more reasonable approach is that used in other societies where community awareness campaigns promote a positive image of adolescent sexual relationships, aimed at empowering them to take responsibility for their actions by using condoms (Williams & Davidson 2004). This is a harm minimisation approach, which has been effective in containing the HIV epidemic in Australia as well as other countries. However, it has not yet been extended to other aspects of adolescent behaviour (Williams & Davidson 2004).

Harm minimisation policies

The harm minimisation approach is structured around a public health or morally neutral approach to policies rather than one that makes moral judgements about such behaviours as alcohol or drug misuse. This approach precludes thinking about substances within the rhetoric of 'good' or 'bad' substances, focusing instead on reducing the harm

associated with risky behaviours (Hamilton 2003). Reducing usage is a goal, but the focus remains on protecting individuals and the community from harm. The philosophy underpinning this approach is that permitting access to the substances and teaching safe usage can reduce the likelihood of a young person progressing to more harmful drugs and habits (Beyers et al 2005). It also protects the community by acknowledging that governments have a responsibility to ensure public safety. For example, this could include protecting injecting drug users by providing them with a separate place to inject their substances, or installing condom dispensaries in places frequented by adolescents.

Tobacco control policies have provided important lessons about the effectiveness of regulation and legislation in creating conditions for better health. The combination of government-mandated smoke-free workplaces, major increases in tobacco taxation, warnings on cigarette packaging and the prohibition of tobacco advertising has dramatically reduced the rate of tobacco smoking in countries like Australia and New Zealand. The returns on government investment in these areas have been extraordinary. Media anti-smoking campaigns have also enjoyed remarkable success, which has made the global anti-smoking movement the most successful of all health promotion interventions, a fitting outcome, given that tobacco causes more deaths than any other substance. The lessons from tobacco control could be extended to such issues as obesity control or other population-wide programs. These involve effective clinical intervention and management; individual and population education strategies; regulatory efforts, especially at school level; and economic approaches, through taxation and other incentive schemes (Mercer et al 2003).

CREATING SUPPORTIVE ENVIRONMENTS

The two most important environments of adolescent health are the school and social environment. Bonding with the school community helps young people stay grounded in what is usually a safe and supportive environment. School is also vital in connecting young people to their peers. Schools with nursing and other health services provide the most timely source of help and guidance for the numerous challenges of adolescent life. For health professionals, communicating with adolescents about behavioural issues can be a challenge. This is a particular problem for those seeking mental health services. Some health service providers have been criticised for being patronising and insensitive to adolescents, especially those with little experience of working with mental health clients. Communicating with young people about sexual health issues can also be confronting, as these interactions focus on sensitive issues such as sexual practices and relationships (Kim et al 2008). School and family health nurses typically approach this type of communication by being visible and accessible (Tkaczyk & Edelson 2009). They create a trusting atmosphere, showing respect, empathy, being patient and maintaining confidentiality (Kim et al 2008).

> **ACTION POINT**
> School-based health promotion programs are an effective means of reaching young people.

School-based programs have been found to be effective in providing a context for health promotion that can be connected to peers. For example, smoking cessation programs are considered most effective when they take place in the school setting (Sherman & Primack 2009). Programs targeting sexual health are also more effective when they are focused on the peer group in the school setting. These also involve the 'other half of the solution' of adolescent pregnancy; young fathers (Reeves et al 2009:19). To be inclusive, school-based health promotion programs should be tailored to the needs of both young women and men, and adopt a flexible and holistic approach. To achieve this, the content of these programs should include an explanation of prevailing concepts of masculinity and peer group pressures that prevent many young men from using condoms. They should also encourage young fathers to attend antenatal classes and consider their involvement in parenting classes after the birth (Reeves et al 2009).

Schools also play a part in personal growth and cultural renewal, both of which can be instrumental to building capacity for social competence. Including activities that help shape students' sense of identity and culture can help connect family and school agendas for learning, and cultural, spiritual

> **ACTION POINT**
> School plays an important role in personal growth and cultural renewal among young people. Facilitate young people's involvement in school activities in order to build resilience.

and moral development (Commonwealth of Australia 2009). One of the most important determinants of whether or not a school environment is able to develop adolescent capacity lies with educational governance. The current worldwide shortage of teachers, partly created by the number of teachers leaving the profession, has drawn attention to the frustration teachers experience when their passion for adolescent development is dampened by restrictive school and government policies. In many cases, teachers would be amenable to extending their role to a stronger focus on mentoring, which would see them using their talents to foster health and wellbeing in adolescents. However, current educational risk management trends have left many good teachers focusing on restrained behaviours around adolescents at the expense of providing the warmth and mentoring that is often needed.

Fortunately, community groups have developed mentoring schemes to pick up the challenge, with programs such as the Smith Family's Learning for Life Program, the Life is for Living program (Commonwealth of Australia 2009), and the School Volunteer Program in Western Australia. These have been successful in helping adolescents towards an enhanced capacity for celebrating life (Hartley 2004). The Achievement in Multicultural High Schools (AIMHI) program is another example of an integrated approach designed to support young people. The AIMHI program targets students at nine high schools throughout New Zealand, and is aimed at improving educational achievement through a range of initiatives such as onsite health and social support services, and improving the links between the school and community (Online. Available: www.aimhi.ac.nz/default.asp [accessed 18 November 2009]).

Another link between school and adolescent behaviour lies in supporting physical activity. An interesting survey in New Zealand suggests a reciprocal relationship between school connectedness and a student's propensity to exercise (Carter et al 2007). The study of over 600 high-school students found that those who were closely engaged with their high school were more than twice as likely as others to be physically active (Carter et al 2007). The implication is clear in terms of the mutual benefit of weight control and school connectedness, both of which are beneficial to the developing adolescent.

Supporting parenting

As mentioned previously, family closeness is also a major feature in mediating risky behaviours, with a number of international studies finding important links between feeling connected to family and sexual behaviour, including condom use (DeVries et al 2009). The family has the most powerful influence on adolescent health. The myriad of changes to adolescent social life can be difficult for family members, especially in the midst of dramatic changes in family lifestyles. When adolescent children have only one parent available, when both parents work, or where adolescents are in the midst of multiple family transitions, this creates an

additional layer of intensity and extra challenges for parents. They, and other family members, need considerable support from nurses and other health professionals, especially where they have no extended family members or other support networks.

> **ACTION POINT**
> The family provides the most powerful support for adolescent health. Health professionals can, in turn, support families as they guide their children towards adulthood.

The major work of parenting includes monitoring, being an appropriate role model and keeping the lines of communication open with their adolescent children (Ford et al 2009). Because many parents do not have time to be closely engaged with the school or social environment, it is important that nurses and family support workers take advantage of every encounter, to assess how they are

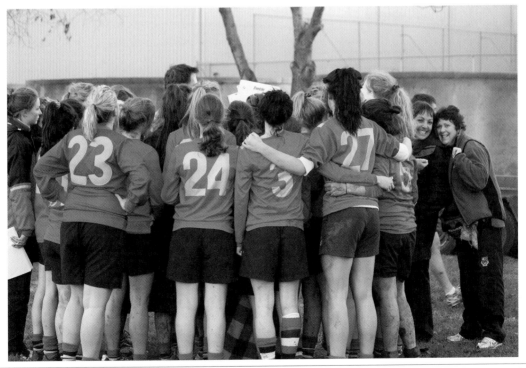

Figure 7.3 Jenny Poppe, school nurse, Ballarat Clarendon College, with teacher/trainer and Girls First Fastball Association Grand Final team (with permission, Ballarat Clarendon College. Photo courtesy of Lisa Panozzo, school nurse, Ballarat Clarendon College, Ballarat, Victoria)

coping with parenting and to keep the channels of communication open. Where clinical interactions occur because of a health issue, the critical elements are non-judgemental support and a positive attitude. Helping parents deal with highly emotional issues such as sexuality, eating disorders, substance abuse or self-harm requires sensitivity towards their needs as parents and the patience to help them through a period of insecurity and conflicting emotions (Honey et al 2008; Rissanen et al 2009; Velleman & Templeton 2007). Some have difficulty accepting that their child may be sexually active and needs protection, or that they are not entirely responsible for other behaviours (Haldre et al 2009). Including parents in their child's care planning and understanding their vulnerability and expectations can help keep the channels of communication open for future contacts (Honey et al 2008).

Parents may also need help in working through their own conflicts, and may be unaware of the impact of family conflict on adolescent emotional development (Herrenkohl et al 2009). In all situations, the best approach is to help them recognise and acknowledge what their children are doing well, rather than focus on their risks and problems (Ford et al 2009). Encouraging a strengths-based sense of promise, rather than risk, may have a long-term impact on parents, and indirectly, on the health of their children. This can be approached by communicating understanding of the complexity of adolescent issues, and of the importance of building family resilience and a harmonious family environment. Resilient children surrounded by resilient families have a greater chance of escaping social and economic disadvantage, lower risks of psychological problems as an adult and smoother transitions along the life course (WHO 2009). When programs to support families are connected with those that provide school support, there is a greater potential to achieve positive outcomes for young people and their families (Velleman & Templeton 2007).

STRENGTHENING COMMUNITY ACTION

The primary community for most adolescents is the school, and therefore this should be the heart of major efforts to strengthen community action. The Health Promoting Schools initiatives were begun as part of the World Health Organization (WHO) 'settings' movement, which identified the most influential places to promote health as those places where people work, live, study and play (Kickbusch 1997). Since the early 1990s networks of health promoting schools have developed worldwide, and these underline the importance of school as an ideal setting for strengthening action in a young person's peer community. As we reported in Chapter 4, healthy schools combine health and education in components that motivate teachers, parents and students to maintain health and to foster learning in relation to key values, appropriate skills and cultural norms.

ACTION POINT
Encouraging personalised communication and connectedness between home, school and community can promote positive health behaviours.

Schools that have the ability and the will to be part of a vibrant community also have a greater capacity to help adolescents in their transitions to adulthood. Interaction with parents and other aspects of community life help young people develop a level of comfort in interacting outside their immediate family or friendship network, while maintaining their sense of place. This type of opportunity is lacking in the lives of adolescents who do not attend school, or who leave school early to seek employment. Integrating protective family, school and community factors has been shown to discourage risky behaviours among adolescents. Other influences on whether or not an adolescent will adopt risky behaviour patterns are derived from a mix of temperament and family relationships (Bond et al 2005). This points to the importance of comprehensive strategies for promoting positive health behaviours that involve personalised communication and connectedness between home, school and community (Bond et al 2005; Fergus & Zimmerman 2005). These strategies should be informed by research that extends beyond single factor studies of drug abuse, delinquent behaviour or criminal activity, to comprehensive investigations of the influence of the social determinants of their lives.

DEVELOPING PERSONAL SKILLS

Adolescents are not a homogenous group, but they do like to conform to group norms of behaviour. Significant others in their immediate environment can have a major influence on their self-esteem and identity formation. Criticism, shaming or humiliating comments can have a long-lasting negative effect on these important developmental tasks (Aslund et al 2009). On the other hand, unconditional support and nurturance can help them develop social competence for adult life.

Adolescent life also changes throughout the adolescent years. Carr-Gregg and Shale (2002) separate adolescence into three stages according to the critical periods of development, each with its own peculiar challenge embodied in the way adolescents question their lives. Early adolescents (age 13–14) ask 'Am I normal?', middle adolescents (15–16) ask 'Who am I?' and late adolescents (age 17–18) ask 'What is my place in the world?' Understanding the subtle differences between the various stages helps frame adult interactions with adolescents in slightly different ways. For example, early adolescents' fears are generated from wanting to conform to this first step towards adulthood. Sensitivity to their loss of childhood and reassurance in the face of their fear of the future can help build self-esteem by reinforcing the fact that their behaviours, thoughts and feelings are normal. Middle adolescence is the stage of identity formation and it is here that adolescents need a guide or mentor. This is also the stage of greatest risk-taking, with adolescents testing who they 'really' are. At this stage, adolescents need safe spaces, a secure and trusted significant friend and they need to be listened to, to establish and confirm their uniqueness. During late adolescence, adolescents confront their developing identity, reinventing themselves in terms of the family, back from the isolation of early and middle adolescence (Carr-Gregg & Shale 2002).

ACTION POINT

Nurses can support parents to recognise loneliness in their adolescent children, and help them develop strategies for supporting the young person to cope with this.

Relationships with school and teachers are important at all three stages. Adolescents develop their capacity to a higher level when they have teachers who engage with them in a meaningful and stimulating way, maintaining high standards for academic learning and conduct, but personalising learning environments (Klem & Connell 2004). Where young people are taught academic content in ways that motivate, engage and involve them, they invest in their own achievement, developing social and emotional, as well as cognitive competence in the process (Catalano et al 2004). Having teachers who are psychologically invested in providing an engaging learning environment helps adolescents develop and expand coping strategies for social as well as occupational endeavours (Klem & Connell 2004). School and public health nurses have an important role in supporting teachers to develop innovative ways of engaging young people in learning about health.

Developing personal skills, especially resilience, is extremely important in countering depressive symptoms in adolescents (Bond et al 2005). Adolescents need to be educated on matters related to their health and supported in changing those they decide to change. This can be nurtured along by helping adolescents integrate functional knowledge (what must be done to improve health or prevent illness), motivational knowledge (how beliefs affect behaviour), outcome expectancy (belief in the effectiveness of preventative action) and self-efficacy (confidence that one can use skills effectively) (Becker 1974).

Many of today's parents of adolescents lead a frenetic life and it is easy to overlook the effect this may have on their adolescents. Most adolescents do not tell their parents how lonely they feel or how important it is to have a sense of belonging to the family. Instead, what is often most visible to parents is a sense that the adolescents are pulling away from the family. Fuller (2002) explains that belonging bridges the gulf between intimacy and isolation. He describes it as an all-embracing feeling that can protect and support the adolescent at each stage of development. He charges parents with recognising the loneliness that adolescents experience in the rush of contemporary life. The violence that creates social toxicity also affects adolescents, even though they often place themselves in situations of high risk. Along with other stressors in adolescents' lives, violence creates a fear of the future as well as confusion about who to be and how to be.

The other aspect of personal development that is not always addressed with adolescents concerns spiritual needs. Many of us get so caught up in achievement and the whirlwind of activity that we suffer from a kind of 'heart hunger' that distances us from others and bankrupts the spirit (Moore 1993). At adolescence, it can create a lifelong template for dissatisfaction and longing. When young people are encouraged to feel connected to family, and to something larger than their own lives, they have a better chance of developing into genuine, good-hearted, compassionate people (Fuller 2002). This helps them see relationships in a more positive light than the way the media distorts them, and helps provide nourishment, energy and solace (Fuller 2002).

REORIENTING HEALTH SERVICES

One of the most important problems of adolescent life can be alienation from societal institutions, including those that provide health care. School health centres are usually designed to be attractive to adolescents and provide an invaluable teaching service. Drop-in centres and neighbourhood health clinics are also designed for easy and confidential access, and these can be designed in collaboration with adolescents themselves. Places where young people congregate should also be the repository of information on health issues, especially to meet the needs of those who have left school. Radio and television stations that attract a large adolescent audience provide an opportunity to reinforce the messages of authority figures, or to have new ones developed by the adolescents themselves that link the ideas of safe behaviour with popular culture. But with today's adolescent lifestyles one of the most effective ways of accessing adolescents for health promotion and health education is via the technologies that have become such an important part of their lives. Technologies such as telephone hotlines have been used for some time for confidential guidance and counselling. However, it

---

BOX 7.2 EYES WIDE OPEN: HONOURING ADOLESCENT PARENTS AND THEIR CHILDREN

The Eyes Wide Open (EWO) project is an initiative of the Peel Youth Program, in Mandurah, Western Australia. The program is aimed at helping adolescent mothers develop realistic expectations of their parenting role and their infant's behaviour, and access existing resources available in the community, including educational opportunities. EWO is also aimed at preventing further unplanned pregnancies for those who had already become adolescent parents by helping them build a trusting network to share their ideas, their fears and their needs.

Many who write about adolescent pregnancy tend to see 'babies having babies', decrying the difficulties and obstacles involved in this situation, instead of seeing the potential for a healthy future. Few celebrate the promise in adolescent life, the 'naturalness' of adolescents, the way a little encouragement can help them develop creative solutions to problems. The EWO project is based on the notion of empowerment as capacity building. From this perspective, sharing the experience of adolescent pregnancy and parenting can be part of the foundation of a cohesive, community-oriented culture. Those facilitating the program provide a venue to get together, safe spaces to solve problems, a non-judgemental network of concerned others, and support for meaningful and therapeutic communication. Talking together lies at the core of healing. It is a way of honouring another person, their situation and their thoughts. The group honours 'birth' with birthday celebrations, exploring the importance of welcoming individuals into the world and other rituals that mark important moments. Working with midwives, child health and community-based nurses, the group learns life skills, emotional skills, child care, creative skills and information relevant to health and fitness to stimulate growth and development. The young women are also given the opportunity to advance their high-school study through online courses offered in the 'Happy Hut' which houses the program. In addition, they are exposed to self-caring strategies, including pampering sessions offered by students from the local beauty school. Another aspect of the program is its outreach to community events such as festivals and various local workshops, which helps nurture pride in pregnancy, motherhood and in oneself. This, in turn, has helped many young girls overcome isolation, low self-esteem, or other residual effects of difficult childhoods.

Young mothers from the initial EWO program have developed a network of peer educators who offer support and advice from their own knowledge and experiences of parenting. This peer support strategy is effective in reducing the sense of isolation so often experienced by adolescent mothers and helping them develop resilience in a caring, supportive environment. Another aspect of the program is a joint initiative of the school and the local community to link young parents back to education. A further element includes group discussion on issues surrounding relationships, conflict resolution, domestic violence and child development. The programs have grown from strength to strength, building the young women's personal capacity and a multidimensional, vibrant community of young adolescents. From the first three adolescents in 1999, the program has now grown to prepare hundreds of young women for motherhood, and for sisterhood, reflecting the basic premise that there is strength in sharing.

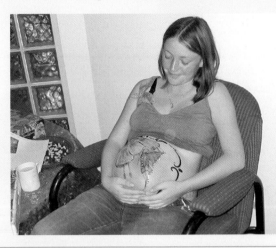

Eyes Wide Open: honouring adolescent parents and their children (with permission)

is only recently that social networking sites and mobile phones have been used for health-related advice and guidance.

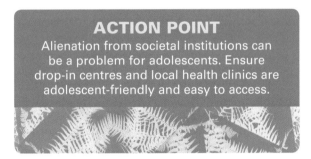

ACTION POINT
Alienation from societal institutions can be a problem for adolescents. Ensure drop-in centres and local health clinics are adolescent-friendly and easy to access.

Electronic media, risk and support

With up to 90% of adolescents communicating online or through instant messaging technologies the potential for health education is considerable (Moreno et al 2009). The notion of 'community' in adolescent life has been transformed by the technologies. Some adolescents interact in virtual communities to a far greater extent than in the real world. This has both advantages and disadvantages. Many users of social networking join health-related groups, which can be useful in communicating information on a variety of topics. For example, researchers found that adolescents with asthma frequently access an asthma site on the internet for information on medication, lifestyle, diagnosis or other issues (Versteeg et al 2009). Some successes have also been reported from online alcohol and smoking reduction interventions (Moreno et al 2009). This type of assistance holds promise for those with confidentiality concerns, or for someone who may find it difficult to access the school health centre or other sources of information. In New Zealand, text messaging has become one of the primary forms of communication among young people (Thompson & Couples 2008). Young people interviewed about their text messaging viewed it as a positive form of interaction, enabling them to create and nurture new friendships and connections with peers in a non-threatening way, as well as an effective means of staying connected with family members (Thompson & Couples 2008). Nurses can support young people as they embrace new communication technologies by growing their own use of technology alongside the young people they work with, using the same technologies to stay in touch with them.

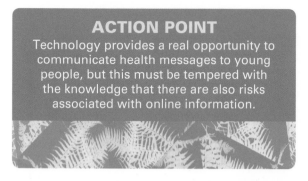

ACTION POINT

Technology provides a real opportunity to communicate health messages to young people, but this must be tempered with the knowledge that there are also risks associated with online information.

On the other hand, there are also risks involved in online information. For those who post sexual references on their personal site, there is an increased risk of being victimised by sexual predators, especially where there is no parental monitoring of online use (Moreno et al 2009). The other risk is related to the accuracy of information. In the asthma study, for example, researchers found that some questions from young people were predictable; such as those involving medication and dealing with family members. They also found harmful responses to queries, such as the person who advised: 'Cocaine helps my asthma …' (Versteeg et al 2009:91). In monitoring the asthma project they found that adolescents do not check the legitimacy of the information. They tend to use trial and error messages and bounce ideas back and forth rather than accessing referenced information (Versteeg et al 2009). This can lead to misinformation. The implications for nurses and other health professionals suggest that the technologies can be useful for practice. Some sites, such as those used to encourage STI screening are effective in enhancing awareness of risks to adolescent health (Lee et al 2009).

Use of the technologies also requires increased vigilance and understanding of what is available and what is being accessed. Since the use of social networking has become so popular, school nurses and others involved in health education have had to shift their assessment style to gather information on the source and types of guidance adolescents are receiving. Many are also establishing networking sites to encourage students to visit them online for appropriate guidance or support. In this respect, social networking can be a valuable tool to provide timely, accurate and individually tailored health advice.

School nurses are also working with young people to help create awareness of the effect sexualised images in the media are having on their decision-making. This issue is also an important topic for child and family health nurses guiding parents on how to deal with early sexualised behaviours. One approach that has proven effective is a classroom and community media literacy component of health education courses. Evaluation of one peer-led media literacy program conducted in several middle schools and community sites in the US found that confronting the influence of sexualised portrayals in class enhanced students' awareness of myths and helped empower their own decision-making (Pinkleton et al 2008).

ACTION POINT

Sexual identity is an issue of great interest to young people, but it can often be a topic causing embarrassment and shyness. Using technology to assist young people to access the information can be one way in which sexuality can be addressed in a non-threatening manner.

Sexual identity is a topic that adolescents frequently discuss using the internet. A large study in the US investigated online construction of identity and sexuality in a sample of conversations from teen chat rooms. Many who participated, communicated information on their gender, physical attractiveness and sexual behaviour. These conversations mirror those that adolescents would be sharing with one another in face-to-face interactions, but the content of their messages were cruder and more explicit, especially in unmonitored chat rooms (Subrahmanyam et al 2006). The researchers explained this in terms of the disinhibition that occurs in text-based interactions, which are anonymous. Discussing explicit sexual image issues would be like wearing makeup or sexy attire in the real world to declare a sexual identity and demonstrate attractiveness. This can provide an opportunity to compensate for what they lack offline. Clearly, adolescents should be aware of the risks inherent in providing such personal information to strangers.

The disinhibition that occurs in virtual networks can also be used as a way to help adolescents alleviate distress, through self-disclosure and social comparison (Whitlock et al 2006). This has been seen in a study of self-harming adolescents who posted messages on sites related to self-harm, and received calming advice and support to help alleviate their distress (Whitlock et al 2006). These studies suggest that social networking and other mobile technologies offer a viable opportunity for interaction to those who feel marginalised (Whitlock et al 2006). Young people find support by forming a virtual community around internet sites, hanging out socially, having multiple simultaneous conversations with others, or participating in instant messaging with smaller groups (Whitlock et al 2006). This helps them practise social skills without the risks of face-to-face encounter.

> ### ACTION POINT
> The internet can also be used to provide stress management courses and emotional counselling.

Another way the internet can be used to support adolescents is through internet-based stress management courses and emotional counselling. An Australian web-based stress management course was implemented across six schools to provide knowledge and support for Year 8 students (Van Vliet & Andrews 2009). Evaluation of the course revealed that it was effective in providing valuable knowledge about stress, and improving wellbeing scores in the young people who attended. The course also had a beneficial effect on mood and helped reduce psychological distress (Van Vliet & Andrews 2009). Similarly, a course provided via text messaging by the Samaritans in the UK was found to have a powerful effect on students' emotional health. Students at risk of self-harm or suicide were encouraged to contact the program anonymously, which students found more beneficial

> ### ACTION POINT
> Nurses who encounter young people in their practice can use the opportunity to assess them for some of the more difficult health issues facing young people, such as sexual risk and depression.

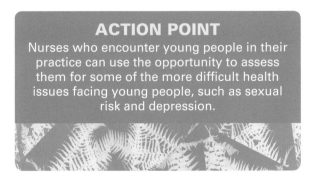

than telephone calls because of the increased confidentiality. They also found it helpful to be able to send a text message or response in their own time rather than be tempted to hang up on the counsellor in a live telephone call (Ferns & Schmidt 2008).

The rapidly evolving and varied uses of the internet draw our attention to the need for vigilance in social networking, especially when so many adolescents are online without parental filtering mechanisms. It also suggests a role for nurses and health professionals in ensuring the accuracy of information that is guiding adolescents in health-related decision-making. Some nurses are also using the internet as a way to counter bullying. A program in the UK, CyberMentors, provides a nationwide online peer mentoring social networking site supported by nurses (Henshaw 2009). They have also developed a mental health toolkit to guide non-specialist nurses in helping adolescents with mental health issues. This is an example that fits well with the ethos of PHC; use of appropriate technology and effective collaboration to work with young people where they live and play: on the internet.

Adolescents' lack of knowledge about their bodies, particularly in relation to sexual health, underlines the need for screening programs. These can provide the basis for anticipatory guidance for disease prevention, family planning and parenting (Denny-Smith et al 2006). In many cases, practice nurses play a valuable role in promoting safe sex. They are usually able to provide written information and guidance when young people come to the practice for STI treatment (Dean 2009). Practice nurses (PNs) can also broach the subject of risk and assess sexual risk with adolescents who attend general practice for other reasons. However, this is not a consistent aspect of general practice, in some cases, because GPs and practice nurses do not feel they have the skills, time, appropriate educational preparation or knowledge of mandatory reporting requirements (Thompson et al 2008; Williams & Davidson 2004). A further barrier is the lack of funding for STI screening in general practice (Williams & Davidson 2004).

To gain access to screening and comprehensive treatment options, adolescents need to access sexual health clinics, which are usually available in major cities. Rural youth in Australia and New Zealand are often excluded from care because of the difficulties in accessing designated clinics. This creates a double disadvantage because they may delay treatment, and also have no alternative source of information and guidance. In New Zealand a program of free GP sexual health consultations was introduced in several practices to reach under-served populations, such as adolescents, Maori and Pacific Island peoples. The program was effective in increasing screening and testing for STIs, especially in detecting *Chlamydia* among young women (Morgan & Haar 2009). Holland is another country that has adopted an adolescent-friendly, cost-free service with convenient opening hours, aimed at promoting sexual health (Williams & Davidson 2004). In Australia, dramatic reductions in the number of GPs who bulk bill to Medicare continues to create financial and access difficulties for adolescents, especially in rural and outer metropolitan areas.

ACTION POINT

Adolescent-friendly health services are needed in all contexts: rural, urban, school, community.

Mental health service provision has always been fraught with some degree of fragmentation, especially when services are not integrated with other community health services. A further difficulty arises when services are not tailored to the needs of adolescents with disabilities (Kingsnorth et al 2007). A strengths-based approach to services for adolescents should focus on self-esteem and validating an adolescent's ability to make decisions. This approach can be empowering and help them feel confident in dealing with challenges in the future. Strategies will also be more effective if they are linked to peers. Most young people want to feel that their experiences are unique yet have something in common with others their age. Providing youth-friendly

BOX 7.3 CREATING EVIDENCE FOR PRACTICE

The Youth2000 project was set up by the Adolescent Health Research Group at the University of Auckland to provide accurate and timely information about youth health to policy-makers, health and education professionals, schools and parents. The overall goal of the Youth2000 project is to improve the health and wellbeing of all young people in Aotearoa New Zealand. Two national health and wellbeing surveys have been undertaken with young people in 2000 and 2007. The results from both surveys have been published widely, providing data on a wide range of health and wellbeing topics affecting young people. The 2009 reports address issues on the health and wellbeing of young people attracted to the same or both sexes (Rossen et al 2009), the health and wellbeing of young Maori (Clark et al 2008), young people attending teen parenting units (Johnson & Denny 2007) and secondary school students (Adolescent Health Research Group 2007). Research of this type provides a solid foundation for developing evidence-based health promotion projects and nursing and midwifery initiatives that meet the specific needs of young people.

services and accommodating variable schedules to fit with study and social activities sends a message of understanding to those in need of support services. This approach also creates awareness of their need for belongingness. It is also important to connect young people's needs and treatment goals with family expectations. Adopting an approach that is inclusive of parents will help build trust between the health professional and young person. It can also be more effective in ensuring there is family support for whatever intervention has been required. This also conveys the message that the health and wellbeing of the adolescent is everyone's concern.

Case study

In Sydney, Maria's niece, Susie, is 15 and has been feeling unwell. She visits the school nurse who assesses her general health and takes a brief sexual history, then together, they visit the website www.checkyourrisk.org.au. The nurse guides Susie in responding to the prompts, then they discuss the fact that Susie may be at risk of an STI. Following the nurse's suggestion, Susie attends a women's health clinic, where she can be screened for STIs. On the return visit to the nurse the following week Susie reports that she has been cleared of any infection, but that the clinic staff have tested her for pregnancy, with a positive result. The nurse explores with Susie how she will consider the various options. She has already told her boyfriend about the pregnancy and they are undecided about the next steps. One option would be to try to finish the school year and then spend the latter part of her pregnancy with her aunt, Maria.

REFLECTING ON THE BIG ISSUES

- Adolescents are generally healthy but often have psychosocial issues that create risks to their health.
- Adolescents can be seen as 'at promise' as well as 'at risk'.
- Adolescents 'at risk' often engage in a cluster of risky behaviours.
- From a social ecological perspective, home, school and the social environment are closely connected in adolescents' lives.
- The principles of primary health care can be used to ensure that adolescents have access to health and other services, that they develop in equitable life conditions and have culturally sensitive guidance that makes the most appropriate use of technology.
- Although there is considerable research into norms of adolescent behaviour many gaps remain in the nursing research agenda.

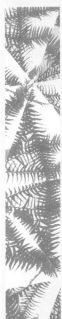

Reflective questions: how would I use this knowledge in practice?

1 Explain the main risks of adolescence and how these can be addressed by nurses using a variety of strategies.

2 Describe health promotion resources available to adolescents in your community.

3 Outline a set of strategies for a program to develop resilience in adolescents based on the social ecology of adolescent life.

4 Design an adolescent suicide prevention program for a local school based on the principles of primary health care.

5 Using the HEADSS assessment (Appendix G) identify some of the needs that you believe would be revealed by an adolescent. Explain how you would promote a sense of community connectedness for this person.

6 Explain the health literacy needs of a typical adolescent.

7 Identify one research question that would guide an important aspect of adolescent health research.

8 Outline what strategies you would employ to support Susie as she works through the choices she now faces.

Research-informed practice

Read the article by Waters et al (2009) 'Social and ecological structures supporting adolescent connectedness to school: a theoretical model'.

- How could you use the theoretical model to guide a research study into the social determinants of adolescent health?

- Identify three specific research questions you could investigate using the model.

References

Adolescent Health Research Group 2008 Youth'07: The Health and Wellbeing of Secondary School Students in New Zealand. Initial Findings. University of Auckland, Auckland

Anderson Moore K 2009 Teen births: examining the recent increase. Child Trends Research Brief. Online. Available: www.childtrends.org (accessed 16 April 2009)

Aslund C, Leppert J, Starrin B, Nilsson K 2009 Subjective social status and shaming experiences in relation to adolescent depression. Archives of Pediatric Adolescent Medicine 163(1):55–60

Atkins R, Hart D 2008 The under-controlled do it first: childhood personality and sexual debut. Research in Nursing & Health 31:626–39

Australian Institute of Health and Welfare (AIHW) 2008 Australia's Health 2008 Cat No. AUS 99, AIHW, Canberra

—— 2009 A picture of Australia's children 2009. Cat No. PHE 112 AIHW, Canberra

Australian Research Alliance for Children & Youth (ARACY) 2009 Action for young Australians report. Online. Available: www.aracy.org.au (accessed 12 November 2009)

Bandura A 1977 Self-efficacy: toward a unifying theory of behavioral change. Psychological Review 84:191–215

Beale Spence M, Tinsley B 2008 Identity as coping: assessing youths' challenges and opportunities for success. The Prevention Researcher 15(4):17–21

Becker M 1974 The Health Belief Model and Personal Health Behavior. Charles B Slack, New Jersey

Benson J, Kirkpatrick Johnson M 2009 Adolescent family context and adult identity formation. Journal of Family Issues 30(9):1265–86

Beyers J, Evans-Whipp T, Mathers M, Toumbourou J, Catalano R 2005 A cross-national comparison of school drug policies in Washington State, United States, and Victoria, Australia. Journal of School Health 75(4):134–40

Bond L, Toumbourou J, Thomas L, Catalano R, Patton G 2005 Individual, family, school, and community risk and protective factors for depressive symptoms in adolescents: a comparison of risk profiles for substance use and depressive symptoms. Prevention Science 6(2):73–88

Borders M 2009 Project hero: a goal-setting and healthy decision-making program. Journal of School Health 79(5):239–46

Bourke L, Humphreys J, Lukaitis F 2009 Health behaviours of young, rural residents: a case study. Australian Journal of Rural Health 17:86–91

Braun V 2008 'She'll be right'? National identity explanations for poor sexual health statistics in Aotearoa/New Zealand. Social Science & Medicine 67:1817–25

Bronfenbrenner U 1986 Alienation and the four worlds of childhood. Phi Delta Kappan 67:430–6

Bursztein C, Apter A 2008 Adolescent suicide. Current Opinions in Psychiatry 22:1–6

Carr-Gregg M, Shale E 2002 Adolescence: A Guide for Parents. Finch Publishing, Sydney

Carter M, McGee R, Taylor B, Williams S 2007 Health outcomes in adolescence: associations with family, friends and school engagement. Journal of Adolescence 30(1):51–62

Cassidy W, Jackson M, Brown K 2009 Sticks and stones can break my bones, but how can pixels hurt me? School Psychology International 30(4):383–402

Catalano R, Haggerty K, Oesterle S, Fleming J, Hawkins D 2004 The importance of bonding to school for healthy development: findings from the social development research group. The Journal of School Health 74(7):252–61

Chandra A, Martino S, Collins R, Elliott M 2008 Does watching sex on television predict teen pregnancy? Findings from a national longitudinal survey of youth. Abstract, Pediatrics 122(5):1047

Clark T, Robinson E, Crengle S, Herd R, Grant S, Denny S 2008 Te Ara Whakapiki Taitamariki.

Youth'07: The Health and Wellbeing Survey of Secondary School Students in New Zealand. Results for Māori Young People. The University of Auckland, Auckland

Commonwealth of Australia 2008 Living is for Everyone (LIFE): Research and evidence in suicide prevention. Online. Available: www.livingisforeveryone.com.au/Research-and-evidence-in-suicide-prevention.h (accessed 4 November 2009)

—— 2009 Family-school Partnerships Framework. A Guide for Schools and Families. Australian Government Department of Education, Employment and Workplace Relations, Canberra

Craig E, Jackson C, Han D, NZCYES Steering Committee 2007 Monitoring the Health of New Zealand Children and Young People: Indicator Handbook. Paediatric Society of New Zealand, New Zealand Child and Youth Epidemiology Service, Auckland

Dean L 2009 Promoting safer sex in young people. Practice Nurse 37(9):28–9

DeLeel M, Hughes T, Miller J, Hipwell A, Theodore L 2009 Prevalence of eating disturbance and body image dissatisfaction in young girls: an examination of the variance across racial and socioeconomic groups. Psychology in the Schools 46(8):767–75

Denny-Smith T, Bairan A, Page M 2006 A survey of female nursing students' knowledge, health beliefs, perceptions of risk, and risk behaviors regarding human papillomavirus and cervical cancer. Journal of the Academy of Nurse Practitioners 18:62–9

DeVries K, Free C, Morison L, Saewyc E 2009 Factors associated with the sexual behavior of Canadian Aboriginal young people and their implications for health promotion. American Journal of Public Health 99(5):855–62

Duke N, Skay C, Pettingell S, Borowsky I 2009 From adolescent connections to social capital: predictors of civic engagement in young adulthood. Journal of Adolescent Health 44:161–8

Eckersley R 2004 Separate selves, tribal ties, and other stories. Family Matters 68:36–42

Erikson E 1963 Childhood and Society (2nd edn). Norton, New York

Estevez Lopez E, Murgui Perez S, Musitu Ochoa G, Moreno Ruiz D 2008 Adolescent aggression: effects of gender and family and school environments. Journal of Adolescence 31:433–50

Fairburn C, Harrison P 2003 Eating disorders. The Lancet 361(9355):407–16

Faulkner G, Adlaf E, Irving H, Allison K, Dwyer J 2009 School disconnectedness: identifying adolescents at risk in Ontario, Canada. Journal of School Health 79(7):312–18

Feinberg T, Robey N 2009 Cyberbullying. Online. Available: www.eddigest.com (accessed 2 November 2009)

Fergus S, Zimmerman M 2005 Adolescent resilience: a framework for understanding healthy development in the face of risk. Annual Review of Public Health, 26:399–419

Ferns J, Schmidt T 2008 Getting the msg across. Mental Health Today, July–Aug:14–16

Ford C, Davenport A, Meier A, McRee A 2009 Parents and health care professionals working together to improve adolescent health: the perspective of parents. Journal of Adolescent Health 4:191–4

Franko D, Thompson D, Affenito S, Barton B, Striegel-Moore R 2008 What mediates the relationship between family meals and adolescent health issues? Health Psychology 27 Supp (2):S109–S117

Fulkerson J, Story M, Mellin A, Leffert N, Newmark-Sztainer D, French S 2006 Family dinner meal frequency and adolescent development: relationships with developmental assets and high-risk behaviors. Journal of Adolescent Health 39:337–45

Fuller A 2002 Valuing boys, valuing girls: celebrating difference and enhancing potential. Presentation to the Excellence in Teaching Conference, Fremantle, Western Australia, 14 November. Online. Available: www.andrewfuller.com.au (accessed 20 December 2005)

Gardner F 2008 Analysis of self-harm. Community Care 1725:22

Goldenring J, Cohen E 1988 Getting into adolescents' heads. Contemporary Paediatrics: 75–90

Haegerich T, Tolan P 2008 Core competencies and the prevention of adolescent substance use. New Directions for Child and Adolescent Development 122:47–60

Haldre K, Rahu K, Rahu M, Karro H 2009 Individual and family factors associated with teenage pregnancy: an interview study. European Journal of Public Health 19(3):266–70

Halpern-Felsher B 2009 Adolescent decision-making: an overview. The Prevention Researcher 16(2):3–7

Hamilton H, Noh S, Adlaf E 2009 Perceived financial status, health, and maladjustment in adolescence. Social Science in Medicine 68:1527–34

Hamilton M 2003 Drugs: a contested policy area. In: Liamputtong P, Gardner H (eds) Health, Social Change & Communities. Oxford University Press, Melbourne, pp 306–27

Hartley R 2004 Young people and mentoring: time for a national strategy. Family Matters 68:22–7

Hayman F 2009 Kids with confidence: a program for adolescents living in families affected by mental illness. Australian Journal of Rural Health 17:268–72

Heaven P, Ciarrochi J 2008 Parental styles, gender and the development of hope and self-esteem. European Journal of Personality 22:707–24

Henshaw P 2009 Supporting victims of cyber-bullying. British Journal of School Nursing 4(3):110–11

Herman K, Reinke W, Parkin J, Traylor K, Agarwal G 2009 Childhood depression: rethinking the role of the school. Psychology in the Schools 46(5):433–46

Herrenkohl T, Kosterman R, Hawkins J, Mason W 2009 Effects of growth in family conflict in adolescence on adult depressive symptoms: Mediating and moderating effects on stress and school bonding. Journal of Adolescent Health 44:146–52

Holland J, Klaczynski P 2009 Intuitive risk taking during adolescence. The Prevention Researcher 16(2):8–11

Honey A, Boughtwood D, Clarke S, Halse C, Kohn M, Madden S 2008 Support for parents of children with anorexia: what parents want. Eating Disorders 16:40–51

Johnson R, Denny S 2007 The Health and Wellbeing of Secondary School Students Attending Teen Parent Units in New Zealand. The University of Auckland, Auckland

Jui-Han W, Miller D 2009 Parental work schedules and adolescent depression. Health Sociology Review 18(1):36–49

Kickbusch I 1997 Health promoting environments: the next step. Australian & New Zealand Journal of Public Health 21(4):431–4

Kim Y, Heerey M, Kols A 2008 Factors that enable nurse-patient communication in a family planning context: a positive deviance study. International Journal of Nursing Studies 45:1411–21

Kingsnorth S, Healy H, Macarthur C 2007 Preparing for adulthood: a systematic review of life skill programs for youth with physical disabilities. Journal of Adolescent Health 41:323–32

Klem A, Connell J 2004 Relationships matter: linking teacher support to student engagement and achievement. The Journal of School Health 74(7):262–73

Kuntsche E, Kuendig H, Gmel G 2008 Alcohol outlet density, perceived availability and adolescent alcohol use: a multilevel structural equation model. Journal of Epidemiology Community Health 62:811–16

Leather N 2009 Risk-taking behaviour in adolescence: a literature review. Journal of Child Health Care 13(3):295–304

Lee D, Fairley C, Kit Sze J, Kuo T, Cummings R, Bilardi J, Chen M 2009 Access to sexual health advice using an automated, internet-based risk assessment service. Sexual Health 6:63–6

Lim M, Aitken C, Hocking J, Hellard M 2009 Discrepancies between young people's self-reported sexual experience and their perceptions of 'normality'. Sexual Health 6:171–2

Major-Wilson H, Sanchez K, Maturo D 2008 A collaborative approach to providing care for HIV-infected adolescents. Journal of School and Pediatric Nursing 13(4):295–6

Martyn-Nemeth P, Penckofer S, Gulanick M, Velso-Friedrich B, Bryant F 2009 The relationships among self-esteem, stress, coping, eating behavior, and depressive mood in adolescents. Research in Nursing & Health 32:96–109

May A, Kim J, McHale S, Crouter A 2006 Parent-adolescent relationships and the development of weight concerns from early to late adolescence. International Journal of Eating Disorders 39(8):729–40

McDonald G, O'Brien L, Jackson D 2007 Guilt and shame: experiences of parents and self-harming adolescents. Journal of Child Health Care 11(4):298–310

Mental Health Foundation 2006 Truth Hurts: Report of the National Inquiry into Self Harm Among Young People. Mental Health Foundation, London

Mercer S, Green L, Rosenthal A, Husten C, Khan C, Dietz W 2003 Possible lessons from the tobacco experience for obesity control. American Journal of Clinical Nutrition 77 Suppl (4):S1073–S1082

Ministry of Health New Zealand (MOHNZ) 2002 Youth Suicide Facts: Provisional 2000 Statistics (15–24 year olds). New Zealand Health Information Service, Wellington

—— 2006 An Analysis of the Usefulness and Feasibility of a Population Indicator of Childhood Obesity. MOHNZ, Wellington

—— 2008 A Portrait of Health. Key Results of the 2006–07 New Zealand Health Survey. MOHNZ, Wellington

Moore T 1993 Care of the soul: the benefits and costs of a more spiritual life. Psychology Today 26(3):284–8

Moreno M, VanderStoep A, Parks M, Zimmerman F, Kurth A, Christakis D 2009 Reducing at-risk adolescents' display of risk behavior on a social networking web site. Archives of Pediatric Adolescent Medicine 163(1):35–41

Morgan J, Haar J 2009 General practice funding to improve provision of adolescent primary sexual health care in New Zealand: results from an observational intervention. Sexual Health 6:203–7

Nakhaee F, Black D, Wand H, McDonald A, Law M 2009 Changes in mortality following HIV and AIDS and estimation of the number of people living with diagnosed HIV/AIDS in Australia 1981–2003. Sexual Health 6:129–34

Norman A 2009 First impressions count: finding ways to support self-harmers. British Journal of School Nursing 4(3):141–2

Pinkleton B, Weintraub Austin E, Cohen M, Chen Y, Fitzgerald E 2008 Effects of a peer-led media literacy curriculum on adolescents' knowledge and attitudes toward sexual behavior and media portrayals of sex. Abstract, Health Communication 23(5):462

Price B 2009 Body image in adolescents: insights and implications. Paediatric Nursing 21(5):38–43

Ramjan L 2004 Nurses and the 'therapeutic relationship': caring for adolescents with anorexia nervosa. Journal of Advanced Nursing 45(5):495–503

Reeves J, Gale L, Webb J, Delaney R, Cocklin N 2009 Focusing on young men: developing integrated services for young fathers. Community Practitioner 82(9):18–21

Rissanen M, Kylma J, Laukkanen E 2009 Helping adolescents who self-mutilate: parental descriptions. Journal of Clinical Nursing 18:1711–21

Rodgers R, Chabrol H 2009 Parental attitudes, body image disturbance and disordered eating amongst adolescents and young adults: a review. European Eating Disorders Review 17:137–51

Rossen F, Lucassen M, Denny S, Robinson E 2009 Youth'07 The Health and Wellbeing of Secondary School Students in New Zealand: Results for Young People Attracted to the Same Sex or Both Sexes. The University of Auckland, Auckland

Schilling E, Aseltine R, Glanovsky J, James A, Jacobs D 2009 Adolescent alcohol use, suicidal ideation, and suicide attempts. Journal of Adolescent Health 44:335–41

Sheeder J, Tocce K, Stevens-Simon C 2009 Reasons for ineffective contraceptive use antedating adolescent pregnancies Part 1: an indicator of gaps in family planning services. Maternal Child Health Journal 13:295–305

Sherman E, Primack B 2009 What works to prevent adolescent smoking? A systematic review of the National Cancer Institute's research-tested intervention programs. Journal of School Health 79(9):391–400

Shochet I, Dadds M, Ham D, Montague R 2006 School connectedness is an underemphasized parameter in adolescent mental health: results of a community prediction study. Journal of Clinical Child and Adolescent Psychology 35(20):170–9

Sparrow M 2009 A mad abortion debate. Christchurch Press Online. Available: http://thehandmirror.blogspot.com/2009/03/mad-abortion-debate-by-dr-margaret.html (accessed 16 November 2009)

Subrahmanyam K, Smahel D, Greenfield P 2006 Connecting developmental constructions to the internet: identity presentation and sexual exploration in online teen chat rooms. Developmental Psychology 42(3):395–406

Thompson K, Casson K, Fleming P, Dobbs F, Parahoo K, Armstrong J 2008 Sexual health promotion in primary care — activities and views of general practitioners and practice nurses. Primary Health Care Research & Development 9:319–30

Thompson L, Couples J 2008 Seen and not heard? Text messaging and digital sociality. Social and Cultural Geography 9:95–108

Thunfors P, Collins B, Hanlon A 2009 Health behavior interests of adolescents with unhealthy diet and exercise: implications for weight management. Health Education Research 24(4):634–45

Tkaczyk J, Edelson A 2009 School nurses a bridge to suicide prevention. NASN School Nurse doi. 10.1177/1942602X09333894:125–7

Van Vliet H, Andrews G 2009 Internet-based course for the management of stress for junior high schools. Australian and New Zealand Journal of Psychiatry 43:305–9

Velleman R, Templeton L 2007 Substance misuse by children and young people: the role of the family and implications for intervention and prevention. Paediatrics and Child Health 17(1):25–30

Versteeg K, Knopf J, Posluszny S, Vockell A, Britto M 2009 Teenagers wanting medical advice: is MySpace the answer? Archives of Pediatric Adolescent Medicine 163(1):91–2

Waters S, Cross D, Runions K 2009 Social and ecological structures supporting adolescent connectedness to school: a theoretical model. Journal of School Health 79(11):516–24

Whitlock J, Powers J, Eckenrode J 2006 The virtual cutting edge: the internet and adolescent self-injury. Developmental Psychology 42(3):407–17

Williams H, Davidson S 2004 Improving adolescent sexual and reproductive health. A view from Australia: learning from world's best practice. Sexual Health 1:95–105

World Health Organization (WHO) 2009 Mental Health, Resilience, and Inequalities. WHO Regional Office for Europe, Copenhagen

Useful websites

http://www.aifs.gov.au — Australian Institute of Family Studies

http://www.sane.org/information/factsheets — mental health information

http://www.nzhis.govt.nz — New Zealand Health Information Service

http://www.spinz.org.nz — New Zealand Youth Suicide Prevention

http://www.plunket.org.nz — Plunket nurses

http://www.myd.govt.nz — Youth affairs

http://www.mindnet.org.nz — New Zealand mental health promotion

http://www.mhc.govt.nz — Strengthening Families, Family Start programs

http://www.youthbeyondblue.com — Information for Australian youth on depression, emotions and bullying

http://www.reachout.com — Help for young people in tough times

http://www.kidshelp.com.au — Kids helpline

http://www.lifeline.org.au/service_index — Lifeline service finder

http://www.ncab.org.au/about/— Australian National Centre Against Bullying

http://www.mentalhealth.org.nz — Mental health promotion NZ

http://www.checkyourrisk.org.au — Melbourne Sexual Health Centre advice on sexual screening and testing

http://www.aimhi.ac.nz/default.asp — Achievement in Multicultural High Schools — collaborative program aimed at educational achievement among multicultural young people

http://www.youth2000.ac.nz/default.htm — Youth health in New Zealand — a profile of their health and wellbeing

http://www.vibe.org.nz — Youth Health Service in New Zealand

http://www.evolveyouth.org.nz/default.aspx — Youth health service in New Zealand

http://www.nobully.org.nz — New Zealand Police and Telecom website on bullying

http://www.netsafe.org.nz — Internet safety website

Chapter 8

Healthy adults

INTRODUCTION

By the time most people have reached adulthood, they have usually experienced at least one illness or injury serious enough to seek medical help. For the majority of adults these are acute episodes of short duration that are resolved without major intervention or residual effects. For others, however, chronic, disabling conditions cause either premature mortality or compromise the quality of their lives. The difference between these two groups is related to biological, social, cultural and environmental influences and how a person has learned to respond to these influences. Adult health and wellbeing also reflect the culmination of the policy environments that have circumscribed people's lives and constrained or facilitated their choices for health and lifestyles. These include a wide range of policies; for example, those governing taxes on alcohol or tobacco, or workplace policies permitting sick leave when workers are ill, or family leave when children need to be cared for. Besides these influences, health in adult life is also a product of family structure, ethnicity, education, employment and place of residence. How an individual has learned to cope with any of these influences, as well as historical illness, injury, disabling conditions or various stressors may be indicative of whether (s)he is able to cope with unexpected events in adult life. Stress and coping are therefore central elements in sustaining health in adult life. Coping strategies are also indicative of how well an adult is able to continue on the pathway to older age. These issues will be outlined in relation to various health outcomes throughout the chapter.

The environments surrounding adult life remain critical to health. This is particularly evident in the effects of the social environment on health and quality of life. A growing body of research linking health to socio-economic disparities, cultural and economic factors sets the stage for greater knowledge of adult health than was available in the past. This chapter will address the effect of these environments on lifestyle choices, especially in relation to the cluster of behaviours that contribute to the burden of ill health from type 2 diabetes, cardiovascular disease and mental illness. The physical environment will also be discussed as part of the ecology of health and wellbeing in adult life. Some aspects of the environment are a cause for urgent concern, with the health effects of climate change, and other global changes, having a major effect on the way we live our lives in the 21st century. Contemporary lifestyles are also influenced by new developments in research and technology. Unique programs of research are forging ahead in informing disease treatments, particularly since the mapping of the human genome and the development of stem cell therapies to respond to errant genes and their expression in the human body. This 'translational' body of research knowledge is an important part of the toolkit for guiding adults towards better health, and it is discussed here in the context of creating and sustaining healthy communities.

THE HEALTHY ADULT

Adulthood is the time of a person's life when the intersecting influences of biology, the environment and lifestyle are most apparent. The years between age 20 to around 50 are concerned with finding one's place in the family, work environment and society, reconciling the needs of various roles and expectations. By the time people

Point to ponder

Adult health and wellbeing reflect the culmination of the policy environments that adults have experienced from birth to adulthood. Adulthood is often characterised by the first experience of a chronic or disabling condition.

Objectives

By the end of this chapter you will be able to:

1 identify the main influences on health and illness in adulthood

2 explain the social determinants of health, illness, injury and disability among adults

3 examine the cumulative effects of interactions between physical, social and cultural environments along the pathway to adult life

4 outline a health promotion intervention for adults focused on reducing multiple health risks through health literacy

5 explain how the health of adults can be improved using the strategies of the Ottawa Charter for Health Promotion

6 identify gaps in research knowledge that could be reduced by nursing and midwifery research.

have become adults, their innate predispositions combine with their past and current lifestyles and a variety of life circumstances to establish relatively stable patterns for the future. For most, the prospect for a long life free of the burden of illness and disability is good. However, other people achieve less than optimal health because of genetic predisposition, the social determinants of their childhood or current circumstances. Fortunately for most adults in Australia and New Zealand, the environment provides considerable potential for overcoming vulnerability to ill health and achieving high levels of health and wellbeing. Unlike some other parts of the world, most people in this part of the world have access to nutritious food, clean air and water, good housing, education and employment possibilities, scientific and technological expertise, relatively low levels of community violence, and accessible and appropriate health care and social support services. However, environmental factors in Australia and New Zealand also create risks emanating from climate change, which is one of the defining challenges of this century, making it a public health priority (Campbell-Lendrum et al 2009). Climate change risks worsening the health of those already disadvantaged, especially Indigenous people, through natural disasters such as drought, floods and fire, and worsening social inequity. As the impact of climate change cascades through daily life, we will have to work intersectorally to understand the health implications of policies such as carbon pricing, the increased cost of living from energy, power generation, transport and agriculture, and a need for heightened surveillance of community

life (Campbell-Lendrum et al 2009). The discussion to follow addresses the strengths, weaknesses, opportunities and threats of adult life in this part of the world, and the effect of global influences on health risks and potential.

RISKS TO HEALTH

A number of factors have been identified as the top 10 causes of mortality throughout the world. These are road traffic accidents, suicide, violence, falling, drowning, poisoning, fire, war, alcohol and drug overdose (Online. Available: www.socyberty.com/death/worlds-top/10-killers-non-disease-related-causes-of-deaths [accessed 30 October 2009]).

Point to ponder

The most common causes of adult mortality in Australia and New Zealand are cancer, heart disease and cerebrovascular disease (stroke).

The 10 categories represent dramatic, non-disease causes of death, many of which occur in catastrophic circumstances. They are of significant concern to nurses and midwives because they provide an overarching guide to goals for preventative nursing interventions. In addition, priorities for interventions are based on the major causes of the burden of disease. In Australia and New Zealand, as in many other countries, the burden of disease is calculated on the basis of the disability-adjusted life year (DALY), representing each year of potential healthy life lost to disease or injury (Australian Institute of Health and Welfare [AIHW] 2008; New Zealand Ministry of Health [NZMOH] 2009a). This is linked to population norms for certain conditions and demographic groups. So, for example, if a male has a fatal heart attack at age 50 and the 'norm' for heart attack for men with his genetic predisposition and health history is age 70, his *individual* burden of disease is 20 DALYs. In terms of the *total* burden of disease among adult Australians, cancers contribute 19% of DALYs, followed by cardiovascular disease (17%), neurological and sense disorders (12%), chronic respiratory diseases and injuries (7% each) (AIHW 2008). The most frequent causes of deaths in Australia are coronary heart disease, lung cancer and cerebrovascular disease (stroke), other cancers, suicide and diabetes (AIHW 2008).

New Zealand also uses a summary measure of population health called Independent Life Expectancy (ILE) — defined as the number of years expected to be lived free of functional limitation needing assistance. ILE extends our understanding of population health from life expectancy to health expectancy. Health expectancy indicators offer the opportunity for policy-makers in the developed world to focus on population health gain, rather than on the traditionally narrow preoccupation on extension of life (New Zealand Ministry of Health & Statistics New Zealand 2009). In New Zealand, the leading causes of death are cancer (28.5% of deaths) and ischaemic heart disease (20.8%), followed by cerebrovascular disease and chronic obstructive pulmonary disease (NZMOH 2009b).

ADULT MORBIDITIES

The number of deaths from cancers has declined in recent years, because of early detection and better treatment. Colorectal and cervical cancers have shown significant declines, however, lung cancer remains an ongoing problem because it is a preventable cause of death, and because there is a long latency period between the cause (smoking) and the outcome (the disease). Lung cancer is the second most frequent cause of cancer deaths in Australia and the leading cause of cancer deaths in New Zealand, followed by colorectal cancer (AIHW 2008; NZMOH 2009b). Prostate and breast cancers are significant sex-specific cancers causing premature deaths in adults. Breast cancer is the leading cause of death in women aged 45–64

in Australia representing 15% of all deaths for this group (AIHW 2008). It is the second leading cause of death after lung cancer among New Zealand women (NZMOH 2009b). Reductions in the mortality rates have left many adults living with cancer in the community, which has major implications for their quality of life. Breast cancer in particular, is affecting more young women between 20 and 40 than in the past, perhaps because of better surveillance and detection. These younger women have more aggressive forms of disease and lower survival rates than postmenopausal women. They face not only a shorter life span, but longer treatment consequences and the possibility of infertility and premature menopause (Shaha & Bauer-Wu 2009). Like others who are diagnosed with cancers they are confronted with the finiteness of their life; feelings of uncertainty, loss of control and the transitory nature of life (Shaha & Bauer-Wu 2009). This presents a major challenge for nurses working in the home and community to ensure that their psychosocial needs are given as much attention as their physical needs, which are considerable.

> **Point to ponder**
> Nurses have a responsibility to ensure that both psychosocial and physical needs of an individual who is diagnosed with cancer are met.

Road traffic accidents and suicide are the major causes of injuries and represent the leading preventable cause of death and disability (AIHW 2008). Alcohol, fatigue, sleepiness and speeding are the main causes of motor vehicle accidents, with young men over-represented among the victims, especially those from rural areas (AIHW 2008). Over the past decade, Australia, New Zealand and other Western nations have had significant declines in the rate of motor vehicle injuries due, in part, to improved public education programs, better law enforcement, stricter penalties, better roads and improvement in vehicle safety design. There is also increasing recognition that risky driving behaviours are embedded in a pattern of risky behaviours, as we discussed in Chapter 7. This indicates that the most effective approach for accident prevention is by addressing the cluster of risky behaviours within the context and structures that support them.

Point to ponder

Long-term or chronic conditions are common among Australian and New Zealand adults. Many of these are linked to lifestyle factors and are amenable to change.

Although nursing interventions in the community include injury management, especially in occupational health and rehabilitation settings, most revolve around the more insidious conditions of daily life; the risk factors that cause diseases, premature deaths and reduced quality of life. These include cardiovascular disease, chronic obstructive pulmonary disease (COPD), cancers, asthma and other respiratory conditions, type 2 diabetes, arthritis, sensory impairments (vision and hearing), back pain and mental illnesses (AIHW 2008). Approximately 77% of Australians and 66% of New Zealanders have at least one of these long-term conditions lasting six months or more (AIHW 2008; NZMOH 2008). Some conditions are more common in different age groups; for example, asthma in younger adults and arthritis in older people. At a population level, these compromises to health are disabling for 20% of the population, many of whom live with chronic pain or restricted mobility (AIHW 2008). Many of these conditions and diseases have a biological component in their web of causation, but most are also linked to lifestyle factors. This means that there are modifiable aspects of people's environments that are amenable to change.

STRESS IN ADULT LIFE

Stress, especially workplace stress, is one of the most significant sources of ill health, which may be modifiable through individual, community and social interventions. A variety of workplace stressors affect members of socio-economic groups differently, but workplace stress is becoming more prevalent across all categories of workers. This is linked to changing social conditions. Life in the 21st century has become fast-paced for many adults, with resounding effects on the family, the workplace and society. The 'busyness' of lifestyles has therefore become a public health issue (Bryson et al 2007). It is of particular concern to nurses not only in planning nursing interventions for community living adults, but in dealing with their own work stress, which is among the highest of

all occupations. Helping others cope with existing stress or preventing stress from causing unhealthy behaviours is therefore personal. This requires attention to the harmful combination of poor diets, inactivity, alcohol and tobacco consumption (Umberson et al 2008), as well as the social determinants that can either provoke or minimise these behaviours.

Point to ponder

Stress is one of the most significant sources of ill health among adults.

The sources of workplace stress are numerous, but globalisation and technological innovations have transformed workplaces today. Where once it was necessary for workers to be completely engaged and active during their work day, current processes often involve passive, monitoring-type activities. Away from the workplace, adults' busy lives also leave little time for the requisite physical activity levels that would help prevent cardiovascular disease and alleviate stress. A further issue is transportation. The lack of public transportation in many cities has created an automobile-dependent society, where taking the car even to the corner shop is commonplace. Growing urbanisation has also created shrinking spaces for parks and bicycle pathways that would encourage people to cycle to work. As a population group, many urban dwellers also consume too many high-salt, high-fat meals, especially those obtained at fast-food outlets, and this has led to an epidemic of overweight and obesity (Aranceta et al 2009; Laforest et al 2009). Although there have been some improvements in lifestyle behaviours such as alcohol and tobacco consumption, many adults in Australia and New Zealand continue to smoke and drink alcohol at excessive levels. The links between these behaviours, poor nutrition, low levels of activity and the escalating rates of chronic illness are cause for concern (AIHW 2008).

LIFESTYLE AND CHRONIC DISEASE

Throughout the world, there are many different causes of disease. Among poorer, developing countries, infectious diseases remain a major cause of morbidity and mortality, despite some improvements over the past few decades (WHO 2008). In the industrialised nations, diseases linked to modern lifestyles continue to rise, to where 25% of adults are affected by at least two chronic health conditions, and this rate increases to 50% for those over age 80 (WHO 2008). Tobacco-related illness alone accounts for nearly 10% of all deaths worldwide (WHO 2008), which is the highest burden of disease and injury. Yet, 18% of Australians continue to smoke (Kirby 2009; NZMOH 2008). The second highest risk to health is physical inactivity, with more than one-third of Australians reporting that they undertake little or no regular physical activity (Street et al 2007). Half of all New Zealanders also fail to meet recommended daily physical activity recommendations (NZMOH 2008).

In Australia, chronic conditions account for 70% of all health expenditures and constitute 50% of all GP consultations (Commonwealth of Australia 2009; Kirby 2009). New Zealand data on the cost of chronic or long-term conditions is limited, however it is known that chronic conditions create a significant economic burden for New Zealand, with more than 20% of all visits to a GP being for long-term conditions (NZMOH 2008, 2009a). As we discussed previously, the social environment creates conditions within which people make healthy lifestyle choices, so it is not helpful to blame the victim of ill health. However, research indicates that most of these chronic conditions are preventable through modification of risk factors such as smoking, excessive alcohol consumption, lack of physical activity and low consumption of fruit and vegetables (Cardi et al 2009). So there must be some rearrangement of circumstances that allows people access to, and encouragement for, healthier lifestyles. This is a challenge for those living in poverty or marginalised by social exclusion; the two most important factors in precipitating chronic diseases such as type 2 diabetes (McDermott 1998). Poverty and social exclusion are both community problems, as individuals and families require an enabling community to develop the capacity to maintain the resources for good health. Two strategies for rearranging environments for better health include first, ensuring that local communities are working towards enabling health for the disadvantaged, rather than constraining people's attempts to lead healthy lives, and second, strengthening workplace-based health promotion programs for those trying to sustain their ability to remain employed.

In recent years, there has been a worldwide decline in heart disease and strokes, which are strongly linked to behavioural risk factors

(Commonwealth of Australia 2009). Reductions in morbidity and mortality can be attributed to public awareness, improvements in treatments and increases in the number of people adopting certain healthy behaviours. Paradoxically, the improvements in disease outcomes are accompanied by dramatic increases in the prevalence of overweight and obesity (Rosengren 2009). In 2009, 54% of adult Australians and 63% of adult New Zealanders were overweight or obese, which places them at risk of type 2 diabetes, heart disease and cancer. The increase in obesity among the population is expected to result in three-quarters of the population being overweight or obese by 2020 (Commonwealth of Australia 2009; NZMOH 2008). This mirrors the situation in the United States and Canada and many parts of Europe, where similar patterns of lifestyle behaviours have seen exponential growth in overweight and obesity across all age groups (Aranceta et al 2009; Cardi et al 2009; Lee et al 2009; Penn et al 2009).

Point to ponder

In 2009, 54% of adult Australians and 63% of adult New Zealanders were overweight or obese.

The 'obesity epidemic' is placing large numbers of adults at risk for metabolic syndrome, type 2 diabetes and cardiovascular disease (CVD) as well as some cancers (Aranceta et al 2009; Brown et al 2008; Cardi et al 2009; Lee et al 2009; Martinez-Gonzalez et al 2009). CVD includes coronary artery disease (CAD) and stroke, which are responsible for the largest proportion of deaths throughout the world, including Australia and New Zealand (AIHW 2008). The cluster of factors that create the highest risk for CVD includes hyperlipidaemia (high LDL cholesterol), high plasma glucose, hypertension and type 2 diabetes (Deambrosis et al 2009; Grundy et al 2005; Jones 2008). Metabolic syndrome, which often precedes type 2 diabetes, is a particular problem, as it represents a constellation of inter-related metabolic risk factors for CVD (Grundy et al 2005). The prevalence of these risk factors in the adult population is alarming, and they are rapidly increasing in younger adults (Lee et al 2009). Establishment of new drug therapies, such as statin treatment to lower LDL cholesterol for those with existing risk factors, has reduced the incidence of cardiovascular events

(Korber 2008). But although this treatment is seen as clinically effective, it is also associated with increased liver- and muscle- related adverse outcomes (Morrissey et al 2009). Attempts to address the risk through early detection and intervention include cardiovascular risk assessment such as those implemented by many primary health organisations (PHOs) in New Zealand (for example, see www.nzgg.org.nz/guidelines/0035/CVD_Risk_Summary.pdf).

Point to ponder

Early detection of those identified as at risk allows nurses to provide appropriate interventions to reduce the impact of cardiovascular disease and diabetes on individuals, families and communities.

Behaviour changes in relation to better diets and less smoking have been responsible for a continuing decline in mortality from CAD (Rosengren 2009). However, these improvements have not been experienced evenly across the population. Disadvantaged people continue to have a higher rate of smoking, especially among those with lower education, lower income, unskilled workers or the unemployed, or those on social welfare benefits (Tsourtos & O'Dwyer 2008). This is also the population group with high levels of stress, which often act as a deterrent to quitting smoking, or adopting other healthy behaviours (Raphael et al 2003). Studies have also found that smoking tobacco may actually ameliorate stress. This occurs through the action of the anti-stress hormone dehydro-epiandrosterone (DHEA) which has positive effects against stress and anxiety (Tsourtos & O'Dwyer 2008). Many disadvantaged people also live in neighbourhoods with a high concentration of convenience stores where they can purchase cigarettes. So they experience more barriers than others to quitting smoking through a combination of biological, environmental and social factors (Tsourtos & O'Dwyer 2008).

Unlike smoking, obesity remains problematic across all socio-economic groups (Chaturvedi 2004; Lee et al 2009). Obesity is not only a constraint on the health, wellbeing and quality of life of the population, but also presents a significant drain on health care resources (WHO 2000a). This is expected to worsen with higher rates of obesity among children and younger adults creating longer-term,

and therefore more costly, treatment (Aranceta et al 2009; AIHW 2008). The need for behavioural interventions to help stem the epidemic of overweight and obesity is clear, particularly in balancing exercise and a healthy diet. However, as with smoking, the environment cannot be overlooked. Obesity is considered a product of obesogenic environments, where calorie-dense foods are marketed and accessible throughout the community, and lifestyles require low physical exertion (Aranceta et al 2009; Rosengren 2009). This needs to be recognised by health professionals as well as the general public, to counter the stigma attached to obese people in the community. Discriminatory hiring practices and ongoing denigration or ridicule of obese people have been described as 'civilised oppression' (Maclean et al 2009:89). Stigmatising people for being overweight is based on a common view that weight is easily controlled by disciplined individual decisions to exercise more and eat less, which misinterprets the role of environmental determinants (Maclean et al 2009). Even though personal resources for behaviour change and social support can act as buffers for socially patterned stressors, stigmatisation can constrain an obese person's attempt to conform to behavioural norms (Meyer et al 2008; Umberson et al 2008).

The diet industry has some responsibility for marketing appropriate foods, but there is considerable public misinformation about diets, particularly in purveying the idea that low-fat products will solve the problem of overweight. In fact, a person's diet is influenced by a range of biological, cultural, economic and social factors, not just marketing by food producers (Coveney 2007). A large body of evidence points to the healthful effects of a Mediterranean diet. This consists of high consumption of olive oil, legumes, unrefined cereals, fruits and vegetables, moderate consumption of dairy products (cheese and yoghurts), moderate to high consumption of fish, low consumption of meat, and moderate wine consumption (Martinez-Gonzalez et al 2009).

Point to ponder

Nutrition counselling needs to be tailored to meet individual needs. Cultural imperatives and the social context of eating and motivation influence the ability of individuals to make the dietary changes they need to maintain good health.

The Mediterranean diet is known to have a higher protective effect against CVD risk factors compared with a low-fat diet. Equally as important is the fact that those who consume a Mediterranean diet tend to have greater adherence than those who eat low-fat diets, perhaps as a function of family lifestyle, which also illustrates the cultural context of healthy eating (Martinez-Gonzalez et al 2009).

Nutrition counselling is often a first step in helping people with lifestyle improvements once they are diagnosed with chronic illness. This needs to be tailored to individual needs, as a one-size-fits-all prescription for healthy eating may present barriers for certain individuals. Any of the chronic conditions may change a person's appetite and attitude to food as well as their access to preferred products. Some diabetics, for example, have difficulty with the constant food vigilance. Some do not feel comfortable eating with others, which changes their social circumstances (Telford et al 2006–07). Treatment regimes can also be a problem. Statin treatments come with contraindications for certain foods because they effect changes to metabolism. Motivation can also be a challenge. Individuals who suffer from loneliness, anxiety or depression as well as diabetes or CVD can experience low motivation to eat a nutritious diet (Haddad 2009). In these cases, the combination of decreased functional abilities, limited financial resources, psychological responses to deprivation such as feeling worthless or disempowered, can mitigate against a whole range of healthy behaviours, including good nutrition.

Social and environmental factors are also important in promoting exercise, and health education strategies are often planned around the social environment. Organised physical activities provide opportunities to develop supportive social networks as well as helping manage obesity (Street et al 2007). Group recreation has been found to enhance value, belongingness and attachment to others. Community activities can also help reduce violence in the neighbourhood and promote social capital (Raphael 2009; Street et al 2007). At a personal level, exercise boosts immune functions, enhances anti-tumour activity and has shown positive effects on depression, anxiety, stress, self-esteem, Alzheimer's disease, pain and premenstrual syndrome (Street et al 2007). For this reason, 'sweat' has been called the natural antidepressant.

Point to ponder
Exercise programs need to be socially contextualised and fun.

However, much remains to be learned about exercise, as research into the dose, intensity and environments for exercise has shown mixed results among different groups (Gillison et al 2009; Street et al 2007). One meta-analysis of quality-of-life improvements from exercise interventions showed that exercise had less effect on those with chronic disease than rehabilitation patients or well adults (Gillison et al 2009). Factors such as lack of time, motivation, health and weight restrictions, cost and disinterest can be deterrents to regular exercise, especially for men (Burton et al 2008). Interestingly, Australian men reported one barrier to adult exercise as being less enjoyable than sports, especially compared with the team spirit and obligation to team-mates they had enjoyed in younger years (Burton et al 2008). The implication for health promotion suggests that even for older persons, exercise programs need to be socially contextualised and fun.

RURAL LIFESTYLE RISKS

The relationship between health and place is relevant to the level and type of risks to adult health. People living in regional or rural areas are at significantly higher risk of being overweight or obese than urban dwellers, particularly Indigenous residents (National Rural Health Alliance [NRHA] 2009a). Some of the factors related to high rates of obesity in rural areas include poor health literacy, inherited behaviours, low levels of education, poor access to fresh foods with a disproportionate amount of processed foods, a shortage of dietitians and other health professionals, insufficient resources for maternal and child health, and a lack of funding and personnel available to run exercise and other health promotion activities (NRHA 2009a).

Responses to these issues require political commitment to ensure that adequate nutritious foods are not only available but affordable in rural areas. Health promotion strategies that revolve around health literacy and empowering people to take control over their lifestyles are sometimes moderated by access to resources. For example, the 'digital divide' between those with and without access to internet information can worsen inequities. Although internet information is gaining favour with older people, it is not always available for rural people (Wilson et al 2007). In addition, many regional towns and rural areas do not have access to green parks, exercise playgrounds for children or safe walking trails to school. Rural people have also experienced substantial stress due to economic pressures and environmental degradation (NRHA 2009a). Those who suffer from cancers are also disadvantaged by having to travel long distances for specialised treatment. As a result, many cancers among rural people are diagnosed later than those in urban dwellers (NRHA 2009b).

Point to ponder

High rates of obesity in rural areas can be linked to poor health literacy, a shortage of dietitians and other health professionals, inherited behaviours and low levels of education.

Rural people also have considerable lifestyle stress due to their occupations. Living and working on the land offers rural families few opportunities for respite (NRHA 2009c). Stress from the constancy of their work life is compounded by droughts, floods and bushfires as well as the economic uncertainty of their lifestyles (NRHA 2009c). For young adults, the loneliness of life in rural and regional areas can be problematic. This can lead to relationship breakdown and depression, which can set individuals on a path to over-consumption of alcohol or other substances (NRHA 2009c). Rural residents with same-sex preferences can also be alienated from others in the community, especially given the cultural dominance of values such as masculinity and rugged individualism. Mental health issues emanating from these situations are often ignored by rural residents who tend to be stoical, believing they can take care of things themselves. The lack of counsellors or health professionals who could provide support also leaves many without mental health care. A further deterrent to help-seeking lies in the desire to avoid being stigmatised by seeking help in a small community, where others would take note of their actions. In some cases, unacknowledged depression and other mental health issues can lead to suicide, especially where firearms and poisons such as pesticides are readily available. These reasons are often cited as explanations for the relatively high rate of suicide among rural males (NRHA 2009c).

STRESS, MENTAL HEALTH AND THE SOCIAL DETERMINANTS OF HEALTH

As we have discussed previously, the social gradient and income inequality are major elements of the social determinants of health (SDOH). Analysis of population data from 60 million people in 30 OECD countries has confirmed unequivocally, that the health of any society is better when wealth is more equally distributed (Kondo et al 2009). Educational, economic and social inequality and unequal distribution of resources lead to higher risks for mortality for those who are disadvantaged (Kondo et al 2009; Wilkinson 1996). The impact of inequality is profound in low-income families (Raphael & Farrell 2002). Low income leads to material deprivation, chronic stress, adoption of unhealthy coping behaviours, poor mental health, and exposure to unhealthy environmental conditions at home and at work (CSDH 2008; Feldman et al 2009; Raphael & Farrell 2002; WHO 2009). Stress is even greater for those with chronic conditions, disabilities or those without transportation, as they rely more heavily than others on local services and facilities. For these groups, the effects of incivilities, such as neighbourhood crime, vandalism and conflict, are also experienced more intensely than others (Raphael 2009; Warr et al 2009).

Point to ponder

When the gap between the rich and the poor can be reduced in an empowering way, there is a greater likelihood that social pathways to health will have a protective effect on the whole population.

To redress the disadvantage of inequitable societies and neighbourhoods, redistributing wealth to provide better food, housing and material resources for those who are disadvantaged seems like an appropriate solution. However, simply providing resources would not be effective without opportunities for disadvantaged people to achieve equitable social status, friendship, social capital and a sense of control (Pickett & Wilkinson 2009;

Raphael 2009). These factors are instrumental to mental health as they provide the resilience, health assets, capabilities and capacity for adaptation that help people cope with adversity and realise their full potential and humanity (WHO 2009). This is the basis of arguments for reversing Indigenous disadvantage, which we will address in Chapter 11. When conditions can be rearranged to reduce the gap between the rich and poor in an empowering way, there is a greater likelihood of social pathways that will have a protective effect on the whole of the population. This can help reduce the prevalence of violence, bullying, teenage births, rates of imprisonment, low educational attainment, social mobility and trust, and longer working hours (Pickett & Wilkinson 2009). The impact can be felt at both the individual and community level.

At the individual level, chronic stress 'gets under the skin' through the neuro-endocrine, cardiovascular and immune systems (WHO 2009:iii). This occurs through disruptions to neuro-endocrine and metabolic systems from the constant stress of living disempowered lives (Raphael 2009).

Point to ponder

How people think, feel and relate to one another is crucial to good health and is socially determined.

These responses can elevate cortisol, cholesterol, blood pressure and inflammation. Psychosocial reactions such as anger and despair related to occupational insecurity, poverty, debt, poor housing, exclusion or other indicators of low status can lead to health-damaging behaviours such as smoking, excessive alcohol consumption or poor dietary habits. These impact on intimate relationships, self-care and the care of children, and they can be either a cause or consequence of anxiety and depression (WHO 2009). This insight into the psycho–biological pathways to ill health, highlights the integral nature of mental and physical health.

> Mental health is a feeling of wellbeing, perceived self-efficacy, autonomy, competence, intergenerational dependence and recognition of the ability to realise one's intellectual and emotional potential. It has also been defined as a state of wellbeing whereby individuals recognise their abilities, are able to cope with the normal stresses of life, work productively and fruitfully, and make a contribution to their communities.
>
> (WHO 2003:7)

How people think, feel and relate to one another is crucial to good health and it is socially determined. It is linked to their social position and sense of coherence or meaning in life, as well as their cognitive, emotional and social relations with others. Unequal life conditions therefore have a major impact on mental health, if how they think, feel and relate causes low self-esteem, shame and disrespect (Raphael 2009; WHO 2009). Psychosocial factors such as mood disorders, lack of social support and isolation create the same level of risk to health as smoking, high blood pressure and elevated cholesterol (WHO 2009). This represents a multiplier effect, placing people with mental health conditions at greater risk of CVD, stroke, metabolic syndrome, diabetes, infections and respiratory diseases (WHO 2009). The way these conditions are intertwined is widely recognised today, with global figures showing that mental illness, including suicide, is responsible for 30% of the total burden of morbidity and disability (WHO 2009).

POSITIVE MENTAL HEALTH AND WELLBEING

Positive mental health has a powerful effect on individuals and the community. People with positive mental health tend to be more socially connected, to volunteer, to have better social networks and high health assets, or quality of life. Those who have developed positive mental health skills such as resilience, optimism, self-esteem and self-efficacy are better able to buffer stress, resulting in high emotional and cognitive capital. They do so within resilient neighbourhoods and communities with high social and environmental capital, which also buffers the cumulative effects of deprivation with feelings of hope, trust and social support (WHO 2009). In addition, mental wellbeing has a powerful effect on job performance, worker productivity, creativity and absenteeism (WHO 2009). Workers who feel in control of their work life, and who feel they are treated fairly at work have been found to have lower stress levels (Fujishiro & Heaney 2009; Lawson et al 2009; WHO 2009; Ylipaavalniemi et al 2005). This has a reciprocal effect on the workplace, as individual employees feel empowered to participate in decision-making, provide mutual support, engage in employee health promotion programs and work towards achieving team goals.

Point to ponder
People with positive mental health are more socially connected, are more likely to volunteer in the community and have higher quality of life.

Education is one of the most valuable assets for positive mental health. Education plays a powerful role in mediating social inequalities and in creating a pathway to better physical and mental health in adult life. This occurs because individuals with better health are more likely to achieve higher levels of education. The reverse is also true. Having an education leads to better health (Topitzes et al 2009). Being educated helps those at the lower end of the health gradient alter their life course to a higher socio-economic level in society. This can lead to better adult lifestyle behaviours. Those in higher socio-economic groups tend to smoke less, achieve better rates of smoking cessation, consume less alcohol and have lower levels of depressive disorders (Topitzes et al 2009). This begins in childhood. Participating in school programs and activities during the developmental years facilitates cognitive growth, social adjustment and school commitment, all of which foster social and emotional maturity for a stable, healthy adult life (Topitzes et al 2009). As we mentioned in Chapter 7, having a high-quality preschool experience and staying in the education system plays a role in emotion regulation, which reduces the propensity for tobacco smoking and substance use. Education is therefore empowering, and provides the preparation to function as a healthy adult.

SOCIAL EXCLUSION AND MENTAL ILL HEALTH

Some social conditions surrounding adult life can cause stress and stress-related disease for disadvantaged individuals not only through economic deprivation, but also through structures that allow disproportionate exposure to prejudice and discrimination (Meyer et al 2008). Obvious examples of discrimination are perpetrated on the basis of race, gender or other personal characteristics. In the absence of social support, some people are socially excluded on a number of fronts. They may be *marginalised* through exclusion from certain social activities in their local community because of non-conformity or personal behaviours. At a societal level, they may be excluded from secure, permanent employment, sufficient earnings, access to credit or land; housing and adequate consumption of necessities; education, skills and cultural capital; welfare, citizenship and legal equality; democratic participation, public goods, family and sociability, humanity, respect, fulfilment and understanding (Meyer et al 2008).

Point to ponder
Prejudice and discrimination can result in marginalisation and exclusion of individuals from their communities, in effect compounding the impact of socio-economic disadvantage.

All of these aspects of social exclusion constitute structural stressors. In addition, many individuals experience the added burden of acute stressors, which can range from unemployment to prejudice-related life events (Meyer et al 2008).

In some cases, cultural norms may exacerbate states of mental ill health. Certain cultures recognise anxiety, depression, grief, stress or worry as merely problems in living, and therefore they do not warrant help-seeking (Tyson & Flaskerud 2009a). Those who seek help may be devalued and *stigmatised*, considered to have brought shame on the family (Tyson & Flaskerud 2009b). Other cultures have a broader perspective on mental health and ill health. An Australian study of people's perceptions of mental health found that the three most common factors contributing to positive mental health were having good friends to talk problems over with, keeping an active mind and having control over one's life (Donovan et al 2007). The same cohort described being mentally *unhealthy* in terms of excessive use of alcohol or drugs, having no friends or support network, and life crises or traumas (Donovan et al 2007). At the extreme end of the continuum is homelessness, where those disadvantaged by a lack of employment and housing live in a vicious circle of vulnerability to ill health, injury, violence and a lack of social support.

What's your opinion?
Culture and cultural beliefs can have a profound impact on mental health. Is this a positive or negative impact or both?

In 1997, New Zealand began a publicly funded campaign called Like Minds Like Mine. The campaign was one of the first in the world aimed at reducing discrimination and stigma associated with mental illness. Using a combination of community action at a local level with nationwide strategies and media advertising, the campaign has led to increased acceptance and openness in the community about mental illness (NZMOH 2007). Although change has occurred in people's attitudes towards those with mental health issues, the campaign continues today to ensure changes in behaviour, policies and practice follow the changes already achieved in attitudes (NZMOH 2007).

The unhealthy coping behaviours people use to deal with stress can reverberate throughout the adult life course, having a cumulative effect on health and causing mental illness (Umberson et al 2008). Behaviours such as consuming high-fat diets, increased alcohol consumption and lower levels of physical activity may help alleviate psychological and physiological arousal and regulate mood (Umberson et al 2008). On the other hand, stress can also lead some people to engage in healthier behaviours, such as physical activities to buffer stress. As a person ages, the coalescence of psychological, physical and social factors may change their coping style, making them less reactive to stress and allowing existing stress to dissipate (Umberson et al 2008). In some cases, this is because, as adults age, they may begin to focus less on themselves and more on others. It has also been explained on the basis that behaviours such as eating, drinking and smoking may be less effective in reducing the arousal of stress among older age groups (Umberson et al 2008).

FAMILY STRESS

Among the most pronounced sources of stress in adult life are those related to family events. These include separation, divorce, death or illness of a family member, abuse or economic hardship. Early family life can have a cumulative effect across the adult life span. As we mentioned in Chapter 5, adults exposed to inter-parental violence, poor parent–child relationships or parental psychopathologies in childhood can experience serious negative impacts on health in their adult lives that become chronic conditions (Nicolaidis & Touhouliotis 2006; Roustit et al 2009). As adults, marital quality plays an important role in psychosocial functioning. Poor relationships can have a

negative influence on cardiovascular, endocrine, immune and neurosensory function, while positive relationships can provide a supportive context for dealing with stress or illness (Windsor et al 2009). This underlines the importance of social support in health and wellbeing. Close relationships, such as marriage, can moderate health, overcoming some of the negative aspects of earlier years (Windsor et al 2009).

> **Point to ponder**
> Family events such as separation, divorce, death or illness of a family member, abuse or economic hardship are among the most pronounced sources of stress in adult life.

For spouses with a good relationship, health and wellbeing tend to become similar over time, acting as a protective mechanism in controlling stress or external forces in their environment (Windsor et al 2009). Adults in marriage and de facto relationships tend to have fewer mental health issues and a lower rate of suicidal thoughts and behaviours than those who live their adult lives alone (Johnston et al 2009). This is related to the *interdependency*, rather than *dependency* of the relationship, wherein people are able to develop a sense of control or mastery over their environments (Windsor et al 2009).

STRESS IN THE WORKPLACE

Workplace stress is a serious problem in today's society, incurring a cost to industry and the health system, as well as the personal costs of distress. Because it affects adults at all stages of their working life, it is also becoming an increasing issue for nurses working in home, family and community settings. Job strain and stressful working conditions, can create multiple pressures for the individual, especially where they are worried about job security (Lander et al 2009). Studies have shown that job strain, and its consequent stress, is a risk factor for major depression, which is the most prevalent mental disorder in the working population (Wang et al 2009). Sources of job stress can include overwork or shiftwork as well as workplace relationships.

Shiftwork, especially with irregular work schedules, is a problem for many nurses, as well as other health professionals. The combination of excessive workloads and shiftwork can create conflict in the workplace that can have an effect on family life (Yildirim & Aycan 2008). Shiftwork has the additional disadvantage of compromising workers' lifestyle behaviours, by reducing access to good nutrition and opportunities for physical activity, and creating sleep disturbances, fatigue, digestive problems and stress-related illnesses (Bambra et al 2008; Zhao & Turner 2007). Shiftwork can also cause psychological and social desynchronisation, where the worker experiences disharmony, or is 'out of sync', within the body, as well as in external relationships (Bambra et al 2008).

Many contemporary workplace cultures have changed the nature of work and working conditions. In the interests of flexibility and productivity, changes include abnormal working hours, working from home and compressed work schedules, where a person can undertake their week's work in fewer, but longer days (Bambra et al 2008). Some of these conditions can cause or worsen states of health, especially where they conflict with family obligations or time pressures (Roxburgh 2006). Home-based work requires clear demarcation between the boundaries of work and family life, which works well for some people trying to balance the two, but can also cause stress if there is no respite from the combination of both.

Point to ponder
While stress at work or the threat of unemployment can affect the entire family emotionally, positive work experiences can enhance physical and psychological wellbeing.

High workloads and work stressors can place pressure on family relationships, especially where the worker comes home stressed or where (s)he receives little social support from a spouse or partner (Michel et al 2009; ten Brummelhuis et al 2008). Likewise, family conflicts can cause problems in the workplace by influencing organisational performance (Beauregard & Henry 2009). Workplace policies also affect home life. Some, but not all countries, have flexible workplace policies, where employers are obliged to continue a person's employment if they have experienced illness. Without workplace policies that provide income security, workers hesitate to take sick leave, even

in the face of severe illness or injury. This creates additional stress, especially with the threat that the worker may be dismissed without explanation or financial compensation (Lander et al 2009). Stress at work and the threat of unemployment can affect the entire family, emotionally, through spill-over from work to family life, as well as financially (Bambra et al 2008; Michel et al 2009; Roxburgh 2006; Yildirim & Aycan 2009). On the other hand, positive work experiences can have an additive effect on physical and psychological wellbeing, and help buffer the effects of personal stress. This can occur through role enrichment that flows from being satisfied with both the work role and family relationships (Bourne et al 2009).

Point to ponder
Workplace incivility such as bullying is becoming increasingly common in Australian and New Zealand workplaces due to casualisation, job insecurity, and work intensification due to staff shortages.

Some stressors in the workplace arise from interpersonal behaviours, such as bullying and intimidation. These are antisocial behaviours that reflect a power imbalance in the working relationships, where an employee may be victimised by co-workers or a supervisor. A broader construct for this type of effect is commonly referred to as *incivility*, which refers to unfairness or insensitivity of supervisors to employees (Cortina & Magley 2009). It constitutes behaviours that violate norms of interpersonal respect, workplace morality and a sense of community (Cortina & Magley 2009). Employees subjected to uncivil treatment in the workplace experience high levels of stress, cognitive distraction, lower job satisfaction, higher levels of sickness absence and reduced creativity (Cortina & Magley 2009; O'Donnell et al 2010). Incivility is increasing in many workplaces, partly because of casualisation and job insecurity, and as a reaction to the work intensification caused by staff shortages and/or employer competitiveness.

Uncivil behaviours such as bullying are often the result of multi-layered work systems where each layer of management tends to micro-manage the next level down, keeping tighter and tighter control over each person's work. Micro-managing leaves little room for creativity or lateral thinking.

Instead, the objective of the day's work becomes appeasement of the person above. This occurs in hospitals and health organisations, as well as in other workplaces. Bullying seems to occur more frequently in organisations with rigid hierarchical lines of responsibility, such as in the public service. In Australia, the public service has proliferated at all levels to where state, territory and Commonwealth government departments constitute many layers of bureaucrats working towards endless circles of reporting. Bullying is rife, and, in some cases, it has transformed into an insidious epidemic of 'mobbing' behaviour (Shallcross et al 2008).

Workplace mobbing is where several people in the workplace 'gang up' on someone, usually to try to bring about their expulsion or resignation. It can begin with gossip, innuendo and malicious accusations about a person, intended to discredit them or their work. Because this type of behaviour has created toxic work environments that threaten employees' mental health, mobbing is an important topic for workplace research (Shallcross et al 2008). The behaviour tends to move through five phases. First there is a conflict or critical incident, followed by a campaign of psychological abuse. The next phase involves reporting negative comments to the person's manager with the objective of further isolating her/him from the work group. As the target person, usually a relatively weak female employee, reacts, they are accused of being difficult or even mentally ill. The fifth phase culminates in the employee's resignation, as (s)he finds the workplace unbearable.

Point to ponder

Occupational health nurses have a key role to play in reframing a toxic workplace culture into one that embraces equity, diversity and tolerance.

One of the relevant issues uncovered in the research on mobbing is related to diversity and gender roles in the workplace. In workplaces with high levels of diversity and gender balance, mobbing is less likely (Shallcross et al 2008). However, where there is high occupational segregation with gender and ethnic power imbalances, conformity rules. This has been identified as part of the problem in Australian public sector workplaces. Australia ranks highest among all OECD countries for occupational segregation, where males and females tend to work in different sectors (Shallcross et al 2008). Women are frequently in the lower paid ranks of education, health, social welfare, and more often than males, are casual staff, especially in those sectors experiencing downsizing. Women are therefore easier targets for bullying and mobbing, scapegoating and manipulating, especially if they are seen to be different from the norm, or if they try to assume masculine management behaviours. The issue is not always gender based, as women managers can also be perpetrators as well as victims. But it is an important part of workplace culture, and therefore workplace health.

Reframing a toxic workplace culture into one where equity, diversity and tolerance are pre-eminent is a challenge for occupational health nurses. At the primary level, the objective is to identify, reduce or eliminate the causes of stress in the working environment. Secondary interventions involve teaching employees coping strategies, and where necessary, tertiary interventions include psychological therapy and guidance (Bamber & McMahon 2008). Another aspect of the role is networking with other community-based nurses to provide continuity of care for the family, and referral to community resources and support. All of these roles merge into a common need for nursing advocacy, for workers, their families and a socially cohesive community.

OTHER WORKPLACE HEALTH AND SAFETY ISSUES

Because 80% of the adult population is employed, health and safety in the workplace is a major risk to adult health (AIHW 2008). Illness and injury at work has the potential for long-term disability, which can affect not only the worker, but his/her family and community. Workplace events also cause losses in worker productivity which, in cases where a worker does not have job security, can exacerbate socio-economic disadvantage. Accidents and injuries also incur costs to businesses and the health care system. Workplace accidents are highly variable, depending on the type of work and the workplace culture, particularly in terms of safety and support. Most are sprains and strains of joints and muscles, primarily back and hand injuries. Musculoskeletal injuries are the most common work-related injuries, with around 20% affecting

BOX 8.1 VITAL@WORK

One of the main sources of workplace stress is related to age. With the baby boomers on the verge of retirement many employers are trying to persuade as many as possible to remain in the workplace. This will help sustain an economically viable workforce who will be able to support younger workers across a range of industries. Although some workers prefer to retire early, others feel that while they enjoy good health during their 50s and 60s, they would like to remain a viable part of the workforce. However, many who work after age 55 often find the physical and mental demands more stressful than when they were younger. Employers concerned about the drain on resources from large numbers of retirees are actively seeking to renew older workers' quality of work life through a range of programs to help them remain working. One such program, called the 'Vital@Work' project, was developed as a research program to test the effects of workplace health and wellbeing programs on worker vitality (Strijk et al 2009). These Dutch researchers are investigating whether, over time, interventions aimed at enhancing older workers' vitality will prolong their employment. The group characterise vitality as having 'high levels of energy, feeling strong and fit, mental resilience while working, willingness to invest effort in their work, and persistence in the face of difficulties' (Strijk et al 2009:412). Their program consists of yoga for relaxation at work, as well as strength training, aerobic exercises and fresh, healthy foods available in the workplace. The program is currently being evaluated in a randomised clinical trial, with results expected in 2011. It is highly likely to provide a model for employers in other countries who are interested in the mix of factors that would lead to greater worker satisfaction, better health and wellbeing, and longer workforce participation.

BOX 8.2 ACC

New Zealand's Accident Compensation Corporation (ACC) provides comprehensive no-fault personal injury cover for all New Zealanders including for accidents that occur at work. In Australia, each state has an agency that provides a similar service. In 2009, a new statutory body called Safe Work Australia was created to compare performance and worker's compensation outcomes across states. The ACC and various state programs also provide comprehensive injury prevention programs to support employers to prevent workplace injuries, and help return injured employees back to work as soon as possible.

Other factors affecting health and safety in the workplace include the type of work undertaken, the pressures placed on the workers to meet productivity targets and exposure to hazardous substances or safety risks. Productivity pressures can cause biologic, physical or psychosocial risks or a combination of these. For this reason, primary prevention activities include a hazard or risk assessment in the workplace. This begins with an ergonomic assessment of the workplace and the working conditions. Ergonomic assessment involves examining the engineering aspects of the relationship between the worker and her/his work environment. Ergonomic hazards are those that induce fatigue, boredom, glare, or tasks that must be conducted in an abnormal position. Examples include work that causes vibration, repetitive motion, poor workstation–worker fit and lifting heavy loads. Biologic hazards can include exposure to bacteria, moulds, insects, viruses or infectious co-workers. Chemical hazards can include exposure to dangerous liquids, gases, dust, vapour or fumes. Examples of physical hazards are extremes of temperature, noise, radiation, poor lighting or exposure to unprotected machinery.

Stressful working conditions

Psychosocial hazards are those that produce an inordinate amount of stress. As a response to the competitiveness of global markets, downsizing, rightsizing and streamlining work processes have become the norm. Performance-based human resource policies and management structures have increased job demands, task reorganisation, restructuring of work teams and work intensification, all

long-term health (AIHW 2008). Another prevalent work-related injury is hearing loss, caused by excessive noise in the workplace. In some cases, workplace injuries are linked to individual worker characteristics as well as the work environment, including the worker's commitment to health and safety. For example, the consumption of alcohol or illicit substances, either during or before work, can interfere with jobs that require the operation of machinery or intense concentration.

of which create pressures on the family as well as the worker (Beauregard & Henry 2009; Crouter & Helms-Erikson 2000; Dragano et al 2005; Fujishiro & Heaney 2009). These demands are not always accompanied by supportive co-workers or managers, which can erode workers' respect and dignity as well as other indicators of psychosocial health (Lawson et al 2009). The problems become worse for casual employees or those without long-term contracts, as well as for those with the added stress of family responsibilities.

In addition, many workers are at the mercy of electronic intrusion into their work life from email, text messaging and other instant communications media that creates a further layer of stress, and precludes any respite from the job. This has become a major source of stress, especially when responses to messages are expected even after the formal day's work. Home-based access, which for many, was established to make work more efficient, has severely compromised work–life harmony, extending workers' connection to their workplace beyond most people's expectations. Unlike other countries, there is no cap on working hours in Australia, and workers now work an average of 70 minutes unpaid overtime per day, which is among the longest working hours in the Western world (The Australia Institute 2009). In New Zealand, three out of 10 full-time workers work 50 or more hours per week, again, very high by international standards (Families Commission 2009).

> ### Point to ponder
> Stressful working conditions can have a profound impact on workers' health. Technology has increased workplace stress, decreasing the ability of workers to achieve work–life harmony.

One of the most stressful workplaces is the health care workplace, in which workers have to contend with the stresses common to other workplaces, as well as violence from patients, and exposure to allergens and infectious agents. All of these risks can be life threatening. They require workplace vigilance, and often, rapid responses, which is even more dangerous in the face of staffing shortages (Bamber & McMahon 2008; Yassi et al 2005). Ylipaavalniemi et al's (2005) Finnish study of health care personnel, 50% of whom

were nurses, investigated workplace factors that predicted clinical depression among staff. The strongest predictor was found to be poor team climate, where work objectives were unclear, unattainable, not shared or visionary, and where workers were not involved in decision-making. These characteristics created a major hazard for workers, which was worsened by unfair and impolite supervisor behaviours. This type of stressful environment pervades hospital environments throughout the world and it has implications for patient care. Overwork, work intensification and stress can interfere with surveillance and monitoring of patient condition, early detection of adverse events and measures that would prevent complications (West et al 2009).

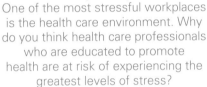

> ### What's your opinion?
> One of the most stressful workplaces is the health care environment. Why do you think health care professionals who are educated to promote health are at risk of experiencing the greatest levels of stress?

One effort designed to address the impact of poor working environments on patient care is the Magnet Recognition Program. This American initiative is designed to recognise health care organisations that provide excellence in nursing care. Characteristics of a Magnet hospital include nurse participation in hospital affairs, nursing foundations for care, nursing management ability, support and leadership, adequate staff and resources, and collaborative nurse–doctor relationships (Armstrong et al 2009). Hospitals achieving Magnet hospital recognition clearly demonstrate better patient outcomes than non-Magnet hospitals (Aiken et al 2009), and a number of Australasian hospitals have sought and achieved Magnet recognition including Hutt Hospital in New Zealand and Princess Alexandra Hospital in Queensland.

The WHO has done significant work in supporting the development of healthy workplaces, developing a set of criteria for a healthy workplace (see Box 8.3). The imperative to address the health needs of workers was reinforced at the World Health Assembly in 2007. The Assembly endorsed the WHO Global Plan of Action on Workers' Health 2008–2017 (WHO 2007), which emphasises the need to address all aspects of workers' health, including health promotion at work, protection of workers' health and primary prevention of occupational hazards.

ENVIRONMENTAL FACTORS AFFECTING ADULT HEALTH

Among the most important factors affecting adults' health are the necessities of clean air, water and food. These remain issues of major concern in the 21st century, where there is renewed concern about the natural environment, particularly land and water quality, and climate change (AIHW 2008). The previous century revealed harmful effects of overpopulation, and new knowledge of environmental threats to health. These include microbial contamination of food and water, especially in drought conditions, diseases transmitted by insects such as mosquitoes, respiratory and cardiac diseases from air pollution and workplace chemicals, other chemically induced conditions, and damage from noise and heat (AIHW 2008). High levels of water pollution in many areas have increased the prevalence of food-borne infections. Air pollution has also increased from larger motor vehicle usage, mining, energy production and agriculture and bushfires. Indoor pollution continues to affect health from cooking, heating and tobacco smoking (AIHW 2008). Most members of the general public are aware of the need to monitor levels of ozone in the environment, which is a major problem for cities like Sydney and Melbourne, which exceed the maximum safe levels of ozone (AIHW 2008). The significant depletion of ozone in Australia and New Zealand is linked to the fact that they have the highest rates of melanoma in the world, with sun exposure in childhood

and adolescence, also key contributors to its development (Garbe & Leiter 2009).

Point to ponder

Although the health impacts of climate change are not pre-destined, health professionals must work with communities to preserve current environments in order to safeguard the future.

Besides the depletion of stratospheric ozone, other environmental changes that affect human health are deforestation, land degradation, loss and damage to wetlands, loss of biodiversity, depletion and contamination of fresh water and urbanisation (AIHW 2008). The environmental issue attracting most attention globally, as well as in Australia and New Zealand, is climate change. Since 1910, the annual average temperature in Australia has risen about 0.9 degrees Celsius. The effect of this global warming is that it has altered wind patterns, sea levels, and the frequency and/or intensity of extreme weather events, such as heatwaves, droughts, floods and tropical storms (AIHW 2008). These effects have the potential to reduce food production through crop, livestock and fisheries yields, and increase pollutants into the air, including infectious agents. Heat stress has also caused illness and injuries from floods, storms, cyclones and bushfires, with some events, particularly bushfires, causing deaths (AIHW 2008).

Global warming displaces people, causing poverty through loss of their livelihood, malnutrition or diseases. It places pressure on global migration, especially among people from countries that are ravaged by weather events or where their own environment has already been damaged beyond sustainable levels (AIHW 2008). This is a problem for some 200 million international migrants, who all live in unhealthy environments for varying periods of time (WHO 2008). Climate change is therefore a cause for concern for all health professionals advocating for communities. The health impacts of climate change are not pre-destined; in fact, there are many outcomes that are as yet speculative. What is known, however, is that there is an urgent and unconditional need to work towards preservation of current environments to safeguard the future. Together with reduction in unhealthy and unsafe behaviours, sustainable environments will ensure the next generations have at least the potential to achieve the state of health to which they aspire.

The ecology of adult health also includes attention to new biotechnologies that are changing patterns of risk and potential. Since the Human Genome Project (HGP), there has been a clearer understanding of the influence of genetic factors on health, which is helping to inform some people's treatment decisions. Stem cell research has reached the stage where in future, an individual's genes will be transformed for therapeutic advantage in treating certain long-term disease states, such as Parkinson's disease.

Point to ponder

Biotechnology will have an increasing role to play in future health outcomes, as more work is done to understand the impact of genetic factors on health.

As knowledge provides greater clarity on how nature and nurture interact at the cellular level, families and communities will have many decisions to make about their ecosystems and exposures, the risk/reward ratios of different activities and even whether and when to alter their genetic makeup (Fielding et al 2000). Some of these developments have been rapid, challenging people's level of health literacy. A major role for nurses will therefore involve staying well informed to keep abreast of the new developments so that they can make informed choices. As Omenn (2000:10) suggests, wise choices for future generations will depend on 'excellent science, compassionate values, effective communication, appreciation of diverse cultures and preferences, openness to new knowledge and alternative views, commitment to disease prevention and health promotion'. The first challenge lies in reframing goals for health within both visionary perspectives and creative approaches to identifying and defending scientific evidence as a basis for community health research.

HEALTHY ADULTHOOD

The best approach for adult health is community participation in all matters concerning health and wellbeing, irrespective of whether the objective is to overcome risks or enhance the quality of people's lives. The most pertinent issues in

planning for healthy adulthood are social: to overcome inequity and inequality. The focus of today's health promotion agenda for adults should be to reduce risk, to improve the quality of work and family life, to prevent and better manage chronic diseases, including mental health, and to respond capably to current and future threats including both infectious diseases and threats to the environment. To address these issues requires public awareness of the seriousness of each, and dissemination of accurate information that will be both instructive and supportive. The focus should remain on communities in creating and maintaining health to decrease the incidence of chronic diseases, develop safer workplaces, living spaces and societies, and provide greater opportunities for people to achieve better physical, mental, spiritual, environmental and culturally sensitive health.

Goals for adult health

The major goals for adult health include:

- ensuring an appropriate balance between comprehensive and selective primary health care (PHC), particularly in addressing chronic conditions for disadvantaged populations
- providing political support for health in all policies
- integrating primary, secondary and tertiary intervention for adult health in the workplace and community
- adopting a life course approach for the prevention of chronic conditions
- promoting an ecological risk reduction approach by focusing on the environments for good health
- using intersectoral collaboration to address health issues
- ensuring cultural sensitivity in all interactions
- designing health promotion strategies that are empowering, with people and families as partners at the centre of care
- using health resources efficiently and effectively, eliminating boundaries between professionals
- using the Ottawa Charter as a guideline for health promotion.

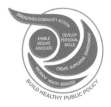

BUILDING HEALTHY PUBLIC POLICY

Public policies to support adult health should be comprehensive, and aimed at addressing the social conditions and structures that either enhance or prevent environments and conditions that are optimal for health and wellbeing. This is based on the understanding that healthy environments will promote opportunities for community engagement, health literacy and capacity development. It is also a more holistic approach to policy development than policies for individual risk factors or health issues. A multidimensional, comprehensive approach to policy development has a greater chance at being effective at the population level than single agencies working from single government departments on single issues. In 2009, the Australian National Preventative Health Taskforce made a series of policy recommendations to promote healthier lifestyles (Kirby 2009). These included increasing taxes on cigarettes and alcohol, and eliminating advertising for both. Another recommendation was for eliminating media promotion of unhealthy food, especially during children's viewing hours, and new pricing strategies to promote healthy eating. These policy recommendations are congruent with similar policy developments being initiated in other countries concerned about obesity and chronic conditions that begin in childhood (Aranceta et al 2009). Like all health promotion policies, they are also intended to be inclusive, with full community participation. In New Zealand calls are being made to address obesity issues in the same way that smoking has been addressed — with a multi-pronged approach to prevention, including public policy changes, taxation, and creating environments that support people to make healthy food choices (Pearson 2009).

Besides comprehensive, population-level policies, some public policies target health and wellbeing in specific settings. For example, occupational health and safety policies in Australia and New Zealand are aimed at the working population. These policies are governed by national agencies such as Safe Work Australia (Online. Available: www.australia.gov.au/topics/health-and-safety/occupational-health-and-safety [accessed 24 November 2009]) and the New Zealand Workplace Health and Safety Council (NZ Department of Labour 2007). The national organisations coordinate government legislation, standards, policies and practices, and provide information for workers and their representatives, including the trade unions. One of the historical problems with occupational health and safety policies is that they have tended to have a singular biomedical focus rather than linking workplace health and safety to the social determinants of workers' health and lifestyle balance. This reflects a wider problem in policy development in Australia and New Zealand, where health promotion has focused on the quick fix of behavioural change and individual persuasion, rather than the SDOH (Bauman et al 2007).

ACTION POINT
Nurses have a key role in advocating for inclusion of the SDOH in all policies.

Nurses have a role to play in ensuring that the SDOH are included in all policies, especially those that inform occupational health and safety. They also play an important role in advocating for workers to become empowered to provide feedback to agencies, either individually or through worker advocates, such as the unions. Policies that reflect understanding of the SDOH are those that provide income security and appropriate wages, housing for those with disabilities, employment, adequate provision for carers, and cross-cultural and gender considerations in helping people cope with their life situations (Raphael 2009). A further challenge in today's work environment is to ensure the sustainability of the workforce, by long-term planning for workers once the baby boomer generation retires. This is a major issue for the health workforce, with existing shortages of health professionals (Forbes & While 2009).

Mental health policy development is another area that has attracted considerable attention in Australia, which has one of the highest rates of suicide in the world. The national framework presented in Chapter 7 'Life: A framework for preventing suicide and other self harm in Australia' (Commonwealth of Australia 2009), and the National Mental Health Strategy, provide examples of bipartisan collaboration in addressing a problem of national significance (Parham 2007). These policies, like the chronic illness initiatives, have a PHC focus. They target general practice, the media, schools, workplaces, community groups and organisations to gather intersectoral collaboration that will cut across population groups and areas of influence.

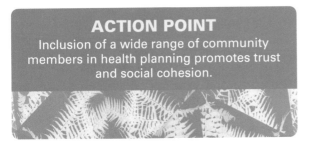

Nurses working in the community play an important role in informing policy development, particularly practice nurses (PNs), and those working in home care settings. Because they have knowledge from the operational level, their voices should be heard at the policy table. These groups can lobby policy–makers to shift the overall focus to population-wide initiatives for better health, rather than simply targeting individual behaviours that could risk blaming the victims of illness (Bauman et al 2007). Mental health policy remains a classic example of where too much segregated planning has failed to place the person and their community at the centre. If mental health policies were integrated with policies for physical health, there would be a better chance of ensuring that interventions and the evidence base that informs these are cognisant of the lived experience of people (Bryant et al 2007). However, some conditions will need selective attention and policies to support the allocation of resources to support interventions. For example, those with psychiatric conditions trying to live as part of the wider community will sometimes require acute crisis intervention. Unless mental health advocates lobby for protective resources such as medical emergency teams to attend to their needs, their care may be absorbed into inappropriate models of care.

CREATING SUPPORTIVE ENVIRONMENTS

Supportive environments are those that promote equitable access to resources at the local level, where people live, work and play. They are also sustainable across the life course and across generations. To sustain community life, as well as personal health and wellbeing, children and their families need access to safe spaces for family life, adequate education and opportunities for community engagement. Safe, vibrant, inclusive spaces for living, working and playing require multisectoral, inter-agency partnerships and collaboration with the focus on community residents (WHO 2009). Supportive environments are also designed to help the most vulnerable in the community access better working conditions and supports for healthy living. Support for the adult population also involves health and safety programs focused on creating a healthy work environment. They also include providing individual and group support for personal crises or mental health needs, whether these needs become evident at work or in the neighbourhood (WHO 2009).

> **Point to ponder**
> Increased urbanisation has led to decreased levels of exercise. There is a growing need for urban planners and health providers to work together to create environments that encourage people to gain the exercise they need for health.
> For a number of interesting readings on urban planning and health, see: www.phac.health.govt.nz/moh.nsf/pagescm/7558/$File/rethinking-urban-environments.pdf.

Working towards sustaining the community also brings a set of personal values to the community. These enrich the community–health professional partnership with respect, support and mutual caring (Hill 2009). Helping the community sustain what is valued recognises the need for integration of personal, social, spiritual and ecological issues within a social ecological approach (Hill 2009). At the centre of all issues is a commitment to preserving and celebrating community strengths. The social–ecological approach also includes recognition of the individuals who are at the vanguard of community life; the volunteers and informal caregivers. These are the individuals who make a difference to the quality of life of those most in need. As carers, they need ongoing encouragement and support from others, and a healthy environment within which they can undertake their important roles.

Many carers are also living in economically disadvantaged situations, with no chance of improving their circumstances because of their caring responsibilities (AIHW 2009; Fremstad 2009). Like those they care for, they often have reduced earnings, no opportunity for self-improvement through education and no income security. As with many other groups in the community, carers can become socially isolated. This is a particular problem for those without access to transportation (WHO 2009). Rearranging environmental conditions may involve collaboration with community planning agencies, or working with local government or community agencies to bring these people together. Inclusive approaches to planning bring members of different ethnic groups or migrant groups together with long-term residents. This type of connectedness promotes trust, norms of reciprocity and social cohesion, all of which contribute to social capital as well as culturally competent care (Peckover & Chidlaw 2007).

A major focus for environmental planning concerns the obesogenic environments that are problematic in most cities. School and workplace lifestyle supports can help counter the effect of unhealthy environments by restricting the type of food available at school, and worksite interventions can include strength training, exercise programs and health education (Aranceta et al 2009). Population-based approaches to dealing with obesity should be aimed at making healthy choices easy and accessible. Research indicates that parks and green spaces in the city help promote social contacts (Cattell et al 2009; Maas et al 2009). However, city planners are not always aware of the health benefits or liabilities in the way they approach plans or modifications. This leaves an important advocacy role for health professionals working closely with community members. Environmental supports also extend to community based programs, or modifications to the built environment to keep adults active. Public transportation encourages walking rather than taking the car. Providing friendly, open stairs in public places can encourage people to take the stairs rather than the lift, as can better lighting in public places (NRHA 2009a).

STRENGTHENING COMMUNITY ACTION

Community action is necessary to support people in working towards community sustainability.

This can be guided by the strengths, weaknesses, opportunities and threats (SWOT) analysis we introduced in Chapter 3 to assess community strengths and weaknesses. It begins with helping members of the community assess environmental assets such as infrastructure for health, education, transportation and community facilities. Next, it involves identifying which community leaders will help with the planning and engagement of others, then analysing the potential in terms of cultural, social and economic features of the community (NRHA 2009d). This type of foundation for planning can be invaluable to strengthening community action. As the 'guide on the side', nurses need to acquire local knowledge of the community, as well as awareness of current research, including knowledge of effective action and intervention strategies generated by other disciplines. This information can then be translated into plans that will suit the local context. Plans for community action should also be based on current awareness of what is being disseminated in the media, to clarify any public misperceptions or expectations. This helps strengthen health literacy, particularly critical health literacy.

> **ACTION POINT**
> Use the community assessment process outlined in Chapter 3 to guide plans for community action.

Some members of the community may need help to understand the politics of health. Because urbanisation and technology have created an overwhelming amount of information for the average family to sift through, translating research findings to the community can help promote discretion and fully informed choice. At the community level, for example, it makes no sense to teach people about the need for good dietary practices, and then have them confronted with blatant commercial messages urging them to eat kilojoule-dense, low-nutrient foodstuffs. To be empowered to take action, it is important that they understand both the products being advertised, and the powerful vested interests that shape their lives (Choi et al 2005). They also need to know the practicalities of nutrition, where to access healthy foods that are affordable, and what lifestyle supports may be available through the local council. Providing accurate and appropriate information will help ensure a level of authenticity of information that extends beyond the 'bytes' offered to them in the popular media.

Many people are also unaware of the policies that govern the health care system and how to access appropriate services. This may be particularly important for the large number of people who live alone at all stages of adult life. They may not have opportunities to engage with others or they may be hesitant to seek advice, yet they need to know the potential impact of current government debates on various health initiatives, treatments and pharmaceuticals, and how these affect their health and treatments. Members of the public also need to understand the impact of political lobby groups who may be more inclined to encourage spending health funds on new hospitals and monopoly services, rather than on programs for families, or continuing care for those with illnesses or disabilities. This type of information can promote the type of citizen engagement that leads to community action. It can also help assure quality interventions from appropriate health professionals, such as PNs or nurse practitioners. When members of the community are drawn into health care service discussions and planning, there is a greater chance of achieving the PHC goals of appropriate technologies and community empowerment.

DEVELOPING PERSONAL SKILLS

Providing support for people to improve their health literacy is one of the most important ways nurses can help them develop personal capacity. Some community residents may have moderate levels of health literacy, but generally, low levels of health literacy are found among those who have migrated from non-English-speaking countries, and those with advanced age, lower educational attainment, poorer health and less social participation (Barber et al 2009). Homeless people also have a need to develop sufficient health literacy to survive, and to navigate informal, as well as formal systems, that can help them cope with chronic illness, injuries and mental illness. The role of nurses in supporting them includes being sensitive to the shame, embarrassment and discrimination they experience when they attempt to secure care and support (Fetter 2009). This is also a problem for other hard-to-reach groups. Despite the barriers

to bringing disenfranchised people such as the homeless into care, neighbourhood-based nursing activities have been found to be effective by providing primary care and social support (Poulton et al 2006).

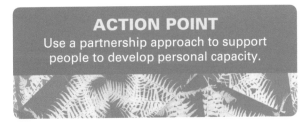

ACTION POINT
Use a partnership approach to support people to develop personal capacity.

For those who have been stigmatised by being poor, or discriminated against on the basis of being from a visible ethnic minority, the sensitivity of health professionals can be the most important step towards personal capacity building (Maclean et al 2009). This is also an issue for those suffering from family violence, which is not always considered a chronic condition. In reality, many women suffer a plethora of impacts from living in a chronically violent household, or having done so in the past. Supporting them in the community includes breaking down organisational barriers to care, and helping them, and the community, develop a level of understanding about family violence issues (Nicolaidis & Touhouliotis 2006).

Helping people develop personal capacity is a central goal of PNs and others working with adults who attend general practice or community clinics. A partnership approach works well with people seeking lifestyle changes, and this begins with an exploration of their personal health goals. Assessing their preferences allows a program to be customised to their needs. It also acknowledges their need for autonomy in working towards health improvements, or maintenance of ongoing conditions. When their needs for autonomy and relatedness are incorporated into health promotion initiatives they will be more likely to engage in positive health behaviours, such as increasing activity patterns or improving their diets (Lauver et al 2008). Tailoring the health education components to their individual preferences can also help ensure the appropriateness of the mode of delivery of health messages. Studies have found that adults tend to prefer the face-to-face approach for advice, despite the fact that they could access information on the internet. People report that the individual approach helps foster trust and a closer therapeutic partnership (Lauver et al 2008). There are a number of models that can guide nurses in their work with adults to develop personal skills, including the Flinders Model and the Chronic Disease Self-Management Program (CDSMP), both of which were discussed in Chapter 4.

REORIENTING HEALTH SERVICES

The quality of a health care system can be judged on how well or how badly its services address inequalities, how they respond to people's expectations and to what extent dignity, personal rights and freedoms are respected (WHO 2000b). There has been a worldwide shift in health services from episodic care to chronic disease management and this is entrenched in national initiatives such as the PHC strategies of the Australian and New Zealand governments. The PHC approach is responsive to the community, particularly in the role encompassed by PNs and those working in home and family care (Haddad 2009). To date, many health services have been organised on the basis of a separation of the needs of those with chronic physical illnesses, and those with mental health problems such as depression. These conditions are now co-morbid in many people, indicating the need for better integration of services and better continuity of care. Family caregivers in particular, find service discontinuities challenging.

Nurses' interventions in helping people with chronic conditions are increasingly complex. Nurses working in the community tend to approach managing care for those with chronic conditions on two levels: horizontally and vertically. Horizontal care accommodates people's needs between systems and settings, to ensure continuity of care. Vertical care management involves preventative care, self-care support and education. This includes identification of problems, managing care across the continuum of different therapies, and establishing ongoing support and rehabilitation, which can involve case management in complex cases for people with multiple needs (Forbes & While 2009). This model of care is integrated and collaborative. It represents a multidimensional approach that has been used across many settings. For example, the combination of education, collaborative problem-solving and instruction in coping has been found to be effective in helping community residents coping with cancer (van der Feltz-Cornelis 2009) and type 2 diabetes (Atak et al

2008–09). In the workplace, integrated programs that include exercise, stress management training, health information and workplace assessment have also shown improvements in health, physical fitness, and management of pain, stress and the work situation (Tveito & Erikson 2008). Community mental health nurses working in collaboration with other specialists have also been effective in helping those living with mental illness cope with their needs (Elsom et al 2009).

Many of these nursing roles have adopted a

> **ACTION POINT**
> An integrated and collaborative approach to care allows nurses to manage complex cases and support people with multiple needs more effectively.

comprehensive, primary, secondary and tertiary approach to health promotion. For example, occupational health nurses balance individual and population-based strategies for healthier workplaces. This begins with assessment and surveillance of the work environment, often in collaboration with the safety officer. At the primary level, occupational issues and problems are assessed and triaged, identifying strengths, weaknesses, opportunities and threats. This is called a hazard audit. Primary prevention for reducing stress includes attention to ergonomics, work and environmental design, and organisational and management development. At the secondary level, the nurse can help identify appropriate interventions for modifying the environment to support worker health and safety. To counter employee stress, secondary prevention can involve worker re-education and training as well as guidance on coping strategies (WHO 2003).

> **ACTION POINT**
> Assessment of workplace risk is one of the more important roles of a nurse working with adults. Take an approach that considers primary, secondary and tertiary prevention strategies.

Extensive liaison with others is the key to tertiary level activities. These can be aimed at reducing the impact of stress through more sensitive and responsive management and occupational health and safety programs (WHO 2003). Tertiary interventions can also include collaboration with general practitioners, PNs, nurses working in family and community roles, and other rehabilitation personnel involved in planning. A major part of tertiary interventions is liaison with management to ensure successful implementation of programs, and ongoing evaluation of effectiveness.

Health professionals have always been challenged by the need to help individuals develop strategies to foster better personal health and well-being. In our market-driven economies, weight loss, for example, has become a major growth industry and it has become the norm for people to outlay large sums of money to be urged to lose weight and take up physical activity. This has created a decline in health education services offered by governments and community agencies. It would seem fairer to society if members of the public were offered supports for living healthy lives. This could include public health assistance for trying to achieve health and fitness, rather than punitive initiatives to cast blame. This type of approach represents a de-commodification of health, which places community needs at the heart of the community, instead of at the centre of the health services bureaucracy (Raphael 2009).

Case study

Jim, who is part of the marketing department of an investment company, is concerned about the impact of the global financial crisis on his employment. This has affected some of his co-workers who, like him, work on commission instead of a predictable salary. The investment company has suffered from some bad publicity in the media about financial planners and the fact that they have been unregulated until recently.

Jim has not been sleeping well. He suffers from chest pain and reflux. After having the chest pain checked out, and providing reassurance that his heart was strong, his GP sent him to the practice nurse for assessments of his cholesterol and blood lipids. The lab tests revealed that he does, in fact, have elevated LDL cholesterol. The nurse reported back to the GP who prescribed statins for Jim. The nurse then made an appointment for him to come in for lifestyle counselling. In preparation for this appointment, she prepared an outline of a diet and activity plan, and asked Jim for permission to contact the occupational health nurse employed by his company. The occupational health nurse saw Jim in her office, and enrolled him in a stress management program that she conducts onsite weekly. Jim has agreed to attend. He has also given permission for the two nurses to liaise with one another and his GP.

REFLECTING ON THE BIG ISSUES

- Adult health is socially determined and needs to be seen in the context of a person's life course development.
- Adult health can be compromised by unhealthy behaviours.
- The physical environment has a major influence on health behaviours, suggesting an important relationship between health and place.
- The major burden of disease in the 21st century comes from lifestyle factors such as poor nutrition, inactivity and stress.
- Chronic physical conditions are often co-morbid with chronic mental health problems.
- Equity is a major factor in adult health, with chronic illnesses experienced more intensely by those who are disadvantaged.
- As most adults spend the majority of their time in the workplace, the health of both worker and workplace is a major focus for intervention.
- The work–home life nexus can create major stress, especially for women trying to lead a balanced life.
- Workplace relationships can be a source of psychological ill health.

Reflective questions: how would I use this knowledge in practice?

1 What would be the most important priorities for Jim's health and wellbeing? What would you include in a health care plan for him and the family?

2 What information would you need to conduct a comprehensive workplace health assessment of a 50-year-old administrative officer with clinical depression?

3 Identify five important issues that must be addressed in a program to encourage positive mental health among 40–50-year-olds with a family history of cardiovascular disease?

4 Design a set of strategies for guiding someone who has been victimised by workplace bullying.

5 What components would you include in a health literacy project designed to help empower residents of a migrant community?

6 In the research on balancing family and home responsibilities, no mention is made of the triple responsibility of work–study–home balance. What research does this suggest to you? How would you go about such a study? What variables do you think should be included?

7 How do you think nursing education programs can help prevent incivility in the health workplace?

Research-informed practice

Read the article by Forbes and While (2009) 'The nursing contribution to chronic disease management: a discussion paper'.

- Using their idea of the horizontal and vertical integration of care planning, how would you go about developing a research program to ensure that chronic conditions were managed on the basis of evidence for practice?
- What variables would you need to measure? For which groups of people?
- How would you accommodate varying environmental conditions? Social situations?

References

Aiken L, Havens D, Sloane D 2009 The Magnet Nursing Services Recognition Program: a comparison of two groups of Magnet hospitals. Journal of Nursing Administration 39 Supp (7):S5–S14

Aranceta J, Moreno B, Moya M, Anadon A 2009 Prevention of overweight and obesity from a public health perspective. Nutrition Reviews 67 Supp (1):S83–S88

Armstrong K, Laschinger H, Wong C 2009 Workplace empowerment and magnet hospital characteristics as predictors of patient safety climate. Journal of Nursing Care Quality 24(1):55–62

Atak N, Gurkan T, Kose K 2008–09 The effect of education on knowledge, self-management behaviours and self efficacy of patients with type 2 diabetes. Australian Journal of Advanced Nursing 26(2):66–74

Australian Institute of Health and Welfare (AIHW) 2008 Australia's Health 2008. Cat. No. AUS 99, AIHW, Canberra

—— 2009 Australia's Welfare Online. Available www.aihw.gov.au (accessed 20 November 2009)

Bamber M, McMahon R 2008 Danger—early maladaptive schemas at work!: the role of early maladaptive schemas in career choice and the development of occupational stress in health workers. Clinical Psychology and Psychotherapy 15:96–112

Bambra C, Whitehead M, Sowden A, Akers J, Petticrew M 2008 'A hard day's night?' The effects of compressed working week interventions on the health and work–life balance of shift workers: a systematic review. Journal of Epidemiology Community Health 62:764–77

Barber M, Staples M, Osborne R, Clerehan R, Elder C, Buchbinder R 2009 Up to a quarter of the Australian population may have suboptimal health literacy depending upon the measurement tool: results from a population-based survey. Health Promotion International 24(30):252–61

Bauman A, O'Hara L, Signal L, Smith B, Ritchie J, Parker E, Rissel C 2007 A perspective on changes in values in the profession of health promotion. Health Promotion Journal of Australia 18(1):3–6

Beauregard T, Henry L 2009 Making the link between work–life balance practices and organizational performance. Human Resource Management Review 19: 9–22

Bourne K, Wilson F, Lester S, Kickul J 2009 Embracing the whole individual: advantages of a dual-centric perspective of work and life. Business Horizons 52:387–98

Brown R, Bylund C, Kline N, De La Cruz A, Solan J, Kelvin J, Gueguen J, Eddington J, Kissane D, Passik S 2009 Identifying and responding to depression in adult cancer patients: evaluating the efficacy of a pilot communication skills training program for oncology nurses. Cancer Nursing 32(3):E1–7

Brown W, Hockey R, Dobson A 2008 Physical activity, body mass index and health care costs in mid-age Australian women. Australian and New Zealand Journal of Public Health 32(2):150–5

Bryant T, Raphael D, Travers R 2007 Identifying and strengthening the structural roots of urban health: participatory policy research and the urban health agenda. Promotion and Education 14(1):6–11

Bryson L, Warner-Smith P, Brown P, Fray L 2007 Managing the work–life roller-coaster: private stress or public health issue? Social Science & Medicine 65:1142–53

Burton N, Walsh A, Brown W 2008 It just doesn't speak to me: mid-aged men's reactions to '10 000 steps a day'. Health Promotion Journal of Australia 19(1):52–9

Campbell-Lendrum D, Bertollini R, Neira M, Ebi K, McMichael A 2009 Health and climate change: a roadmap for applied research. The Lancet 373:1663–5

Cardi M, Munk N, Zanjani F, Kruger T, Warner Schaie K, Willis S 2009 Health behavior risk factors across age as predictors of cardiovascular disease diagnosis. Journal of Aging and Health 21(5):759–75

Cattell V, Dines N, Gesler W, Curtis S 2009 Mingling, observing, and lingering: everyday public spaces and their implications for wellbeing and social relations. Health and Place 14:544–61

Chaturvedi N 2004 Commentary: socioeconomic status and diabetes outcomes; what might we expect and why don't we find it? International Journal of Epidemiology 33:871–3

Choi B, Hunter D, Tsou W, Sainsbury P 2005 Diseases of comfort: primary cause of death in the 22nd century. Journal of Epidemiology and Community Health 59:1030–4

Commission on the Social Determinants of Health (CSDH) 2008 Closing the Gap in a Generation. Health Equity Through Action on the Social Determinants of Health. Final report of the CSDH. WHO, Geneva

Commonwealth of Australia 2008 Living is for Everyone (LIFE): Research and evidence in suicide prevention. Online. Available: www.livingisforeveryone.com.au/Research-and-evidence-in-suicide-prevention.h (accessed 4 November 2009)

—— 2009 A healthier future for all Australians — final report of the National Health and Hospitals Reform Commission, Publications No. P3-5499 AGPS, Canberra

Cortina L, Magley V 2009 Patterns and profiles of response to incivility in the workplace. Journal of Occupational Health Psychology 14(30):272–88

Coveney J 2007 Food and trust in Australia: building a picture. Public Health Nutrition 11(3):237–45

Crouter A, Helms-Erikson H 2000 Work and family from a dyadic perspective: variations in inequality. In: Milardo R, Duck S (eds) Families as Relationships. John Wiley, Chichester, pp 99–115

Deambrosis P, Terrazzani G, Walley T, Bader G, Giusti P, Debetto P, Chinellato A 2009 Benefit of statins in daily practice? A six year retrospective observational study. Pharmacological Research 60:397–401

Donovan R, Henley N, Jalleh G, Silburn S, Zubrick S, Williams A 2007 People's beliefs about factors contributing to mental health: implications for mental health promotion. Health Promotion Journal of Australia 18(1):50–6

Dragano N, Verde P, Siegrist J 2005 Organisational downsizing and work stress: testing synergistic health effects in employed men and women. Journal of Epidemiology and Community Health 59:694–9

Elsom S, Happell B, Manias E 2009 Informal role expansion in Australian mental health nursing. Perspectives in Psychiatric Care 45(1):45–53

Families Commission 2009 Finding time: parents' long working hours and time impact on family life. Families Commission, Wellington, New Zealand. Online. Available: www.familiescommission.govt.nz/research/work-life-balance/finding-time (accessed 26 February 2010)

Feldman P, Warr D, Tacticos T, Kelaher M 2009 People, places and policies — trying to account for health inequalities in impoverished neighbourhoods. Australian and New Zealand Journal of Public Health 33(10):17–24

Fetter M 2009 Promoting health literacy with vulnerable behavioral health clients. Issues in Mental Health Nursing 30:798–802

Fielding J, Lave L, Starfield B 2000 Preface. Annual Review of Public Health 21:v–vi

Forbes A, While A 2009 The nursing contribution to chronic disease management: a discussion paper. International Journal of Nursing Studies 46:120–31

Fremstad S 2009 Half in Ten. Why taking disability into account is essential to reducing income poverty and expanding economic inclusion. Center for Economic and Policy Research, Online. Available: www.cepr.net (accessed 20 November 2009)

Fujishiro K, Heaney C 2009 Justice at work, job stress, and employee health. Health Education and Behavior 36(3):487–504

Garbe C, Leiter U 2009 Melanoma epidemiology and trends. Clinics in Dermatology 27:3–9

Gillison F, Skevington S, Sato A, Standage M, Evangelidou S 2009 The effects of exercise interventions on quality of life in clinical and healthy populations: a meta-analysis. Social Science & Medicine 68:1700–10

Grundy S, Cleeman J, Daniels S, Donato K, Eckel R, Franklin B, Gordon D, Krauss R, Savage P, Smith S, Spertus J, Costa F 2005 Diagnosis and management of the metabolic syndrome. Circulation 112:2735–52

Haddad M 2009 Depression in adults with a chronic physical health problem: Treatment and management. International Journal of Nursing Studies 46:1411–14

Hamilton M 2003 Drugs: a contested policy area. In: Liamputtong P, Gardner H (eds) Health, Social Change and Communities, Oxford Press, Melbourne pp 306–27

Hill S 2009 Social ecology as future stories: an Australian perspective. University of Western Sydney, Sydney

Johnston A, Pirkis J, Burgess P 2009 Suicidal thoughts and behaviours among Australian adults: findings from the 2007 National Survey of Mental Health and Wellbeing. Australian and New Zealand Journal of Psychiatry 43:635–43

Jones P 2008 Expert perspective: reducing cardiovascular risk in metabolic syndrome and type 2 diabetes mellitus beyond low-density lipoprotein cholesterol lowering. American Journal of Cardiology 102 Supp:41L–47L

Kirby T 2009 Australia considers string of preventive health measures. The Lancet 374:963

Kondo N, Sembajwe G, Kawachi I, van Dam R, Subramanian S, Yamagata Z 2009 Income inequality, mortality, and self rated health: meta-analysis of multilevel studies. British Medical Journal 330:b4471 doi.10.1136/bmj.b4471

Korber K 2008 Statin therapy works for patients who have type 2 diabetes. JAAPA 21(10):58 Online. Available: www.jaapa.com (accessed 26 September 2009)

Laforest L, Van Ganse E, Ritleng C, Desamericq G, Latrilliart L, Moreau A, Rosen S, Mechnin H, Chamba G 2009 Correlates of quality of life of pre-obese and obese patients: a pharmacy-based cross-sectional survey. BMC Public Health 9:337–48

Lander F, Friche C, Tornemand H, Anderson J, Kirkeskov L 2009 Can we enhance the ability to return to work among workers with stress-related disorders? BMC Public Health 9:372–378. Doi: 10.1186/1471-2458-9-372

Lauver D, Worawong C, Olsen C 2008 Health goals among primary care patients. Journal of the American Academy of Nurse Practitioners 20(3):144–54

Lawson K, Noblet A, Rodwell J 2009 Promoting employee wellbeing: the relevance of work characteristics and organizational justice. Health Promotion International 24(3):223–33

Lee D, Chiu M, Manuel D, Tu K, Wang X, Austin P, Mattern M, Mitiku T, Svenson L, Putnam W, Flanagan B, Tu J 2009 Trends in risk factors for cardiovascular disease in Canada: temporal, socio-demographic and geographic factors. Canadian Medical Association Journal 181(3–4):E55–E66

Maas J, van Dillen S, Verheij R, Groenewegen P 2009 Social contacts as a possible mechanism behind the relation between green space and health. Health and Place 15:586–95

Maclean L, Edwards N, Garrard M, Sims-Jones N, Clinton K, Ashley L 2009 Obesity, stigma and public health planning. Health Promotion International 24(1):88–93

Martinez-Gonzalez M, Bes-Rastrollo M, Serra-Majem L, Lairon D, Estruch R, Trichopoulou A 2009 Mediterranean food pattern and the primary prevention of chronic disease: recent developments. Nutrition Reviews 67 Supp (1):S111–S116

McDermott R 1998 Ethics, epidemiology, and the Thrifty Gene: Biological determinism as a health hazard. Social Science & Medicine 47(9):1189–95

Meyer I, Schwartz S, Frist D 2008 Social patterning of stress and coping: Does disadvantaged social status confer more stress and fewer coping resources? Social Science & Medicine 67:368–79

Michel J, Mitchelson J, Pichler S, Cullen K 2009 Clarifying relationships among work and family social support, stressors, and work–family conflict. Journal of Vocational Behavior doi:10.1016/j.jvb.2009.05.07

Morrissey R, Diamond G, Kaul S 2009 Statins in acute coronary syndromes. Journal of the American College of Cardiology 54(15):1425–33

Mudur G 2005 World needs fresh research priorities and new policies to tackle changing patterns of chronic disease. British Medical Journal 331:596

National Rural Health Alliance (NRHA) 2009a Obesity and Nutrition in Rural Australia. NRHA. Online. Available: www.nrha.org.au (accessed 8 November 2009)

—— 2009b Cancer in Rural Australia. NRHA. Online. Available: www.nrha.org.au (accessed 8 November 2009)

—— 2009c Suicide in Rural Australia. NRHA. Online. Available: www.nrha.org.au (accessed 8 November 2009)

—— 2009d Sustainable Small Communities. NRHA. Online. Available: www.nrha.org.au (accessed 8 November 2009)

New Zealand Department of Labour 2007 Workplace Health and Safety Council, Wellington

New Zealand Ministry of Health (NZMOH) 2007 Like minds, like mine national plan 2007–2013: Program to counter stigma and discrimination associated with mental illness. NZMOH, Wellington

—— 2008 A Portrait of Health. Key Results of the 2006–07 New Zealand Health Survey. NZMOH, Wellington

—— 2009a Report on New Zealand Cost-of-illness Studies on Long-term Conditions. NZMOH, Wellington

—— 2009b Mortality and Demographic Data 2006. Ministry of Health, Wellington

New Zealand Ministry of Health & Statistics New Zealand 2009 Longer life better health? Trends in Health Expectancy in New Zealand 1996–2006. Statistics New Zealand, Wellington

Nicolaidis C, Touhouliotis V 2006 Addressing intimate partner violence in primary care: lessons from chronic illness management. Violence and Victims 21(1):101–15

O'Donnell S, MacIntosh J, Wuest J 2010 A theoretical understanding of sickness absence among women who have experienced workplace bullying. Qualitative Health Research 20(40):439–52

Omenn G 2000 Public health genetics: an emerging interdisciplinary field for the post-genomic era. Annual Review of Public Health 21:1–13

Parham J 2007 Shifting mental health policy to embrace a positive view of health: a convergence of paradigms. Health Promotion Journal of Australia 18(30):173–6

Pearson J 6 December 2009 Fags and fat: nutrition sector looks to learn from smoke-free successes. Press release. Online. Available: www.obesityaction. org.nz/media/091206FagsandFat.pdf (accessed 8 December 2009)

Peckover S, Chidlaw R 2007 The (un)-certainties of district nurses in the context of cultural diversity. Journal of Advanced Nursing 58(4):377–85

Penn L, White M, Oldroyd J, Walker M, Alberti K, Mathers C 2009 Prevention of type 2 diabetes in adults with impaired glucose tolerance: the European Diabetes Prevention RCT in Newcastle upon Tyne, UK BMC Public Health 9:342 doi:10.1186/1471-2458/9/342

Pickett K, Wilkinson R 2009 Greater equality and better health. Editorial, British Medical Journal 339:b4320 doi:10.1136bmj.b4320

Poulton B, McKenna H, Keeney S, Hasson F, Sinclair M 2006 The role of the public health nurse in meeting the primary health care needs of single homeless people: a case study report. Primary Health Care Research and Development 7:135–46

Raphael D 2009 Restructuring society in the service of mental health promotion: are we willing to address the social determinants of mental health? International Journal of Mental Health Promotion 11(3):18–31

Raphael D, Anstice S, Raine K, McGannon K, Rizvi S, Yu V 2003 The social determinants of the incidence and management of type 2 diabetes mellitus: are we prepared to rethink our questions and redirect our research activities? International Journal of Health Care, Quality Assurance Incorporating Leadership in Health Services 16(3):x–xx. doi 10.1108/13660750310486730

Raphael D, Farrell S 2002 Beyond medicine and lifestyle: addressing the societal determinants of cardiovascular disease in North America. Leadership in Health Services 15(4):i–v

Rosengren A 2009 Declining cardiovascular mortality and increasing obesity: a paradox. Canadian Medical Association Journal 181(3–4):127–8

Roustit C, Renahy E, Guernec G, Lesieur S, Parizot I, Chauvin P 2009 Exposure to interparental violence and psychosocial maladjustment in the adult life course: advocacy for early prevention. Journal of Epidemiology and Community Health 63:563–8 doi:10.1136/jech.2008.077750

Roxburgh S 2006 'I wish we had more time to spend together …' The distribution and predictors of perceived family time pressures among married men and women in the paid labor force. Journal of Family Issues 27(4):529–53

Shaha M, Bauer-Wu S 2009 Early adulthood uprooted: transitoriness in young women with breast cancer. Cancer Nursing 32(3):246–55

Shallcross L, Sheehan M, Ramsay S 2008 Workplace mobbing: experiences in the public sector. Journal of Organisational Behaviour 13(2):56–70

Street G, James R, Cutt H 2007 The relationship between organised physical recreation and mental health. Health Promotion Journal of Australia 18(3):236–9

Strijk J, Proper K, van der Beek A, van Mechelen W 2009 The Vital@Work study. The systematic development of a lifestyle intervention to improve older workers' vitality and the design of a randomized controlled trial evaluating this intervention. BMC Public Health 9:408–28 doi:10.1186/1471-2458-9-408

Telford K, Kralik D, Isam C 2006–07 Constructions of nutrition for community dwelling people with chronic disease. Contemporary Nurse 23(2):202–15

ten Brummelhuis L, van der Lippe T, Kluwer E, Flap H 2008 Positive and negative effects of family involvement on work-related burnout. Journal of Vocational Behavior 73:387–96

The Australia Institute 2009 Something for Nothing. Unpaid overtime in Australia. Policy Brief No. 7, Online. Available: www.actu.asn.au (accessed 23 November 2009)

Topitzes J, Godes O, Mersky J, Ceglarek S, Reynolds A 2009 Educational success and adult health: findings from the Chicago Longitudinal Study. Prevention Science 10:175–95

Tsourtos G, O'Dwyer L 2008 Stress, stress management, smoking prevalence and quit rates in a disadvantaged area: has anything changed? Health Promotion Journal of Australia 19(1):40–4

Tveito T, Erikson H 2008 Integrated health program: a workplace randomized controlled trial. Journal of Advanced Nursing 65(10):110–19

Tyson S, Flaskerud J 2009a Cultural explanations of mental health and illness. Issues in Mental Health Nursing 31:650–1

—— 2009b Family and community responses to mental illness. Issues in Mental Health Nursing 30:718–19

Umberson D, Liu H, Reczek C 2008 Stress and health behaviour over the life course. Advances in Life Course Research 13:19–44

van der Feltz-Cornelis C 2009 A nurse delivered management programme for depression in cancer patients reduces depressive symptoms compared with usual care. Evidence-Based Mental and Health 12(1):9

Wang J, Schmitz N, Dewa C, Stansfield S 2009 Changes in perceived job strain and the risk of major depression: results from a population-based longitudinal study. American Journal of Epidemiology 169(9):1085–91

Warr D, Feldman P, Tacticos T, Kelaher M 2009 Sources of stress in impoverished neighbourhoods: insights into links between neighbourhood environments and health. Australian and New Zealand Journal of Public Health 33(1):25–33

West E, Mays N, Rafferty A, Rowan K, Sanderson C 2009 Nursing resources and patient outcomes in intensive care: a systematic review of the literature. International Journal of Nursing Studies 46:993–1011

Wilkinson R 1996 Unhealthy Societies: The Afflictions of Inequality. Routledge, London

Wilson C, Flight I, Hart E, Turnbull D, Cole S, Young G 2007 Internet access for delivery of health information to South Australians older than 50. Australian and New Zealand Journal of Public Health 32(20:174–6

Windsor T, Ryan L, Smith J 2009 Individual wellbeing in middle and older adulthood: do spousal beliefs matter? Journal of Gerontology: Psychological Sciences 64B(5):586–96

World Health Organization (WHO) 1999 Regional Guidelines for the Development of Healthy Workplaces. WHO, Manila

—— 2000a Obesity: Preventing and Managing the Global Epidemic. Report of a WHO consultation, Technical report series 894. WHO, Geneva

—— 2000b The World Health Report 2000: Health Systems, Improving Performance. WHO, Geneva

—— 2003 Investing in Mental Health. World Health Organization, Geneva. Online. Available: www.who.int/mental_health/en/investing_in_mnh_final.pdf (accessed 18 November 2009)

—— 2007 Workers health: global plan of action. Online. Available: http://apps.who.int/gb/ebwha/pdf_files/WHA60/A60_R26-en.pdf (accessed 14 December 2009)

—— 2008 World Health Report 2008 Primary Health Care, Now More Than Ever. Online. Available: www.who.int/whr/2008/whr08_en.pdf (accessed 14 July 2009)

—— 2009 Mental Health, Resilience and Inequalities. WHO Regional Office for Europe, Copenhagen

Yassi A, Gilbert M, Cvitkovich Y 2005 Trends in injuries, illnesses, and policies in Canadian health care workplaces. Canadian Journal of Public Health 96(5):333–9

Yildirim D, Aycan Z 2008 Nurses' work demands and work–family conflict: a questionnaire survey. International Journal of Nursing Studies 45:1366–78

Ylipaavalniemi J, Kivimaki M, Elovainio M, Virtanen M, Keltikangas-Jarvinen L, Vahtera J 2005 Psychosocial work characteristics and incidence of newly diagnosed depression: a prospective cohort study of three different models. Social Science & Medicine 61:111–22

Zhao I, Turner C 2007 The impact of shift work on people's daily health habits and adverse health outcomes. Australian Journal of Advanced Nursing 25(30:8–22)

Useful websites

http://www.asthma.org.au — Asthma

http://www.diabetescontrol.com — Diabetes

http://www.beyondblue.org.au/index.aspx? — Beyondblue Depression site (Australia)

http://www.justask.org.au — Lifeline's rural mental health information service (also their help line 1300 131 114)

http://www.vibe.com.au — Vibe Australia — services by location

http://www.health.gov.au/internet/main/publishing.nsf/content/pq-arthritis — Arthritis

http://www.healthinsite.gov.au — Variety of topics on Australia's health

http://www.heartfoundation.com.au/sepa/index_fr.html — Supportive Environments for Physical Activity — SEPA

http://www.inclusivecities.ca — Inclusive cities

http://www.moh.govt.nz — Ministry of Health, NZ

http://www.obesityaction@xtra.co.nz — Sport and recreation, NZ

http://www.sparc.org.nz — Obesity Action Coalition, NZ

http://www.worklifebalance.com.au/ — Work–life balance site

http://www.business.gov.au — Business topics, occupational health

http://www.worksolutions.com.au — Occupational health and safety services

http://www.likeminds.org.nz — Reducing the stigma and discrimination associated with mental illness

http://www.acc.co.nz — New Zealand accident insurance scheme

http://www.phac.health.govt.nz/moh.nsf/pagescm/7558/$File/rethinking-urban-environments.pdf — Useful readings on urban planning and health

Chapter 9

Healthy ageing

INTRODUCTION

This chapter addresses the health of older persons in the context of community. The central challenge for healthy ageing lies in creating the conditions for people to age with optimal health and well being and a good quality of life. But what is ageing? In the 21st century, social commentators quip that 40 is the new 20, and 60 the new 40. Does this make 80 the new 60, and if so, what does that mean for the way we nurture health and wellbeing along the latter stages of life's pathway? We know that the quality of ageing depends on the cumulative effects of social determinants in the earlier years. But there are also developmental changes that occur in the years from 65 to 90, and these have not often attracted the attention of health care planners. Instead, planning has tended to revolve around population trends towards disease states, and how to prevent, treat and palliate these. These are important aspects of health care for older people, especially for those trying to cope with the cumulative effects of lifelong disadvantage. But nursing care for older people in the community also includes health promotion activities that focus on healthy environments within which older people can enjoy good health into the years of the 'oldest old', and engage in healthy lifestyles.

Communities for healthy ageing need to acknowledge the extent to which older persons contribute to the social, cultural and geographical life of the community. People over the age of 65 are vital to child care and other aspects of family life, particularly for their grown children who may be living in busy, dual-earner families. Many older persons are also carers for family members with disabling conditions. Importantly, older citizens are also a viable economic force. Some continue in the workplace longer than their forebears, bringing wisdom to a wide range of industries, including health care. Older adults also have the potential to dominate shifts in the economy through their spending, investments and service requirements.

They are a political force through the sheer weight of numbers, capable of swaying the policy climate for health, the environment, and their grandchildren's educational future. In some communities, older people help calm the social climate through their understanding, and by having a more emotionally balanced perspective that comes with the patience of ageing. Others' lives may be destitute and lonely. The combination is unique for every person and experienced differently, depending on social and environmental supports. This chapter examines the continuum of ageing across different experiences and contexts, with a view towards establishing community and societal goals for health and wellbeing in the latter stages of life.

> **Point to ponder**
> The most important challenge for healthy ageing is creating the conditions for people to age well.

AGEING AND SOCIETY

The terms 'ageing' and 'elderly' were once used to indicate that a person had begun the journey to the end of life. Yet, today, as the world experiences a proliferation in medical and health-sustaining knowledge and technology, ageing has taken on a new connotation, that of unexplored possibilities. Many people over the age of 65 in Australia and New Zealand lead healthy and productive lives, some thriving in ways they could not during their middle years, when their life circumstances prevented them from achieving a balance between work, recreation and family responsibilities. A large number of older people are also unwell, suffering from chronic diseases or conditions that limit their mobility or sense of wellbeing. But these two groups are not polar opposites. There are numerous older people whose health lies between the extremes of high-level wellness and immobility.

Objectives

By the end of this chapter you will be able to:

1 describe the most important influences on health and wellbeing among the ageing population
2 discuss the stereotype of ageism and its implications for health care
3 explain the implications of understanding older adults' experiences of life and life transitions
4 outline the major contributions older people make to the health of the community
5 identify older people's health literacy needs
6 identify health promotion strategies for the ageing population using the Ottawa Charter for Health Promotion
7 identify the most important gaps in nursing research knowledge related to older persons.

The challenge for nurses and other professionals working with older persons, is to see each person in terms of individual strengths and needs, and the environments that support or constrain health and wellbeing. This includes understanding their individual journey, and what it has meant for the way they experience health. From this understanding, plans can then be implemented to provide community supports that enable the highest level of health and capacity possible.

This generation of older people born in Australia and New Zealand live in relative peace and harmony. The lives of most of those approaching their 70s in the 21st century have not been without conflicts, including the Vietnam war of the 1960s–1970s. Conflicts and disrupted living circumstances have also affected the earlier years of immigrants who are ageing in both countries, and who are the most rapidly growing group of older citizens (Crisp & Taylor 2009). But most people between age 65 and 75 are ageing well, perhaps because they have not lived in the deprivation of World War I and World War II, like the oldest old in society. For this, and other reasons, they tend to have a more optimistic outlook on life than their parents.

As a group, today's over 65s have lived their lives around values of hard work and industriousness. Many have a strong spiritual connection to place, either to the land, or to the community and its ability to provide employment. In their younger years, they entered married life to raise a family, then went through some of the most dramatic social changes of any generation before them. They were the first generation to experience the women's movement and the subsequent changes to marriage and family life. Their relative prosperity meant that they were well nourished, but often with too many high-fat, high-salt foods, and perhaps too much meat. Most smoked and many drank alcohol. Some also experimented with marijuana and other drugs that created altered states of consciousness. But somewhere along their adult lives, they likely discovered the error of their ways and stopped smoking. Many began to eat yoghurt, a habit that would have been unheard of among their parents. Some also adopted new ways of thinking and got in touch with their feelings, taking up meditation, Tai Chi and a plethora of techniques to create harmony in their lives. These too are aspects of social life that were not part of their parents' generation. Yet, despite being unique, interesting, socially engaged, balanced, yet rebellious at times, they are often the subject of discrimination and ageist attitudes.

> **Point to ponder**
> Despite today's older adults having grown up in an era of experimentation, dramatic social change and relative prosperity, they are still subject to ageist attitudes, behaviours and stereotyping from those younger than themselves.

Ageism is a type of discrimination against older adults on the basis of misconceptions about their characteristics, attitudes, abilities and capacity. Describing older persons as a 'demographic time bomb' or as universally and exclusively needy, dependent and ill negates their diversity and varied outcomes (Garner 2009). The global state of alarm at population ageing may therefore be the most 'pernicious' example of ageism (Garner 2009:5). With so much attention drawn to population ageing, it is common to hear younger people make disparaging comments about older people being non-productive, resistant to change, or a liability to society. This type of comment causes older people to wonder about health-related decisions that might affect their future, including the possibility that a younger generation might ration their health and social services (Fairhurst 2005). Insensitive comments often draw undue attention to an older person's memory slip, labelling it as dementia or Alzheimer's disease, when it may be due to other factors such as motivation, the saliency of remembering, or personal interest (Wilkinson 1996). In many cases, where ageist remarks are made, there is little consideration of personality characteristics, or personal responses to provocation, pain, disability or recent life events. Instead, the older adult's concerns are often stereotyped as if they were typical of the entire demographic group.

Stereotypes of older persons include negative impressions of their cognitive function (senile vs wise), physical functions (decrepit vs spry) and social lives (boring perhaps) (Levy & Leif-heit-Limson 2009; Sanchez Palacios et al 2009). Stereotypes include assumptions that being older causes illness, irritability, that older people are lonely and devoid of affective links, or that they are disinterested in sexual activity (Sanchez Palacios et al 2009). These negative stereotypes can be insulting to older people. If they are commonly held perceptions by others in the community, they can also be barriers to adequate care and support (Reyna et al 2007). Garner (2009:6) notes that there is 'greater individual variability between 70 year olds than among 17 year olds'. Older people also continue to develop and evolve into their oldest years. Some do not cope well with ageing because of negative beliefs about self-efficacy, but others thrive, especially those who remain connected to social activities in the community (Sanchez Palacios et al 2009).

Although people age and mature in different ways, many begin to develop a more balanced perspective of life as a function of getting older. Psychological changes include a greater capacity for delayed gratification, and a greater valuing of relationships (Garner 2009). These traits evolve through acquired knowledge, and the recognition that internal resourcefulness and a sense of humour are critical to ageing well and maintaining a high quality of life. Placing a high value on relationships also fosters greater tolerance of difference, which is important in an era where there is such diversity in community life. In the cities, especially, older people can be an anchor for newcomers such as migrants, with the time and tolerance to help ease their transitions and changes in the social fabric of their community. Clearly, it is important to recognise the strengths older people bring to community life, to balance the perspective purveyed in policy debates and the media that population ageing is a threat to Western society.

POPULATION AGEING

With longevity at an all-time high, the world is ageing rapidly. Population ageing is also linked to the fertility rate. With fewer babies being born and older people living longer, the largest group in society is older people. The WHO (2008) estimates that by 2050, the world will contain 2 billion people over the age of 60, around 85% of whom will be living in today's developing countries, mostly in urban areas. Throughout the world, thousands of older people live in poverty and conditions of disadvantage, particularly in countries where infectious diseases like HIV/AIDS and malaria have caused deaths in family members. In families ravaged by disease there are fewer middle-aged adults to guide and support younger generations through their transitions into adult life. Older people in these families may be the only ones available to care for young children. As is the case in many developing countries, their lives may be difficult not only from caregiving, but also overwork, a lack of food security, civil conflicts or family displacement (WHO 2008).

GLOBAL AGEING PERSPECTIVES

Any analysis of ageing trends should include a cross-national or cross-cultural perspective, as population ageing is of major consequence throughout the world.

Migration and other environmental concerns are relevant to the global dialogue on ageing, especially with so many families being displaced and relocating with their elders. Comparing health and social life between countries also illuminates the strengths, weaknesses, opportunities and threats of ageing in different environments, especially in planning for social policies that will govern people's lives and the health care systems that will sustain them. It is important to know, for example, how successful communities help their elders financially and socially, and it is equally important to see the areas where intervention is required to rearrange circumstances for those living more challenging lives. This is a major part of citizenship in today's society, and it requires intergenerational sensitivity, as older people's needs are accommodated differently in various communities and workplaces.

Point to ponder

Despite dramatic increases in the oldest old and the 'baby boomers' leaving the workforce in growing numbers, fears of decreased tax intake and increasing health care costs may be exaggerated.

The dramatic effects of population ageing have evoked strong responses throughout the world (Castles 2000). Two distinct demographic trends are acknowledged by all sides of the debate. First, because people are living longer the future will see a dramatic increase in the 'oldest old' proportion of the population. Second, the children of the post-World War II generation, the 'baby boomers', are leaving the workforce and reducing their contribution to the economy through taxes. This has caused widespread uneasiness about the declining capacity of the remaining workforce to provide for the health and social security of older citizens. Public debates have therefore revolved around the needs and potential of the older generation and the effect of a shrinking workforce having to pay for a growing number of pensioners (Brockmann et al 2009). These discussions need to shift the focus from the 'disability' rhetoric of ageing to an emphasis on older people's capacity and abilities, particularly in retirement.

One solution to the imminent retirement of the baby boomer generation is to adjust the official retirement age upwards, through policies that would keep people working longer. Some policy experts have argued that retirement is a risk factor for illness or frailty, while others have mounted a counter-argument, that leaving the stress of the workplace and assuming a healthier lifestyle during retirement has major health benefits. Brockmann et al's (2009) research conducted on a large cohort of retirees indicates that early retirement lowers mortality risks. Those with poorer health self-select themselves out of the workplace, leaving a healthier workforce behind, thereby reducing their risk for mortality or further morbidity. Retired life also provides more opportunities for healthy lifestyles, which improves health and quality of life. This is often more likely for those of higher socio-economic status. Those wealthy enough to retire early, enjoy healthier ageing because of their opportunities for healthy lifestyles as well as the protective effect of financial security (Brockmann et al 2009).

The main public concerns about the exit of the older generation from the workplace are centred on skills shortages, a lack of mentors for young people and erosion of the tax base, as retired people pay much less in tax than those employed in paid work. However, these concerns may be exaggerated by younger people. The current generation of older people have greater wealth than their parents, and many will be self-funded retirees, rather than relying on government support in their older years. In addition, many also enjoy better health than their age group has in previous eras, so the strain on health care systems may not be as great as some imagine. Financial security also permits greater opportunities for social engagement, which is a critical element for both retirees and those who choose part-time employment in their older years. Social engagement in the workplace is a lifeline for many older people who, like a large proportion of others in the population, may be living alone. For some older people the family remains the centre of their social life, but for others, the freedom that comes from retiring and having fewer family responsibilities can open up new social networks, which are fundamental to health and wellbeing.

Point to ponder

Maintaining social connectedness is a priority for older adults.

As we mentioned previously, the generation of people who are approaching their 70s in the second decade of the 21st century are unique in their social and marital history, and this affects their patterns of social activity. They were the first generation of married couples to be offered and, in some cases, encouraged by no-fault divorce. As young adults, their lives were bombarded by the 1970s public media that promoted self-involvement and constant questioning of the status quo. Some resisted and lived their mid-adult lives as married couples, but others have experienced multiple divorces and family combinations. As older citizens, members of this group tend to be more self-aware, more adaptable to new situations and capable of living independently. Others, who have lived a more conservative lifestyle, may experience social life in their older years entirely differently. But for both groups, maintaining social connectedness is a priority.

RISK AND POTENTIAL IN OLDER PERSONS

The experience of ageing is typically characterised by some or all of the following:

- normative declines in health, physical and cognitive abilities and the likelihood of developing ill health or chronic diseases
- greater salience of health concerns in life
- diminishing time left to live
- the experience(s) of bereavement
- having more restricted but intense social relationships and networks
- being perceived or treated in ageist ways
- increasing interiority (looking inward), desire for integrity and search for meaning in life
- greater acceptance of what cannot be controlled and greater fear of losing control over one's life.

(Settersten 2005:S175)

Despite the inherent declines of ageing, older people in the 21st century have the potential for a long life, and better health status than the generations before them. Australians over age 65 comprise 13% of the population, and this is expected to double over the next 4 decades (AIHW 2008; Commonwealth of Australia 2008). Their life expectancy is second only to Japan, at 81.4 years. In New Zealand, 12% of the population are over age 65, and this is expected to rise to 19% by 2021 (Ministry of Health New Zealand [MOHNZ] 2006). Life expectancy in New Zealand, at 80.1%, does not quite match Australia's, although there is a 4.2-year difference between male and female life

BOX 9.1 GRANDPA'S GIRLFRIEND

Two 11-year-old girls are walking through the markets on a Saturday morning, a few steps behind the grandfather of one of them. Grandpa only buys his vegetables at the farmers' markets, a habit he has maintained for years. On Saturday mornings he picks up his granddaughter for a brisk one-hour walk and a trip to the markets, lifestyle habits he is hoping will inspire her life choices. He is fit, healthy, 70, and conscious of his weight and general health. On this day his granddaughter, Cassie, has brought her friend, Ella.

'What should we do today?' asks Cassie.

'I have to go shopping with my mum after this,' says Ella.

'Maybe we can hook up in the afternoon then,' says Cassie. 'I have to go shopping too. I need to get a birthday present for Grandpa's girlfriend. We are going to her place, then I have to go with my mother to my step-grandma's apartment and pick up a big pot for my gran. She's getting ready to bake the wedding cake for Louise's wedding.'

'Whatever … Who's Louise?' asks Ella.

'Louise is my step-sister from my dad's second marriage. She's going to get married in a park and come to my grandpa's house for the reception. That way we won't have to go to a church.'

'Why don't they want to get married in a church?'

'We don't want to mix up Grandpa, Grandpa's girlfriend, and Gran. Also, my dad doesn't want his girlfriend to argue with Grandpa's girlfriend, which always happens. As if … so my mum and I are getting the stuff to bake the cake at Gran's and everyone can stay away from each other. So I need to get the present over to Grandpa's girlfriend before I go over to Gran's.'

This is an actual conversation overheard on a Saturday at the markets. It reflects the reality of some of the older people in contemporary life, and the multi-generational impact of their social lives. We present this to provoke reflection on stereotypical thinking about the lives of older persons, and to underline the need to assess individual needs in the context of existing lifestyles and family dynamics.

expectancy, with males lagging behind females (MOHNZ & Statistics New Zealand 2009). Most people over age 65 consider themselves to be in good health, with a large proportion of older women rating their health as excellent (Commonwealth of Australia 2008). Despite better prospects for healthy ageing, some changes are predictable in the latter part of a person's life. Physical changes reduce the body's physiological reserve, presenting a range of obstacles to healthy ageing, more serious for some than others. All older people experience some loss of skin resilience and moisture. Most develop more pronounced facial features from the loss of subcutaneous fat and skin elasticity. Changes in vision and hearing are typical. Respiratory muscle strength tends to decrease, and there may be decreased cardiac output due to decreased cardiac muscle strength. There may also be changes in mass, tone and elasticity of breasts, the abdomen, and the reproductive system. The urinary and musculoskeletal systems function less efficiently, and there may be some loss of balance, due to neurological changes. Some problems affect quality of life more profoundly than others. Incontinence, for example, can be a major problem for older people, as it is surrounded by stigma and can rapidly lead to social isolation, with those who are incontinent becoming less inclined to venture out of their homes. Separately, none of these conditions may be life threatening, but in combination they can work against a person's attempts to stay young and vital.

Point to ponder

Life expectancy in Australia is currently at 81.4 years — up from 77.1 years in 1990. In New Zealand, life expectancy has increased from 75.3 years in 1990 to 80.1 years in 2010.

Many older people live with the burden of social disadvantage and disabling chronic diseases. Urbanisation, ageing and globalised lifestyle changes have combined to make chronic and non-communicable diseases — including depression, diabetes, cardiovascular disease and cancers — and injuries the most important causes of morbidity (WHO 2008). Among those aged 65–84 cancer, cardiovascular disease and stroke are the most common causes of death, with cardiovascular disease dominating the over 85 age group (Commonwealth of Australia 2008; MOHNZ 2006). As many as 25% of 65–69-year-olds and 50% of 80–84-year-olds in Western countries are affected by two or more chronic health conditions simultaneously.

BOX 9.2 COMMON CHRONIC DISEASES OF AGEING

- Cardiovascular disease
- Hypertension
- Stroke
- Diabetes
- Cancer
- Chronic obstructive pulmonary disease
- Musculoskeletal conditions (arthritis, osteoporosis)
- Mental health conditions (dementia, depression)
- Blindness and visual impairment.

(AIHW 2008)

These are the same group of chronic diseases as are manifest in adulthood (see Chapter 8). The nine most common of these are identified in Box 9.2

Chronic diseases, such as type 2 diabetes, can lead to visual impairments and the risk of falling, which is the most frequent injury-related cause of death, especially among those over age 75 (AIHW 2008). Injuries from falls have a major effect on people's lifestyles, often precipitating admission to hospital or residential care (AIHW 2008). Those in residential care have a greater risk of falling for a number of reasons. These include pre-existing conditions that affect their balance or lower limb strength, psychotropic medications, wearing slippers, or the environmental conditions of residential care facilities. Another chronic condition that impedes people's lifestyle is poor oral health, especially the loss of teeth, which affects many older adults and often has a long-term effect on their nutritional status, self-confidence and quality of life (AIHW 2008).

Point to ponder

The most common causes of morbidity in older adults in Australia and New Zealand are depression, diabetes, cardiovascular disease, cancer and injuries.

The main health concerns for older people include day-to-day adjustments required to cope with disability and chronic conditions (Westaway 2009; WHO 2008). For some, disabilities are a result of the cumulative effect of lifelong exposures to various environmental factors (Commonwealth of Australia 2008). As mentioned earlier, in the industrialised world, as many as 25% of 65–69-year-olds and 50% of 80–84-year-olds are affected by two or more chronic health conditions simultaneously. When conditions such as type 2 diabetes, hypertension and obesity occur together they can have a compound detrimental effect on health (Westaway 2009). Although these diseases may not cause death they can impair a person's physical function, severely limiting their quality of life (Lang et al 2008).

People over age 65 have the highest proportion (35%) of hospitalisations, with males being hospitalised more frequently than females. Although many of these are short-stay hospital visits, their highest expenditures arise from joint replacement surgery for hips and knees replacements or revisions. Other major causes of problems among the over 65s include adult-onset hearing loss, Parkinson's disease in males, and falls and osteoarthritis in females (Commonwealth of Australia 2008; MOHNZ 2006). One out of every five Australians and New Zealanders lives with at least one disability, and these are more frequent among the older age groups (Commonwealth of Australia 2008; MOHNZ 2008).

WEIGHT AND MOBILITY IN OLDER AGE

Illness and lack of sleep can also cause people to eat more than usual, and antidepressants can stimulate the appetite, cause water retention or slow metabolism. Joint pain, decreased mobility and activity intolerance can also contribute to an inactive lifestyle, and lead to overweight or obesity (Newman 2009). Obesity, in particular, creates a cycle of disadvantage for those who are trying to maintain a healthy lifestyle. Obesity in older age is often related to a decrease in energy expenditure, with hormonal changes causing an accumulation of fat, and metabolic changes that decrease a person's ability to regulate appetite (Newman 2009). In addition, environmental and social factors include concerns about safe places to walk, a lack of recreational spaces, safety fears because of neighbourhood hazards, and the tendency to eat out or from vending machines, for those without someone to share mealtimes (Newman 2009). Being overweight or obese can exacerbate arthritis and osteoarthritis by increasing the load on knee and hip joints, causing deterioration of the cartilage. Arthritis is the most chronically disabling condition, particularly for those over age 75, but joint and mobility problems also affect those under age 75 (AIHW 2008). Although mobility in joints should be maintained by stretching and strengthening exercises, these may cause pain that often prevents older persons with even mild levels of joint deterioration from continuing to be active (Newman 2009).

Point to ponder

Ageing, genetics, intergenerational effects and the cumulative effects of lifelong exposure to environmental factors contribute to an increased risk of developing joint and mobility problems in older people.

PHYSICAL ACTIVITY AND AGEING

Maintaining physical activity is one of the greatest challenges of ageing. Although joint pain and a lack of muscle strength can be a deterrent to regular exercise it is important to help maintain joint mobility. Combined with pain management techniques, regular exercise can help sustain quality of life throughout the older years. Strength training and Tai Chi are particularly effective for older persons to help with balance and muscle integrity. Strength and balance, together with safe home and environmental modifications, can help prevent falls, which are the most common cause of injuries in older adults (Comans et al 2009). Physical activity also provides social opportunities, whether through interactions at a gym or other facility, walking or cycling groups. Maintaining 30 minutes of exercise a day helps prevent physical deterioration and prevent lifestyle-related diseases in all adults. International studies have shown that this level of exercise has been responsible for reducing coronary artery disease, some cancers, type 2 diabetes, obesity, osteoporosis and injury from falls (Kolt et al 2009). Regular activity also improves quality of life and psychological function, reduces the risk of dementia, and facilitates independent living (Kolt et al 2009).

Most countries have introduced national guidelines for 30 minutes of exercise per day for all adults, including older people. Because older people are at risk of physical inactivity, New Zealand has also introduced the 'Green Prescription', which is an activity prescription provided by primary care providers, including nurses (Elley et al 2003; Kolt et al 2009; NZ Ministry of Social Policy 2001; Sinclair & Hamlin 2007). Prescribing the exercise regime helps motivate a person to achieve the requisite level of activity by drawing attention to the benefits of exercise at the primary care visit, then intermittent telephone support by exercise professionals from the Regional Sports Trust. The program has already been deemed effective in terms of maintaining physical fitness, and it has proven cost effective (Dalziel et al 2006; Elley et al 2003, 2004; Kerse et al 2005). Researchers are now instituting a 12-month trial that will add a prescription for the over 65s, encouraging the participants to add a minimum level of steps to their daily exercise, measured through a pedometer-based study. Evaluation of the trial is expected to show even greater benefits for heart health, quality of life and functional status (Kolt et al 2009).

MENTAL HEALTH ISSUES

Many older people have mental health issues, the most common of which are Alzheimer's disease and other forms of dementia. Dementia is a brain syndrome caused by abnormal accumulation of proteins around the neurons of the brain. These clump together, interfering with brain cell function and connections, eventually leading to cell death (Alzheimer's Australia 2008). The disease results in an impaired level of arousal affecting at least three areas of mental activity. These can include language, memory, visuo-spatial skills, personality or emotional state, and cognitive functions such as planning, abstraction or judgement (Alzheimer's Australia 2008; Flood & Buckwalter 2009). Memory loss tends to be the first sign of dementia, and this can cause enormous stress as the person tries unsuccessfully to retrieve something elusive from their memory (Alzheimer's Australia 2008). For those with Alzheimer's disease the memory loss is followed by language dysfunction and problems with spatial orientation (Alzheimer's Australia 2008). Dementia can be caused by Alzheimer's disease or other factors, such as vascular disease, HIV infection, neurological disease, chronic alcoholism or head trauma (Flood & Buckwalter 2009). Alzheimer's disease often has no genetic cause but, like other dementias, it can be instigated by conditions that cause vascular damage, such as type 2 diabetes, hypertension, high cholesterol and smoking (Alzheimer's Australia 2008).

Dementia is the most significant cause of disability at older ages, but it can also affect people under age 65 (Alzheimer's Australia 2008). It is a progressive, incurable condition that is highly disabling as it affects activities of daily living and can lead to the need for long-term high-level care (Chang et al 2009). The condition is more prevalent in over 85s, with older females having higher rates because they tend to live longer than males. But with the increase in life expectancy for both women and men, it is an important population health issue (Nepal et al 2008). Even moderate dementia can cause severe impairments in judgement and the ability to function independently, which renders the condition a major cause of stress for both the person suffering and their carers. It is also a major expense for the health care system and for family members who absorb the expenses of caregiving, either in the home or when institutional care is required. Caregivers also have to deal with the challenges of mobility and communication difficulties that accompany dementia, especially when these cause difficult behaviours (Moniz-Cook et al 2008). Some people with dementia develop psychotic symptoms and aggressive behaviours. Often this is a response to being placed in an alienating environment, or because of the frustration of not being able to communicate their needs. Although anti-psychotic drugs are frequently prescribed to older adults with dementia, recent research suggests that the potential benefits of their use are outweighed by their adverse effects. Recommendations suggest that further research be undertaken into non-pharmacological methods of treating behavioural problems in dementia and that health professionals need to be up-skilled in managing the complexity, co-morbidity and severity of people with dementia (Banerjee 2009).

Point to ponder

Developing effective approaches to managing the complexity of dementia is a research imperative.

Other mental health issues affecting older people include anxiety and depression, which can be a cause or a consequence of loneliness or social isolation. Depression can also be caused by functional and sensory impairment, incontinence, loss of mobility and/or pain (Dening & Milne 2009). The depressed person typically shows persistent symptoms of being sad, anxious, loss of interest or feelings of guilt, worthlessness and hopelessness (Dahle & Ploeg 2008). The condition often impacts on physical health through disrupted eating and sleeping patterns, which cause malnutrition and decreased energy as well as difficulties in concentrating (Dahle & Ploeg 2008). Depression is an interesting phenomenon in older people, thought to arise from the cumulative effects of chronic stressors and negative life events, including both health- and non-health-related events. However, depression may also arise as a response to behaviour patterns established in earlier life stages that trigger stressors. This works like a feedback loop, in that stressors trigger depressive symptoms, which continue to elicit behaviours such as antagonistic interpersonal interactions that generate more stressors. Once this self-perpetuating loop is set in motion, it may endure for years, because of relatively stable personality and interaction patterns among older adults.

Point to ponder

Person-centred care refocuses the provision of health care on effective interpersonal relationships rather than medical diagnoses.

Coping strategies are an important concern for those dealing with the changes associated with ageing, or those helping others deal with these changes. Self-efficacy, believing in one's ability to overcome difficulties, is crucial to positive coping. A sense of humour can reinforce self-efficacy, especially if social support is also available (Marziali et al 2008). Cultural considerations also play a part in coping with ageing. Some families may not encourage help-seeking because of a cultural value of self-sufficiency, while others may be more inclined to seek assistance early for any difficulties. Because of wide variation in family responses, it is important that nurses interacting with older persons and their families reinforce the need for 'personhood' and person-centred care, especially for those with dementia (Adams & Moyle 2007:159). Person-centred care places the emphasis on relationships rather than whatever medical condition might be present. This type of approach can help reframe caregiving in terms of empowerment, diversity and choice, rather than predetermined assumptions of a person's needs, many of which are influenced

by their environment (Price 2009). Trying to cope with depression is a pervasive challenge for those in long-term care (Dahle & Ploeg 2008; Dening & Milne 2009). When a person moves into long-term care they often lose touch with friends and distant family members, who may have remained in touch while they lived at home. The sense of loss of all that is familiar can lead to a loss of control over a person's life, and their sense of the future. This underlines the importance of place and the difficulties of displacement, especially for older persons who have lived in relatively stable environments throughout their lives.

HEALTH AND PLACE

People develop ways of adjusting to the challenges of their lives in a variety of ways. Some of these differ by gender, or other factors, but some differ according to the environmental or circumstantial aspects of their lives. 'Place' holds a preeminent position in the lives of many older adults, beyond the space where they live. The place or setting where people grow old usually has meaning for them, in that it shapes the intimate relations between people, and the broader processes of social relations that comprise society (Wiles 2005). As they go through the many transitions of ageing, their places, whether these are homes or institutional environments, are constantly being negotiated as a kind of personal geography. This includes where they live, how they move about and how they experience and understand their surroundings (Wiles 2005).

The most visible influence of place on health is in rural–urban comparisons. Ageing in the city has unique challenges. Independent-living older people with the financial means to be selective often gravitate to inner-city living, where services such as the medical practitioner, pharmacist, physiotherapist, grocer or newsagent are readily available. Safety and accessibility are the most important issues for these people, so the features they look for if they are choosing a neighbourhood are well-maintained footpaths, lighting, safe traffic conditions and shelter. Other independent-living people may wish to remain in their more suburban homes. Their environmental concerns may be focused on transportation, and ensuring there is someone to monitor their health and wellbeing, especially if they live alone.

Rural people have even greater needs for safety, access to services and health monitoring because of distance, and the sparse distribution of services. Few people are able to live alone throughout their entire older years in their home because of the isolation. Like people in urban areas, safety and access to services are paramount. Rural living also carries a higher risk for families caring for older people. This is related to a lack of transportation and assistance to move older family members when they need care, a lack of emergency or specialist services, or the type of supports for various disabilities that may be available in the cities or regional areas. In addition, carers usually have no access to respite services in rural or remote areas. Their burden is multiplied when they have to move older family members into residential aged care, which may be at a great distance from home (National Rural Health Alliance [NRHA] 2009).

Point to ponder

The 'place' where people grow old has significance to an individual beyond its physical boundaries, providing meaning to the older person, through the creation and maintenance of broader interpersonal and intergenerational relationships.

Many older adults experience 'displacements' through multiple relocations; from their own home to the residence of a family member and sometimes back and forth between the homes of family members. They may also experience relocations between residential facilities, health care institutions and their usual residence. Each of these moves adds stress to older adults' lives, especially if they have been forced by illness or family circumstances to leave a home in which they have spent a substantial portion of their lives. For some, the stress is exacerbated by the unpredictability of the move, either because of its location or duration, or because it signals that the family has become scattered, and there may be no one to take care of them. Relocation stress is influenced by several factors: the person's characteristics prior to the move, their attitude towards moving, their preparation for the move, their physical and cognitive status and the extent to which they feel they have control over the move.

At some point, most people experience a loss of place in both the material and emotional sense. Some have an extended period of grieving, which can be a very intense personal experience. Besides losing the material comforts of their home, they may also be grieving for the symbolic meaning of their sanctuary, the place where they have established and sustained the family. Home is often a source of satisfaction in having provided a protective environment for loved ones. It is where possessions and personal touches mark significant family moments and memories. Dislocation from the family home because of financial peril causes extraordinary stress for some people, and brings with it concerns about becoming homeless, or dependent on institutionalised care. Some people also worry about losing their home if it will leave their children financially liable, or in difficult circumstances following their death.

The relationship of personal geographies to health and wellbeing has implications for both home and community care. Home care may violate a person's sense of personal space by the intrusion of caregiving devices and external caregivers, or it may be readily accommodated and help define a person's sense of place. These reactions are variable. Models of shared care involving one or more outsiders and someone in the family setting may be received differentially, depending on the older person's connection with others, and how they choose to negotiate the relationships involved in both care and domestic living (Sebern 2005). The nurse–client relationship is often pre-eminent. Older people attending general practice or other primary health care (PHC) settings typically rely on nurses for advice and support for their self-management of chronic conditions. Nurses also provide the first line of support for caregivers, particularly in the context of home visiting. Home visiting nurses may be the most trusted health professional in an older person's network of support because of their skill in bridging the gap between the formal and informal health care context. This requires a respectful attitude, diplomacy, and a commitment to working in partnership with the older person and/or family to identify strengths and needs in the home that will provide protection from harm, and promote health and wellbeing. Most nurses approach home visiting by tailoring their communication, assessment, health education and advocacy skills to individual needs and preferences.

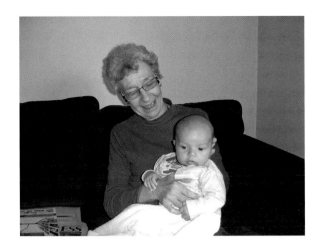

SAFE ENVIRONMENTS FOR AGEING

Safety is a priority in home, community and residential care. Protecting older people from harm throughout ageing begins with attention to the community environment, and the structural features of their lives. Maintaining a safe environment at home includes falls prevention strategies, ensuring the home is safe and secure from intruders, and assessing the need for physical supports. Home visits can be an opportunity for surveillance of the immediate home environment and the neighbourhood, with a view towards determining whether they need mobility supports to prevent falls, or any modifications that would help with any hearing or vision problems. Safety surveillance outside the home includes ensuring safe walkways, transportation systems, and measures to ensure road safety. Well-maintained parks and footpaths with good lighting are crucial to keeping older people mobile and independent as well as providing an incentive for exercise.

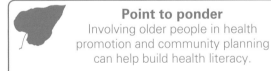

Point to ponder

Involving older people in health promotion and community planning can help build health literacy.

Evaluating health literacy is also a component of safety surveillance. Identifying information needs can help promote self-awareness of any strengths or constraints that may influence a person's capacity for independent living. This includes helping them understand any physical or mental condition that might influence their ability to continue driving, or engaging in other activities of community life. Older people also need information and

support to take precautions against violence, or other community crimes that may place them at risk. This information can be shared with others in community planning forums, gathering input from those with a wide variety of needs for services and support. Sharing information is invaluable for older people who may be unaware of how to access services or manage liaison across services, from primary care to acute and home care. Their involvement in planning can help promote awareness of the type and location of services available, and how they can be accessed.

An important objective of assessing the home and community environments is to help people stay in their own homes as long as possible. This is also the focus of various government support programs for healthy ageing. These include the Australian National Injury Prevention and Safety Promotion Plan (NPHP 2005) and the New Zealand ACC (Online. Available: www.acc.co.nz/preventing-injuries/at-home/older-people/index.htm [accessed 20 December 2009]), both of which outline measures for falls prevention, and support national and state-run programs. These preventative programs are intended to keep older people on their feet at home and in the community, to prevent hospital admissions for falls injuries. All provide information for older people and their carers. Some programs, such as the Western Australian program Healthy@Home (Online. Available: www.health.wa.gov.au/HealthyatHome/home [accessed 20 December 2009]), provide in-home services such as chronic disease support, falls assessment, physiotherapy services, telehealth, assistance with wound management, and hospital in the home (HITH) interventions for acute care needs. Others, such as the New South Wales program, Healthy at Home (Online. Available: www.health.nsw.gov.au/initiatives/healthyathome/index.asp [accessed 20 December 2009]), provide rapid response and fast-track diagnosis and elder care (within 48 hours) through integration of services and individual case management.

Other government initiatives for health and safety in ageing in Australia and New Zealand are aimed at extending health protection and risk management by promoting positive and active ageing (Online. Available: www.health.gov.au/internet/ministers/publishing.nsf/Content/mr-yr08-je-je099.htm [accessed 8 December 2009]; and MOHNZ 2002, 2002). The goals and initiatives of the Australian government program include supports for older people maintaining their health, physical activity, and recreational and community engagement, as well as their contribution to the paid and unpaid workforce. The New Zealand Positive Ageing Strategy extends this type of commitment to monitoring older people's living standards, health, housing, transport, cultural diversity, access to services, especially in rural areas, and employment circumstances. The New Zealand strategy is also expansive in promoting community attitudes towards positive ageing, valuing older people's wisdom and providing opportunities for personal growth and community participation (Online. Available: www.osc.govt.nz/positive-ageing-strategy/index. html [accessed 8 December 2009]).

ELDER ABUSE

One of the most concerning issues facing older people in society is the risk of abuse. Elder abuse/neglect is the abuse and/or neglect of older people aged over 65, by a person with whom they have a relationship of trust (Ministry of Social Development 2002). Elder abuse can occur for many reasons. There may be a history of family violence, caregivers may be struggling to cope with their role, and dementia, substance abuse or mental health problems may compound the likelihood that abuse may occur. It is estimated that between 2% and 5% of the population over the age of 65 years may be victims of elder abuse (Glasgow & Fanslow 2006). The most common types of elder abuse are financial and psychological, and these are most likely to be perpetrated by a family member (Families Commission 2009), however, other forms of physical and/or sexual abuse and/or neglect may also occur (Glasgow & Fanslow 2006). Most elder abuse occurs in the older person's own home, and most victims are female, however, abuse also takes place in residential care facilities, hospitals and private homes, and victims can be male (Families Commission 2009). There are a range of features that can suggest abuse or neglect is occurring and these are outlined in Box 9.3.

Point to ponder

Elder abuse may occur in up to 5% of the older adult population.

Nurses may be the first to recognise signs or symptoms of abuse and are in a key position to provide support, guidance and resources to the

BOX 9.3 INDICATORS FOR ELDER ABUSE

- There is discrepancy between observations made by the health professional and information from the older person.
- There is discrepancy in perceptions of the older person and the suspected abuser.
- There is incongruity between an injury and the history.
- There are unexplained injuries, conflicting stories, vague or bizarre explanations, or denial.
- There are frequent requests for care or treatment for relatively minor conditions.
- There is a delay in seeking care or reporting an injury.
- The older person is described as 'accident prone' or has a history of injury, untreated injuries and multiple injuries.
- There are repeated accident or emergency attendances of the older person from the same care setting.
- There are manifestations of inadequate care, including poor hygiene or nutritional status, poorly controlled medical conditions, frequent falls or confusion.
- A relative or carer appears overly protective or controlling, or the older person displays unexplained anger or fear towards the carer or relative.
- There is an apparent inability to be able to afford food, clothing, housing or social activities or questionable use of the older person's possessions/property/funds.

(Adapted from Glasgow & Fanslow 2006:34–5)

older person. Important first steps in supporting an older person experiencing abuse include establishing a trusting relationship, and conveying respect and a non-judgemental attitude. Nurses also have a role in developing evidence-based policies and procedures within their organisations to ensure older adults experiencing abuse are identified and supported.

SOCIAL AND SPIRITUAL SUPPORT

Social support is the most fundamental need for all age groups, but especially those who may have protracted difficulties over a long period of time. Sustained engagement with others can help a person manage pain, distress, anxiety, loneliness and loss (Marziali et al 2008). Family interdependencies are also important in managing difficulties in the older years, which is an advantage for those who have had children. A strong parental role can help an older person retain cohesive relationships that provide respect, recognition of their experiences and meaningfulness (Zunzunegui et al 2009). Spirituality is another mediating factor that helps many older people cope with the stresses of ageing (Marziali et al 2008; Price 2009). Private expressions of spirituality, or the communal sharing of religious rituals, such as attending church services, can be a source of comfort and hope for those with disabling conditions, whether these are physical or emotional (Marziali et al 2008).

Faith-based communities promote common bonds of hope and faith, which can be integral to preventing or recovering from illness. Church groups can also act as a buffer for the adverse effects of stress, anger, disappointment, loss and bereavement (Chatters 2000; Levin 1994). Collective worship promotes a sense of community, in helping people feel they are not alone, even when life circumstances seem to leave them feeling abandoned. This type of communal activity, warmed by positive interpersonal behaviours, can be a source of solace to older adults. Many therefore turn to religion in their older years, to work through life's transitions within a community of people who are spiritually similar, comfortable and caring. In some cases, use of the word 'reconciliation' in the religious context is used to introduce spiritual compatibility, or consistency in thoughts and deeds. This helps shape interpersonal behaviours that promote warmth, friendliness, love, compassion, harmony, tolerance and forgiveness (Chatters 2000).

Point to ponder
Respecting older peoples' spiritual needs and beliefs helps maintain their dignity.

Faith-based communities can also be instrumental in shaping behaviours that determine risk-taking or health maintenance, which may include dietary restrictions, prohibition against alcohol or tobacco, or promoting healthy patterns of activity and the values of moderation and conformity (Chatters 2000). However, some aspects of the relationship between religion and health remain ambiguous. For some people, religion seems to enhance peacefulness, self-confidence and sense of purpose, while others are beset by guilt, self-doubt, shame and low self-esteem. These responses may be a result of the interaction between personal belief systems, and those that flow from a religious affiliation (Levin 1994). Irrespective of the source of comfort, there is a need to respect older people, and ensure that all care is provided in a way that maintains their dignity.

MAINTAINING DIGNITY IN COPING
Dignity is also an issue for those ageing in conditions of social disadvantage. Being poor increases a person's vulnerability to the effects of ageing, and constrains their coping ability. Clearly, it is easier for those with sufficient resources to access the social activities they need. For people living in disadvantaged circumstances, being able to connect with others in the community can be a greater challenge. With adequate financial resources there are more opportunities to access social support, which helps people develop a sense of mastery over their lives (Gadalla 2009). Social disadvantage creates even more difficulties in coping with ageing for women, and those with low educational levels (Rueda et al 2008). Many women continue to have responsibility for the household into old age, and this can place a burden on their health. Those without transportation are also at a disadvantage in not being able to get out and interact with others. Another layer of disadvantage for women occurs among those living in rural areas. As high users of health services, older, rural women have poorer health and lower survival rates from disease because of their lack of access to services (NRHA 2009; Vagenas et al 2009).

Personal coping behaviours can also be problematic. Some older adults regularly use alcohol in combination with other drugs to manage pain, the frustrations of disabling conditions, and loneliness. In many cases, the alcohol consumption remains hidden unless it is detected in diagnostic tests, which may not occur until later in life. For some, consuming alcohol may be a lifelong coping mechanism. Overconsumption of alcohol is responsible for a large proportion of the burden of cirrhosis of the liver, primarily in men (AIHW 2008). Alcohol also has a compound effect if it is mixed with other medications, and this is often the case with older people. Many older people suffering from even mild depression are treated with antidepressants. Others may be on analgesics for pain relief, and also on medications for metabolic disorders or cardiovascular conditions. This 'polypharmacy' creates the risk of overdosing when alcohol is added to the daily intake of substances. Being in an altered state from alcohol can also create a risk of falling, losing awareness of the immediate environment, or having an accident such as a burn injury, because of a lack of attentiveness. Many people who consume alcohol also ignore their diet, which compounds their level of risk for illness.

> **Point to ponder**
> Being poor increases an older person's vulnerability to the effects of ageing, and may result in ineffective coping strategies.

The attraction of alcohol is that it works so well. For those with sleep problems, as often occurs in older people, alcohol has a relaxing effect, helping a person get to sleep, even though it is usually a restless sleep. When mixed with antidepressants or other medications alcohol becomes antagonistic to sleep, and can start a cycle of sleeplessness that is difficult to resolve. However, alcohol can help numb the pain of aching joints, and alleviate loneliness where this is an issue. So although it is a perverse solution, it remains a constant in many older people's lives, especially if it has played a major role in a person's social life in their younger years. One of the dangers of continuing to drink large amounts of alcohol during the older years is that a person's tolerance may change. Smaller amounts

of alcohol can cause headaches, frequent memory lapses and reduction of mental abilities (Flood & Buckwalter 2009). Those particularly at risk are those who are trying to cope with a transition such as retirement, relocation, or the loss of a spouse, friend or family member.

CRITICAL PATHWAYS TO AGEING

By the time a person reaches age 65, the cumulative risks from all earlier stages of life are usually evident. These risks accumulate from hereditary predispositions and conditions in the womb; childhood illnesses and injuries; immunisation status; access to education; growth and developmental issues; coping styles; diet and activity patterns; obesity, smoking, other risky behaviours; exposure to harmful substances or traumatic events; socio-economic status in childhood, adolescence and adult life; and a host of circumstances in the home, family, community and occupational environments. Just as these can be mapped across the pathway of childhood development, they also provide a pathway to healthy ageing, as depicted in Figure 9.1.

The 'critical pathways across the life course' model illustrates the parallel influences on achieving health and wellbeing at either end of the developmental continuum. From this perspective, ageing can be seen as a process incorporating events and predispositions from a person's earlier life, rather than a specified stage of life. This 'long view' of ageing seeks to understand accumulated risk and potential from childhood throughout the life course. Tracking the effects of the many

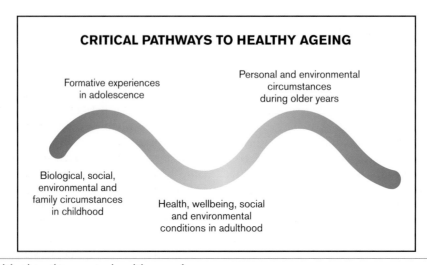

CRITICAL PATHWAYS TO HEALTHY AGEING

Formative experiences in adolescence

Personal and environmental circumstances during older years

Biological, social, environmental and family circumstances in childhood

Health, wellbeing, social and environmental conditions in adulthood

Figure 9.1 Critical pathways to healthy ageing

and varied influences on a person's life provides insight into the social meanings they hold in their later years and how these have been shaped by their biological, psychosocial and environmental experiences. An individual's journey along the pathway is also indicative of how their personal history affects the world around them as they continue to make transitions to the end of life.

TRANSITIONS: CHALLENGES AND OPPORTUNITIES

The critical pathway approach to ageing incorporates various views of ageing. Erikson's (1963) model of human lifecycle stages contends that we all have certain characteristic 'crises' to resolve at various stages of development. In the context of this theoretical framework, the major life crisis of old age is the struggle between integrity and despair, the resolution of which is expected to produce wisdom. But this may be a generalisation of what actually occurs because of wide variability among people's individual responses to the circumstances of their lives (Wilkinson 1996). Some older individuals experience entirely different life crises. Attitudes vary widely, and while some people do not consider themselves old at 80, others believe they are old at age 50. Others do not experience transitions as 'crises', but as opportunities to refresh their lifestyle.

Workplace and retirement transitions

A large, but not exclusive, component of adults' self-esteem is developed in the context of work roles. Occupational roles give people a sense of presence and place. For this reason, the sting of ageism in the workplace cuts deep, and some feel it for a period of years leading up to their actual retirement, and beyond. It is also surprising to ponder ageist attitudes in the workplace given widespread recognition of our need for the skills and wisdom of older adults in many fields of work. Despite the need for older adults' mentorship, and a general recognition that older workers are honest, dependable and stable, many workplaces continue to discriminate against older workers (Berger 2009). Some employers stereotype older workers as being inflexible, in poor health, less productive, prone to accidents, less creative and disinterested in technology (Berger 2009). These attitudes become a self-fulfilling prophecy where older workers are overlooked for employer training programs and promotion. Being relegated to a passive, rather than active, role in the workplace threatens the capacity of older workers to remain socially engaged, especially for those whose lives have revolved around their work role. For those over age 65 the risk of being displaced from the workplace can be traumatic because of the lack of mobility, education and training (Berger 2009).

One of the major challenges for employers of older workers is to rearrange health and safety aspects of the workplace to accommodate employees' needs. Older workers may need to work at slower speeds, with fewer extremes of posture and less cardiovascular stress. They can also have lower tolerance to extremes of temperatures and may need intermittent breaks throughout their shift. However, studies have shown that even though work tasks may take more time, workers in their 60s tend to have equivalent or superior decision-making and other cognitive skills. They are also exposed to the same stressors as younger workers, which, as we mentioned in Chapter 8, are considerable. Some older workers are content to stay in the workplace and plan a slow, graduated transition into retirement. They tend to anticipate retirement as a reward for growing older, embracing retirement without looking back wistfully, as if they were losing a major part of their lives. Many seek this transition as an opportunity to engage in desirable and valued non-work activities, which can balance a number of different dimensions of a person's life and promote personal self-esteem, a sense of social engagement or belongingness, and greater satisfaction with life.

Transitions to single ageing or widowhood

The most significant transition for many older people is the change from a long-term partnership to being alone. In some cases this occurs because of a partner's death, while in other cases it may arise from divorce or a partner's placement in long-term care. Although couples have varied life histories, many older people in this generation have been partnered for most of their adult life, and find the transition from being part of a couple to being alone devastating. It is unknown whether this is more difficult the longer a couple has been together because couples go through variable adaptations in their lives. Some older people grow comfortably content with one another, while others find their relationship more difficult with the passing of time. The latter situation can occur if a couple has enjoyed an active life together, then experience a dramatically changed lifestyle because of ill health in one partner. The healthy partner may actually anticipate the loss of their partner because of the demands of caregiving, seeing the closure that comes with the definitive moment of loss as a step toward a better quality of life. Another dramatic transition occurs in older singles who, after many years alone, have partnered, only to find the relationship short-lived, because of the death or disablement of their new spouse or partner. Included in the anguish of these two situations is the loss of intimacy and sexuality.

Transitions in intimacy and sexuality

Intimacy is an important aspect of self-esteem. For many people, intimacy includes romance, companionship, communication, touching, affection, and a sense that they are attractive and sexually desirable (Rheaume & Mitty 2008). For others intimacy may simply mean feeling close to another, irrespective of the type of relationship. The loss that comes with widowhood is often an intense loss of intimacy.

Both widows and widowers suffer loneliness from losing their partner, but the cause and consequences differ for each. The 'widowhood effect', where a widowed spouse is likely to die soon after losing their partner, is a well known social phenomenon. Even though there are differences between men and women in the widowhood effect, the lack of social support seems to play a role in the demise of the widowed partner (Elwert & Christakis 2008). Bereavement may have a profound effect, creating social isolation or lifelong loneliness after a long-term marriage or partnership. Social isolation is typically experienced as minimal contact with others and low involvement in community life, and some people are content to live socially isolated lives without feeling lonely (Grenade & Boldy 2008). Loneliness is a more subjective state, wherein a person feels his/her level of social engagement is deficient in some way (Grenade & Boldy 2008). The presence of friends or a confidant, children, good health, and a social network are protective factors against loneliness (Grenade & Boldy 2008). Conversely, having no family or surviving children, living alone or having poor health can all be risk factors for loneliness.

> **Point to ponder**
> Men and women cope with loneliness and loss differently. Men tend to rely on long-standing friendships for support, while women rely on a network of relationships.

People cope with loneliness in different ways, depending upon factors such as their personality, self-esteem, capacity for resilience, and their style of relating to others. Access to friends, self-help support groups, home visiting services, or community social activities can be helpful, especially if a person is bereaved (Grenade & Boldy 2008). Men and women experience sources of help differently, and tend to cope with loss and loneliness in the way they have coped with other stressors in their lives. The marital relationship tends to provide the closeness and support men need throughout their married life, and they are often more devastated by their partner's death than women, who nurture a range of relationships throughout their adult lives (Hall et al 2007). However, men's long-standing friendships with other men have been found to be as important to their coping as women's networks (Hall et al 2007). Becoming engaged in meaningful activities after bereavement can help both. Volunteer activities are often helpful. So too, are activities with some economic or social benefit. People who have been in the workforce most of their life tend to gravitate to participating in community activities that are closely aligned with their previous roles. These often reflect the need to respond to expectations of success and competency, just as they have done in the workplace (Hall et al 2007). This type of activity can also provide an incentive to adjust to the lack of intimacy.

An important element of the loss of intimacy is the loss of sexuality and its contribution to a sense of personhood. Not all older people are as interested in sexual expression in the same way as they may have been in their younger years, but their desire for closeness and intimacy is usually unchanged (Rheaume & Mitty 2008). People have a right to intimacy and sexuality throughout the life span. The WHO defines sexuality as follows (in Rheaume & Mitty 2008:342):

> Sexuality is a core dimension of life that incorporates notions, beliefs, facts, fantasies, rituals, attitudes, values, and rights with regard to gender identity and role, sexual acts and orientation, and aspects of pleasure, intimacy, and reproduction.

According to this definition, everyone has a right to intimacy and sexuality throughout their life span. What nurses can do to support healthy sexual expression in older people is support their right to a pleasurable sexual relationship without fear, shame, violence or coercion (Rheaume & Mitty 2008). In residential care, this can be challenging, especially for those with cognitive impairment, but in the community, nursing interventions may be more focused on permission-giving and health literacy. People who may have grown up in a culture where sexuality was suppressed often find ageing confusing, in terms of understanding their bodily changes, and what they believe is appropriate behaviour. Nurses working in primary care or community settings are the first person with whom they can discuss these issues, usually in the context of a home visit. A holistic health assessment may reveal a need for information about sexual behaviour or changing sexual function. This can often include information on the effects of chronic conditions, normal hormonal changes, and/or medications on sexual desire or performance. Any of these factors may affect the health of one or both partners, and their goals for a continuing sexual relationship (Rheaume & Mitty 2008).

Point to ponder
Intimacy and sexuality are as important at older age as they are at younger ages.

For many older people, having a partner become dependent on them for caregiving represents a loss of intimacy, sexuality, self-identity and a sense of the future. In New Zealand 11.8% of people aged over 65 years provide unpaid care for a family member in their own household who is ill or disabled (Statistics New Zealand 2007). In Australia more than 2.6 million Australians care for others because of disability or old age, most (78%) in their own homes (AIHW 2008). More than half of these carers are women, many of whom have care needs themselves. Caring

often takes up to 20 hours a week, which severely compromises carers' financial status as well as the opportunity to engage in paid work outside the home. It is a demanding role, often causing difficulties with physical, mental and emotional health and wellbeing because of caring responsibilities (AIHW 2008).

Caregiving is therefore a frequent source of chronic stress among women, who often go through transitions from child carer to parent carer without respite. Many of these 'sandwich carers' combine caring for both children and parents at the same time, often with few resources (Pinquart & Sorensen 2006). When caregiving is replaced by widowhood, the caregiver's health risks may be compounded by loneliness. Loneliness can cause depression or anxiety, or a sense of worthlessness. At the time of widowhood and beyond self-esteem tends to suffer. Some people neglect their health or discontinue healthy behaviours they may have shared as part of a couple. This is the period when grieving, or lonely, people may also be at greatest risk of allowing their health and fitness to decline. Their needs at this time revolve around social support, and regaining a sense that there is a future to look forward to, and opportunities to continue developing physically, emotionally and spiritually.

Point to ponder
Many women in both Australia and New Zealand societies become 'sandwich carers', caring for both children and parents simultaneously.

Transitions to the end of life

Nurses play an important role in helping older persons at the end of their lives. This requires considerable knowledge and judgement as nurses are often called upon to help people make complex care decisions (Allen et al 2008; Chang et al 2009). These can include decisions about symptom management for pain, physical, psychosocial, spiritual or socio-legal issues, and those related to palliative care. In many cases this type of support is provided in home care visits. Palliative care can begin whenever a person's condition is no longer amenable to cure. It consists of any measure to improve a person's comfort and function, which should be responsive to their unique combination of needs (Chang et al 2009). Palliative care is aimed at improving quality of life in those with a life-threatening illness by relieving suffering, and early identification and treatment of pain and other problems — physical, psychosocial and spiritual (WHO 2002). The palliative care movement has seen the development of palliative care homes or hospices in many communities. These offer an attractive alternative to hospital care at the end of life, but they are not widely available in some settings (Payne 2009). Some people also choose to die at home, especially those who live alone or who have no family caregiver available to assist them (Aoun et al 2008).

The objective of palliative care is to work towards close engagement with the patient and family for healing and harmony at the end of life, especially in accommodating family members' burden of care and cultural needs (Chater & Tsai 2008). Palliative care nurses are highly trained in psychosocial skills, to respond to anger and a range of emotions that might occur from family members who are hesitant to let go of their loved one (Pavlish & Ceronsky 2009). They can help enhance personal growth for the surviving family members if they are treated as partners in care, rather than as merely visitors, throughout this stage of their elder's illness (Whitaker 2009). Because palliative care nurses are specialists in family relationships they can act as a resource for others to ensure that a partnership model is implemented. This type of approach to care includes teaching, caring, coordinating, advocating and mobilising resources (Pavlish & Ceronsky 2009). These outcomes are accomplished with personal attributes that include maintaining clinical expertise, honesty, having a family orientation, perceptive attentiveness, being present, calm and connected, collaborating with others in a way that would provide a cohesive plan for care, and being purposeful and deliberate in their preparation (Pavlish & Ceronsky 2009).

Point to ponder

A partnership approach to palliative care supports both the older adult and their family as the older adult reaches the end of his/her life.

Palliative care is also guided by a set of ethical and cultural principles, as identified in Box 9.4.

BOX 9.4 ETHICAL AND CULTURAL ISSUES IN PALLIATIVE CARE

- Respect for the patient's and family's choices.
- Advanced care planning.
- Integrity and selflessness in caring.
- Open communication; relevant, appropriate message at the right pace.
- Agreed goals of care negotiated between patient, family and multidisciplinary team.
- Attentiveness to bereavement concerns, cultural differences in the requirement for religious and spiritual support.
- Regular assessment and review of goals and preferences.
- Inclusion of those who are resource poor.
- Consideration of rural populations and those without access to care.
- Providing care for the caregivers, such as those who are caring for orphans or children caring for children.
- Tailoring care to the needs of children where appropriate.
- Meeting special requirements of those with special needs such as those with learning difficulties, mental health problems, refugees, prisoners, internally displaced people.
- Addressing the needs of minority and ethnic groups.

(Adapted from Payne 2009)

RESILIENCE AND HEALTH IN OLDER AGE

Resilience in ageing can be part of the developmental continuum if adequate and appropriate supports are provided. From a health promotion perspective, the emphasis in helping people remain active and vital in a community should focus on individual experiences and perceptions. Many adults cope well with normative declines as they grow older, particularly when they occur gradually. The experience of pain, of not being able to navigate the environment or interact with others, are the adversaries of healthy ageing, because these are seen as signs that the body is deteriorating. Pain, in particular, has a profound impact on quality of life. Pain changes a person's lifestyle as it can cause, or exacerbate, immobility and dampen chances of remaining physically active. Effective pain management strategies can support older people to overcome the impact of pain on their lives and develop the resiliency needed to age well.

The most significant societal-level challenge for the next decades will be how to best care for the over-85 age group, which is the fastest-growing group globally (Commonwealth of Australia 2009). Population ageing will require adjustments in pension and income security schemes to support the ageing population. Health care systems will also have to accommodate changing needs. Acute care hospitals will be populated by a large proportion of the oldest old, many of whom will experience multiple health problems. With shortened hospital stays, nurses practising in the community have already begun to provide the bulk of care across extended periods of time for a wide range of acuity. In the near future, evolving technologies and therapeutic techniques will transform home care. Nurses will be part of the rapidly developing models of care that will see treatments customised to individual needs. Their roles will be central to caring for the communities where ageing takes place, supporting health promoting behaviours, and advocating for environmental supports for lifestyle modifications.

Goals for healthy ageing

Healthy and successful ageing provides:
- access, equity, empowerment and cultural safety
- physical, emotional and spiritual health
- adequate financial and health care resources to sustain the latter stages of life
- social engagement
- intersectoral collaboration for services and resources based on individual needs and strengths
- a balance between independent living and adequate service provision based on appropriate technologies
- acknowledgement of the relationship between health and place
- a place to feel safe and comfortable in living a dignified life.

Once again, the strategies of the Ottawa Charter for Health Promotion provide a guide to implementing these health goals.

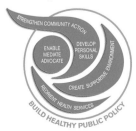

BUILDING HEALTHY PUBLIC POLICY

Involving older persons as partners in health is crucial to developing age-appropriate health care systems and healthy ageing. Older persons consume more health care than any other demographic group. They carry the major burden of chronic diseases and primary care services. But they also contribute to the overall care of the population, especially for those with disabilities. This unpaid work should warrant a greater voice in health care planning, and some older persons do participate in this type of planning. But, far too often, older people are excluded from participating in meaningful ways for service improvements. As a numerically dominant group they should be given greater opportunities to influence models of health care based on their experiences and needs. This will become even more important in future, with the development of personalised therapies from genomics and molecular biology on the horizon. Today's older people may be the first trial recipients of stem cell transplants and other new therapies.

> ### ACTION POINT
> Providing links for older people to connect with organisations that advocate for older people's rights, can empower them to become involved in policy-making.

Like children, older adults are often dependent on others and this does not always offer them a voice at the policy table. One of the most important outcomes of this dependency is that their health, wellbeing, security and wishes are often subjected to the decisions of others. Policies governing the way older adults will spend the last years of their lives should be inclusive, equitable and participatory. Some progress has been made in this direction over the past two decades, particularly with the development of global organisations such as the Associations of Retired Persons, Age Concern, Grey Power and others, to advocate for their rights. The Australian Department of Health and Ageing has also developed a number of policy initiatives to support older people. One is the National Injury Prevention and Safety Plan 2004–2014

(NPHP 2005). Another is the National Palliative Care Program (Commonwealth of Australia 2004) that recognises the specialty of palliative care and advocates adoption of such a model for aged care facilities.

New Zealand's Positive Ageing Strategy (New Zealand Ministry of Social Policy 2001) and Family Violence Intervention Guidelines: Elder Abuse and Neglect (Glasgow & Fanslow 2006) along with a range of publications from the New Zealand Families Commission (Online. Available: www.familiescommission.org.nz/category/topic/older-adults/grandparents [accessed 22 December 2009]) also support the promotion of positive experiences for older people as vital to healthy communities. Policies affecting the older population should also be intergenerational. As Settersten (2005) suggests, policies must move away from the 'zero-sum logic' of political decisions which see expenditures for one age group construed as competing with, or draining support from, another. Having a voice at the policy table may help ensure this perspective is maintained.

Health policies for older people also include those governing safe food and water, clean air and safe accommodation. One of the most important policy decisions impacting on the health of the ageing population relates to housing and other types of accommodation for the elderly. Many older adults move from home to a hospital, hostel or palliative care environment and back to home. These multiple transitions and relocations have distressing effects, particularly if financial support for accommodation is inadequate. Some government schemes have persuaded older adults to sign away their homes to secure residential care. Imbalances in services and funding arrangements have placed many older adults at risk of chronic illness and impoverished large numbers of families. The lack of personal financial security will place an indeterminate burden on society in the future as larger numbers of people require care that is effective, age-appropriate and allows maximum levels of health with minimal risk to both health and finances.

CREATING SUPPORTIVE ENVIRONMENTS

The emphasis in health care has shifted from stemming the tide of disability to examining what will help older people develop their potential for health and wellbeing. Today, society is gradually becoming aware of the need to value older people as instrumental to sustaining community capacity. Older people themselves are also more inclined to consider the potential of modifying their environments and engaging in robust personal behaviours for healthier lives. These include healthy nutrition, physical exercise, low-risk personal habits and coping styles, and a general refocusing on what can enrich rather than compromise their health and happiness in the later years.

ACTION POINT
Spend time advocating for the development of environments that support older people to maintain healthy lifestyles.

Healthy lifestyles among older people are visible in communities that provide environmental supports, such as the beach communities on Queensland's Gold Coast, which attract a large number of retirees. The local Gold Coast Council has established walking trails alongside the beaches, with exercise stations approximately every 10 metres. The stations are equipped with weather resistant gym equipment that is shared by young and old people on a daily basis. The equipment represents a small investment in the health and fitness of citizens that might otherwise be precluded from exercising because of a lack of transportation or finances.

One of the most important areas for supportive intervention is the workplace. Programs like the Vital@Work program, outlined in Chapter 8 (Box 8.1), should be extended to those over age 65 who continue to be part of the paid workforce. As people remain in the workforce longer, employers will need to accommodate any declines in older workers' capacity, including work content or physical loading, stressful work environments and the psychosocial elements of good work practices. They will also need to ensure there is a culture that supports worker interaction and social engagement. Vulnerable groups among older generations in need of supportive environments include the migrant population, the rural population, the economically disadvantaged and those attempting to fulfil casual employment positions.

Another group at risk of unhealthy ageing is the rural community. The shrinking of the rural sector is an issue that has caused many older rural people considerable stress. Away from their familiar space and sense of independence, many experience the crowding and financial stress of the cities for the first time, during and after retirement. Many of these people have led self-reliant and independent lives, yet find their preferences subsumed within lifestyles unfamiliar to them, and they often have the added misfortune of suffering from dementia, depression or other chronic diseases. Often it is these chronic and long-term conditions that contribute to older people making the move from their rural homes to cities to be closer to health services. Age-friendly community networks can help them remain engaged and feeling viable until the end of life.

STRENGTHENING COMMUNITY ACTION

The greatest community asset in many cities and communities today is the vast array of volunteer networks that often provide a critical link to social life and social services. These networks often comprise numerous people having reached older age themselves. Their guidance is often invaluable in helping others make the transitions from rural to urban, home to community or residential care, or to services and facilities they need. Volunteering is one of the most rewarding activities for older adults, as it helps build a strong sense of control. Often volunteers have a deep understanding of older adults' problems from first-hand experience, and they often recognise the type of information or assistance that is needed. They may also have the time and patience to listen when it is most needed, especially for people who may be suffering from depression or other mental illness. Volunteers also develop a sense of self-esteem through their actions, especially knowing the extent to which their input is valued.

ACTION POINT
Encourage older people to volunteer or take up educational opportunities as a means of increasing self-esteem and maintaining cognitive ability.

One of the most vital movements of current times is the response to widespread recognition of the need for lifelong learning, through courses such as those in the University of the Third Age (U3A). Older students are often willing to share life experiences, integrating their insights into course material. Older people also approach learning in unique ways, using new knowledge to forestall deterioration of their cognitive abilities, eager to build linkages between old and new knowledge. Studying and learning helps build cultural bridges, linking personal and public perspectives, and blending emotional insights with enhanced awareness of the world (Wainwright & Williams 2005). The advent of the internet has also provided some older persons with a thirst for even more knowledge, and different ways of exploring the world. Organisations such as SeniorNet (www.seniornet.org.nz) provide opportunities for older people to learn internet skills at a pace that is appropriate to their needs. A recent evaluation showed that SeniorNet has not only enhanced older people's use of the internet to find information and to engage with organisations and agencies online, but has also decreased the sense of isolation older people can feel as they age, increased mental stimulation and improved contact with family and friends (Federation of New Zealand SeniorNet Societies 2009). Some organisations for older people focus on advocacy. For example, non-governmental agencies in New Zealand, such as Age Concern and Grey Power, advocate for older people's rights in health, social, economic and human rights arenas (Online. Available: www.ageconcern.org.nz/ and www.greypower.co.nz [accessed 20 December 2009]).

One way to promote connectedness within the ageing community is to reinforce the value of religious institutions, where this is appropriate to community members. Relocation to a different environment may cause older adults enormous stress if they are unable to retrieve the familiarity of the church, temple, mosque or synagogue, or those who provide religious support. Our role as health advocates should include assessing older community members' needs for communication and spiritual worship. This may involve arranging transportation, social networks of lay people with similar religious affiliations, or visits by members of the church, especially for older adults who are incapacitated and cannot meet the obligations of their faith.

DEVELOPING PERSONAL SKILLS

Building personal health capacity in the later years should be multidimensional, addressing psychosocial health issues, as well as any risks related to disability or poor general health. Priority areas are heart health, diet, exercise, fears or concerns about mental health, substance use and social engagement (Runciman et al 2006). Promoting healthy behaviours at this stage of life can be more effective if the social rewards are emphasised, particularly for those who may be living alone or isolated (Runciman et al 2006). There are many ways older people continue to develop personal skills. When confronted with a serious illness, some will change their lifestyle habits, not always for the better. For some individuals, their decision to become inactive, or to drink alcohol or engage in other risky behaviours, may be a result of loneliness. Some older adults, especially men, shy away from close connections and withdraw from social activities after losing a partner or family member. They often have fewer activities to distract them when they are trying to make major lifestyle changes, and also have a longer history of the behaviour(s) than young people.

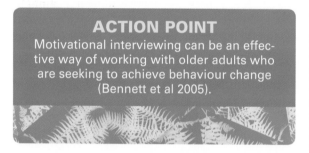

ACTION POINT
Motivational interviewing can be an effective way of working with older adults who are seeking to achieve behaviour change (Bennett et al 2005).

It is difficult to understand the challenges and obstacles involved in trying to unlearn, then relearn ways of behaving. Patience is crucial, and this helps older adults feel that they are being taken seriously. For some, massage, therapeutic touch and alternative therapies provide a remedy to counter unhealthy lifestyles or loneliness. Others respond to a more cognitive, rational approach and can be convinced to reframe the negative lifestyle practice as a threat to their longevity or to the quality of their life. The most successful techniques to help build personal strengths capitalise on both the unique and shared characteristics of people attempting to change. They also place at least equal emphasis on community infrastructure that would support the change. The most important

determinant of change is a sense of control: believing you can change, and that the community is there to support you. Supportive communities are empowering and aimed at nurturing health literacy. Understanding an older person's need for knowledge to maintain personal capacity begins with a comprehensive assessment of personal strengths and barriers to change. This information can then be used to validate their existing knowledge and direct them to access any further information that will help support choices for health and wellbeing.

REORIENTING HEALTH SERVICES

Older people are often inappropriately admitted to acute hospitals due to delays in diagnostic tests, specialist consultations and discharge, and the lack of appropriate post-acute and community care services. The widespread attention to acute health care for older adults has also deflected attention from their health promotion needs. For years, community health professionals have been relentlessly urging governments to deploy resources into community and home supports for healthy ageing, but still, most resources continue to go to the hospital sector. In Australia, it is estimated that close to 20% of those in public hospitals would be more appropriately cared for elsewhere (Commonwealth of Australia 2009). The emphasis on hospital and specialist care has a profound effect on those ageing in rural and remote areas. As we have mentioned previously, community services are often absent in rural areas, leaving them at a disadvantage (NRHA 2009; Vagenas et al 2009). Nurses and other health professionals working with older people in the community need to be vigilant to ensure that rural voices are heard, and that policies include strategies for implementation with a focus on the specific needs of elders (Shaw 2008).

ACTION POINT
Applying a primary health care approach to nursing practice in any setting will help reorient health care provision away from an acute care focus to one that recognises the impact of the socio-ecological environment on individuals', families' and communities' health and wellbeing.

One area where community-based care is well serviced is falls prevention. In Australia, state and Commonwealth governments have deployed significant resources to keep older people mobile, especially the frail elderly. Government initiatives in both Australia and New Zealand are listed in Box 9.5 (below).

Mental health services for older people continue to be sporadic, and community mental health nurses remain the best source of assistance for families trying to manage dementia-related behaviours. These nurses are also an ideal support for family members trying to manage their own anxieties related to caregiving (Moniz-Cook et al 2008; Thompson et al 2008). Working as specialist practitioners, community mental health nurses adopt an evidence-based approach to care. For example, they use validated assessment tools to screen for mental health problems as a basis for care planning. A systematic review reinforced this approach to care, indicating that it can improve the effectiveness of interventions. The authors concluded that without screening tools mental health disorders could be under-detected and under-treated (Thompson et al 2008). Using tools to gather accurate data can provide the evidence for a personalised, solution-focused approach to care. Solution-focused care includes the perspectives of the individual and family members to ensure that their preferences and needs are acknowledged (Adams & Moyle 2007). This information can then provide a foundation for creative and imaginative solutions.

An important role for nurses working in home and community care is to help older people manage chronic conditions and prevent deteriorating health (Mason 2009). Ideally, this is achieved in collaboration with practice nurses and others practising from a PHC perspective. Managing chronic conditions should also include attention to patient safety, especially surrounding medication management. A multi-professional, collaborative team approach by nurses, pharmacists and dietitians is considered best practice (Horgan et al 2009). This approach can focus more comprehensively on risk reduction, educating people about diet and exercise, monitoring and adjusting drug therapy, and helping motivate them to adhere with prescribed medications (Horgan et al 2009; Mason 2009). The multi-professional approach should also extend across the continuum of care, to include acute care episodes and palliative care, involving the older person and family members as partners in care (Hickman et al 2007; Payne 2009). Nurses and/or nurse practitioners are also among the most frequent visitors to long-term care homes. In this capacity they often coordinate care, promoting continuity between services and caregivers (Dening & Milne 2009). Another important function is to draw long-term care staff's awareness to the range of psychosocial issues that may be challenging in care, including the need to provide opportunities to develop new, meaningful relationships (Dahle & Ploeg 2008).

BOX 9.5 FALLS PREVENTION PROGRAMS

- ACT: Falls Prevention — www.health.act.gov. au/c/health?a=&;did=10135884
- NSW: Healthy At Home — www.health.nsw. gov.au/initiatives/healthyathome/index.asp
- Queensland: Stay on your feet — www.health. qld.gov.au/stayonyourfeet/collaborative/ default.asp
- South Australia: Falls Prevention — www. fallssa.com.au/
- Victorian Government Falls Prevention:—www. health.vic.gov.au/agedcare/maintaining/falls/ index.htm
- Western Australia: Healthy@Home — www. health.wa.gov.au/HealthyatHome/home/
- New Zealand: ACC Falls Prevention — www.acc.co.nz/preventing-injuries/at-home/older-people/index.htm

---

ACTION POINT
Use a collaborative approach in supporting people to manage chronic or long-term conditions.

Another aspect of service provision demanding attention is the need to tailor services to the needs of subgroups that lie beyond 65. Older adults are not a homogenous group, nor do they represent a common culture, or common experiences of illness or disability. It is therefore important to assess people's individual needs before assigning them to one type of care. Care facilities are already being redesigned to accommodate various subgroups within residential and semi-residential care, and this is a step in the right direction. Home to residential care will probably be the most problematic transition for the oldest old, and current initiatives for 'ageing in place' need to be customised to individual preferences and needs. Ageing in place is an international initiative designed to allow someone to move to residential care, and then access various levels of care as they age, and their needs change. This type of care will work for some but not all people and services should accommodate a range of preferences and choices where possible. Recent research into the types of skills nurses need when working with older people in residential care settings resulted in the need for advanced assessment skills, the ability to manage complex care, and a focus on PHC and keeping people well (Clendon 2009). Older adults living in residential care settings are, in essence, at 'home'. Nurses working in these settings must ensure the care they provide is based on a PHC approach that meets the complex needs of older adults who have transitioned into this environment, resulting in support for these people to age well.

In an era of protracted economic restraint, increasing emphasis has been placed on community and home care, which increases the burden on family caregivers. These people need ongoing support and education that provides a base of information on rehabilitation strategies, as well as the intervention technologies planned for their family member. There is also a significant need for respite care to prevent situations where they are overcome by the stress of caregiving. Caring for our ageing population requires careful deliberation of the mix that constitutes optimal conditions for health enhancement. This includes access and equity in service provision, empowerment for older adults and their families, and a physical and social environment within which health can be achieved until the end of life within a milieu of encouragement and caring. Australia has made improving older people's health a national research priority, with the interface between residential aged care and acute care a major area for aged care policy and research (Commonwealth of Australia 2008). Our nursing research agenda should also include evaluation studies that link health promotion activities with health gains (Runciman et al 2006).

Case study

In New Zealand, Harold has recovered from his fractured ankle (see Chapter 4), but is still struggling to cope with retirement. He is being treated for late onset depression, and with a little encouragement from Millie he has joined the local gym and started Tai Chi classes. Millie has also had a few problems. She is not managing her diabetes well. She has an appointment to attend the specialist diabetes clinic one and a half hours' one and a half' drive from her home at Nelson Hospital. Neither Harold nor Millie are comfortable driving this far, and they have already missed the first appointment. A second appointment is made, and the local primary health care nurse arranges for them to access a regular health shuttle to and from the clinic.

REFLECTING ON THE BIG ISSUES

- Although there are some common influences on ageing, it is an individual experience, dependent on a person's social, physical and psychological history.
- Older people are often the subject of stereotypical age discrimination in the workplace, in social life and in health care.
- Older people need to be valued for their wisdom, calmness and ability to see life in perspective.

- An older person's health and wellbeing is the product of cumulative experiences, indicating the need for a life course approach in evaluating health and wellness.
- Older people undertake a disproportionate amount of family caregiving and community volunteer work.
- Nursing research has primarily focused on illness and disability in ageing, leaving gaps in our knowledge of healthy ageing and health promotion for older people.

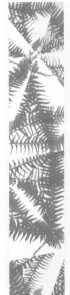

Reflective questions: how would I use this knowledge in practice?

1 What social, physical and psychological influences have the most important effects on healthy ageing?
2 How does the environment affect older people's risk and potential?
3 Discuss the relationship between health and place for older people.
4 Develop a strategic plan for the prevention of falls in community-living older people.
5 How can primary health care principles be used to guide a holistic assessment of an older person's health needs?
6 What are the unique health literacy needs of older people living alone?
7 How would you promote healthy ageing in the community using the Ottawa Charter for Health Promotion as a guide?
8 Outline the types of strategies you may use to support Millie to manage her diabetes.

Research-informed practice

Read Runciman et al's (2006) article 'Community nurses' health promotion work with older people'. These nurse researchers surveyed community nurses in Scotland about their work with older people.

- Do you think the findings would be similar if you interviewed nurses in Australia and New Zealand about their roles?
- The Scottish nurses found a disproportionate emphasis on biomedical care rather than health promotion. If this was the case in your community, how would you go about changing that to provide more health promotion and illness prevention for older people?

References

Adams T, Moyle W 2007 Transitions in aging: a focus on dementia care nursing. In: McAllister M Solution-focused Nursing: Rethinking Practice. Palgrave Macmillan, Basingstoke, pp 154–62

Allen S, Chapman Y, O'Connor M, Francis K 2008 The evolution of palliative care and the relevance to residential aged care: understanding the past to inform the future. Collegian 15:165–71

Alzheimer's Australia 2008 Quality dementia care series: understanding younger onset dementia. Online. Available: www.alzheimer's.org.au (accessed 3 December 2009)

Aoun S, Kristjanson L, Oldham L, Currow D 2008 A qualitative investigation of the palliative care needs of terminally ill people who live alone. Collegian 15:3–9

Australian Institute of Health and Welfare (AIHW) 2008 Australia's Health 2008. AIHW, Cat. No. AUS 99, Canberra

Banerjee S 2009 The Use of Anti-psychotic Medication for People With Dementia: Time for Action. Online. Available: www.dh.gov.uk/en/Publicationsandstatistics/Publications/PublicationsPolicyAndGuidance/DH_108303 (accessed 17 December 2009)

Bennett J, Perrin N, Hanson G, Bennett D, Gaynor W, Flaherty-Robb M, Joseph C, Butterworth S, Potempa K 2005 Healthy ageing demonstration project: nurse coaching for behavior change in older adults. Research in Nursing & Health 28:187–97

Berger E 2009 Managing age discrimination: an examination of the techniques used when seeking employment. The Gerontologist 49(3):317–32

Brockmann H, Muller R, Helmert U 2009 Time to retire — Time to die? A prospective cohort study of the effects of early retirement on long-term survival. Social Science & Medicine 69:160–4

Castles F 2000 Population ageing and the public purse: Australia in comparative perspective. Australian Journal of Social Issues 35(4):301–16

Chang E, Daly J, Johnson A, Harrison K, Easterbrook S, Bidewell J, Stewart H, Noel M, Hancock K 2009 Challenges for professional care of advanced dementia. International Journal of Nursing Practice 15:41–7

Chater K, Tsai C 2008 Palliative care in a multicultural society: a challenge for Western ethics. Australian Journal of Advanced Nursing 26(2):95–100

Chatters L 2000 Religion and health: public health research and practice. Annual Review of Public Health 21:335–67

Clendon J 2009 Enhancing Preparation of Undergraduate Students for Practice in Older Adult Settings. Nelson Marlborough Institute of Technology, Nelson

Comans T, Brauer S, Haines T 2009 A break-even analysis of a community rehabilitation falls prevention service. Australian and New Zealand Journal of Public Health 33(30):240–5

Commonwealth of Australia 2008 Families in Australia: 2008. Department of the Prime Minister and Cabinet, Canberra

—— 2009 A Healthier Future for all Australians. Final Report, National Health and Hospitals Reform Commission. AGPS, Publication No. P3-5499, Canberra

Commonwealth of Australia Department of Health and Ageing 2004 Guidelines for a palliative approach in residential aged care: The national palliative care program. Department of Communication, Information Technology and the Arts, Canberra

Crisp J, Taylor C 2009 Older Adulthood. In: Crisp J, Taylor C (eds) Fundamentals of Nursing (3rd edn). Elsevier, Sydney, pp 219–42

Dahle R, Ploeg J 2008 On the outside looking in: nurses in gerontology. A qualitative descriptive study of the lived experiences of older women with depression living in long-term care. Perspectives 33(1):5–12

Dalziel K, Segal L, Elley C 2006 Cost utility analysis of physical activity counselling in general practice. Australian and New Zealand Journal of Public Health 30:57–63

Dening T, Milne A 2009 Depression and mental health in care homes for older people. Quality in Ageing 10(1):40–6

Elley C, Kerse N, Arroll B, Robinson E 2003 Effectiveness of counselling patients on physical activity in general practice: cluster randomised controlled trial. British Medical Journal 326:793–6

Elley R, Kerse N, Arroll B, Swinburn B, Ashton T, Robinson E 2004 Cost-effectiveness of physical activity counselling in general practice. New Zealand Medical Journal 117(1207):1–15

Elwert F, Christakis N 2008 The effect of widowhood on mortality by the causes of death of both spouses. American Journal of Public Health 98(11):2092–8

Erikson E 1963 Childhood and Society (2nd edn). Norton, New York

Fairhurst E 2005 Theorizing growing and being older: connecting physical health, well-being and public health. Critical Public Health 15(1):27–38

Families Commission 2009 Family Violence Statistics Report: A Families Commission Report. Families Commission,Wellington

Federation of New Zealand SeniorNet Societies 2009 Improving our Understanding of Older Person's Needs in Learning New Technologies. Online. Available: www.seniornet.org.nz/researchreport.asp (accessed 22 December 2009)

Flood M, Buckwalter K 2009 Recommendations for mental health care of older adults Part 2 — An overview of dementia, delirium, and substance abuse. Journal of Gerontological Nursing 35(2):35–47

Gadalla T 2009 Sense of mastery, social support, and health in elderly Canadians. Journal of Aging and Health 21(4):581–95

Garner J 2009 Considerably better than the alternative. Quality in Ageing 10(1):5–8

Glasgow K, Fanslow J 2006 Family Violence Intervention Guidelines: Elder Abuse and Neglect. Ministry of Health, Wellington

Grenade L, Boldy D 2008 Social isolation and loneliness among older people: issues and future challenges in community and residential settings. Australian Health Review 329(3):468–78

Hall C, Brown A, Gleeson S, Zinn J 2007 Keeping the thread: older men's social networks in Sydney, Australia. Quality in Ageing 8(4):10–17

Hickman L, Newton P, Halcomb E, Chang E, Davidson P 2007 Best practice interventions to improve the management of older people in acute care settings: a literature review. Journal of Advanced Nursing 60(2):113–26

Horgan S, LeClair K, Donnelly M, Hinton G, MacCourt P, Krieger-Frost S 2009 Developing a national consensus on the accessibility needs of older adults with concurrent and chronic, mental and physical health issues: a preliminary framework informing collaborative mental health care planning. Canadian Journal on Aging 28(2):97–105

Kerse N, Elley C, Robinson E, Arroll B 2005 Is physical activity counseling effective for older people? A cluster randomized, controlled trial in primary care. Journal of the American Geriatric Society 153:1951–6

Kolt G, Schofield G, Kearse N, Garrett N, Schluter P, Ashton T, Patel A 2009 The Healthy Steps study: A randomized controlled trial of a pedometer-based Green Prescription for older adults: trial protocol. BMC Public Health 9:204 doi:10.1186/1471-2458-9-404

Lang I, Llewellyn D, Alexander K, Melzer D 2008 Obesity, physical function, and mortality in older adults. Journal of the American Geriatric Society 56:1474–8

Levin J 1994 Religion and health: is there an association, is it valid, and is it causal? Social Science & Medicine 38(11):1475–82

Levy B, Leifheit-Limson E 2009 The stereotype-matching effect: greater influence on functioning when age sterotypes correspond to outcomes. Psychology and Aging 24(10):230–3

Marziali E, McDonald L, Donahue P 2008 The role of coping humor in the physical and mental health of older adults. Aging & Mental Health 12(6):713–18

Mason C 2009 Preventing coronary heart disease and stroke with aggressive statin therapy in older adults using a team management model. Journal of the American Academy of Nurse Practitioners 21(1):47–53

Ministry of Health New Zealand (MOHNZ) 2002 Health of Older People Strategy. New Zealand, Wellington

—— 2006 Older People's Health Chart Book 2006. New Zealand, Wellington

—— 2008 Disability Services Draft Strategic Plan for July 2008 to June 2010. Ministry of Health, Wellington

Ministry of Health New Zealand and Statistics New Zealand 2009 Longer life better health? Trends in health expectancy in New Zealand 1996–2006. Statistics New Zealand, Wellington

Ministry of Social Development 2002 Te Rito New Zealand Family Violence Prevention Strategy. Ministry of Social Development, Wellington

Moniz-Cook E, Elston C, Gardiner E, Agar S, Silver M, Win T, Wang M 2008 Can training community mental health nurses to support family carers reduce behavioural problems in dementia? An exploratory pragmatic randomized controlled trial. International Journal of Geriatric Psychiatry 23:185–91

National Public Health Partnership (NPHP) 2005 The National Injury Prevention and Safety Promotion Plan: 2004–2014. NPHP, Canberra

National Rural Health Alliance (NRHA) 2009 Ageing in Rural, Regional and Remote Australia. Online. Available: www.ruralhealth.org.au (accessed 20 November 2009)

Nepal B, Brown L, Ranmuthugala G 2008 Years of life lived with and without dementia in Australia 2004–2006: a population health measure. Australian and New Zealand Journal of Public Health 32(6):565–8

New Zealand Ministry of Social Policy 2001 The New Zealand Positive Ageing Strategy. New Zealand, Wellington

Newman A 2009 Obesity in older adults. The Online Journal of Issues of Nursing 14(1) manuscript 3, Online. Available: www.nursingworld.org/Main MenuCategories/ANAMarketplace/ANAPeriodicals? OJIN/TableofContents/Vol142009/No1Jan09/Obesity-in-Older-Adults.aspx (accessed 4 May 2009)

Pavlish C, Ceronsky L 2009 Oncology nurses' perceptions of nursing roles and professional attributes in palliative care. Clinical Journal of Oncology Nursing 13(4):404–12

Payne S 2009 The role of the nurse in palliative care settings in a global context. Cancer Nursing Practice 8(5):21–26

Pinquart M, Sorensen S 2006 Gender differences in caregiver stressors, social resources, and health: an updated meta-analysis. The Journals of Gerontology, 61B(1):P33–P45

Price B 2009 Supporting patients' dignity in the community. Primary Health Care 19(3):38–45

Reyna C, Goodwin E, Ferrari J 2007 Older adult stereotypes among care providers. Journal of Gerontological Nursing 33(2):50–5

Rheaume C, Mitty E 2008 Sexuality and intimacy in older adults. Geriatric Nursing 29(5):342–9

Rueda S, Artazcoz L, Navarro V 2008 Health inequalities among the elderly in western Europe. Journal of Epidemiology Community Health 62:492–8

Runciman P, Watson H, McIntosh J, Tolson D 2006 Community nurses' health promotion work with older people. Journal of Advanced Nursing 55(1):46–57

Sanchez Palacios C, Trianes Torres M, Blanca Mena M 2009 Negative aging stereotypes and their relation with psychosocial variables in the elderly population. Archives of Gerontology and Geriatrics 48:385–90

Sebern M 2005 Shared care, elder and family member skills used to manage burden. Journal of Advanced Nursing 52(2):170–9

Settersten R 2005 Linking the two ends of life: what gerontology can learn from childhood studies. The Journals of Gerontology, 60B(4):S173–S180

Shaw A 2008 Do socio-economic factors, elderly population size and service development factors influence the development of specialist mental health programs for older people? International Psychogeriatrics 20(6):1238–44

Sinclair K, Hamlin M 2007 Self-reported health benefits in patients recruited into New Zealand's 'Green Prescription' primary health care program. Southeast Asian Journal of Tropical Medicine & Public Health. 38(6):1158–67

Statistics New Zealand 2007 New Zealand's 65+ population: a statistical volume. Statistics New Zealand, Wellington

Thompson P, Lang L, Annells M 2008 A systematic review of the effectiveness of in-home community nurse led interventions for the mental health of older persons. Journal of Clinical Nursing 17:1419–27

Vagenas D, McLaughlin D, Dobson A 2009 Regional variation in the survival and health of older Australian women: a prospective cohort study. Australian and New Zealand Journal of Public Health 33(2):119–25

Wainwright S, Williams C 2005 Culture and ageing: reflection on the arts and nursing. Journal of Advanced Nursing 52(5):518–25

Westaway M 2009 The impact of chronic diseases on the health and well-being of South Africans in early and later old age. Archives of Gerontology and Geriatrics doi: 10.1016/j.archger.2009.03.012

Whitaker A 2009 Family involvement in the institutional eldercare context: towards a new understanding. Journal of Aging Studies 23:158–67

Wiles J 2005 Conceptualizing place in the care of older people: the contributions of geographical gerontology. International Journal of Older People Nursing 14(8b), in conjunction with Journal of Clinical Nursing 14(8b):100–8

Wilkinson J 1996 Psychology 5: implications of the ageing process for nursing practice. British Journal of Nursing 5(18):1109–13

World Health Organization (WHO) 2002 Active Ageing: A Policy Framework. WHO European Office: Copenhagen

—— 2008 World Health Report 2008 Primary Health Care, Now More Than Ever. Online. Available: www. who.int/whr/2008/whr08_en.pdf (accessed 14 July 2009)

Zunzunegui M, Beland F, Sanchez M, Otero A 2009 Longevity and relationships with children: the importance of the parental role. BMC Public Health 9:351 doi:10.1186/1471-2458-9-351

Useful websites and helplines

http://www.alzheimers.org.au — Alzheimer's Australia website

National Dementia hotline — 1800 100 500

http://www.carers.net.nz — Carers New Zealand

http://www.dementiacareaustralia.com — Dementia Care Australia

http://www.depression.org — National Foundation for Depressive Illnesses

http://www.health.gov.au/ — Office for An Ageing Australia

http://www.vuw.ac.nz/ageing-institute/nzag/nzag.htm — New Zealand Association of Gerontology

http://whqlibdoc.who.int/trs/WHO_TRS_898.pdf — WHO Home-Based Long Term Care

http://www.nscchealth.nsw.gov.au/services/hornsby/hkhs/hahmain.htm — Healthy at Home NSW

http://www.health.wa.gov.au/HealthyatHome/home — Healthy@home Western Australia

http://www.nphp.gov.au/publications/a_z.htm — Australian National Injury Prevention Strategy

http://www.nps.org.au/ferh — National prescribing service new resources

http://www.osc.govt.nz/positive-ageing-strategy/index.html — NZ Positive Ageing

http://www.health.gov.au/internet/ministers/publishing.nsf/Content/mr-yr08-je-je099.htm — Australian Positive and Active Ageing Strategy

http://www.moh.govt.nz/moh.nsf/indexmh/greenprescription — Green Prescriptions

http://www.greypower.co.nz — Political lobby group for those 50+

http://www.ageconcern.org.nz — Organisation supporting older people in New Zealand

Section 3

Inclusive communities and societies

Chapter 10 **Health and gender: healthy women, healthy men**

Chapter 11 **Cultural inclusiveness: safe cultures, healthy Indigenous people**

Chapter 12 **Building the evidence-base: research to practice**

Chapter 13 **Inclusive policies, equitable health care systems**

INTRODUCTION TO THE SECTION

This section begins with an explanation of what is meant by an inclusive community and society, and how these concepts are integral to primary health care (PHC). Social inclusion and social exclusion lie at two ends of the same continuum. Along this continuum, people have varying opportunities to achieve health. Social *exclusion* leaves many members of society without the support and resources they need for health and wellbeing. Social *inclusion* creates social capital, trust, norms of reciprocity and cohesion; the essence of a healthy community. These vital elements of community life are important to any discussion of the power relations that exist in society. Gender, race, ethnicity and other issues that impact on social participation are fundamental elements of the social determinants of health. Gender has been identified as a separate social determinant of health, yet the gender relationships in a family and community may be intensified by the intersection of racial or ethnic issues, family conflict or societal norms of behaviour. In Chapter 10, we focus on healthy men and healthy women in the context of these social determinants of health, and in relation to the PHC tenets of empowerment, equity, and equality.

Too often, gender issues have tended to polarise health services and health promotion activities towards either females or males, sometimes at the expense of the other. In discussing these issues within the same chapter, distinctions and areas of congruence are illuminated. This helps our understanding of how approaches to improving women's health, for example, can be used to improve men's health. Although their history differs, parallels can be drawn between men's health and women's health. Both intersect boundaries between various diseases and states of health. Each has issues of sensitivity that both men and women look for in service provision, to retain the personal, private issues that they choose not to share with one another. Discussing men's and women's health from a distinct, but common conceptual framework, such as social inclusion, provides opportunities to identify areas of differentiation and similarity in experiences of health and illness, which often can be relevant to treatment and health promotion strategies.

The feminist movement has experienced almost 30 years of visibility, whereas the nature of the men's movement remains idiosyncratic. A substantial base of research evidence has now been generated to inform strategies for women-friendly service provision, and to preserve the health and wellbeing of women and their children. Despite this relative historical advantage, we continue to live in an inequitable world. Women and children are more vulnerable than men for longer periods of their life span, by virtue of their greater longevity compared with men. They continue to earn less, and undertake most of the domestic work surrounding family life. Women are also excluded from aspects of social life, especially in the developing world, where male infants are privileged over female infants, and deprived of the education and resources that would help them reach their potential. Men, on the other hand, suffer disadvantages because of their socially sanctioned behaviours and attitudes, from risk-taking, to ignoring threats to health. The central theme of this chapter is inequity and exclusion, and the need to draw health professionals' attention to the special needs of men and women respectively, and to the gendered nature of health, and its social determinants. The ultimate objective for society is to ensure equity of access to education, social supports and the environmental structures within which women and men can achieve the level of health to which they aspire.

Chapter 11 addresses the need for communities to provide the foundations for cultural safety, especially in relation to Indigenous people's health, risk, and potential. International reports indicate that there has been little progress in redressing the culturally constructed inequities in societies that have left a legacy of illness, injury and disability among Indigenous people, and those from minority cultures. The factors constraining their capacity for health and wellness are well known. Cultural disadvantage is socially embedded. Redressing the social conditions that create disadvantage is a matter of urgency. We therefore focus on Indigenous people's health as a critical element of cultural inclusiveness. Our discussion revolves around the need to share both the risks and wisdom of each of our nations with one another for mutual benefit and capacity enhancement. The end-point of the chapter is a renewed call to create an ethos of community and social life built on equitable foundations. Perhaps with cross-fertilisation of good ideas, and the cautionary tales of barriers to equity, we can draw into clearer focus, strategies for achieving inclusive communities and social justice.

Chapter 12 provides an exploration of research, its major elements and strategies. Evidence-based practice is outlined as important to informing community health strategies, but evidence is generated and used in many forms. These range from conventional notions of evidence-based practice from comparative, controlled trials of interventions to a broader base of evidence on nursing, midwifery, health management, education, policy-making and implementation. This suggests that everyone working with communities has some level of obligation to be research-minded. We have undertaken a major scan of the nursing and midwifery publications over the past several years, to develop a sense of what gaps remain in the growing knowledge base for community practice. Reporting on this body of knowledge in Chapter 12 is intended to inspire further participation in research by practitioners as well as students. In some cases, research participation will be undertaken by contributing information on the realities of practice to researchers. In other cases, researchers may provide evidence for practice from their investigations. Both are crucial to generating knowledge for practice and translating this knowledge into strategies for promoting health and wellbeing. The challenge to nurses and midwives is therefore to accept a role as proponent, instigator, funder, investigator, or consumer of research to advance community health. When research is integral to planning, implementing and evaluating the merits of community level interventions, we will all be speaking in a language that helps create enthusiasm for change, and incremental development of rational, justified and defensible community health and wellbeing policies and strategies.

Chapter 13 represents the coalescence of research and policy-making, addressing contemporary gaps in our knowledge and areas where this needs to be translated into practice. The chapter provides a culmination of the policy discussions from previous chapters, particularly in Section 2. The chapter includes a critique of the strengths and weaknesses of selected health policies, with recommendations for strengthening existing policies and developing new ones. The convergence of policies also informs an analysis of health care systems. It is instructive to examine the strengths and weaknesses of system-level factors in relation to the needs of communities, to inspire more creative ways of understanding the mechanisms that support or inhibit good health in the community. We address recent initiatives in Australian health care management aimed at developing a PHC approach. This follows a similar approach implemented in New Zealand over the past decade. Although there have been some strengths and weaknesses in PHC initiatives to date, PHC remains an appropriate approach for focusing health planners' attention on the critical needs of a community; access, equity, empowerment, cultural sensitivity and cultural safety, and intersectoral collaboration. Our discussion culminates in a list of characteristics of an ideal health system, so that we can all strive beyond today, to create a better policy environment, more responsive systems and healthier communities for tomorrow.

Chapter 10

Health and gender: healthy women, healthy men

INTRODUCTION

This chapter focuses on gender, the roles of women and men in society, and how this is linked to social inclusiveness. Attention to gender issues is important for several reasons. Gender is a pivotal social determinant of health (SDOH). A person's gender can determine the extent to which they have opportunities to achieve health and wellbeing. People are also assigned relatively different positions in society depending on their gender, particularly in being granted differential education, work opportunities or social support because of their gender. Gender influences can be cumulative along the life course. As individuals develop along the critical pathways from birth to older age, gender, like other SDOH, shapes not only biology, but experiences and opportunities that become reinforced over time. Because men and women occupy different social positions in the household, the workplace and in the community, they are exposed to different risks and potential. Along the pathways of women's and men's life course, gender differences are apparent at every stage, and this is the case in different countries and contexts. These gender differences interact with other life circumstances to create complex webs of factors affecting health and wellbeing.

Environmental conditions play a large part in gender relations, in determining the physical and social geographies of people's lives, and the effect of 'place' on their lives, especially their access to material resources and support. Rurality, for example, operates as a determinant of inequity, affecting men and women in different ways, limiting opportunities for women outside the home and causing considerable health risks for men. Rural communities, such as the one pictured (French Pass, Marlborough Sounds, New Zealand), may be several hours by road, boat or plane from health care.

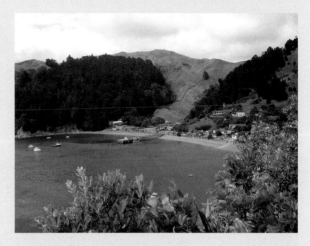

Urban life also creates different outcomes for men and women, most notably in their relative access to sufficient income, appropriate housing and employment. In any environment, parenting is enacted in different roles for women and men, and, combined with socio-economic status, tends to leave women in a more inequitable position than their male counterparts, both within and beyond marriage. At the extreme, poverty affects men and women differentially, with more profound effects for women who are caring for children. This creates a 'feminisation of poverty', as we mentioned in Chapter 5. Women are typically those with the fewest resources, and have the least involvement in the type of health and social decision-making that would help them improve their current situation and their potential for the future. We discuss this in relation to their roles as partners and mothers.

The community is an ideal place to address inequities that arise from social exclusion, particularly in the process of unravelling constraints and facilitating factors involved in developing capacity. Gender equity and differential access to childhood education, health literacy, prevention, care and economic opportunities are pivotal to community

Objectives

By the end of this chapter you will be able to:

1 explain the importance of social inclusion and social exclusion

2 describe the social determinants of health, illness, injury and disability according to gender relations

3 identify the societal factors that impinge on the health of women and men, and how these could be modified to achieve greater equity in health for both

4 explain the central issues that have to be considered to achieve equitable health outcomes for men and women

5 identify the health literacy needs of men and women, respectively

6 develop a community strategy for improving the health of women and the health of men using the Ottawa Charter for Health Promotion.

development, community competence and building social capital. Support for gender equity must therefore begin in the community; otherwise, in this rapidly changing global world, civilisations will grow stagnant. To flourish, societies need to address the way gendered relations interact with other social determinants of ill health, and to seek ways of creating more harmonious, socially just communities.

INEQUALITY, SOCIAL EXCLUSION AND GENDER

In previous chapters we have addressed the link between socio-economic disadvantage and poor health. Social exclusion plays an important role in this relationship. Socially excluded people are unable to access opportunities to become educated, earn a living, receive social support for their personal needs, live in safe houses and neighbourhoods with a secure food supply and a viable physical environment, raise their children in a non-violent home, cultivate friendships, or participate in social and political life.

Point to ponder

Gender, race and ethnicity are important social determinants of health. Social exclusion on the basis of any of these can be detrimental to health.

Social exclusion affects men, women and children in a wide variety of ways. For example, children living in a jobless household grow up with

the risk of becoming socially excluded through a lack of education and other opportunities to change the course of their lives (Commonwealth of Australia 2008a). Women confined to physical work from an early age, such as occurs in many developing countries, are socially excluded by virtue of having no opportunities to become educated or to change their status. Men working in isolated circumstances may be socially excluded because they have few opportunities to find a partner, raise a family or gain employment in a geographic area with social amenities. Members of sexually diverse minority groups such as lesbian, gay, bisexual or transgender (LGBT) are also at risk of social exclusion, especially young gay men who live in environments where there are strict norms of socially determined heterosexual behaviour. Racial minorities are often socially excluded from some of the most significant aspects of the dominant culture, with profound negative impacts on their health and wellbeing. People with disabilities can also be excluded from social participation on the basis of a perceived lack of capabilities. Although social exclusion can arise from a lack of capabilities, it is often the result of a denial of resources, rights, goods and services that are available to the majority of people in society. It affects the quality of life of individuals and equity and cohesion in the community and society (Levitas et al 2007).

Cultural norms can play a major role in social exclusion, particularly in ascribing roles on the basis of gender. In some cultures women's domination by men is responsible for major traumatic events throughout their life course, and sometimes, systematic violence against them. Family violence and sexual abuse contribute to social exclusion, in some cases, pushing young people into self-exile, and, for those who were vulnerable before the violence or abuse occurred, worsening their experience of being marginalised (Commonwealth of Australia 2008a). Men can also be disadvantaged by cultural norms. Rural stoicism and resignation to the hardships of being a family breadwinner is deeply embedded in rural culture, to the extent of being a health risk. The intersection of gender and culture can, in these cases, create health risks that are embedded in societal structures, especially power structures and processes (Kickbusch 2008). Because gender relations are part of social structures, processes, and the interactions people have in their everyday lives, gender is dynamic. This means that a person's gender is not simply a static attribute, or simple assignment of a sex role. Instead, gender is defined in the way it is socially constructed in the context of personal experiences (Emslie & Hunt 2008).

Point to ponder
The division of household labour is one of the most contentious gender issues facing families in today's society.

Life experiences have gendered expectations. For example, the experience and expectations of being a parent differ for men and for women, and these change over time (Vespa 2009). An individual may undergo role transitions to partner, to parent, to divorced person, with each of these transitions shaping the way gender is viewed. For example, researchers have found that the longer single women work, the less they believe they should stay home after becoming a parent (Vespa 2009). This is a reflection of the changes in social life that have evolved with the prevalence of the dual-earner family. Social norms still continue to dictate gender roles, creating pressure on women to nurture, and pressure on men to be breadwinners, with varying outcomes (Loscocco & Spitzke 2007). But as we outlined in Chapter 8, the work–family system is out of synchrony with the way people actually live their lives. Women are changing faster, and men are changing slower, making the division of household labour the most contentious gender issue (Loscocco & Spitzke 2007). A man's work continues to be the way he accomplishes 'gender', and the accompanying power structure that affords him greater prestige and money than women (Loscocco & Spitzke 2007).

Employers shape understandings of gender by providing greater opportunities to men in the workplace, because of their role as a family provider (Vespa 2009). Yet at the same time that women are moving into new roles as family providers, they continue to be expected to undertake the traditional homemaker role (Loscocco & Spitzke 2007). Within the family, expectations are both gendered and racialised, which can affect the way women or men are treated, and how they come to view their role in society (Vespa 2009). In many places, particularly developing countries, women bring home 90% of their wages for household expenses, while men contribute 30–40% (World Bank 2009). Single-parent households headed by women continue to have a high risk of impoverishment (United Nations Family Planning Association [UNFPA] 2000). If societies were truly inclusive, there would be no discrimination on the basis of gender, race or ethnicity. Instead, members of all groups would be equally empowered to live the life to which they aspire (Sen 1999).

EMPOWERMENT

Empowerment is a term frequently found in the literature on gender and discrimination, but often with ambiguous meanings. In many cases, empowerment is explained as advocacy, the type of actions nurses and others take to help people overcome disempowerment (Kasturirangan 2009). For example, in helping women victims of intimate partner violence (IPV), empowerment may be equated with safe shelter, counselling and other support services. As admirable as these measures are, the term empowerment actually refers to the processes by which people gain *mastery* over their lives. It may be experienced as a perceived sense of control, or an actual increase in control over resources (Rappaport 1987). Empowerment often begins with critical awareness, or participating in activities to create social and political change. Some of those actions may be aimed at fostering 'distributive justice'; that is, the equitable distribution of resources (Kasturirangan 2009).

Point to ponder
Empowerment is when a person perceives they have control over their own life and resources. It is often confused with advocacy, which involves actions a nurse may take to help a person overcome disempowerment.

The extent of empowerment that is possible depends on the situation, and the needs and values of a person who is working towards empowerment. For example, some people can be empowered by information and the development of health literacy. Others would be frustrated by such an approach, given a lack of resources or opportunities to make changes in their lives, even if they had the knowledge to do so. Powerlessness is therefore highly contextualised to a person's life. Ideally, empowerment begins with consciousness raising, understanding the oppressive social forces that are barriers to development, taking intentional action to overcome those forces, and sustaining a belief in the possibility for change (Love, in Kasturirangan 2009).

Disempowerment, especially disempowerment on the basis of gender, lies at the core of social exclusion. This is why the power imbalance between men and women is so important. In Western societies, men typically hold economic, political, organisational and physical power over women, and this affects many aspects of their lives. These societal-level power imbalances create multiple layers of disadvantage for women who may have begun life in vulnerable circumstances through poverty, racism or other forms of marginalisation, or whose pathway to adult life may be stymied by discrimination, and other gender-related barriers to development. In some cases, men can be disempowered relative to women; for example, through the biological power of childbirth. Recent research in New Zealand suggests that most fathers attending antenatal classes prior to childbirth found the courses irrelevant to their needs as fathers (Luketina et al 2009). However, given the right circumstances and support, the quality of parenting may be equal for both a father and a mother. The main issue for nurses and midwives practising in the community is that there are modifiable factors in community life that can change historical gender roles, to promote equity and equality of opportunity. To this end, the following discussion focuses on the experience of being a woman or a man in contemporary society, and how these experiences can shape health and wellbeing.

WOMEN'S HEALTH ISSUES

Women's health issues are influenced by many factors: childbirth, gender-linked health conditions including unique reproductive health risks, women's health behaviours, and their social disadvantage and longevity relative to that of men. Women's innate constitution gives them an advantage over men in terms of life expectancy, but the social realities of being a woman can compromise the quality of her life (Emslie & Hunt 2008). Childbirth is the most recognisable biological event for women. Childbirth risks are a serious concern for women in developing countries, but they are relatively low in Australia and New Zealand. However, there has been an annual maternal death rate of 10–15 Australian women, and up to 10 women in New Zealand over the past 15 years, with several other deaths per year indirectly related to having given birth (Commonwealth of Australia 2009; New Zealand Health Information Service [NZHIS] 2007).

Globally, the two leading mortality risks for women are similar to those of men: cardiovascular disease and stroke. The gender difference lies in the fact that women's symptoms may be different from those of men's and they tend to develop later in life (World Health Organization [WHO] 2009). Because of the age difference in diagnosis, and a greater likelihood of co-morbidities, women have poorer outcomes from cardiovascular disease (Reibis et al 2009). Many die of sudden cardiac death before arrival to hospital, compared to men (Shaw et al 2009). It is interesting that women are also less likely to be treated according to guideline-indicated therapies, such as cardiac rehabilitation programs, despite evidence indicating the advantages of such programs (Lavie & Milani 2009; Shaw et al 2009). When women are referred to rehabilitation programs, it is often for shorter periods of time than their male counterparts (Lavie & Milani 2009; WHO 2006). This under-treatment of women's cardiovascular health has been linked to physicians' lack of awareness of risk factors in women, and options for their treatment (Oertelt-Prigione & Regitz-Zagrosek 2009).

Point to ponder

Globally, the two leading causes of death among women are cardiovascular disease and stroke.

The cumulative effects of different lifestyles and health risks from childhood to ageing also affect women and men differently. Poverty is a major problem for women worldwide. The persistence of poverty among women of wealthy nations seems a social contradiction, given the international declarations to alleviate inequality and discrimination during the 1990s. These included the 1993 Convention on the Elimination of All Forms of Discrimination against Women (CEDAW), ratified by 150 nations, excluding the United States and Afghanistan; the International Conference on Population and Development in Cairo (1994); and the Platform for Action of the Fourth World Conference on Women in Beijing (1995) (Lewis 2005). Yet, discrimination against women and the lack of opportunities for them to develop their capacity is rampant around the world. Poor women are sometimes seen as responsible for their circumstances. Being a poor and dependent woman, particularly where there are children to support, attracts a societal judgement that somehow, a woman has a choice, and has chosen badly (Reid 2004). This kind of thinking helps justify the social exclusion of poor women, which becomes part of an endless cycle of deprivation. A woman may be too poor to access the means to manage her life and that of her children, to gain education, opportunities and resources. Inequity is then transformed into a deprivation of basic capabilities (Sen 1999). The gendered nature of the problem has been known for many years, yet the socio-economic disadvantage of many women in many countries, including the wealthy countries of the West, is not improving, and women remain disempowered around the world (WHO 2005).

A lack of education is another risk to women's health. In every region of the world, educating girls is the single most powerful way to promote equitable personal opportunities, and pathways to health and wellbeing. It is also good for the economy, with a flow-on effect for building social cohesion. Women with access to education tend to marry later than uneducated women. They have smaller families, make better use of antenatal and delivery care, and understand how to use family planning methods. They seek medical care sooner in the event of illness, maintain higher nutritional standards, and raise their daughters to receive sufficient education to keep the cycle of health improvements moving in a positive direction (UNESCO 2000; UNFPA 2000). Educated women typically have the level of health literacy to retain control over their reproductive function. They understand the issues involved, the presence of risk, and the steps that need to be taken to ensure health and safety for them and their babies. It is also widely accepted that education prepares mothers in developing early, enhanced child-rearing practices. Most educated mothers have an appreciation

of the need to foster learning readiness and a good preschool foundation for subsequent stages of a child's development (Karoly et al 2005).

Point to ponder

Educating girls is the single most powerful way to promote equitable personal opportunities and pathways to health and wellbeing in any country of the world.

Other risks for women are linked to conditions that affect their health disproportionately, compared with men. As we reported in Chapter 6, boys have nearly twice as many injuries as girls, while girls have higher rates of asthma in their teenage years than boys (Commonwealth of Australia 2008a). By adulthood nearly twice as many women have asthma than their male counterparts (Valerio et al 2009). The development of asthma is also linked to overweight or obesity, creating a health risk that has been attributed to hormonal and metabolic factors. This correlation is related to increased oestrogen levels that are associated with the effect of obesity on the smooth muscles of the airway, and on inflammatory and immune system function (McCallister & Mastronarde 2008). The combination of these factors can impinge on women's quality of life, and cause low self-esteem. Cervical cancer is another unique risk for women, but screening has seen dramatic drops in mortality from this type of cancer (Commonwealth of Australia 2009). Breast cancer is the most common cancer in women, and, because of earlier diagnosis and treatment, deaths from breast cancer have been decreasing since the 1990s (Australian Institute of Health and Welfare [AIHW] 2009a; Ministry of Health New Zealand [MOHNZ] 2009). Lung cancer continues to be the leading cause of death for women. Lung cancer deaths and chronic obstructive pulmonary disease (COPD) have declined in men over the past few decades, primarily because men who began to smoke tobacco early in the last century have died. However, with women living longer, more die from lung cancer (AIHW 2008).

Another impact of women living longer than men is that they endure more years of illness and severe disability, especially for those with chronic conditions (AIHW 2009b). They also live alone for more of their lives, spending nearly twice as many hours alone per week than men (78% as compared with 37% for men) (AIHW 2009b). Women's higher rate of dementia is also linked to their longevity, and they are more likely than men to be in aged care facilities. On the other hand, men are more likely to be hospitalised for mental illness (AIHW 2008). When women are diagnosed with mental illness such as depression, they tend to be quickly prescribed biochemical solutions, primarily antidepressants, without further investigations. Many remain on this type of medication for years, creating the impression that women's mental health problems do not warrant in-depth discussion or longer-term exploration.

Point to ponder

The longevity of women contributes to them enduring more years of illness, disability and living alone than men.

Protracted use of medications for women's depression can be a mind-numbing solution to a problem that may have a social cause, such as workplace stress. Prolonged workload stress in women can be caused by multiple roles as partner, parent and worker (Kostiainen et al 2009). It can arise from a combination of overwork, a lack of opportunities in the workplace, being the family caregiver, or raising children as the head of a single-parent household (AIHW 2009b). Although paid employment is known to promote psychosocial health and wellbeing, a stressful and demanding job, combined with motherhood and a relationship, can lead to increased strain, psychological distress and burnout caused by exhaustion, depersonalisation and diminished personal accomplishment (Kostiainen et al 2009; ten Brummelhuis et al 2008). Managing the permeable boundaries between these roles, and their combined workload can also prevent women from accessing opportunities for physical activity, or other stress management supports (Coulter et al 2009).

Another area of vulnerability is the heightened risk of poor health outcomes for migrant women. Studies have shown that migrant women can be disadvantaged if their health is not considered as important as that of men, because of culturally determined subservient roles, or when cultural norms emphasise a fatalistic attitude towards illness rather than preventative care (Gholizadeh et al 2008). Some migrant women also have personal misperceptions of risk, especially coronary heart disease, and tend to ignore symptoms, rather than seek help. These misperceptions can also be accompanied by poor lifestyle habits in relation to diet and exercise. In Middle Eastern cultures, for example, the dominant cultural expectation of modesty means that women must dress according to cultural norms and exercise in gender-specific locations. This can act as a deterrent to exercise. Combined with these risks, is the added difficulty for women who are from non-English speaking backgrounds (NESB) trying to cope with employment, or other contexts where communication is important (Syed & Murray 2009). Workplace stress may be added to the stress of migration and the need to adapt to a different culture (Gholizadeh et al 2008). Some migrants also deal with the added stress of racism, placing their health and them in a situation of 'double jeopardy' (Syed & Murray 2009:415). Unless they have the time and opportunity to deal with stress, or neighbourhood supports, they may suffer severe health risks. For those dealing with mental health issues or severe stress, being precluded from exercising adds a layer of difficulty to their situation, particularly in light of the therapeutic value of exercise in preventing, or dealing with, stress and depression.

Point to ponder

Refugee and migrant women have multiple health needs that may not be easily addressed due to cultural mores and poor health literacy skills.

Refugee women have some of the most acute health and social needs of any group in our communities. In Chapter 5, we mentioned the social justice implications of holding refugees in detention centres, and the compromises this causes to health. For women, the experience of many months in detention can cause lifelong mental health trauma, which cannot help but affect their children. In Australia, mandatory detention is enshrined in the Migration Act (Newman et al 2008). The experience is akin to immersing families in a prison culture, where infants and children have no opportunities for education or play, and their mothers' role revolves around protecting them from witnessing the 'mental deterioration, despondency, suicidality, anger and frustration' experienced by their parents and others around them (Newman et al 2008:116). In detention, women and children are exposed to multiple suicide attempts, self-harm and other manifestations of a collective depression syndrome. This causes major psychosocial traumas, which often include multiple losses, post-traumatic stress syndrome, re-traumatisation through detention, severe depression, and the threat of repatriation to a country that was intolerable enough for them to risk their lives leaving (McLoughlin & Warin 2008; Newman et al 2008). As nurses, our obligation to these imperilled women includes political advocacy to restore the fundamental human right to seek asylum, as is the case in New Zealand, where refugee policies are more closely aligned with the UN Charter of Human Rights (see Chapter 5).

WOMEN AND SOCIAL DISADVANTAGE

In all societies, women are disadvantaged by their social position. Their sexual norms of behaviour are dictated by clinicians and sexologists on the basis of cultural expectations rather than the way women themselves interpret sexual needs (Hinchliff et al 2009). This is implicit in the pervasive and dominant heterosexual discourse of male 'need' and female 'response' (Hinchliff et al 2009). As we mentioned above, social exclusion also results from being deliberately excluded from education, which occurs in many parts of the world. In the global labour market, including Western nations, women occupy less prestigious and highly paid positions than men. This makes the workplace the setting where gender inequalities have been described as 'both manifested and sustained, with consequent impacts on health' (WHO 2006:v). Gender inequities can be found in many aspects of women's work. Even though women in Western nations are not as oppressed as their sisters in developing countries, the decline of union power over the past few decades has left many women without solidarity

in the workplace, and increasingly, at the mercy of casual employers.

More women than men are engaged in unpaid domestic work, of low status and with no protective legislation and with only fragmented leisure time (WHO 2006; World Bank 2009). Those who enter non-traditional occupations suffer discrimination and sexual harassment more often than men, and earn less money. Women migrants are at the mercy of employers, who, in Australia, do not see cultural diversity as an important priority (Syed & Murray 2009). They are often exposed to hazards that are more harmful to them than to men, because safety standards have been

Point to ponder

Despite growing levels of education, women still occupy the most poorly paid and least prestigious positions in the workforce, and are still engaged in more unpaid domestic work than men.

BOX 10.1 RESEARCHING COMMUNITY SUPPORTS FOR WOMEN

An important nursing study of how Middle Eastern women migrants in Sydney perceive their health risks found that there is a need for culturally and linguistically competent screening and health literacy programs for migrant women to overcome misperceptions about health and the causative factors for heart disease (Gholizadeh et al 2008). The researchers suggested a health promotion approach that would encourage help-seeking behaviours for mental disorders among immigrants, and support for culturally accepted alternative therapies, as well as strategies for managing stress (Gholizadeh et al 2008). Another Sydney study focused on social and health-related factors that affect women's health when they live in disadvantaged neighbourhoods (Griffiths et al 2009). A nurse-led capacity building initiative provided women in this study with enhanced opportunities for social participation. It was particularly important, given that the neighbourhood where the study was situated has a large proportion of culturally and linguistically disadvantaged NESB women. The researchers found that by providing activities designed to promote friendship, social relations, support networks and social cohesion, the women developed a greater connectedness with their community, and had more positive views of their health and safety (Griffiths et al 2009). Both studies suggest that the community is an ideal context for promoting empowerment and social inclusion. Gathering systematic research evidence to identify women's needs and perceptions is a significant step in the evolving nursing and midwifery research agenda in relation to women's health.

developed on the basis of male models (WHO 2006). Women sex workers throughout the world are also exposed to risks of violence and sexually transmitted infections (STIs) (WHO 2006; World Bank 2009). In the family, they are usually left with little choice but to be the family caregiver, because of men's more privileged position and because gender socialisation encourages women to be gentle, compassionate and nurturing (Spitzer 2005).

Homelessness is a major problem for both men and women, but more so for women. The social context of homelessness leaves many women enmeshed in a network of alcohol and substance abusers (Wenzel et al 2009b). Violence and sexual abuse are frequently perpetrated against homeless women, especially those who are lesbian and/ or bisexual, who are over-represented among the homeless (Wenzel et al 2009a). Women, especially young women, are vulnerable to sexual coercion, which can create long-term poor psychological, physical and sexual health (de Visser et al 2007; Fineran & Gruber 2009). Sexual coercion can establish a cycle of health-compromising behaviours to cope with distress, such as drug or alcohol abuse, cigarette smoking, or other self-destructive behaviours, which often lead to further sexual abuse and disempowerment (de Visser et al 2007). In some cases, women who have fallen into this type of cycle, become further victimised by health and social services, especially where personnel have been ill-prepared to understand the depth or breadth of their distress (Adams Tufts et al 2009; de Visser et al 2007; Postmus et al 2009). A further difficulty can be the threat of having children removed from a violent home, which acts as a deterrent to disclosure (Postmus et al 2009; Terrance et al 2008).

INTIMATE PARTNER VIOLENCE AND EMPOWERMENT

Although we have addressed intimate partner violence (IPV) in the context of family relations in Chapter 5, it is addressed here as one of the most gender-specific causes of women's disempowerment. Gender-based violence is an act, or the threat of an act, intended to hurt or make women suffer physically, sexually or psychologically (Krantz & Garcia-Moreno 2005). Marriage is often used to legitimise a range of sexual and familial violent acts against women, and this varies with different cultures. These acts of violence include practices such as sex-selective abortion, denial of the means to prevent pregnancy or infection, female genital mutilation, treating young girls as a commodity-in-trade by marrying them off before puberty, or offering a girl's sister to the matrimonial home as compensation for her death; providing a girl to a family to ensure an inheritance or fulfil an obligation to produce an heir; acid thrown to disfigure a woman because of dowry disputes; honour killing based on the presumption of infidelity; elder abuse; or various forms of trafficking in women and prostitution (WHO 2002). A large body of research indicates that children living in homes where woman abuse occurs are more likely to be abused themselves, to have behaviour problems, and be at increased exposure to other adversities such as alcohol and drug abuse, crime and other antisocial coping strategies (Holt et al 2008). The risk factors for violence against women vary across cultures, and to date, there remains no definitive pattern for predicting which factors will lead a man to abuse a woman. Those factors that have been identified comprise a multifaceted web of causation, where violence is a result of the interaction between aspects of the individual, the relationship, the community and society, as illustrated in Figure 10.1.

The frequency of violence against women has inspired a WHO global prevention campaign to heighten awareness of what has become a major source of injury among women (WHO 2008). Nurses and midwives throughout the world who work in communities are often best positioned to respond to this. Many already are leading advocates for championing the rights of women and addressing IPV, and its effects on health and wellbeing. The research agenda informing their practice is gradually expanding, creating greater awareness of such issues as the link between IPV and women's failure to access cervical screening (Loxton et al 2009). The move towards screening for violence in health settings is also gaining momentum, particularly with research studies indicating that women appreciate being asked about abuse (Adams Tufts et al 2009; Feder et al 2006; Hathaway et al 2008). Nurse researchers in New Zealand interviewed women who had attended either an emergency department or PHC setting to canvass their views of having been screened for violence, and found that 97% were pleased to have been asked about the issue (Koziol-McLain et al 2008). The women

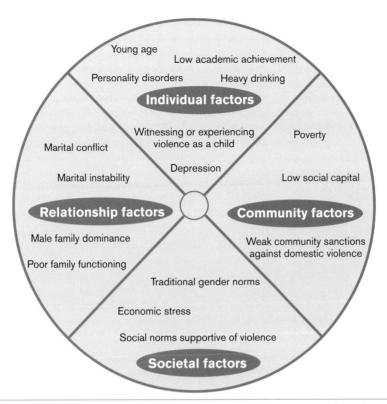

Figure 10.1 Factors associated with a man's risk of abusing his partner (WHO 2002)

reported that being screened afforded them an opportunity to learn about IPV, and the resources available to them. They also saw the screening encounter as giving them permission to talk about abuse in their lives (Koziol-McLain et al 2008).

> **Point to ponder**
> Screening for interpersonal violence is an effective means of reaching women who may be at risk of violence. It also offers the opportunity to provide support and safety as needed.

The New Zealand and other screening protocols are based on empowerment and safety, and ensuring that there are adequately prepared health professionals to be of primary, secondary and tertiary assistance to women. Researchers have found that the services that do have a lasting impact on women's ability to survive abuse such as intimate partner violence (IPV), rape or child abuse, are those that provide for women's immediate needs through welfare benefits, food

and spiritual counselling (Postmus et al 2009). Helping women gain financial independence has also been identified as the strongest predictor of a woman being able to leave the violent partner (Kim & Gray 2008). Economic and social support has been found to be more helpful in the long run, than the punishment law-and-order approach currently used in many places, which often creates more danger for women (Morgaine 2009; Paterson 2009). Financial support and practical services can help women become self-sufficient, and begin to develop self-efficacy and empower them to live their lives in freedom. Once their immediate needs are met, longer-term empowerment can be based on providing them with the opportunity to explore the issues of power and control embedded in their relationships (Boonzaier 2008; Whitaker et al 2007). Support groups, advocacy, shelter, education, legal aid and collaboration between service providers are also important components of service provision (Hathaway et al 2008; Paterson 2009; Postmus et al 2009). Equally as important is the need for mutual support friendship networks, which women often find the most accessible means of support.

> ## BOX 10.2 INTIMATE PARTNER VIOLENCE: THE HIDDEN VICTIMS
>
> Violence against an intimate partner is usually part of a gendered relationship of power and control; typically men attempting to control women. Sometimes gender-related violence is perpetrated on individuals on the basis of their gender expression as an LGBT person. In male to female violence, the male tyrant abuses his power because of an inability to control a female partner. But this may be an oversimplification of a complex set of relations, often defying disentanglement. In some societies where women have low status, men can control their wives through economic dependence, without reverting to violence. In other, more equitable societies where women have well-established economic power and a role in decision-making, violence is also less prevalent. Violence is highest in societies where there is greater economic equality, but where sex role stereotypes prevent women from being decision-makers. Campbell's (2001) research around the world shows that the greatest danger lies in situations where women's status is changing, and in contention with men's status, challenging their control. This often occurs in situations where, after many years of domestic life, a woman chooses to develop her educational and economic capacity by undertaking formal studies, or secures a job that may be beyond her partner's expectations of her.
>
> Another situation that places a woman at risk is family separation. With so many marriages in Australia and New Zealand ending in divorce a large number of households are in upheaval, because of the change to the couple's power relations. Violence in these families, often subjects young children to the conflicts related to family separation. In many cases, they are witness to, or unwitting pawns in episodes of IPV, leading up to family separation, during protracted negotiations, and following the separation. This cycle also repeats itself in many blended families. In the case of culturally sanctioned violence, women and children may also be involved in systematic, patriarchal terrorism in their own homes for a wide range of reasons, usually violating norms of obedience to the perpetrator. For adults, the gender wars of everyday life are difficult. For children, they often have lasting effects. Some child victims of violence grow up to find love and commitment elusive, and often replicate their dysfunctional upbringing with their own children. The cradle of violence in their family lives therefore becomes a cradle of societal violence (Strauss 2001).
>
> In the LGBT community, violence is often perpetrated for no other reason than a person's intolerance of diversity, the inability to control others' sexual identity or expression. Gay relationships have the added difficulty of few available sources of support or assistance. Like women victimised by their partners, the gay victim needs to find a way out of the situation where their life is under the control of someone else. Also like women in an IPV situation, the gay victim may be caught up in a situation from which they can see no way out. Many victims of IPV tend to direct their efforts to reducing the violence, instead of leaving. This is particularly the case for women with children who have no economic resources, and no alternative avenue of assistance. In many violent partnerships, the woman's life becomes dominated by trying to please the abuser/controller. The abuser tries to exploit the relationship, creating further dependency through little acts of treachery; creating a financial debt, or holding her to ransom by excessive neediness or a sense that she is the abusive one. During this time, the situation becomes dysfunctional for both of them, and for the children.
>
> Young children witnessing IPV develop no sense of a woman's experience of self-esteem. They see their mother as a whipping post, and they feel her frustration and defeat. How then can a child of such a household partner develop effective relationships of equal power, characterised by respect, support and a sense of the future? Does this occur because society labels domestic violence a woman's problem, instead of a problem of civilisation itself? If this is society's approach, we pay only lip service to social justice, and the world continues to privilege one gender over another, and prevent alternative forms of gender expression. As nurses and midwives gender-based violence is a human rights issue. Our obligation, like that of other members of society, is to engage in policy debates and let our voices reverberate in the chambers of those who do not appreciate that all people are deserving of a non-violent, harmonious and optimistic future.

MEN'S HEALTH ISSUES

Like women's health, men's health is created in the SDOH, but this is not always recognised. Society is often gender-blind, especially when it comes to the socially determined differences between men and women. It is far easier for most people to relate to men's health, and women's health, in terms of biological factors, categorising health and health needs in terms of their respective reproductive systems or body parts, instead of socially constructed patterns of behaviours. Images of health and wellbeing are also engineered by the media. These images disguise reality, by portraying biologically perfect specimens doing exciting things or, in complete contrast, images of young people engaged in a wide range of antisocial acts. Little wonder that those on the verge of developing their gender identity are uncertain of where to find role models. Some of the most important gender issues for men are bound up in stereotypical roles ascribed by society. Some men acknowledge their androgynous selves (having both male and female characteristics) without a problem, but others experience role strain in dealing with the fact that they have multidimensional, and sometimes complex, character traits.

Will Courtenay (2000), who is one of the leading men's health researchers, argues that social and institutional structures help to sustain and reproduce men's health risks and the social construction of men as the stronger sex. These structures reproduce a *hegemonic* view of gender. Hegemony refers to the fact that men are more culturally valued in Western society, and therefore the dominant sex. Gender, as an SDOH, is one of the most significant influences on health-related behaviour for men, as well as for women, yet common perceptions of gender as a social determinant revolve around women's health. The way men negotiate gender roles actually creates *higher* health risks in comparison to women. The cluster of healthy lifestyle behaviours that men have come to see as synonymous with masculinity are deadly: smoking, drinking and driving, unhealthy diets, avoiding exercise or screening for various conditions. Health is equated with strength and control, illness is not masculine (Nobis & Sanden 2008).

Point to ponder

Men's unhealthy behaviours are due to a combination of social and cultural expectations regarding what is considered to be the 'male ideal'.

MEN'S LIFESTYLES AND HEALTH

Men's lifestyles are also determined by the social gradient, where they sit in relation to socio-economic status, as determined by factors such as education and employment. Men at the lower end of the gradient especially, tend to see their bodies as a work instrument, and large body size as an indication of strength and dominance (Khlat et al 2009). Large body size can also be culturally

mediated. Tongan men, for example, consistently choose larger body sizes as more attractive in both men and women (Coyne in MOHNZ 2008a). Another lifestyle factor impeding exercise lies in men's employment. For many men, strenuous manual work limits their motivation for recreational exercise. Although men at higher levels of the social gradient are more disposed towards physical exercise for recreation, this group also tends to value being physically dominant. This differs from women, who, at higher levels see slimness as a marker of beauty and professionalism, as distinct from those at the lower end of the social gradient, who associate being overweight with femininity, and maternal qualities (Khlat et al 2009). Another distinction between men's and women's 'embodiment' is that in Western society, women's bodies are extensively defined and overexposed, whereas societal forces take men's bodies for granted and exempt them from the same type of scrutiny (Coward in Courtenay 2000).

To some extent men's unhealthy behaviours are due to the greater social pressure to conform, relative to women. Conforming to the male ideal means a man sees himself as not only strong, but independent, self-reliant, robust and tough (Courtenay 2000). In the process, men deny weakness, or vulnerability, assume emotional and physical control, and the appearance of strength. This construction of masculinity has been explained in terms of mastery of self and others (Brown 2009). Men respond to societal expectations by dismissing any need for help, displaying aggressive behaviour and physical dominance, and a ceaseless interest in sex (Courtenay 2000). Although some behaviours are shaped by ethnicity, social class and sexuality, most men also take risks to assert their masculine side. They brag about resisting the need for sick leave from work, boast that drinking does not impair their driving, and dismiss the need for preventative health care, all aimed at maintaining their ranking among other men (Courtenay 2000).

These stereotypes of behaviour can become entrenched in a boy's life from an early age, and subsequently, in the pursuit of power and privilege in relation to women and other members of society. In Western society, boys are often systematically restricted in the amount of access they have to affectionate physical contact. The contact they do have with other boys tends to be either sexualised or furtive, and their sexual expression and intimacy is carefully scripted in terms of heterosexual behaviours (Brown 2009). They are discouraged from expressing grief, and instead, encouraged to suppress all emotions except anger, and to ignore pain (Brown 2009). As a result of this cultural and institutionalised stoicism and the suppression of emotion, boys can develop defensive emotional strategies, and limited capacity for, or discomfort with, empathy (Brown 2009).

To examine men's health issues the question must be asked: what is unique to men that compromises their health and wellbeing, and conversely, what will help men live healthy lives? Most descriptions of men's health issues are problem-based, addressing the 'problems' of being a man, or of having male-specific health hazards. An SDOH approach shifts the problem-orientation, from pathologising men's behaviour as something endogenous, to society (Macdonald 2006). In the context of social determinants we need to reconsider how culturally appropriate, gender-specific health and preventative services can better meet the needs of men, rather than blaming men for their behaviour (Macdonald 2006; Saunders & Peerson 2009). This should be informed by research into the interplay of social determinants, including gender, social class, education, age, employment status, geographical location and community, occupation, marital status, race, ethnicity, sexual orientation and disability and the ways these combine to cause unhealthy outcomes (Saunders & Peerson 2009).

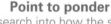

Point to ponder
Research into how the social determinants of health interplay to impact on men's health will enable the development of more culturally appropriate and gender-specific health services for men, moving away from blaming men for their health outcomes.

To some extent, this approach mirrors that of women. For both women and men, low socio-economic status can cause stress, which may impinge on job opportunities, transportation difficulties, social exclusion and the coping behaviours used to cope with these factors. Like women, men can become stuck in dead-end jobs, trying to support a family in difficult circumstances, be relegated to substandard housing, and subjected to discrimination and racism. Their job insecurity

may affect them the same way as women, provoking diminished sense of self and loss of self-esteem. However, unlike women, many men do not have personal support networks, which can further exacerbate their distress, and sometimes lead them to seek support in antisocial ways, such as overconsumption of alcohol or drugs (Macdonald 2006).

MEN'S HEALTH RISKS

The social construction of masculinity does not deny that there are some biological differences. Men have more intentional and non-intentional injuries than women. They die younger than women, with 20% of young men's deaths resulting from suicide, a much larger proportion than women (AIHW 2008). Like women, the main causes of death among men are cardiovascular disease and stroke (AIHW 2008). Deaths from cancers in men are from lung cancer and prostate cancer. Survival rates from prostate cancer are increasing, but this has yet to be linked to increased screening (Commonwealth of Australia 2008b). Because of the persistence of unprotected sexual activity men's rate of STIs is steadily increasing. Tobacco smoking also has an effect on their sexual health, reducing fertility (Commonwealth of Australia 2008b). Alcohol consumption causes the greatest burden of disease among men in Australia and New Zealand. For men over age 18, 62% of Australian men and 65% of New Zealand men are overweight (Commonwealth of Australia 2008b; MOHNZ 2008b). In Australia 58% of men are not physically active, whereas only 45% of men in New Zealand are not physically active (Commonwealth of Australia 2008b; MOHNZ 2008b).

Tobacco smoking contributes to respiratory and heart disease, yet 18% of non-Indigenous and 51% of Indigenous men in Australia and 18% of non-Indigenous and 42% of Maori men in New Zealand continue to smoke. Men are also disproportionately represented in workplace injury statistics, especially in construction and mining. They are also at greater risk of experiencing violence, particularly while consuming alcohol or drugs (Commonwealth of Australia 2008b; MOHNZ 2008b). In summary, the cluster of major risk factors for men's ill health includes obesity, physical inactivity, alcohol and substance abuse, tobacco smoking, injuries and violence. These risk factors, combined with hereditary predisposition and social disadvantage, lead to high rates of type 2 diabetes (especially in the over 55s), cardiovascular disease, cancers and depression (Commonwealth of Australia 2008b).

Psychological health is also a different experience for men and women. In terms of single indicators of psychological health, such as self-esteem, men tend to be favoured, but in the web of factors comprising mental health, men's risks are greater. The social pressures of masculinity, especially in socially dictated norms and roles, create conditions that see many men disadvantaged in psychosocial relationships. Men hesitate to talk about sensitive issues, especially sexual problems, which are often seen as damaging to their identity (Nobis & Sanden 2008). Depression is a major problem for men, especially those in the younger and older age groups, rural men, and those who are veterans or current members of the Australian Defence Force (Commonwealth of Australia 2008b).

Depression is the major risk factor for suicide, and in men, it is often less likely to be diagnosed, due to health professionals' lack of recognition of male-specific symptoms (Men's Health Forum [MHF] 2006). Depression can manifest in aggressive behaviour, obsession about work, substance abuse, destructive thoughts and refusal to seek help. Behind these behaviours may be vulnerabilities that are not well understood, including a predisposition to postnatal depression (PND) in cases where their partner may be suffering from PND (O'Connell-Birns 2009). This context of mental ill health has thus far been virtually ignored in the health care system. Similarly, attention to the psychological and physical health of single fathers has been overlooked, yet the same factors of low income, unemployment, social isolation, and child care affect both men and women as single heads of the household (Janzen et al 2006). Women rely heavily on friends for support, but men's inclination when they are depressed is often to camouflage their need, especially rural-living men. This prevents them from accessing the most important elements that would help develop resilience: social support and a sense of belonging (McLaren & Challis 2009). Men's psychological health is further jeopardised by a lack of appropriate counselling services. Whereas women-only services have been developed to help women feel comfortable in treatment and screening, generally, equivalent services for men have yet to emerge, but where they do exist, they tend to be those of urologists, or sexual dysfunction clinics. This underlines the inverse care law: those who most need help are least likely to receive it (O'Connell-Birns 2009).

Point to ponder

Depression may manifest itself among men in different ways from women. Health professionals need to be able to recognise male-specific symptoms and risk situations in order to be able to provide appropriate care.

MASCULINITY, BEHAVIOUR AND THE MEN'S HEALTH MOVEMENT

As most people are aware, the women's movement was successful in raising consciousness across many societies, which for many years, excluded women from various aspects of everyday life, for no reason other than gender. The women's movement has not succeeded in achieving gender parity in the workplace, and stereotypical behaviours continue. However, the increased awareness has been a major step forward. A similar men's movement began in the early 1990s, and within a decade, there has been a groundswell of support to better understand men and their health needs. Like the women's movement, men themselves have mounted a grassroots effort to draw attention to the issues that affect their health and wellbeing. Their voices are joined by those of health professionals who are trying to help nurture changing perspectives, and help men become empowered to live the lives they seek.

Most agree that men's distinctive characteristics involve risk and risk-taking, and they must deal with the challenges surrounding various notions of masculinity, and how these inform behaviours. In some cases, their risk-taking is scorned; attributed to men behaving badly (Courtenay 2000). In others it is reified, confronted, and men become pushed to extremes. The men's movement is not about entrenching or excusing the old traditional way of using their masculinity for self-aggrandisement. Nor does it revolve around the 'sensitive new age guy' approach, which, in the guise of learning more intimate ways of relating, actually reinforces the masculine privileged power relationship to dominate the emotional agenda by eliciting support from women (Brown 2009:126). Instead, the new men's movement situates men, and their behaviours, within social space and time, and frames their health within an SDOH approach, to create deep understandings of how behaviour is shaped by the environment, and the interactions that take place there.

The men's health movement, and the broader men's movement, has drawn attention to a number of important issues, including issues of masculinity involved in parenting. It has normalised the idea of men being increasingly involved in parenting, albeit without concomitant participation in domestic work. The effect on children is significant, particularly where children have the benefit of close relationships with both parents. Parenting provides an avenue of support for men's health by giving them an opportunity to express human warmth, and to receive positive gains from the affection of their children. This has been the subject of research in New Zealand, where men interviewed about barriers to parenting, felt that society did not recognise the importance of fathers, and that the media portrayed them in a poor light (Luketina et al 2009). Because this negative media portrayal can affect men's relationships with their children, there is a need to ensure that men's health policies are justified, and targeted appropriately (Luketina et al 2009). With an evolving research base, some medical practitioners are developing an increased awareness of men's needs, especially the need for primary prevention (Mao et al 2009). At the societal level, there is widespread recognition of the importance of a holistic view of health, which, for men, would include their psychological and social relations as equally as important as the way they should be taking care of their bodies. The men's movement has not been inspired by the type of oppression that led women to rebel against the system, as men continue to dominate political, economic and social affairs. The campaign for men's health seems more appropriately directed towards the health of individual men, and the social conditions that will enable them to thrive, and co-exist with women, in enabling communities that protect and support both.

THE NEED FOR MEN'S AND WOMEN'S HEALTH POLICIES

Among the positive outcomes of the men's movement in Australia is development of a men's health policy. This was fully developed in 2010, on the basis of four foundation principles: gender equity, a focus on prevention, a strong and emerging evidence-base for men's health, and an action plan to address need across the life course (www.health.gov.au/menshealthpolicy). It is accompanied by national guidelines 'Social Determinants and Key Actions Supporting Male Health' (www.health.gov.au/malehealthpolicy). This first National Male Health Policy will be matched by the new national women's health policy, which is in the process of being redeveloped 20 years after the first version of an Australian women's health policy (Commonwealth of Australia 2008b). The main priorities for the women's health policy are to promote women's participation in health decision-making and management. It is intended to create a social context for women to play a full role in Australian life, in economic, social, psychological and political terms (Commonwealth of Australia 2008c). The women's health policy mirrors the policy for men, in addressing gender equity, prevention, the need for an evidence base, health equity for women, and a life course approach. Both policies are framed within a social inclusion agenda, and each addresses Indigenous disadvantage, as well as issues related to gender, and vulnerability among migrants, and those living in rural areas. A major potential of these policies is the opportunity to accept the recommendations of the Australian Women's Health Unit, to develop a gender health focus at state and Commonwealth government levels, rather than two separate health units focusing on women's and men's health respectively (Australian Women's Health Network [AWHN] 2009).

MEN, WOMEN AND INTIMACY

Gender issues come into full focus around the time of adolescence, when young men and women become sexually active. However, this precarious time in a young person's life is traversed differently for males and females. At adolescence, sexuality and intimacy are often confused, as media images of blatant sexuality often overwhelm young people's attempts to distinguish between the two. It is ironic that today, overt images and actions portrayed on television and music videos, show young men and women acting out sexually

Point to ponder

The men's health movement examines men's behaviour in light of the environmental circumstances of their lives and the interactions that take place in these environments. This should inform the development of new approaches to men's health and wellbeing.

explicit roles, often with the woman as initiator in sexual encounters, when the reality is that many young women today still see themselves as passive objects of male sexual desire (Jackson & Cram 2003). This reflects a double standard that remains unchanged from previous generations.

Intimacy seems to come easier to girls' lives, especially in the closeness of female friendships that have no parallel in the lives of young boys. Boys may become more intimate as they reach adulthood, but for many, especially those without access to a father figure, the risk of idealising a 'tough guy' image is high. Fuller (2002) explains this as a subconscious inner dialogue boys sometimes have with themselves, especially if they are the only male in the household. Their self-talk revolves around the thought that 'If I can't be with Dad, I'll try to be like what I think a real man's Dad should be' (Fuller 2002). Often the consequence of this type of thinking is a tenuous distancing from their mothers, through a combination of rage, misogyny and homophobia. At this time, young boys are in danger of developing lifelong antipathy towards women. This is why they need positive male role models, such as male teachers, male coaches or others in their lives who can provide alternatives to the 'tough guy' persona, and show a more respectful, sensitive side (Fuller 2002).

GENDER ISSUES AMONG SEXUALLY DIVERSE POPULATIONS

The health of members of LGBT populations is a particular challenge, because they are marginalised in Western societies like Australia and New Zealand, by discrimination and social exclusion. Although women and men within these groups have distinctive needs, as a group they have an additional illness burden related to their sexual identities and expressions. The socially patterned discrimination that exists in many aspects of their lives leads to heightened risks of violence, social invisibility and marginalisation, isolation, self-denial, guilt and internalised homo/bi/trans/ phobias (Mule et al 2009).

The negative health effects that arise from the social sanctions on their lives have been documented as high rates of drug and alcohol consumption, elevated risks of STIs from unprotected sexual activity, and high rates of depression and suicide (Mule et al 2009). The social determinants of sexually diverse populations are intensified by the fact

that their education and career opportunities may be affected by the prejudice and phobic reactions they have experienced at school, in the workplace or in the community (Mule et al 2009). As we mentioned previously, many young sexually diverse people become homeless, creating a plethora of health problems. In addition, young gay men are victims of approximately one-third of all sexual assaults in Australia (Commonwealth of Australia 2008b).

Gender inequalities and prejudice can also be multiplied for lesbian and bisexual women, members of racial and ethnic minorities, those with disabilities or those excluded from services and support, such as occurs in rural areas (Mule et al 2009). Another group that suffers from prejudice is the children of sexually diverse parents. Many do not identify as gay, but spend their lives concealing the sexual orientation of their parents as a way of preventing bullying or overt discrimination. Their problems can also be exacerbated where they have a non-resident parent, and they are challenged to communicate across settings and across gender groups (Weber 2009). For many of these children, the school nurse is one of the few sources of support and empowerment, to help them deal with other non-diverse peers, and to help them maintain perspective and mental health (Weber 2009).

> **Point to ponder**
> Lesbian, gay, bisexual and transgender people are at increased risk of a range of mental and physical health manifestations due to the existence of discrimination and social exclusion practices in the wider society.

Mental health issues have a major impact on the lives of sexually diverse people. Gay men aged 18–48 have been found to suffer from anger, anxiety, negative self-esteem, emotional instability and lack of emotional responsiveness, in addition to the depression and suicide tendencies found in other sexually diverse groups (Bybee et al 2009). The effects of discrimination are also worse for gay men than sexually diverse women, who also suffer, but the relationship of sexual orientation to their emotional problems is not as clear. To some extent this is because lesbian women have been regarded as part of the 'gay' community, and invisible in their own right (MacDonnell 2009). Both males and females suffer from the identity confusion and turmoil of adolescence, and adding discrimination to the mix can be a heavy burden. Bybee et al's (2009) body of research has found that chronic shame and guilt underlie many of gay men's problems. As gay men age, they tend to develop greater self-acceptance. Although life gets easier as they age, ageism in some communities can add insult to a lifetime of discrimination.

The years of young, gay adulthood can be guilt-ridden out of shame, guilt associated with deception, or fear of being disowned, fired from a job, or physically attacked (Bybee et al 2009). According to these researchers, the shame they may feel can be destructive. It can arise from multiple factors, parental admonishment, being preoccupied with others' negative evaluation, embarrassment, being belittled, and feeling that they have gone against social norms. Guilt can then emerge from feelings of regret and remorse, as the gay person continues to conceal his sexual identity. Coming-out, or another scarring event such as an HIV-related bereavement, or a personal diagnosis of HIV, can lead a gay person to experience enduring anger and ongoing guilt, which inflicts a major assault on a man's mental health (Bybee et al 2009). These events can establish a vicious cycle of depression, stress, social exclusion and sexual dysfunction (Mao et al 2009).

Because sexually diverse people have not been recognised as an identifiable population group for health care, their health needs are virtually ignored in mainstream service planning (Mule et al 2009). As a group, they under-utilise health services, often because of a lack of confidence and systemic discrimination, which leaves some with sub-standard care. Because of typical patterns of medical history taking, their gender identity, sexual orientation and health-related behaviour or circumstances are often overlooked. This leaves health problems undiagnosed, misdiagnosed, or untreated, especially where risky sexual practices have not been identified. Another issue is that, in treating sexually diverse people the same as others, health professionals do not develop familiarity with some of the most significant issues that may be affecting their health (Mule et al 2009). Current attempts to redress this situation include research and practice debates to help empower members of these groups by educating PHC providers and other members of the multidisciplinary health care team, to provide a more comprehensive approach to their care (Mao et al 2009). Because health services are generally based on the expectation that most clients are

> **BOX 10.3** A PORTRAIT OF THE WHOLE FAMILY
>
> Despite many of the negative health impacts attributable to being LGBT, there have been attempts to explore why some of these occur and how they can be addressed. 'Lavender Islands: A Portrait of the Whole Family', was the first national strengths-based study of the lives of LGB people in New Zealand. The Massey University based researchers consulted widely with LGB people in New Zealand, to develop a survey that explored the everyday lives of LGB people and their families. The study explored aspects of LGB life, including identity and self-definition, families of origin, immigration and internal migration, relationships and sexuality, wellbeing, politics, education, income, community connections, and challenges. In general, findings indicated that the LGB population in New Zealand are a robust, highly educated, relatively high income, politically active community. The study found significant differences in the ways male and female respondents experienced same sex relationships and identity. One of the key areas explored in the study was the perceptions of LGB people of PHC providers. Female participants in particular, indicated that the attitude of their health care provider toward their non-heterosexuality identity was important in their selection of provider. Many health care providers assumed that women presenting for care were heterosexual, and this has major implications for their overall health care and management (Neville & Henrickson 2006). There have been a range of publications from the study and many of them can be found on the Lavender Islands website: http://lavenderislands.massey.ac.nz

heterosexual, it is important that nurses and others ensure that they use inclusive language, and that questions regarding sexuality and sexual orientation are included in assessment processes.

GENDERING SOCIETY: GOALS FOR THE HEALTH OF MEN AND WOMEN

- Eliminating all forms of gender bias.
- Public awareness of the need for gender-sensitivity in health.
- Health literacy, targeting the fundamental issues related to gender equality, such as poverty and social exclusion.

- Equal access to fair conditions and fair remuneration in the workplace.
- Gender equality in power and decision-making in the family.
- Eliminating all forms of discrimination and violation of human rights.
- Heightening awareness of the gender bias inherent in globalisation.
- Gendering the social and political debates on child care, gun control, crime prevention, transportation, education and other forums for intersectoral collaboration.
- Heightening awareness of linkages between health, health care, cultural norms and human rights.
- Promoting the health and safety of all family members, free from violence in the home.
- National child care strategies accommodating the needs of different family types.
- Healthy, just and equitable public policies (UNFPA 2000).
- To overcome the stereotypes that are the basis of many existing health promotion campaigns in our Western societies, it is appropriate to situate health initiatives for both women and men within the broader framework of the Ottawa Charter for Health Promotion (Smith & Robertson 2008).

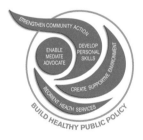

BUILDING HEALTHY PUBLIC POLICY

Gender-sensitive communities emerge from conditions where everyone has an equal opportunity in their daily lives. Affirmative action policies and other policy initiatives aimed at enhancing equality are all steps in the right direction, but to have sufficient impact, gender considerations, as well as policies that promote social participation by vulnerable groups, should be integrated across all policy developments. This is the 'health in all policies' approach. In Europe, every three years, member states report to the European Union (EU)

Commission on what measures they have taken, and are planning to achieve, on common EU objectives for social security and social inclusion. This is a major initiative at a cross-national level to embed social inclusion in all policies. As one of the most socially equitable countries in the world, Sweden's agenda for social inclusion is exemplary. It includes a strong foundation for evaluation of existing policies for social inclusion, and an action strategy that improves social inclusion and reduces exclusion for vulnerable people. The country also has a national strategy for pensions to ensure financial sustainability of older persons, and a national strategy for health care and long-term care for those in need (Swedish Ministry of Health and Social Affairs 2008).

> **ACTION POINT**
> Work to ensure all policy initiatives aimed at enhancing equality integrate gender issues into their framework.

Australia is in the early stages of its social inclusion policy development. In 2009 the Commonwealth government developed a social inclusion committee, with representation from many health policy leaders throughout the country (www.socialinclusion.gov.au [accessed 5 June 2010]). State and territory health departments are also including equity initiatives in some of their policies. In general, healthy policies to accommodate gender disadvantage or social exclusion are those that are designed around distribution justice, redistributing wealth, opportunity and support services where they are most needed, and rearranging structural conditions to create more equitable conditions for health. The public sector can take a lead in reframing workplace policies, for example, around gender issues (Connell 2006).

Policy issues should be developed collaboratively, and focus on education, wage parity, safety, self-respect, parental leave, eliminating discrimination among same-sex couples, providing culturally and gender-sensitive choices for reproductive health, better subsidies for child care, services for supporting parents, and refuge and other supports for those escaping violence in the home. At the community level, men and women would be supported by safe neighbourhoods and adequate housing, crime prevention, and food supplementation and crisis care, especially for the homeless. The current initiatives of the Women's and Men's Health Movements in Australia, to combine gender issues within government departments at the state and Commonwealth levels, provide opportunities to embed gender considerations in all policies. Together, advocates for men's and women's health would be a powerful alliance; one with the potential to advocate for gender equality, and the way gender intersects with other policies that address racism, and other forms of disadvantage. These include policies for occupational health, migration, Indigenous health, mental health, criminal justice, and health and social services.

Policies governing the organisation and delivery of health promotion programs should also incorporate gender sensitivity. This includes drug and alcohol programs, smoking interventions, and programs against violence and sexual assault, all of which need to be cognisant of the special needs of men and women respectively. Likewise, policies that frame preventative screening for certain diseases, such as diabetes, CVD and various types of cancer, should ensure that gender-specific initiatives are developed, funded and evaluated in terms of their applicability for women and for men. To reconceptualise men's health promotion in terms of gender relations requires interdisciplinary collaboration, and synthesis of different disciplinary ideas. The combination of perspectives would help health promotion practitioners to acknowledge diversity and the wide range of influences on identity, such as sexuality, ethnicity, disability and social class (Smith & Robertson 2008).

As mentioned previously, workplace policies should be inclusive, but special emphasis may have to be placed on the needs of migrant and minority group workers, who often neglect their health needs to a greater extent than others. Policies in the workplace can be aimed at integrating health into safety training, and ensuring that occupational health and safety personnel have a broad enough brief to conduct opportunistic assessments of health problems and make appropriate recommendations or referrals. As we mentioned in Chapter 5, family-friendly workplaces should satisfy parental preferences for type and hours of care, with effective quality standards imposed and monitored across all types of care (Adema 2005). Ultimately, healthy public policies also promote

freedom, which is the capability to live a life one has reason to value (Sen 1999).

In civilised societies, policies to overcome domestic violence, especially IPV, are crucial. Humanitarian, as well as economic reasons, indicate the need for renewed interest in policies to reduce violence in any setting where it occurs. Some balance should be struck between zero tolerance policies that are focused exclusively on punitive measures for perpetrators of violence, and taking too lenient an approach, so there are few deterrents to committing acts of violence. A balanced, long-term solution involves government legislation designed to enforce punishment with mandatory retraining for those committing violent offences against intimate partners, children or members of the public. In addition to the punitive measures, policies to protect women need to acknowledge the structural causes of violence. They need the support of both men and women to mobilise resources at the community level that will enhance awareness, and provide not only refuge, but treatment and justice forums, wherein people can address the threats to community life from violence in the family (Paterson 2009). The Family Violence Intervention guidelines for health professionals developed by the New Zealand Ministry of Health provide an example of how an integrated approach to family violence can be achieved (documents available at: www.moh.govt.nz/familyviolence).

CREATING SUPPORTIVE ENVIRONMENTS

Gender equity requires an *enabling*, rather than discriminatory, society (United Nations Development Fund for Women [UNIFEM] 2005). Men's and women's health concerns need to be equally embedded in an ecological perspective. Supportive environments are those that provide material support for those most vulnerable, such as the mentally ill, older persons and the homeless. A supportive environment may begin at birth, with accurate assessments of family need, and then extend through many variations across a child's life course. Environments supportive of early childhood and parenting are typically community-based, informal groups, parents groups or exercise groups that bring young families together. However, many are focused on mothers, and in today's environments, fathers may be the primary caregiver, so there is a need for gender sensitivity in those neighbourhoods where encouragement is necessary to foster the participation of all families.

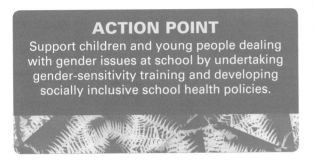

ACTION POINT

Support children and young people dealing with gender issues at school by undertaking gender-sensitivity training and developing socially inclusive school health policies.

Supportive schools are integral to healthy environments, and the expanded role of the school nurse provides a link between health and education that is crucial for young boys and girls. Other sectors can also be brought into the school environment, including the police, social workers, and others involved in providing community support, who are often significant role models for gender-appropriate behaviours. Within the microcosm of the school, gender issues are exposed and, given the right resources, resolved. This requires strong alliances for anti-bullying programs, support for educating teenage girls who become pregnant, and sensitive counselling for children who may be caught in family conflicts over separation, divorce, blended families, child abuse or gender-identity issues. The role of the school nurse is crucial for children of sexually diverse parents. Some of these children have suffered from relationship breakdowns that are very different from those of their friends. For example, the change to family structure precipitated by a separation that leads to gender changes in parenting, such as a change to being parented by a mother and her lesbian partner. This is difficult for children to accommodate, especially if they are young adolescents on the verge of developing their own identity. A supportive school environment can make the difference between whether or not such a child becomes resilient or socially withdrawn (Weber 2009). Research has shown that the main risk for these children is school bullying by same-age peers (Weber 2009). They also experience divided loyalties, especially where they have been exposed to marital separation and custody issues. Gender-sensitivity training can help school nurses become aware of the type and extent of problems they may

experience, and help them develop health literacy and relationship skills (Weber 2009).

Older men and women also have particular needs, which they may only find in the neighbourhood. For example, with older women especially, the safety of public transport systems is an issue. For older men, there is often a danger of becoming recluse, especially older widowers, who tend to grieve for long periods after losing a spouse. In these cases, supportive environments are those in which neighbourhood residents take responsibility for checking on older residents, especially where it is known that no relatives are visiting on a regular basis. With the pace of community life, it is more important than ever for members of the neighbourhood to keep an eye out for the needs of older people, and to understand the gendered health issues that may keep them inside.

STRENGTHENING COMMUNITY ACTION

Community action on gender issues is being implemented at the global and local levels. Global initiatives to address gender issues include a global

---

BOX 10.4 GLOBAL GENDER ACTION PLAN

1 No compromise on global gender equality goals and international commitments.

2 Promote the full integration of gender equality principles into national and regional economic policies.

3 Prioritise girls' education from their earliest years through to adolescence and beyond.

4 Maintain national social protection programs and safeguard social services.

5 Scale up investment in young women's work opportunities.

6 Support young women workers and ensure they get decent pay and conditions.

7 Invest in young women's leadership.

8 Ensure equality for girls and young women in land and property ownership.

9 Count and value girls and young women's work through national and international data disaggregation.

10 Develop and promote a set of practical global guiding principles on girls and young women at work (World Bank 2009).

charter for investment in girls: a 10-point action plan. This is a call for all countries of the world to reduce the disparities and social inequities confronted by women, especially in developing countries. The action plan includes 10 resolutions (see Box 10.4)

A broad, intersectoral network of planning officials in Canada have developed the Inclusive Cities Canada (ICC) initiative, which is a major step forward in providing advice and support on those features of community life that can promote social inclusion (Hancock 2009; O'Hara 2006). The ICC initiative revolves around five dimensions of social inclusion: institutional recognition of diversity, opportunities for human development, quality of civic engagement, cohesiveness of living conditions, and adequacy of community services (O'Hara 2006). These five dimensions all reflect the association between the SDOH, and the need for communities to promote citizenship, solidarity and equality. The ICC is a model for communities in other countries. Its measurable outputs include the effectiveness of policies that address racism and diversity, resources for vulnerable populations, the effectiveness of public participation and shared-decision-making, income and housing indicators, and culturally sensitive policies, programs and strategies adopted by community organisations. These are all applicable to Australia and New Zealand goals for strengthening community action. A similar type of initiative is that developed by the Victorian Health Department, 'A Fairer Victoria' (Online. Available: www.dpcd.vic.gov.au [accessed 17 February 2010]). Although the social inclusion agenda is not quite as pervasive as the Canadian program, the goals of the Victorian initiative have a clear focus on equity and the SDOH.

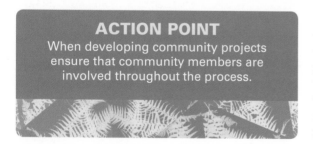

ACTION POINT
When developing community projects ensure that community members are involved throughout the process.

At the community level, collaborative ventures to galvanise people into action can be strengthened by formal and informal community input, whether this is at a sporting venue promoting men's or women's health or an event aimed at encouraging either women or men to participate in screening. Supportive activities range from helping community members organise themselves, to acting as a peripheral resource to community-determined activities. For example, a group from the population sciences division at the University of Waikato in New Zealand have developed a 'cooking at home' program for migrant women. The program is based on the fact that most women are comfortable at home. Cooking, particularly ethnic dishes, is a way of bridging the connection between their old and new home (Longhurst et al 2009). The program captures the link between health and place, supporting them in a context that feels good, which can help them adjust to their new environment. In many cases, the support people require in the community is validation of their feelings and acknowledgement of their strengths and weaknesses. This often relies upon nurses and other health professionals to take the lead in working with community volunteers.

DEVELOPING PERSONAL SKILLS

Developing gender-sensitive personal skills begins in the family. In many communities, the vocal minority is outspoken about the need for respect and tolerance for difference. However, our national agendas strike fear into the hearts of communities, with cautiously disparaging descriptions of those who are different. This is most evident in the dialogue about terrorism and border protection. Personal opinions, and therefore personal behaviours, tend to mimic societal values, as portrayed in daily life and through the media. When communities are led by political notions of respect for others, respect for difference, and a healthy curiosity about the 'real story', there is greater likelihood that individuals will become more thoughtful about events in the world, and make their own decisions on how to behave. The prevailing dialogue on gender identity and gay rights, migration, styles of worship, the right to life and the right to protect oneself, the right to live in a safe home, and the rights of the world's children, provide numerous examples of where personal views are shaped by pre-set opinions set down in the daily newspaper or the nightly news. To break away from the pre-digested version of public opinion requires time, effort and a commitment to social justice. It is made easier when tolerance and respect are role-modelled at the highest level, from global policy-makers, to national, state, and local leaders. Given our knowledge of developmental pathways, it is important to develop the personal skills of mutual respect between genders at an early age, to overcome entrenched behaviours and conditions that lead to violence, discrimination, or systematic inequity and bias.

Changing people's attitudes and behaviour is challenging at any time, especially when the desired change runs counter to family attitudes or entrenched ideas about the way of the world. For boys and young men, attempts to create heightened awareness of gender issues are difficult if they are not reinforced in the home; however, there have been many boys from inequitable home environments who, through education and experience, have transformed their views dramatically. Key intervention points to heighten men's awareness of gender bias occur at primary school age, first-time fatherhood, during significant life transitions, such as when a man is separating or has separated from his partner, and after retirement, when many men stop to reflect on the world and social relations (O'Brien & Rich 2002). Helping men change their risky behaviours, especially those from minorities where personal bravado often masks the need for help and support, is difficult but not impossible.

Nurses, midwives and other health professionals should be aware that gender is an important issue, especially given the history of their subjugation to the medical profession (Pannowitz et al 2009). Understanding policy, legislation and planning is critical to maintaining socially inclusive practice, and overcoming inequalities (McGee 2009). To provide guidance, nurses need to know how men's and women's behaviour is socially constructed, and to understand the differences between their risks and patterns of help-seeking (McGee 2009). Programs designed to foster health literacy, or behaviour change, therefore need to evoke reconsideration of the way society has maintained unequal gender relations, and work towards social and structural change. In some cases, strategies will include helping adolescents and young adults understand the media and how it is shaping social norms. In other cases, health education strategies will focus on drawing women's attention to the vulnerability that results from being brought up to depend on males for social and personal esteem.

Women and men need to recognise the need for a balanced lifestyle, and a woman's right to develop her personal capacity in a way that may differ from her partner's. Because most women are relatively invisible in major decision-making forums, they

ACTION POINT

When providing education or developing health promotion programs, use key intervention points to heighten men's awareness of gender bias, for example, at primary school, first-time fatherhood, and during significant life transitions.

need to be encouraged to learn how decisions are made, so they can participate in securing their preferred future. Interventions to help advance these goals may be focused on garnering support from the community for women's empowerment. It also requires community-level sanctions against abuse of either girls or boys to send a strong message that the community values its young people. To counter domestic abuse, person-centred and problem-focused interventions are essential. These entail programs to help young people develop personal coping strategies and self-esteem, by helping them accept ownership and direction for their own lives. Programs aimed at empowering young people are based on the belief that empowerment is everyone's entitlement; that all people must be able to speak for themselves, and that everyone has a right to dignity and a non-violent lifestyle.

REORIENTING HEALTH SERVICES

In general, and excluding poor women living in vulnerable circumstances, women have gained on males in terms of both longevity and quality of life. Some of this advantage is biological, but there is also a major effect from the services they access. There remains a need to continue offering woman-friendly services, as these have made a major contribution to screening and reducing women's risk. However, there are few men's health services and continual problems attracting men to services because of scheduling difficulties. Men's help-seeking behaviour is remarkably different from women's. They are often ambivalent about seeing a health practitioner, with most seeing a GP three times a year, compared to women's attendance five times a year (Cole 2009). The reasons for their hesitance have been identified as machismo, fear, surgery opening times, and a sense that any information presented will only be female-friendly (Cole 2009). Because of their reticence to seek help, and the difficulties most men face because of work schedules, nurse practitioners have developed outreach health promotion services at barber shops, pubs, bus depots, trade shows, service stations and truck stops (Cole 2009). In New South Wales, nurses have developed a 'Pitstop' program (Russell et al 2006), which has been replicated in the US as well as other states and territories in Australia (Kuhns 2009).

The NSW Pitstop program is aimed at rural men's health risks, and the nurses provide them with information and brief health screening as they wait at the grain elevator to unload the harvest (Kuhns 2009). In Nelson New Zealand, local men's health promoter Philip Chapman has established a men's drop-in centre called The Male Room where men can stop in and discuss issues, gain support or receive counselling over a cup of fresh coffee. The Male Room also provides a location for fathers' groups to meet.

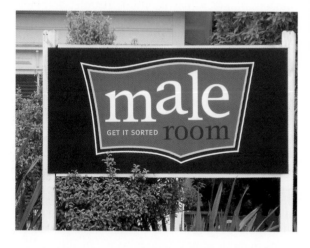

Various researchers have suggested different approaches to promoting men's health. Some argue for supporting programs like 'Pitstop', which uses masculine metaphors for aspects of men's health that may resonate with men's constructions of masculinity. Others suggest circumventing this type of approach, by making the environment more amenable to healthy choices (Saunders & Peerson 2009). The National Male Health Policy background documents emphasise the need to conduct research into men's perceptions of their health, and how diverse masculinities inform men's behaviours and risk-taking (Saunders & Peerson 2009). Another perspective is to develop gender-sensitive health promotion strategies that recognise the key role of gender in socially specific health practices for both men and women. This would help counter the notion that 'gender' refers to women's health, and to overcome the simplistic approach to men's health that has focused on common notions of men's individual behaviours (Smith & Robertson 2008). An alternative approach would seek to understand how men embody gender, experientially and pragmatically, and how men's health issues intersect with women's health issues. This 'relational' approach would incorporate individual and social-structural elements, and their interconnections. For example, men's role in parenting would come to be seen as more than encompassing the provider role, and they would be encouraged to explore their role in both gender and non-gender violence (Smith & Robertson 2008).

> ### ACTION POINT
> In order to develop gender-sensitive health services, use research and tools that move away from the idea that gender is women-specific.

Like women's services, responsive men's services need a man-friendly environment, and an attitude of empathy. Men's hesitancy to freely discuss health issues, and their reticence to explain themselves elicits compassion, especially for men disadvantaged by being members of minority groups. Many men also shy away from any notion of counselling, seeing counsellors as there to fix a specific problem, rather than begin a process of self-discovery. Men also tend to feel uncomfortable with the language and modes of communication used in counselling, which is why counsellors specialising in men's issues will be more effective than those who cater for more general problems (O'Brien & Rich 2002). To develop a man-friendly attitude, there needs to be recognition of how society generalises on the basis of men putting on a good front. To turn this around, there needs to be a commitment to listening to men, allowing them to express themselves, and their needs and preferences. To help men build a repertoire of healthy behaviours, some of the same solutions as are used for women should be used, such as assuring anonymity and privacy, and providing workplace-based services. Gender-specific clinics can achieve positive outcomes for those who are timid or embarrassed about their health needs, particularly if there are health issues of a sexual nature present.

One of the biggest problems for men and women in full-time employment is accessing services after working hours, and this needs to be addressed so that health and preventative care are integral to daily life. The current trend towards providing comprehensive services in PHC organisations will be helpful to both women and men, but there may be a need for satellite clinics to deal expressly with men's and women's health issues, especially mental health issues. Young and older men often hesitate to seek help for depression or anxiety early enough, and are not brought into care until they have come to the attention of criminal investigations or domestic violence programs. Community mentors and role models can help, especially through peer support programs at school. Men's helplines have also enjoyed considerable success, as men tend to view phone conversations as safe and non-threatening. Where gender-sensitive services are funded by governments, and promoted as necessary, there is a greater chance of men and women availing themselves of what is offered. This also reflects the fundamental idea that gender-sensitivity must begin at the top, and filter down through all aspects of society to normalise the importance of mutual respect, human rights and freedom from bias.

Inclusive health services also require considerable transformation to meet the needs of the sexually diverse in the community, establishing goals of access, cultural sensitivity and equity (Mule et al 2009). Clearly, this requires a PHC approach to work towards equity in services, and social inclusion in the community (MacDonnell 2009; Mao et al 2009). Like other community-based services, these work best when there is a team approach, helping individuals develop a core sense of self, the ability to take action based on self-determination, a sense of control over one's life, and a feeling of being connected with others. They should also include community-wide promotion of inclusive approaches and the integration of gender-sensitive materials in all community services.

Case study

Jim's brother Dave, who is 34, is in a stable, supportive long-term partnership with Paul. Paul, who works in a state government department in Sydney has been the subject of emotional bullying and is not coping well. He attended one of the new nurse practitioner clinics in Sydney, and the nurse referred him to a local branch of Relationships Australia where, after two counselling sessions, he was referred to a gay support group.

REFLECTING ON THE BIG ISSUES

- Social inclusion and social exclusion are two points on a continuum of social equity.
- Our society remains unequal, with pockets of systematic discrimination and oppression on the basis of gender, race, ethnicity and sexual diversity.
- Women and men have different health issues, and some common issues related to a combination of biological, behavioural and social factors.
- Women's relative longevity compared to men leaves them suffering more chronic illness and severe disability than men over their lifetime.
- Men's health is often victim to men's notions of masculinity and their need to convey strength, robustness and good health, which leaves many hesitant to seek health care when they need it.
- Intimate partner violence is caused by one person's need to exert power and control over another.
- Primary health care principles can be used to guide inclusive policies for gender relations.
- Every member of society has a right to live in dignity in a non-violent, adequately resourced community without discrimination or fear.

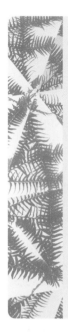

Reflective questions: how would I use this knowledge in practice?

1 What indicators of social exclusion exist in your community?

2 Analyse three gender-sensitive issues in your community in relation to principles of primary health care.

3 What are the advantages and disadvantages of having separate or integrated women's health and men's health policies?

4 What would be the most important issues affecting Dave in his work and community life?

5 What updates will you have to make to the family genogram you have been developing over the course of the last few chapters?

6 What are the most prevalent issues confronting women in today's workplace?

7 What should be included in a comprehensive policy to counter intimate partner violence?

Research-informed practice

Read the article by Griffiths et al (2009) 'Building social capital with women in a socially disadvantaged community'.

Following the social capacity building program led by the nurses, the participants in their study were described as having strong 'bonding' and 'bridging' social capital.

• Review the discussion on social capital in Chapter 1.

• Are there any aspects of social capital that were not reported in the research study?

• What is the strongest evidence that the nurse intervention was successful?

• What research does this suggest for the future?

• How would you design a follow-up study that would distinguish between disadvantaged migrant women and those disadvantaged for other reasons?

References

Adams Tufts K, Clements P, Karlowicz K 2009 Integrating intimate partner violence content across curricula: developing a new generation of nurse educators. Nurse Education Today 29:40–7

Adema W 2005 Babies and bosses. OECD Observer. Online. Available: www.oecdobserver.org/news/fullstory/php/aid/1581/Babies_and_bosses.html (accessed 3 March 2006)

Australian Institute of Health and Welfare (AIHW) 2008 Australia's Health 2008. AIHW, Cat. No. AUS 99, Canberra

—— 2009a Breast Cancer in Australia. AIHW and National Breast and Ovarian Cancer Centre. AIHW, Cat. No. CAN 46, Canberra

—— 2009b Australia's Welfare 2009. Series No. 9 Cat. No. AUS 117, AIHW, Canberra

Australian Women's Health Network (AWHN) 2009 Submission to the Commonwealth government on the new national women's health policy. AWHN, Melbourne

Boonzaier F 2008 'If the man says you must sit, then you must sit'. The relational construction of woman abuse: gender, subjectivity and violence. Feminism & Psychology 18(2):183–206

Brown B 2009 Men in nursing: Re-evaluating masculinities, re-evaluating gender. Contemporary Nurse 33(2):120–9

Bybee J, Sullivan E, Zielonka E, Moes E 2009 Are gay men in worse mental health than heterosexual men? The role of age, shame and guilt, and coming-out. Journal of Adult Development 16:144–54

Campbell J 2001 Global perspectives of wife beating and health care. In: Martinez M (ed.) Prevention and Control of Aggression and the Impact on its Victims. Kluwer Academic/Plenum Publishers, New York, pp 215–27

Cole L 2009 A pro-active approach to men's health. Practice Nurse 37(11):37–9

Commonwealth of Australia 2008a Social Inclusion, Origins, Concepts and Key Themes. Paper prepared by the Australian Institute of Family Studies for the Social Inclusion Unit, Department of the Prime Minister and Cabinet, Canberra

—— 2008b Development of a National Men's Health Policy. Summary of Men's Health Issues. Department of Health and Ageing, Canberra

—— 2008c Developing a Women's Health Policy for Australia — Setting the Scene. Department of Health and Ageing, Canberra

—— 2009 Report of the Maternity Services Review. Pub No P3-4946, Department of Health and Aging, Canberra

Connell R 2006 The experience of gender change in public sector organizations. Gender, Work and Organization 13(5):435–52

Coulter P, Dickman K, Maradiegue A 2009 The effects of exercise on stress in working women. The Journal for Nurse Practitioners 5(6):408–13

Courtenay W 2000 Constructions of masculinity and their influence on men's wellbeing: a theory of gender and health. Social Science & Medicine 50:1385–401

de Visser R, Rissel C, Richters J, Smith A 2007 The impact of sexual coercion on psychological, physical, and sexual wellbeing in a representative sample of Australian women. Archives of Sexual Behaviour 36:676–86

Emslie C, Hunt K 2008 The weaker sex? Exploring lay understandings of gender differences in life expectancy: a qualitative study. Social Science & Medicine 67:808–16

Feder G, Hutson M, Ramsay J, Taket A 2006 Women exposed to intimate partner violence: expectations and experiences when they encounter health care professionals: a meta-analysis of qualitative studies. Archives of Internal Medicine 166:22–37

Fineran S, Gruber J 2009 Youth at work: adolescent employment and sexual harassment. Child Abuse & Neglect 33:550–9

Fuller A 2002 Valuing boys, valuing girls: celebrating difference and enhancing potential. Presentation to the Excellence in Teaching Conference, Fremantle, Western Australia, 14 Nov. Online. Available: www.andrewfuller.com.au (accessed 20 Nov 2005)

Gholizadeh L, Salamonson Y, Worrall-Carter L, DiGiacomo M, Davidson P 2008 Awareness and causal attributions of risk factors for heart disease among immigrant women living in Australia. Journal of Women's Health 18(9):1385–93

Griffiths R, Horsfall J, Moore M, Lane D, Kroon V, Langdon R 2009 Building social capital with women in a socially disadvantaged community. International Journal of Nursing Practice 15:172–84

Hancock T 2009 Act Locally: Community-based population health. Report for The Senate Sub-Committee on Population Health, Victoria BC, Canada. Online. Available: www.parl.gc.ca/40/2/parlbus/commbus/senate/com-e/popu-e/rep-e/appendixBjun09-e.pdf (accessed 17 July 2009)

Hathaway J, Zimmer B, Willis G, Silverman J 2008 Perceived changes in health and safety following participation in a health care-based domestic violence program. Journal of Midwifery & Women's Health 53:547–55

Hinchliff S, Gott M, Wylie K 2009 Holding onto womanhood: a qualitative study of heterosexual women with sexual desire loss. Health: An Interdisciplinary Journal for the Social Study of Health, Illness and Medicine 13(4):449–65

Holt S, Buckley H, Whelan S 2008 The impact of exposure to domestic violence on children and young people: a review of the literature. Child Abuse & Neglect 32:797–810

Jackson S, Cram F 2003 Disrupting the sexual double standard: young women's talk about heterosexuality. British Journal of Social Psychology 42:113–27

Janzen B, Green K, Muhajarine N 2006 The health of single fathers. Demographic, economic and social correlates. Canadian Journal of Public Health 97(6):440–4

Karoly L, Kilburn M, Cannon J 2005 Early childhood interventions: proven results, future promise. Rand Corporation, Santa Monica, Ca

Kasturirangan A 2009 Empowerment and programs designed to address domestic violence. Violence Against Women 14(12):1465–75

Khlat M, Jusot F, Ville I 2009 Social origins, early hardship and obesity: a strong association in women, but not in men? Social Science & Medicine 68:1692–9

Kickbusch I 2008 Healthy societies: addressing 21st century health challenges. Government of South Australia, Department of the Premier and Cabinet, Adelaide

Kim J, Gray K 2008 Leave or stay? Battered women's decision after intimate partner violence. Journal of Interpersonal Violence 23(10):1465–82

Kostiainen E, Martelin T, Kestila LL, Martikainen P, Koskinen S 2009 Employee, partner, and mother. Woman's three roles and their implications for health. Journal of Family Issues 30(8):1122–50

Koziol-McLain J, Giddings L, Rameka M, Fyfe E 2008 Intimate partner violence screening and brief intervention: experiences of women in two New Zealand health care settings. Journal of Midwifery & Women's Health 53:504–10

Krantz G, Garcia-Moreno C 2005 Violence against women. Journal of Epidemiology and Community Health 59:818–21

Kuhns S 2009 Men's health pitstop. American Journal of Nursing 109(7):58–60

Lavie C, Milani R 2009 Secondary coronary prevention in women: it starts with cardiac rehabilitation, exercise, and fitness. Journal of Women's Health 18(8):1115–17

Levitas R, Pantazis C, Fahmy E, Gordon D, Lloyd E, Patsios D 2007 The Multi-dimensional Analysis of Social Exclusion. Department of Sociology and School for Social Policy, University of Bristol, Bristol

Lewis S 2005 HIV/AIDS and women's global health. Network: Canadian Women's Health Network 8 (1–2), Online. Available: www.cwhn.ca/network-reseau/8-12/8-12pg2.html (accessed 13 February 2006)

Longhurst R, Johnston L, Ho E 2009 A visceral approach: cooking 'at home' with migrant women in Hamilton, New Zealand. Transactions: Institute of British Geographers NS34:333–45

Loscocco K, Spitzke G 2007 Gender patterns in provider role attitudes and behaviour. Journal of Family Issues 28(7):934–54

Loxton D, Powers J, Schofield M, Hussain R, Hosking S 2009 Inadequate cervical cancer screening among mid-aged Australian women who have experienced partner violence. Preventive Medicine 48:184–8

Luketina F, Davidson C, Palmer P 2009 Supporting Kiwi dads: role and needs of New Zealand fathers. A Families Commission report. Families Commission, Wellington

Macdonald J 2006 Shifting paradigms: a social determinants approach to solving problems in men's health policy and practice. Medical Journal of Australia 185(8):456–8

MacDonnell J 2009 Fostering nurses' political knowledges and practices. Education and political activation in relation to lesbian health. Advances in Nursing Science 32(2):158–72

Mao L, Kidd M, Rogers G, Andrews G, Newman C, Booth A, Saltman D, Kippax S 2009 Social factors associated with Major Depressive Disorder in homosexually active, gay men attending general practices in urban Australia. Australian and New Zealand Journal of Public Health 33(1):83–6

McCallister J, Mastronarde J 2008 Sex differences in asthma. Journal of Asthma 45:853–61

McGee P 2009 Who says we're all equal? Gender as an issue for nurses and nursing care. Contemporary Nurse 33(2):98–102

McLaren S, Challis C 2009 Resilience among men farmers: the protective roles of social support and sense of belonging in the depression-suicidal ideation relation. Death Studies 33:262–76

McLoughlin P, Warin M 2008 Corrosive places, inhuman spaces: mental health in Australian immigration detention. Health & Place 14:254–64

Men's Health Forum (MHF) 2006 Mind your head. Men, boys and mental wellbeing. National Men's Health Week 2006 Policy Report. MHF, London

Ministry of Health New Zealand (MOHNZ) 2008a Improving quality of care for Pacific peoples. MOHNZ, Wellington

—— 2008b A Portrait of Health. Key Results of the 2006–07 New Zealand Health Survey. MOHNZ, Wellington

—— 2009 Mortality and Demographic Data 2006. MOHNZ, Wellington

Morgaine K 2009 'You can't bite the hand …' domestic violence and human rights. Affilia: Journal of Women and Social Work 24(1):31–43

Mule N, Ross L, Deeprose B, Jackson B, Daley A, Travers A, Moore D 2009 Promoting LGBT health and wellbeing through inclusive policy development. International Journal for Equity in Health 8(18):doi:10.1186/1475-9276-8-18

National Male Health Policy 2010 Social Determinants and Key Actions Supporting Male Health. Online. Available: www.health.gov.au/malehealthpolicy (accessed 20 September 2010)

Neville S, Henrickson M 2006 Perceptions of lesbian, gay and bisexual people of primary health care services. Journal of Advanced Nursing 55(4):407–15

New Zealand Health Information Service (NZHIS) 2007 Report on maternity: Maternal and newborn information 2004. Ministry of Health New Zealand, MOHNZ, Wellington

Newman L, Dudley M, Steel Z 2008 Asylum, detention, and mental health in Australia. Refugee Survey Quarterly 27(3):110–27

Nobis R, Sanden I 2008 Young men's health: a balance between self-reliance and vulnerability in the light of hegemonic masculinity. Contemporary Nurse 29(2):205–17

O'Brien C, Rich K 2002 Evaluation of the Men and Family Relationships Initiative. Commonwealth Department of Family and Community Services, Canberra

O'Connell-Birns K 2009 Men's mental health during the first year postpartum. Journal of Community Nursing 23(7):4–8

O'Hara P 2006 Social Inclusion Health Indicators: a Framework for Addressing the Social Determinants of Health. Edmonton Social Planning Council, Edmonton, Online. Available: www.inclusivecities.ca (accessed 22 October 2009)

Oertelt-Prigione S, Regitz-Zagrosek V 2009 Women's cardiovascular health. Editorial, Archives of Internal Medicine 169(19):1740–1

Pannowitz H, Glass N, Davis K 2009 Resisting gender-bias: insights from Western Australian middle-level women nurses. Contemporary Nurse 33(2):103–19

Paterson S 2009 (Re)constructing women's resistance to woman abuse: Resources, strategy choice and implications of and for public policy in Canada. Critical Social Policy 29(1):121–45

Postmus J, Severson M, Berry M, Ah Yoo J 2009 Women's experiences of violence and seeking help. Violence Against Women 15(7):852–68

Rappaport J 1987 Terms of empowerment/exemplars of prevention: towards a theory for community psychology. American Journal of Community Psychology 15:121–48

Reibis R, Bestehorn K, Pittrow D, Jannowitz C, Wegscheider K, Voller H 2009 Elevated risk profile of women in secondary prevention of coronary artery disease: a 6 year survey of 117 913 patients. Journal of Women's Health 18(8):1123–31

Reid C 2004 The Wounds of Exclusion: Poverty, Women's Health and Social Justice. Edmonton, International Institution for Qualitative Methodology

Russell N, Harding C, Chamberlain C, Johnston L 2006 Implementing 'Men's Health Pitstop' in the Riverina, South-west New South Wales. Australian Journal of Rural Health 14:129–31

Saunders M, Peerson A 2009 Australia's National Men's Health Policy: masculinity matters. Health Promotion Journal of Australia 20(2):92–7

Sen A 1999 Development as Freedom. Alfred A. Knopf, New York

Shaw L, Bugiardini R, Bairey Merz C 2009 Women and ischemic heart disease. Journal of the American College of Cardiology 54(17):1561–75

Smith J, Robertson S 2008 Men's health promotion: a new frontier in Australia and the UK? Health Promotion International 23(3):283–9

Spitzer D 2005 Engendering health disparities. Canadian Journal of Public Health 96(S2):S78–S96

Strauss M 2001 Physical aggression in the family. In: Martinez M (ed.) Prevention and Control of Aggression and the Impact on its Victims. Kluwer Academic/Plenum Publishers, New York, pp 181–200

Swedish Ministry of Health and Social Affairs 2008 Sweden's Strategy for Social Protection and Social Inclusion 2008–2010. Online. Available: www.sweden.gov.se/content/1/c6/11/42/69/1009c964.pdf (accessed 28 October 2009)

Syed J, Murray P 2009 Combating the English language deficit: the labour market experiences of migrant women in Australia. Human Resource Management Journal 19(4):413–32

ten Brummelhuis L, van der Lippe T, Kluwer E, Flap H 2008 Positive and negative effects of family involvement on work-related burnout. Journal of Vocational Behavior 73:387–96

Terrance C, Plumm K, Little B 2008 Maternal blame: battered women and abused children. Violence Against Women 14(8):870–85

UNESCO 2000 Women and girls: education, not discrimination. OECD Observer. Online. Available: www.oecdobserver.org (accessed 14 December 2006)

United Nations Development Fund for Women (UNIFEM) 2005 Enhancing participation of women in development through an enabling environment for achieving gender equality and the advancement of women. Expert Group Meeting, 8–11 November 2005. Online. Available: www.un.org/womenwatch/daw/egm/enabling-environment2005 (accessed 27 February 2006)

United Nations Family Planning Association (UNFPA) 2000 The state of world population 2000. UN, New York

Valerio M, Gong Z, Wang S, Bria W, Johnson T, Clark N 2009 Overweight women and management of asthma. Women's Health Issues 19:300–5

Vespa J 2009 Gender ideology construction: a life course and intersectional approach. Gender & Society 23(3):363–87

Weber S 2009 Policy aspects and nursing care of families with parents who are sexual minorities. Journal of Family Nursing 15(3):384–99

Wenzel S, D'Amico E, Barnes D, Gilbert M 2009a A pilot of a tripartite prevention program for homeless young women in the transition to adulthood. Women's Health Issues 19:193–201

Wenzel S, Green H, Tucker J, Golinelli D, Kennedy D, Ryan G, Zhou A 2009b The social context of homeless women's alcohol and drug use. Drug and Alcohol Dependence 105:16–23

Whitaker D, Haileyesus T, Swahn M, Saltzman L 2007 Differences in frequency of violence and reported injury between relationships with reciprocal and nonreciprocal intimate partner violence. American Journal of Public Health 97(5):941–7

World Bank 2009 Because I Am a Girl. State of the World's Girls. World Bank, New York

World Health Organization (WHO) 2002 World Report on Violence and Health. WHO, Geneva

—— 2005 Make Every Mother and Child Count. The World Health Report. WHO, Geneva

—— 2006 Gender Equality, Work and Health: A Review of the Evidence. WHO, Geneva

—— 2008 Global Campaign for Violence Prevention. WHO, Geneva

—— 2009 Women and Health: Today's Evidence Tomorrow's Agenda. WHO, Geneva

Useful websites

http://www.womenshealthclinic.org — Women's health

http://www.wuhi.org — Women's health

http://www.womenandhealthcarereform.ca/ — Primary health care reform and women

http://www.cewh-cesf.ca/en/publications/awhhrg/index/shtml — Aboriginal women's health and healing research group

http://store.yahoo.com/fvpfstore/healpractool.html — Domestic violence resource for materials

http://www.canadian-health-network.ca/servlet/ContentServer?cid — Men's health

http://www.oecdobserver.org/news/fullstory.php/aid/2367/Babies_and_Bosses:_What_lessons_for_governments_.html — Work and family balance

http://www.oecdobserver.org/news/fullstory.php/aid/432/Lifelong_learning_for_all.html — Lifelong learning

http://www.oecdobserver.org/news/fullstory.php/aid/1664/Does_gender_equality_spur_growth — Gender equality and economic development

http://www.cewh-cesf.ca/healthreform — Primary health care and gender equality

http://www.icn.ch/publications/violence/ — ICN violence statement

http://www.who.int/gender/violence/who_multicountry_study/en — WHO multi-country study on women's health and domestic violence against women

http://www.malehealth.co.uk/ — Men's Health UK

http://www.young-fathers.org.uk — Young father's health

http://www.menshealthforum.org.uk — Men's health information

http://www.workingwithmen.org/ — Working With Men

http://healthinsite.gov.au/topics/Mental_Health_of_Men — HealthInsite — body image, domestic violence, middle age, sexual problems etc

http://www.RaisingtheGlobalFloor.org — Gateway to international labour and work policy data

http://www.socialinclusion.gov.au — National Social Inclusion Committee

http://www.dpcd.vic.gov.au — A Fairer Victoria

Chapter 11

Cultural inclusiveness: safe cultures, healthy Indigenous people

INTRODUCTION

The most compelling mark of an inclusive society is the respect conferred on its Indigenous people. Yet, in many countries of the world Indigenous people are treated as outsiders, the 'other' in relation to the dominant culture. This lack of cultural inclusiveness has an enormous impact on their health and wellbeing, and in some cases, determines whether an Indigenous person is able to live a long life in harmony with the natural and spiritual environment, or whether they suffer premature mortality. In many places, cultural exclusiveness divides citizens by race, ethnicity or affiliation, igniting oppressive actions that, at worst, include violent exchanges and civil wars. In other places, cultural exclusion is more subtle and expressed in racist attitudes, thinly veiled arrogance, and dominant forms of exclusive language. Over time, those who are disadvantaged by ethnicity, race or affiliation, lose not only opportunities to live vibrant, healthy lives, but their sense of place in the world, and in the community. As time goes by, dispossession and hopelessness pervade all aspects of life, and create a self-fulfilling prophecy of vulnerability to ill health and incapacity to change.

> **Point to ponder**
> The most compelling mark of an inclusive society is the respect conferred on its Indigenous people.

Indigenous people in Australia and New Zealand have different histories and experiences. As population groups, what they have in common is a history of colonisation and dispossession that has not yet been fully redressed by non-Indigenous people in either country. New Zealand has made greater progress than Australia in valuing its Indigenous people, particularly since the Treaty of Waitangi, and its mandate for recognition of all New Zealanders as equal before the law. Although Australia has yet to develop a treaty with Indigenous people, there is a renewal of political attention to the need for reconciliation between Australia's Indigenous and non-Indigenous people. This was enshrined in the national public apology to Indigenous people by Australia's Prime Minister in 2008, and Indigenous people are awaiting further action at the community level. Much remains to be done in reshaping Australia as an inclusive society. State, territory and Commonwealth government initiatives to 'control' Indigenous affairs, and therefore Indigenous people's health, have polarised public opinion. Some condone heavy-handed measures to intervene in the way some Indigenous communities live their lives, while others are outraged that non-Indigenous norms and expectations would be placed on Indigenous communities. Australian public opinion is also divided on another issue related to inclusiveness. This issue concerns the plight of refugees from other countries, with some citizens advocating a greater human rights orientation, and others arguing for 'fairness' in the way migrants are processed and/or allowed into the country. As we have mentioned previously, this is one area where New Zealand political will is decidedly clear, supporting a compassionate basis for decision-making.

The relevance of political decisions governing migrants and Indigenous people is of major importance to nurses and midwives working towards community health and wellness. As a basis for any type of intervention, the professions need to be fully informed of how both historical factors and current realities interact to keep some cultural groups, especially Indigenous people, socially disadvantaged, and relegated to disproportionately high levels of disability and disease. Our evolving research agenda has made some progress in helping inform culturally appropriate actions, particularly in providing insights from the perspective of Indigenous people themselves. Understanding Indigenous ways of knowing, and the worldviews of other cultures should lead to change, but it does not always achieve this. The challenge is to advance this knowledge as a basis for informing community awareness, then providing a rationale for policy and practice with the ultimate goal of social justice. Questions for members of our professions revolve around how we can enact our role as advocates to support political enthusiasm for change, and how we can use Indigenous knowledge and skills to inform the direction of change. These questions lie at the basis of sustaining health improvements for all people so that they become entrenched in good and best practice.

We are both members of the non-Indigenous cultures of our respective countries, and we write this chapter drawing on a wide range of Indigenous and non-Indigenous literature, in consultation with members of Indigenous cultures, and on our respective experiences of the health and political environments in which we live and work. We begin this chapter by delving into some of the successes and failures in Indigenous health in Australia and New Zealand. This is explained within a framework that addresses the influences of the historical, social, economic and situational factors that have prevented Indigenous people from achieving good health. From this base of knowledge, we can work together, seeking common solutions that redress past and current barriers to health and wellness. Then we can work towards helping Indigenous people negotiate retention of their culture, and promote equitable, inclusive environments for health and wellbeing.

CULTURE AND HEALTH

Cultural groups are bound together by a tapestry of historically inherited ideas, beliefs, values, knowledge and traditions, art, customs, habits, language, roles, rules, and shared meanings about the world. *Culture* is therefore multidimensional. Cultural influences are often tacit in people's behaviours, as unconscious, shared predispositions, rather than deliberate attempts to be distinctive. Despite the commonalities that bind members of a cultural group, behaviours, cultural traits and predispositions are not always expressed in the same way by all who claim membership in the group. Individual expressions of attitudes, beliefs and behaviours vary according to age, gender, personal histories, and situational factors, and these are, in turn, influenced by family, group and community influences.

Diversity in expressions of culture is also a product of how people relate to their environments. Culture is integral to a person's social life, part of his or her ecological relationship with the world. Cultures are also adaptive, and, in ecological terms, as people in any cultural group interact with their environments, there is a reciprocal effect on the environments and the people themselves (Eckermann et al 2006). The way people respond to, initiate and adapt to changes is therefore a dynamic process, a reflection of the natural,

Objectives

By the end of this chapter you will be able to:

1 explain the influence of culture on health and social justice

2 discuss Indigenous health within the context of primary health care

3 identify risk factors for Indigenous health at the family, neighbourhood and community level

4 explain the importance of historical and cultural knowledge in promoting the health of Indigenous people

5 describe strategies for promoting health literacy in an Indigenous community

6 devise a comprehensive strategy for working with Indigenous families to improve individual, family and community health

7 define cultural safety as a concept and explain its relevance and importance in the provision of health care.

economic, historic, social and political environments; the traditions of their culture, including acquired knowledge, guides to action, language, thoughts and lifestyles; and the way their socialisation has led them to interpret experience and shape behaviour.

Point to ponder

Although there are many commonalities that bind members of a particular cultural group, individual expressions of culture will vary according to the personal characteristics and experiences of the individual.

Cultural behaviours include the way people use language, how they feel and how they learn, what motivates them, how and with whom they interact and express themselves and make decisions (Eckermann et al 2006). Although cultural traditions can bind people together, it is inappropriate to consider members of one or another culture as homogenous, as within cultural groups there is often wide variability.

A critical view of culture seeks to overcome the *monolithic* view that all members are relatively similar. Instead, understanding individuals comes from exploring their history, behaviour, and particular view of the world as it is embedded in their culture, but distinctive in their patterns of attitude and behaviour. Conducting nursing assessments of a person's needs therefore has to include both unique and common strengths and needs. Indigenous 'culture' is not something that can be made explicit, as a formula from which to develop culturally appropriate guidelines and culturally competent care (McMurray & Param 2008). To be authentically inclusive, health professionals have to understand the history and structural factors that have been part of a person's experience, in the context of diversity within, and external to, the group (Culley 2006). This non-stereotypical approach provides insight into people's worldview and their history, and the barriers and strengths that can lead to empowerment and self-determined decision-making. Ultimately, this grants the members of a group the freedom to articulate their lives, and their expectations in the voices of their own language and values (Sen 1999). These choices are embedded in family and

community and the human right to achieve social and cultural capital (see Figure 11.1).

CULTURE CONFLICT

In some cases, the ecological interactions between people, their culture and other cultural groups is mutually beneficial. People of different cultures settling together in a new land often learn from one another, enjoying each other's foods and ways of cooking, lifestyles and folkways, such as festivals and celebrations. Over time, their long-term contact with one another can result in the type of *acculturation* where two cultural groups become integrated; or relatively similar (Beiser 2005; National Health and Medical Research Council [NHMRC] 2005). However, attempts at acculturating two groups can also be fraught with conflict. Berry (1995) describes four different reactions to acculturation. The first is *assimilation*, where one culture abandons their culture in favour of the new or host culture. *Integration* is the creative blending of the two cultures. *Rejection* is a reaction in which the new culture replaces the heritage culture, and *marginalisation* occurs where neither the new nor the old culture is accepted. Clearly, the most desirable option is integration, with marginalisation the least desirable (Beiser 2005).

Culture conflict typically occurs where people are not committed to similar goals or ambitions, and where their decision-making is not based on similar principles and philosophies (Eckermann et al 2006). This occurs often in Indigenous cultures in countries like Australia, Canada, New Zealand and the United States, where discriminatory and often racist attitudes promulgated by media stereotypes portray Indigenous people as a 'problem' rather than showing balanced, positive images of successful Indigenous people and families (Brough et al 2004; Ten Fingers 2005; Toussaint 2003). Even in the health care system, we tend to purvey the impression that non-white populations need to be reconciled within white, Eurocentric models of care, and their behaviours corrected, to conform with disembodied, purified, scientific solutions (Puzan 2003). This perpetuates unresolved issues that continue to plague the lives of Indigenous peoples, adding cumulatively to their unresolved burden of intergenerational trauma and grief (Menzies 2008).

At the community level, culture conflict erodes social and cultural capital by causing disharmony. When this occurs, members of the conflicting groups close ranks, and withdraw from each other, rather than cooperating to build a system of mutual community support. On the other hand, when people from different cultures live with realistic possibilities for the future, they are more likely to work within a type of *cultural relativism*; acceptance of one another's culture as the 'legitimate adaptation of different peoples to various historical, natural, socio-economic and political environments' (Eckermann et al 2006:6). Cultural relativism lies at the centre of tolerance and social inclusiveness. For two cultures to work together, no one culture needs to abandon its traditions or philosophies, but each suspends judgement of the other's beliefs and practices. In this process, each makes a conscious decision to proceed on the basis of their willingness to recognise and respect the beliefs and practices of others, and to continually question their own views and presumptions (Eckermann et al 2006). This is also the first step in maintaining cultural safety.

CULTURAL SAFETY

Cultural safety is a term that grew out of the colonial history of Aotearoa (New Zealand). It was first described in 1988 by Māori nursing students expressing their concern about safeguarding their culture as they were socialised into the world of nursing education, and ensuring the safety of Māori culture among those they would be helping in practice (Eckermann et al 2006). Their concerns were recorded by Ramsden, a Māori nurse who spearheaded the cultural safety movement in Aotearoa, ensuring that cultural safety found its way into the curricula and nursing practice (Eckermann et al 2006). Cultural safety was never meant to catalogue Māori cultural beliefs, but to recognise power imbalances and inequitable social relationships (Anderson et al 2003). As we mentioned in Chapter 2 cultural safety is a concept that refers to exploring, reflecting on, and understanding one's own culture and how it relates to other cultures with a view towards promoting partnership, participation and cultural protection. This notion of cultural safety has now evolved beyond working with Māori to include other ethnic and cultural groups (Wilson & Neville 2009). Cultural safety is a form of cultural relativism, which is concerned with how culture shapes power relations within the social world of the community. It is designed to enable safe spaces for the interaction of all cultural groups, and their understanding of cultural identity. It is absent in the face of actions that assault, diminish, demean or disempower the cultural identity and wellbeing of any individual (Nursing Council of New Zealand [NCNZ] 1992).

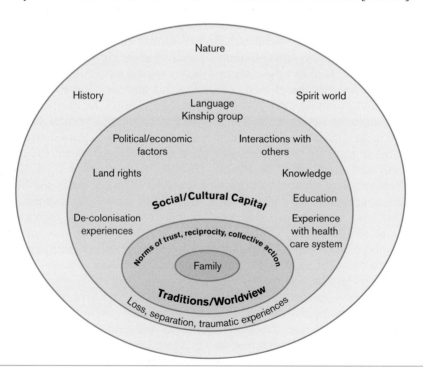

Figure 11.1 Family, culture and social capital

The first step in achieving cultural safety is *cultural awareness*. This includes recognising the fact that any health care relationship is unique, power-laden and culturally dyadic. In other words, there is always the potential for one person (the health provider) to hold power over the other person (someone seeking to access services). When the health care relationship is built on a foundation of *cultural sensitivity*, there is a greater recognition of, and respect for, cultural differences. People develop cultural sensitivity when they begin to engage in self-exploration of their own life experience and realities, and the impact these may have on others. The final stage in developing cultural safety is a conscious commitment to ensuring preservation and protection of others' cultures. Cultural safety is therefore a type of advocacy informed by a recognition of self, the rights of others and the legitimacy of difference (NCNZ 1996). It is integral to all nursing and midwifery interactions, which means that our practice must be culturally competent. *Cultural competence* is the process of ensuring that all nursing and midwifery interactions are cultural interactions (Duke et al 2009).

MULTICULTURALISM

Multiculturalism is a value-laden term that has sometimes been used as a panacea for intolerance. The term has been used to camouflage feelings of superiority of one culture over another. It has also been used to salve the consciences of many people, believing that because they live in a community containing many cultures, the community must be inclusive, when this may be disputed by the realities of daily life. In its truest sense, multiculturalism means 'that people are in fact linked in many more ways than their birthplace divides them' (Wilding & Tilbury 2004:3). Globalisation has brought multiculturalism under close scrutiny because of the spurious arguments used by the most dominant cultures to maintain their position of power over those who are economically dependent on them for survival. In advancing the global economic development agenda, Indigenous people have often been ruthlessly ignored or dismissed, which is discriminatory and adds to their level of disadvantage. Languages have disappeared and cultural characteristics have gradually withered, as people try to minimise feelings of 'difference', and find ways of coping with feeling excluded from mainstream society. These psychosocial outcomes have been accompanied by widening gaps in health, favouring the dominant culture and disempowering those already disadvantaged. Cross-border or multinational decisions take little account of local needs and local voices with little negotiating power, and this exacerbates the cycle of disempowerment by invalidating cultural traditions, eroding the cultural scaffolding that supports health and wellbeing. When this occurs there is a polarised society; one group dominates and the other is left to feel like the 'other'.

> **Point to ponder**
> Although progress has been made towards acknowledging the role of culture in health, this has only resulted in small improvements in health outcomes for Indigenous people.

Although small steps have been made towards heightening public awareness of the role of culture in health, these have been only marginally effective in improving health outcomes. To advance multiculturalism, societies need to institutionalise understanding and tolerance of one another's cultural beliefs and practices in the context of daily living, and in planning for a future in which all cultures will be sustained. Not many societies achieve this level of equity, but it is seen to be an aspiration worthy of just and civil societies. Canada is the only country in the world to have a national multiculturalism law, which was devised in 1971 as an attempt to legitimise the need for harmony among Indigenous and non-Indigenous groups and those who migrated to Canada from other countries (Kulig 2000). This law enshrined equality, diversity and dignity for all people, and confirmed the rights of Canada's Indigenous peoples and the status of the country's two official languages: French and English. Although some have criticised the state of multiculturalism in Canada on the basis that mandating tolerance does not create real understanding, establishing the legal framework was an important step in creating awareness of the need to understand and embrace diversity for the benefit of all society (Kulig 2000).

ETHNOCENTRISM TO RACISM

Ethnocentrism is the tendency to view the world through one's own cultural filters, perceiving and interpreting others' behaviours according to our belief system and behaviours (Matsumoto & Juang

2004). Each of us views the world through the cultural lens with which we have been socialised, and this is why it takes a conscious effort to really 'see' other cultures. When people develop an aversion to the very notion of tolerating other cultures, they are described as *xenophobic*; fearing and despising those who differ. Xenophobia is often used synonymously with *racism*, which is a belief in the distinctiveness of human races, usually involving the idea that one's birth-ascribed race or skin colour is superior to another (Eckermann et al 2006; O'Brien 2006). Maintaining feelings of superiority about another race, or another group, is called *stereotyping*. These feelings can lead to *prejudicial attitudes*, which, when acted upon, result in *discrimination*. Discrimination is shown by speaking against the other person or group, excluding or segregating them, committing acts of violence against them, or, at its extreme, exterminating them as occurred in World War II and in other wars and conflicts.

Today, because of numerous inquiries into historical examples of aggression against one culture by another, we have come to recognise *ethnic cleansing* as an offensive, prejudicial, act of violent discrimination. This is also *racist*. When offensive behaviours are entrenched in socio-legal structures or scientific research, the notion of biological inferiority can lead to *scientific racism*. This occurs when one group is attributed with inferiority on the basis of race, often justified by comparative studies that seek to investigate differences, rather than commonalities (Browne 2005; Eckermann et al 2006; Puzan 2003). It is important that students, academics and practitioners who either generate, or use scientific evidence, recognise this type of racism as embedded in research approaches that are conducted from a 'white' standpoint (Fredericks 2008; Martin-McDonald & McCarthy 2007; Puzan 2003; Wilson & Neville 2009). Systemic bias occurs where research is conducted 'on' instead of 'with' Indigenous people. This research approach perpetuates inequality and imbalanced power relations, and we discuss this further in Chapter 12 in relation to research approaches. *Institutional racism* operates at the level of legal, political and economic organisation in a society, and it creates the impression that, because power dominance is exerted by essential and respected forces in society, it is somehow tacitly acceptable (Eckermann et al 2006). *Systemic bias* allows one group to dominate another through the predominant social order, where organisational and communication skills, financial resources, and commitment of those involved in running a system, are able to exclude others, making them dependent on the powerful group rather than allowing them full participation (Eckermann et al 2006; Toussaint 2003).

> **Point to ponder**
> When the health of Indigenous people is analysed according to norms established in non-Indigenous populations, the health care system is at risk of perpetuating systemic bias.

Health care systems are often accused of systemic bias. This can occur when the health of Indigenous people is analysed according to norms established in the non-Indigenous population, or when the blame for social and health problems is attributed to cultural characteristics instead of inequities in the health care system (Browne 2005). Explaining Indigenous ill health on the basis of culture can lead to health decision-making that stereotypes and therefore excludes some Indigenous people from certain treatments because they have multiple risk factors. It can also be detrimental to health; for example when a person's refusal of treatment is described as a lack of adherence, when it could be due to communication difficulties, or when a child is refused treatment because of a lack of consent from her/his parent, in a case where the child may be in the custody of relatives (Australian Medical Association [AMA] 2007).

A common stereotypical pattern of systemic discrimination lies in the way women victims of violence and child victims of sexual abuse are dealt with in the health care system. In many cases, the injuries and need for ongoing therapy and emotional support are dismissed by broad-brushing the problem as a cultural one, when the victim's needs for protection and care are personal and intense. When victims of violence are differentiated on the basis of Indigenous versus non-Indigenous, the media screams 'culture', and cycles of discrimination are re-launched by conflating culture and race (Anderson et al 2003). This socially exclusive differentiation leads to *alienation* of the victim and her people. Another group of Indigenous people are then disempowered and disengaged from society, leading to disorientation, helplessness, powerlessness and 'normlessness' (Durie 2004; Eckermann et al 2006). The lack of a treaty for Australian Indigenous people is also an anomaly that has left Indigenous people feeling alienated. Without a legal status that entrenches rights and responsibilities, there is no framework for progress and no recognition of their contribution to society (Couzos 2004).

ABORIGINALITY, CULTURE AND HEALTH

The term *Aboriginal* refers to the initial, or earliest, inhabitants of a place. They are also described as *First Nations*, or *Indigenous*, people. However, as mentioned previously, Indigenous people have diverse subcultures and worldviews. Members of different groups also have different influences on their lives, many as a result of their environment. Like non-Indigenous people, those who live in a remote area have substantially different experiences of health from their kin in urban, or other rural settings. Likewise, those who live inland have different health opportunities from those who live close to the sea. The influences on their health are shaped by different determinants beyond biology, age, gender, education, socio-economic status, family membership or neighbourhood. In some groups, cultural knowledge may prescribe diet and eating habits, child-rearing practices, reactions to pain, stress and death, a sense of past, present and future, community and economic structures, responses to health care services and practitioners, and which behaviours are considered a violation of social norms.

The most distinctive feature of Indigenous cultures is a holistic, ecological, spiritual view of health and wellbeing. This encompasses physical, mental, cultural, and spiritual dimensions of health, and the harmonised inter-relationships between these and environmental, ideological, political, social and economic conditions (Eckermann et al 2006; Lutschini 2005). At the centre of Indigenous people's relationship with each dimension of health is a fundamental spiritual connection with land, symbolising the ecological connection between health and place.

Point to ponder

The physical, mental, cultural and spiritual dimensions of health are fundamental to Indigenous understandings of health and wellbeing.

Indigenous people's relationships between health and place

The spiritual relationship with land is a metaphysical connection, governing all other inter-relationships. The land is typically described by Indigenous Australians as 'Country', which is the place that gives and receives life and is part of the support cycle of life–death–life (Kingsley et al 2009). Indigenous Australians 'talk about Country in the same way that they would talk about a person, they speak to Country, visit Country, worry about Country, feel sorry for Country and long for Country' (Australian Heritage Commission, in Kingsley et al 2009:291). For Indigenous people, the spiritual connotation of caring for Country links people with their ancestors. This is a different concept of land from the non-Indigenous understanding, where land is considered an empty space to be 'tamed' or worked (Kingsley et al 2009). New Zealand Māori also articulate a connection with the land. The land historically provided the sustenance necessary for life, but it is also the spiritual, cultural and ancestral home for Māori. This relationship is based on the worldview that ranginui (sky father), and papatuanuku (earth mother), are the primal parents from whom all Māori descend. Māori refer to themselves as tangata whenua (people of the land), which captures the spirit of this kin relationship making the people and the land inseparable (www.foma.co.nz/about_māori/māori_land.htm [accessed 26 February 2010]). Platforms for Māori health are considered to be:

> … constructed from land, language, and whānau; from marae and hapū; from Rangi and Papa; from the 'ashes of colonisation'; from adequate opportunity for cultural expression; and from being able to participate fully within society.
>
> (Durie 2001:35–6)

What Indigenous and non-Indigenous people have in common is the concept of 'biophilia', a construct that reflects how human beings are innately connected and attracted to the natural environment (Kingsley et al 2009). This connection gives meaning and purpose to life, and it can improve health and wellbeing (Kingsley et al 2009). Kingsley et al's (2009) interviews with traditional custodians of their lands revealed that for some people, this connection is vital in fostering mental and spiritual health. One of the custodians reported that the land 'speaks to you … allowing you time to look within yourself … to be grounded … to hear'. Another explained her connection as an affinity towards the land, a sense of belonging. Others described the land as being intrinsic to identity, a way of connecting with culture with a sense of pride, and engendering a sense of responsibility to preserve traditional lands. Importantly, this group of people advocated a return to Country for young people having difficulties in urban living. They felt that working on Country was good therapy for those who were 'numb from the city', dislocated from society' or needing empowerment (Kingsley et al 2009:296).

The close connection with land is what distinguishes the Indigenous 'holistic' view from other common perceptions of holism (Lutschini 2005). Holism is acknowledged in the biomedical literature and its scientific foundations, typically referring to an all-encompassing, comprehensive set of factors that contribute to health. An Indigenous worldview with its connection to Country is where an Indigenous person's life is steeped in the events and stories of their lives (Belfrage 2007). The uncritical way non-Indigenous policy-makers and health planners understand Indigenous 'holism' is problematic when it is seen as a biomedical concept, and translated into strategies for health and health services without deeper understandings of this holistic worldview (Lutschini 2005; Richmond & Ross 2009). Yet, few explanations have emerged in the research literature as to how removing Indigenous people from their lands (environmental dispossession) can undermine and reduce the quality of other social determinants of health (Richmond & Ross 2009).

Colonisation and disconnection between health and place

In many nations, including Australia, New Zealand, Canada and the US, Indigenous people were displaced from their lands by colonising invaders. Colonisation, and the subsequent political decisions that followed, have disrupted Indigenous people's connection between health and place, leaving generations of Indigenous people feeling dispossessed of their place, symbolically, geographically, and politically (Eckermann et al 2006; Pomaika'I Cook et al 2005; Richmond & Ross 2009). Breaking the bond that connected Indigenous people to their traditional lands and environments eroded their identity, their culture, and ultimately, their health and wellbeing. This disconnection has created an imbalance that threatened the health of the community (Richmond & Ross 2009). A further level of disconnection was experienced by those who were subjected to intensive missionary activity and taken to residential schools to enforce assimilation into the dominant culture. Part of this assimilation was to extinguish cultural practices by punishing certain behaviours, including dances, ceremonies, language and songs, many of which tied Indigenous people to features of their lands, and the symbolic importance of water, animals and plants (Richmond & Ross 2009). Where once they had been self-governed, colonial laws forced them to abandon their traditions and self-determination, and become subservient to colonial institutions and laws (Richmond & Ross 2009). Dispossession from land and Country is therefore one of the most critical issues that must be dealt with meaningfully if Indigenous people are to develop and enhance their capacity for health.

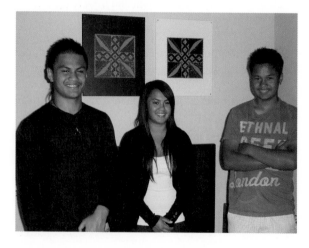

> **Point to ponder**
> Displacement from the land by colonising invaders has had a profound impact on the connections Indigenous people have with their environment, resulting in an imbalance that threatens health.

The colonisation history of Africa, Australia, New Zealand, Canada and the US reveals a belief by their white European conquerors in their superiority over the native people. In most cases, this view was so extreme that the early explorers dismissed the very presence of Aboriginal people as irrelevant, because they failed to use the land in a way that would be expected in a civilised country. The colonisers thus declared the respective countries *Terra Nullius* — an empty, uninhabited land, belonging to no one (Australian Council for Aboriginal Reconciliation [ACAR] 1994; Aboriginal and Torres Strait Islander [ATSI] Social Justice & Australian Human Rights Commission 2010; Eckermann et al 2006). In Australia, this belief represented institutionalised racism, given the colonisers' view that land not cultivated represented a failure of Indigenous people to use the land, a mark of 'civilisation' according to British/European culture. Their colonisers were therefore able to claim the land without having to conquer Indigenous people or negotiate a treaty with them (Eckermann et al 2006). This is different from the situation in North America and New Zealand, where treaties have been established as a mark of socio-legal commitment between Indigenous and non-Indigenous people.

The Treaty of Waitangi, signed in 1840 but not honoured and recognised until the 1970s, was established to protect Māori cultural beliefs, practices and intellectual life and provide equitable access to the benefits of modern life (Turale & Miller 2006; Wilson & Neville 2009). Treaties established in Canada and the US, have also enshrined mutual obligations between Indigenous people and the governments, although these were originally developed as a foundation for assimilation and colonial control (Richmond & Ross 2009). The lack of a treaty and the difficulties surrounding land rights are significant issues for Australian Indigenous people. Native title, that is, acknowledgement that Indigenous people were the original owners and custodians of various lands in Australia, was granted after a 10-year legal battle by Eddie Mabo. Mabo's legal challenge disputed the doctrine of *Terra Nullius*; that the country was unsettled prior to the Europeans coming (Eckermann et al 2006). As a result of the native title acknowledgement, Indigenous people's spiritual connection to land remains *inalienable*, which means the land cannot be sold. However, native title also prevents individual Indigenous people from using land as an asset from which to build economic capital or bargain authentically in the economic arena. Tortuous government red tape continues to mitigate against resolving the issue of land rights, with successive governments lacking

the political will to honour the original inhabitants of the country.

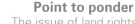

> **Point to ponder**
> The issue of land rights for Indigenous people is being addressed in different ways by different countries but the commonality is a persistent attempt by non-Indigenous cultures to limit the rights of Indigenous cultures to make claim to the land.

The land rights issues in Australia are different from the New Zealand situation. In New Zealand, the Māori Land Court holds much of the written information on Māori land ownership and the historical connections that exist between iwi, hapū, whānau and the land. The Māori Land Court was established as the Native Land Court in 1865 in order to define the land rights of Māori and to translate those rights into land titles recognisable under European law (www2.justice.govt.nz/māorilandcourt/pastpresent.htm [accessed 26 February 2010]). The functions of the Māori Land Court today are to promote the management of Māori land by its owners by maintaining the records of title and ownership information, to contribute to the administration of Māori land, and to preserve taonga Māori (www2.justice.govt.nz/māorilandcourt/pastpresent.htm [accessed 26 February 2010]).

Colonisation also brought environmental destruction from over-grazing, and the destruction of grasslands and forest, with its edible seeds, roots and fauna, all of which have been a personal affront to Indigenous people. The destruction of Indigenous habitats destroyed the metaphysical connections between people, their Country and their family. As in ancient history, Indigenous systems of resource ownership and exchange were intended to provide the opportunity to develop autonomy and mastery over life, and to help young men especially with culturally appropriate identity formation and social integration (Burgess et al 2005; Mignone & O'Neil 2005; Pomaika'I Cook et al 2005). Destroying their ability to accomplish these connections, and to manage natural resources in an Indigenous way has disrupted cultural continuity for young people and adolescents, and the very essence of Aboriginality. It has also created a 'cultural trauma syndrome', a violation of self-hood where disenfranchised individuals take on the role of perpetrator, inflicting cultural wounds on others, leading to intergenerational transference of their grief rather than resolving it in culturally appropriate healing (Pomaika'I Cook et al 2005:119).

Culture blindness and the Stolen Generations

In 1997 the Human Rights and Equal Opportunity Commission (HREOC) published a report of the National Inquiry into Separation of Aboriginal and Torres Strait Islander Children from their Families (HREOC 1997). The Inquiry found that approximately 8% of Indigenous Australians age 15 or over had been forcibly removed from their natural family. The result was mass undermining of Indigenous social organisation, dispersal of geographic groupings and the capture of Indigenous women (Eckermann et al 2006). Their displacement was accompanied by sexual abuse, the introduction of alcohol, and economic and environmental exploitation, which was further demoralising. Then, ludicrously, Indigenous people were blamed for being demoralised and living in squalor — a classic case of what we now call 'victim blaming' (Adelson 2005; Eckermann et al 2006). The dislocation of the 'Stolen Generation' has been linked to a range of negative outcomes, including higher rates of emotional distress, depression, anxiety, heart disease, and diabetes, as well as cultural detachment (Trewin & Madden 2005). Many have had contact with mental health services, or lived in households where there were problems caused by gambling, or overuse of alcohol. An intergenerational effect is evident in the fact that the children of those who had been forcibly removed from their homes were more than twice as likely to be at high risk of clinically significant emotional or behavioural difficulties, and approximately twice as likely to use alcohol and other drugs compared with those who had not been forcibly separated from their family (Zubrick et al 2005).

Point to ponder

Approximately 8% of Indigenous Australians over the age of 15 years were forcibly removed from their natural families.

The separation of Indigenous children from their families has also perpetuated racism and culture-blindness. Removing young Indigenous children from their parents, and sending them to 'white' schools to gain what was considered to be 'appropriate' educational preparation was a culture-blind policy that traumatised Indigenous people and the place of family as the epicentre of life. When this occurred in the last century, Australian Indigenous children who were light-skinned were primary targets for removal, conceivably to protect them from abuse by their family members and other Indigenous people who rejected them as being neither black nor white. The children who were removed grew up in white missions and schools presuming that no such family existed, and often were subjected to inter-racial aggression. Women and children became victims of exploitation and sexual abuse, and most suffered the emotional cost of being confined for prolonged periods, whether in institutionalised housing, or hospitals. The parallel situation with refugees being held in detention is remarkable. Both groups suffer ongoing, severe, intergenerational traumatisation. The consequent loss of freedom and space has a lasting effect that is not easily resolved.

THE HEALTH OF INDIGENOUS PEOPLE THROUGHOUT THE WORLD

There are approximately 350 million Indigenous people in the world, representing more than 5000 cultures in 72 countries (WHO 2007). For all of these groups, life expectancy at birth is approximately 10–20 years less than the rest of the population; infant mortality is 1.5–3 times greater than the national average, and a large proportion suffer from malnutrition and communicable diseases (WHO 1999). In many regions of the world, the health of Indigenous people is also threatened by damage to their habitat and resource base (Harlem Brundtland 1999). Indigenous people's burden of illness, injury and disability is so disparate from that of non-Indigenous people, that in 1999, the WHO convened a meeting with Indigenous representatives from many countries, to develop the Geneva Declaration on the Health and Survival of Indigenous Peoples (WHO 1999). The objective of the declaration was for Indigenous people throughout the world to reaffirm their right of self-determination, and to remind states of their responsibilities and obligations under international law to help address these. Their statement placed responsibility for Indigenous ill health on colonial negation of their way of life and worldview, the destruction of their habitat, the decrease of bio-diversity, imposition of substandard living and working conditions, dispossession of traditional lands and the relocation and transfer of populations (WHO 1999). The Geneva Declaration was followed by the United Nations (UN) Declaration on the Rights of Indigenous Peoples (UN 2007). The WHO's commitment to Indigenous people was reaffirmed in the 2008 report 'Primary health care: now more than ever', which reminded health service providers that many Indigenous people continue to be disadvantaged by their remoteness and lack of health services (WHO 2008).

Point to ponder

In 2007, the United Nations affirmed their commitment to the rights of Indigenous people with the signing of the Declaration on the Rights of Indigenous Peoples. Interestingly, among those nations not signing the Declaration were Australia, New Zealand, Canada and the United States. Australia and New Zealand subsequently ratified the Declaration, but controversy over ratification continues in New Zealand.

One of the most common outcomes of the dispossession and demoralisation of Indigenous people is incarceration. The destructive effect of confinement on the balance of Indigenous family and community life has always been under-estimated, and only recently has become recognised as a powerful and enduring influence on Indigenous people's sense of alienation from their land and erosion of their spiritual identity (Kingsley et al 2009; Richmond & Ross 2009). Until colonial powers established prisons, Indigenous people enacted their own form of tribal justice. Imprisoning people to try to deal with violence, and fighting violence with violence, have had a backlash effect. They have failed to reduce crime or conflict, and instead, have left many families fatherless (Cripps & McGlade 2008). Attempts at assimilation have also failed. Trying to force non-Indigenous culture on Indigenous people in the guise of protecting them, has been utterly destructive around the world, and has led to dispossession and displacement (Adelson 2005; Eckermann et al 2006).

As a result, Indigenous people continue to be the most disadvantaged and marginalised members of the community. Although we have just drawn attention to the fact that these groups are widely diverse, it is important to draw the attention of health planners and policy-makers to the extraordinary constraints on their capacity to become empowered and achieve the health status to which they are entitled.

THE HEALTH OF AUSTRALIAN INDIGENOUS PEOPLE

Of the nearly 20 million people in Australia, close to half a million (2.5%) are Indigenous; Aboriginal or Torres Strait Islanders (AIHW 2008). Compared to non-Indigenous Australians, Indigenous Australians are less healthy, die at a much younger age, have more disability and a lower quality of life (AIHW 2008). More than twice as many Indigenous infants die at birth, or are born with low birth-weights. Morbidity and mortality rates for Indigenous people are imprecise, because of the potential to misclassify or under-report Indigenous status, but, compared with non-Indigenous people, the mortality figures for Indigenous people are startling (Draper et al 2009). Existing data show twice the all-cause rates of death for both men and women, with many more deaths occurring before age 65 (AIHW 2008). The gap in life expectancy between Indigenous and non-Indigenous Australians has drawn considerable attention from the Commonwealth government, with 'closing the gap' becoming a centrepiece of policy development. In 2008 the gap was declared to be 11 years, a reduction from the figure of 17 years used by the previous government. However, according to the Australian Bureau of Statistics (ABS), the figures are dubious, given a radical change in the calculation methods (Hudson 2009). As a result, it is unclear whether the reduced 'gap' in life expectancy is real, or an artefact of the counting method. Irrespective of which figure is used as a benchmark, closing the gap continues to be a major focus of Australian government policy, and a stimulus for health planners.

Point to ponder

More than twice as many Indigenous Australian infants die at birth or are born with low birth-weights than non-Indigenous Australian infants.

The causes of illness and disability for Indigenous Australians are similar to that of non-Indigenous people, including cardiovascular diseases, mental disorders, chronic respiratory disease, diabetes and cancer. Indigenous people are also over-represented in the incidence of chronic illness, not only because of the difficulties of accessing health services, but because of the lack of a healthy start to life. Many Indigenous people who are now middle aged were low birth-weight infants, and therefore have lived their lives with both biological and social disadvantage. The disproportionate distribution of these, largely preventable causes of ill health, contributes 77% to the difference in life expectancy between Indigenous and non-Indigenous people (Zhao et al 2008). In addition, one-quarter of Indigenous Australians live in remote or very remote areas of the country, which adds another level of risk to their burden of ill health, because of a lack of health services, and exposure to some communicable diseases prevalent in remote communities (AIHW 2008). Remoteness also affects older people. Indigenous Australians enter aged care at a younger age than non-Indigenous Australians because of their poorer health status.

As a group, Indigenous people have lower incomes, higher rates of unemployment, lower educational attainment, and lower rates of home ownership than non-Indigenous Australians. A high level of socio-economic disadvantage creates greater health risk factors, such as smoking, alcohol misuse and exposure to violence. These factors are also linked to overcrowded housing conditions, particularly in remote areas. Overcrowding is a challenge for those who wish to refrain from smoking or alcohol use, when others are engaging in these behaviours. Crowding and poorly maintained homes also prevent people from engaging in the fundamental elements of hygiene that would help prevent infections, especially in young children (McDonald et al 2009). Substandard living conditions also present barriers to developing parenting practices that would help reduce the high rates of childhood infectious disease, poor growth and low cognitive outcomes that have plagued Indigenous children in many remote areas (McDonald et al 2009). Living closely with others also makes it difficult for parents to go against traditional social norms of hygiene, or other parenting practices. Consequently, families living in these conditions have neither the freedom to protect their living space from the poor hygiene of others, or appropriate role models to secure even the basic healthy living practices outlined below in Box 11.1 (McDonald et al 2009).

BOX 11.1 HEALTHY LIVING PRACTICES IN REMOTE AREAS

Inadequate housing and overcrowding have attracted few effective interventions. A multidisciplinary team of researchers from South Australia attempted to analyse the issues surrounding housing problems, compiling a list of basic healthy living practices that are linked to housing safety and the environments within which people are expected to keep their families safe and healthy in remote areas (Torzillo et al 2008). These are as follows:

1 washing people, especially children
2 washing clothes and bedding
3 removing waste safely
4 improving nutrition
5 reducing the impact of crowding
6 reducing the impact of animals (dogs) as vectors of disease
7 reducing the impact of dust
8 improving temperature control
9 reducing minor trauma (Torzillo et al 2008:7).

The research team adopted an ecological approach, investigating the 'health hardware' and maintenance processes available in the environment to support healthy living practices. They found that electricity was unsafe. It was impossible to wash a child in a tub or bath. A functioning shower was available in only 35% of houses. Only 6% of houses had adequate facilities to store, prepare and cook meals. Their data dispelled the myth that it is Indigenous people who create damage, and 'house failure'. They developed a set of recommendations for regionally planned housing projects with maintenance processes integrated into funding mechanisms. Their logical conclusion, supported by other researchers, is that health education and health promotion programs will not be successful, unless combined with sustainable developments in health hardware that will help enable a healthy home environment (Commonwealth of Australia 2007; McDonald et al 2009; Torzillo et al 2008). This important study underlines the need to peel back the layers of environmental factors that support or prevent people's attempts to achieve health and wellbeing.

THE HEALTH OF NEW ZEALAND MĀORI

At the last New Zealand Census (2006), people identifying with the Māori ethnic group made up 15% of the total population — up 7% since the previous census in 2001. Māori are a youthful population, with a median age of 23 years, compared to 36 years for the total population. Māori predominantly live in urban areas of the North Island, although are more likely to live in minor urban areas, with a population between 1000 and 9999, than non-Māori. Māori life expectancy also varies substantially from non-Māori. Māori women have a life expectancy of 75.8 years compared to 82.8 years for non-Māori, and Māori men have a life expectancy of 71.2 years, compared with 78.8 years for non-Māori men. This gap has been reducing, moving from 9.8 years in 1995–97 to 7 years in 2006 (Ministry of Health New Zealand [MOHNZ] and Minister of Health 2008). Despite these improvements in life expectancy, on average, Indigenous Māori have the poorest health status of any ethnic group in New Zealand (King & Turia 2002). Compared to non-Māori, inequalities in health status and mortality are large and increasing, with conditions such as coronary heart disease occurring at an earlier age, and with higher fatality rates (Tobias et al 2009). Major causes of mortality for Māori include cardiovascular disease (33% of all Māori deaths), cancer (25%), respiratory disease (8%), accidents (8%), diabetes (7%) and suicide (3%) (Robson & Purdie 2007).

Large disparities exist between Māori and non-Māori determinants of health. In 2005, 49% of Māori secondary school students left school without a qualification, compared to 22% of non-Māori; unemployment rates remain three times higher than that of non-Māori; the median annual income for Māori in 2006 was $20 900 compared with $24 400 for the total population. In 2004, 40% of Māori families were living in hardship, compared to 19% of non-Māori families. Māori are also more likely to be living in overcrowded housing environments than non-Māori (Robson et al 2007a). Young Māori men are more likely to be arrested for minor offences than non-Māori, and are more likely to be referred to the courts, rather than directly for family group conferences (Robson et al 2007a). These factors, along with evidence of the existence of differential access to health care, and of racial discrimination in health care (Reid

& Robson 2007a), serve to further disadvantage Māori as they attempt to redress the factors that contribute to poor health.

The Treaty of Waitangi provides the basis from which Māori have the right to self-determination, and the right to name themselves as tangata whenua (people of the land), and be recognised as such (Reid & Robson 2007). As mentioned previously, it was not until the 1970s that the New Zealand government acknowledged that significant breaches to the Treaty of Waitangi had occurred. As a result, the Crown began to implement a number of policies that sought to address some of the inequities suffered by Māori since the arrival of European settlers in the early 1800s. These included revamping the Māori Land Court, as mentioned previously, and establishing the Waitangi Tribunal. The Waitangi Tribunal was established in 1975 in order to make recommendations on claims brought by Māori relating to actions or omissions of the Crown that breached the promises made in the Treaty of Waitangi (www.waitangi-tribunal.govt.nz [accessed 26 February 2010]). Claims against the Crown continue to this day, and although the Waitangi Tribunal does not have final authority to decide points of law, it has made recommendations in over 100 reports on claims and a range of settlements have been made (www.waitangi-tribunal.govt.nz/reports [accessed 26 February 2010]).

> **Point to ponder**
> Māori have a life expectancy of 73.5 years at birth compared to 80.8 years for non-Māori.

Efforts to address the inequities that exist for Māori also extend into the health care sector. There has been significant growth in health service provision since the mid 1980s of 'by Māori for Māori' health services. Such Māori health services recognise and implement a Māori-centred approach to health care (kaupapa Māori services), which have been demonstrated as effective in reaching Māori whānau (King & Turia 2002; MOHNZ 2006b). There are now over 240 Māori health providers in New Zealand offering 'by Māori for Māori' health services (Māori Health Directorate 2008). Findings from the National Primary Medical Care Survey in 2001–02 suggest that such Māori providers are increasing access to care for Māori, and are frequently cheaper than traditional primary medical services such as GPs (Crengle 2007). Many of the services provided through kaupapa Māori health providers are also provided by nurses. Although numbers of Māori nurses are still not representative of the number of Māori living in New Zealand, many Māori nurses are working with Māori models of care providing effective and appropriate care for Māori individuals and families/whānau. The family or whānau is seen as the principal source of strength, support, security and identity for Māori and plays a central role in Māori wellbeing both individually and collectively (King & Turia 2002). Nurses working with kaupapa Māori models of care draw on this knowledge to provide culturally appropriate care.

BEHAVIOURAL RISK FACTORS

Health risks among Indigenous people also emanate from behavioural factors. Approximately 50% of Australian Indigenous people continue to smoke tobacco daily, a rate that has remained unchanged

BOX 11.2 KAUPAPA MĀORI HEALTH SERVICES

Te Hauora O Ngati Raru was established as a Māori health provider in 1996 and is located in Marlborough in the South Island of New Zealand. In 2005, a Māori diabetes nurse educator was appointed to provide a mix of one-on-one nursing care, in combination with a six-week education program to Māori clients and their whānau living with diabetes. Nursing care is provided to approximately 18 clients per week in both clinic and home environments and is supported by two other staff members in health support roles. Not only is care provided in a Māori-centred way, the nurse works intersectorally to ensure that clients and their whānau receive coordinated care from the variety of health providers with whom they interact. Evaluation of the nurse-led diabetes program demonstrated that clients maintained short-term improvements in physiological status, but most were unable to maintain this once the program ended. However, it was clearly demonstrated that using a Māori-centred approach to nursing care served to keep clients engaged with the service. As the service moves to including long-term family/whānau support meetings, it is anticipated that clients may be able to maintain the improvements seen in physiological status during the shorter program of care currently offered (Janssen 2009).

since figures were first collected in 1994 (Thomas et al 2008). This lies in contrast to the dramatic reduction of tobacco smoking in Australia to 16.6% of those over age 14 (Thomas 2009). In New Zealand, 42% of Māori smoke. Of greatest concern is the fact that Māori women are twice as likely to smoke than non-Māori women, which is one of the highest rates of smoking among any Indigenous group in the world. Māori men are 1.5 times more likely to smoke than non-Māori men (MOHNZ 2008). The poorest and most disadvantaged Indigenous people, those with low levels of education, employment and home ownership, are those most likely to take up smoking (Thomas et al 2008). People who have suffered prolonged mental distress also have a high risk of becoming smokers (Thomas et al 2008). Social disadvantage clearly constrains individual choices in terms of beginning or quitting smoking, including the disadvantage of being excluded from home ownership because of a lack of land rights. These factors and the difficulties of quitting, contribute to disproportionate rates of cancer deaths among Indigenous people in North America, New Zealand and Australia (Shahid & Thompson 2009).

Point to ponder

Approximately 50% of Indigenous Australians and 42% of Māori smoke, increasing their risk of conditions such as cardiovascular disease and lung cancer.

Overall, Indigenous Australians are less likely to consume alcohol than non-Indigenous Australians. For those who do, their consumption tends to be at high-risk levels. In New Zealand, Māori women are twice as likely as non-Māori women to have potentially hazardous drinking patterns. Māori men are 1.5 times more likely to have a hazardous drinking pattern than their non-Māori counterparts (MOHNZ 2008). Illicit drug use has been reported as approximately twice the rate of that of non-Indigenous people (AIHW 2008). Obesity is also a problem for many Indigenous people in Australia and New Zealand. Indigenous Australian women are more likely to be overweight or obese than non-Indigenous women, whereas among males the rates are similar. Māori children are 1.5 times more likely to be obese than non-Māori children in New Zealand, and Māori adults, both men and women, are 1.7 times more likely to be obese than non-Māori adults (MOHNZ 2008). These factors are not spread evenly throughout the population, but are disproportionate in rural and remote areas because of a lack of access to local produce, inappropriate storage facilities and the prohibitive costs of transportation (AIHW 2008). As mentioned previously, remoteness also affects access to hospital and other health services. Where Australian Indigenous people do have access to hospital care, the most common reasons for hospitalisation are dialysis treatment (14 times greater than non-Indigenous people), endocrine diseases such as diabetes (three times greater than non-Indigenous people), respiratory and digestive diseases, and treatment for injuries and mental health issues (AIHW 2008).

Māori adults are significantly more likely to be admitted to hospital than non-Māori and this is increasing across time (MOHNZ 2008). The most common reasons for admission to hospital for Māori were pregnancy and childbirth (41% higher than non-Māori), injury and poisonings (27% higher than non-Māori), and respiratory disease (65% higher than non-Māori). Admissions for endocrine, nutritional and metabolic disorders are 89% higher for Māori than non-Māori (Robson et al 2007b). Among New Zealand women, there are large disparities between Māori and non-Māori mortality rates for cervical and breast cancers, and both rates have increased for Māori women since 2005 (MOHNZ 2009a, 2009b). The inter-relatedness of the various risk factors is significant, as illustrated in an analysis of cancer mortality among Indigenous people (Shahid & Thompson 2009). Indigenous people are more likely to smoke, have lower rates of screening uptake, and be diagnosed with cancer at a later stage of the disease, again, in some cases, because of remoteness from services. These factors contribute to Indigenous people's lower survival rates, compared with non-Indigenous people. Other factors that contribute to the problem are a lack of culturally appropriate health education materials, and the possibility that some Indigenous people believe cancer is associated with shame, or that it will cause social or emotional isolation, and these act as deterrents to help-seeking or screening (Shahid & Thompson 2009).

MENTAL HEALTH AND HEALING

A large proportion of Indigenous Australians, and New Zealand Māori of every age group, report high levels of psychological distress (AIHW 2008; MOHNZ 2008). However, like members of other cultures, the experience of distress is often linked to the way individuals manage their embeddedness in social groups, how they preserve the social order, and their relationship to the social and natural environment (Fisher 2006). For many Indigenous people, seeking outside help for psychological distress is a source of shame and embarrassment, and often not seen as culturally appropriate (Anderson 2008). For Māori, if psychological distress is perceived by the family to be associated with makatu (a penalty for the infringement of tapu or sacredness), regardless of the severity of the illness, all effort will be made to avoid medical intervention (Durie 2001). This has implications for counselling, given that counselling practices would be inadequate without a holistic, spiritual and cultural understanding of the contextual realities of a person's life, family context and past experiences (Stewart 2008; MOHNZ 2006b). Indigenous health and counselling differs from the 'health crisis' perspective of Western medicine, instead moving through a circular process of healing (Stewart 2008).

For Indigenous Australians having a close connection to Country affects assessment and treatment. Indigenous people need to feel that their social world and their health care are connected to their lives, and the way they experience their world, which is a reciprocal relationship between individual and community (Belfrage 2007). Healing conversations therefore need to be inclusive of the cultural construction of their knowledge, language and styles of communication, and the way experiences are understood in the context of community (Stewart 2008). In addition, there is a profound effect on many Indigenous Australian people from a history of loss, separation, traumatic experiences, and previous experiences with mental health services, all of which frame the way new events are experienced. Another issue involved in assessment is that, rather than seeing a mental illness as a parallel experience to becoming physically ill, in a similar way to the Māori concept of makatu outlined above, an Indigenous Australian person might see it as payback for a previous transgression. The person may believe they are being 'sung' by an aggrieved party, married the 'wrong way', 'caught out' by the law, or 'crying for Country'. Because there is often little understanding of the concept of holism as it is understood by Indigenous people, health professionals may misdiagnose expressions of mental distress. Assessment strategies often overlook the fact that healing and therapeutic approaches have to be based on understanding of the cultural meanings of kinship, the land, spirituality and heritage (O'Brien 2006; Vicary & Bishop 2005). The Whare Tapa Wha Māori Model of Health developed by Mason Durie in New Zealand articulates a concept of holism that has been adopted by many Māori and non-Māori, as a means of understanding the way in which Māori conceptualise health. The four cornerstones of the Whare Tapa Wha Model are hinengaro (mental wellbeing), tinana (physical wellbeing), whānau (family wellbeing) and wairua (spiritual wellbeing). Each cornerstone is interlinked, and health may not be achieved without a balance between all four cornerstones (Durie 1994).

> ### Point to ponder
> Indigenous models of health such as Whare Tapa Wha depict holistic wellbeing, which is essential to Indigenous health. Understanding this can assist non-Indigenous providers to work alongside Indigenous cultures to achieve improved health outcomes.

As a spiritual journey, healing requires time and a culturally safe, capacity building approach to assist in the recovery from past traumas, addictions or other problems. The journey is aimed at cultural renewal and strengthening identity, often through language, dance and song, all of which can help a person reconnect with family, community, and culture (Commonwealth of Australia 2009b). The 'by Māori for Māori' health services in New Zealand, as outlined above, has been one approach to addressing many of the cultural needs of Māori as they seek to address their health needs. These services are based in both traditional settings, such as hospitals, and in non-traditional settings, such as on Marae (a Māori meeting ground). Importantly, past traumas, such as those experienced by the Stolen Generations, cannot be resolved until there is government and societal acknowledgement of the source of these problems. Left unresolved, the history of trauma can lead people to internalise shame and guilt, and whole communities can begin to think that pain and chaos is normal (Commonwealth of Australia 2009b).

A study by Vicary and Bishop (2005) revealed that some Indigenous people can fall into a depressed and anxious mood state, needing to go to Country, restless to connect with their land in a way that a non-Indigenous person would not experience depression. In this study, male research participants explained that Indigenous men were more likely to be predisposed to mental ill health, because of the weakening of their traditional role as a provider. This caused the men to have low self-esteem, depression and an inability to see practical alternatives, whereas the women felt they could not afford to become ill, because they had taken over the key family functions (Vicary & Bishop 2005). One of the implications of this study is that healing should take place 'on Country' in the context of gender-sensitive, culturally appropriate conversations, rather than in the type of health facilities or therapeutic approaches used by non-Indigenous people. This is also the approach advocated by Noel Pearson (2009), an Indigenous leader, who suggests that restoring culturally and economically sustainable homelands provides an ideal context for strengthening the cultural transmission of values, language and a sense of the future. Stronger bonds with the land provide a grassroots opportunity to foster confidence and help Indigenous people develop resilience and cultural identity, which can act as protective factors against mental ill health.

Identity is integral to understanding people's responses to health and ill health (Stewart 2008). Kickett-Tucker (2009) explains that Australian literature confuses racial identity with cultural identity, group identity, collective identity, ethnic identity and self-concept. Racial identity can be a source of confusion and conflict, especially in the context of racism in society, and this can, in turn, compromise an individual's self-esteem (Kickett-Tucker 2009). Kickett-Tucker's (2009) interviews with young Aboriginal children were designed to investigate racial identity as a social construct, shaped by their interactions with others, and with social structures surrounding their lives. The children revealed that a strong sense of self, connection to family and kin, Aboriginal language, culture, inheritance, appearance and friends, all were important contributors to their racial identity, which was the centre of their health and wellbeing. This sense of identity has a protective function, helping children learn to deal with stressors such as racism in their environment, and providing them with a circle of strength, love and support (Kickett-Tucker 2009). Clearly, primary prevention for mental health in Indigenous people requires major, interdisciplinary initiatives by child care, education, health and social service professionals, to ensure the secure development of identity formation.

Point to ponder

Indigenous Australian and New Zealand Māori women are significantly more likely to be victims of intimate partner violence than non-Indigenous women.

INJURY AND FAMILY VIOLENCE

Indigenous Australians and Māori also suffer from a greater intentional and non-intentional burden of injury than non-Indigenous citizens, some from habitual subsistence activities, and for those in remote areas, injuries from road trauma, because of unchecked automobile safety standards and poor road conditions (Plani & Carson 2008). The rate of injury or deaths from road trauma among Australian Indigenous people is 2–5 times higher than in the general population, and in New Zealand it is 1.5 times higher. One of the most significant causes of injuries is domestic and family violence, with hospitalisations for assault among Indigenous women 30 times that of non-Indigenous Australian women (Plani & Carson 2008). Māori women are three times more likely to be victims of intimate partner violence (IPV) than non-Māori women (Families Commission 2009). There are numerous programs to counter this type of violence, 131 in Australia focusing on Indigenous people. These provide support, counselling and advocacy. Some focus on strengthening identity, behavioural reform, community policing and monitoring, and many provide shelter, protection and legal support (Plani & Carson 2008). As we reported in Chapters 5 and 10, many assaults against women and children are fuelled by alcohol and have variable levels of follow-up. There is also a lack of appropriate preparation for those providing emergency care and support, and inconsistent screening for violence. Because many Indigenous victims of violence live in remote areas, they are also disadvantaged by distance from services, especially where specialist intervention is required. The onus is often on ambulance paramedics and police to provide emergency life-saving treatment, to manage their trauma and minimise transfer problems. These tasks are frequently undertaken in collaboration with local elders, who can help ease the tension between family members or family groups.

Health professionals and nurses working in remote areas of Australia have also attempted to contend with the problem of child sexual assaults, which has attracted considerable media attention, especially in the Northern Territory, where television reports have declared this problem an epidemic. It is a serious issue, as is any case of oppression against children, but solutions are often masked by the media hysteria that has not recognised the effective interventions that have been quietly taking place in communities confronting sexual violence (Cripps & McGlade 2008). Part of the problem is the lack of evaluative data that would provide benchmarks for successful interventions. The other aspect of the problem that has not been widely publicised is the context in which violence is regularly occurring. Cripps and McGlade (2008) categorise the contextual realities of violence in Indigenous communities in two groups. Group 1 factors include colonisation, policies and practices, dispossession, and cultural dislocation, including removal of families. Group 2 factors include marginalisation as a minority, direct and indirect racism, unemployment and welfare dependency, previous history of abuse, poverty, destructive coping behaviours, addictions, physical and mental health issues, and low self-esteem and a sense of powerlessness. Research findings have shown that a disproportionate number of victims of violence are people who have been removed from their families, those with disabilities, and people who are living in low-income households or unemployed (Cripps & McGlade 2008). In New Zealand the Te Rito New Zealand Family Violence Prevention Strategy is aimed at reducing the incidence of family violence among both Māori and non-Māori families through a variety of approaches, including the development of practice guidelines, extensive training for health professionals, and the appointment of family violence intervention coordinators in all District Health Boards.

ADDRESSING THE PROBLEMS THROUGH HEALING AND EMPOWERMENT

To date, programs to tackle violence in Indigenous communities have not yielded positive results, although there are some improvements. The problems surround 'law and order' interventions, which have left women fearful of retribution if their oppressor is released from custody. Restorative justice programs are considered a positive step towards resolution. These include holding offenders responsible for their behaviour, without stigmatising them, giving victims a greater voice in the criminal justice process, having a say in how the offender is treated, devising punishments aimed at repairing the harm done, and restoring community safety (Cripps & McGlade 2008). Cripps and McGlade (2008) describe a 'best practice' example of this type of approach from Canada, where a Community Holistic Circle Healing process has been developed on the basis of the healing power of both the law and the community. The program focuses as much on the abuser as the victim, and requires a long-term commitment to spiritual heagling and restoration. Its success rate has been widely acknowledged, with a low recidivism rate of offending, cost effectiveness and community empowerment. The Community Holistic Circle Healing program is an example of culturally sensitive, community self-determination. It is a model adopted by other Indigenous groups, particularly in North America where the healing circles have been used to help people with the intergenerational trauma of having been removed from their families (Menzies 2008). A similar program has been implemented in South Australia, where a multidimensional community healing project has been successful in developing community capacity to deal with violence (Kowanko et al 2009).

Point to ponder

Programs addressing violence in Indigenous communities in Australia and New Zealand have had limited success to date. Restorative justice programs have been successful internationally, and may provide a way forward in Australia and New Zealand.

These models are a response to the disempowerment that occurs when diagnostic approaches to mental health issues tend to re-traumatise the victims, excluding meaningful discussions of culture that might help them move forward (Menzies 2008). However, critics of this approach argue that it is not consistent with Indigenous tradition or culture, which would severely punish offenders for such crimes as sexual assault. Other criticisms include the risk of powerful members of the community being able to interfere with the healing processes, which could potentially have a negative impact on the victim, especially if these were previous perpetrators of abuse. Cripps and McGlade (2008) contend that the restorative justice approach has a better chance of being effective than the current adversarial legal system, which often subjects sexual assault victims to further abuse from the Australian justice system. They recommend adapting the healing model in culturally appropriate contexts in Australia, in a way that does not cause further discrimination on the basis of gender or race (Cripps & McGlade 2008). This intersection of gender and race that was mentioned in Chapter 10 is a major problem for Indigenous women who have been subjected to institutional racism. For many, identifying with the Indigenous community rather than with other women, exposes them to a different kind of pressure than that experienced by non-Indigenous women (Kowanko et al 2009). In some cases, the way they have been treated in refuges and health services has been re-traumatising, creating new cycles of victimisation (Vincent & Eveline 2008). Clearly, the solutions lie in refraining from discussing family violence as an Indigenous problem, and ensuring that it is included in policies and practices that recognise the gendered power relations between men and women, and the structural factors that perpetuate inequalities in the roles of men and women.

BUILDING CAPACITY AND SOCIAL CAPITAL

The oppression of Indigenous people is indisputable, and it creates enormous challenges for medical practitioners, nurses, midwives, paramedics, health workers, teachers, police and other professionals working in Indigenous communities. For all of these health advocates the objective is to work out ways of helping people retrieve their sense of self, family, culture, community and society. This can begin from a set of behaviours, delving into the root causes of behaviours such as alcohol or substance misuse, that create cycles of risk, then working with individuals and families to see what can be done to reset the pattern for a more optimistic future. Noel Pearson (2004) and members of the Cape York Institute in Australia's Cape York Peninsula have devoted considerable effort to studying risk and potential in Indigenous people. For example, they address the problem of drug and alcohol abuse, criticising some of the ways it has been addressed in the past. They reject most of the common approaches used by those seeking to change behaviour. For example, the 'symptom theory', which sees addiction as a symptom of societal problems, is seen as unhelpful. The theory argues that symptoms can be redressed by understanding social and historical wrongs, and rearranging the person's environment. Likewise, they reject the 'voluntary rehabilitation' perspective. This approach holds the expectation that addicts will eventually seek help for their addiction. Another perspective, the 'normalisation' or 'responsible drinking' view is based on the notion that promoting responsible drinking will effect behaviour change, while the 'harm minimisation' approach is aimed at dealing with the consequences of abuse by trying to minimise harm to self and others. According to Pearson (2004) none of these is as effective as intolerance of abuse.

Point to ponder

An approach to preventing substance abuse among Indigenous young people is to develop community-determined and community-managed strategies that build on family and community strengths to create a place where young people can develop capacity and self-esteem.

Pearson (2004) equates the problems of substance abuse with other risky conditions; tobacco smoking, poor environmental health and poor nutrition, as all of these have a major impact on families and communities. He argues that historical factors such as trauma and dispossession, are not the most significant determinants of substance abuse, or any of the other risky individual behaviours of today's young people. Rather, the responsibility lies in the following five social conditions:

1 availability of the addictive or harmful substance
2 money to acquire the substance is easily accessed
3 spare time to use it
4 others in the immediate environment are engaging in the behaviour
5 there exists a permissive social ideology that reinforces the behaviour (Pearson 2004:8).

Pearson's (2004) solution to the problem is to reduce these precipitating factors, charging that an over-emphasis on alcohol abuse as a health problem obscures the importance of political and social ideology. Rather than minimise the harm by reducing supply or demand, there is a need to deal with the consequences, to manage the situation from within the community, conveying basic convictions, and establishing a sense of the future. Instead of focusing on disadvantage as an outcome of colonial history, he suggests that a community-determined, community-managed strategy would be a better focus to help put hope into people's hearts, and improve governance in their communities. This involves rebuilding tolerance, controlling the supply, managing money and time, instituting treatment and rehabilitation programs, and fixing up homes and the community to restore social and cultural capital (Pearson 2004, 2005). It also involves making the family and community viable, as places where young people can develop their capacity and personal self-esteem. A parallel approach could be applied to violence against women and children. Ideally, this would involve empowering the community from within, modifying environmental conditions so that they are not conducive to violence and abuse, ensuring there is available, viable employment, appropriate role models, strong cultural identity and a sense of self-worth.

The Cape York agenda for change is framed in the language of the Nobel Prize winning economist Amartya Sen. Sen's philosophy, as mentioned earlier in this book, revolves around *substantive freedom*. Indigenous people require a range of choices and having the capabilities to choose a life that they have reason to value (Pearson 2005). This means that resources cannot simply be allocated to people with an expectation that they will improve their lives. Networks of families, communities and businesses do not emerge from bureaucratic power, but from a combination of public order and safety, and the motivation to develop skills, self-confidence and personal responsibility.

This argument posits that Indigenous people need support and resources, but these must be accessed by members of the community seeking to enhance and revitalise their capacity and that of their community in a way that is mutually responsive and accountable. A stable, functioning family is the moral core of a community, the repository of the seeds of social capital. Any resources given to the community are thus *socially invested* and help the community build its own capacity through individuals bonding with one another, bridging together with other communities, and establishing linkages within interactions with institutions. Mignone and O'Neil (2005:S53) explain that this is a 'culture where families can help each other due to strong norms of reciprocity, where different community sectors and leadership offer support to families in need, where youth sense that they can trust adults before or during moments of crisis'. It is also a well-resourced environment where governments ensure land title, and where Indigenous language and culture are seen as national priorities (Pearson 2005:10).

GOALS FOR INDIGENOUS HEALTH

- Eliminate racism and all forms of discrimination against Indigenous people.
- Address the social determinants of disadvantage for Indigenous people.
- Improve child and youth health and wellbeing through perinatal and early childhood intervention and prevention strategies.
- Recognise the uniqueness and importance of Indigenous family and extended family networks.
- Promote public acceptance of the unique needs and sensitivities of Indigenous people.

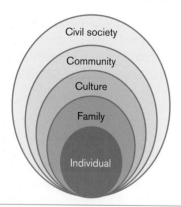

Figure 11.2 Protecting, preserving, empowering self, family, culture, society

- Improve responsiveness of mainstream services and programs to Indigenous people by increasing transparency and accountability.
- Recognise the impact of environmental degradation on Indigenous people, and create genuine opportunities for affected communities to participate in decision-making for environmental restoration.
- Acknowledge the uniqueness of Indigenous systems of knowledge in caring for Country.
- Maintain the health of Indigenous people as the highest priority for health planning.
- Support the development of economic, social and cultural capital to foster self-determinism, and strategies for culturally appropriate, sufficiently resourced education and skill development.
- Adopt strategies for intersectoral collaboration in all policies and planning strategies at all levels.
- Ensure cultural safety in all service provision for all people.
- Enshrine diversity and culture in the laws and social processes of the country.

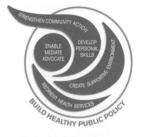

BUILDING HEALTHY PUBLIC POLICY

Healthy public policies are those that ensure access and equity of different cultural groups, and that guide action on inequalities (NHMRC 2005). This begins with acknowledging the interrelatedness of health, place and economic viability. At the international level, the Geneva Declaration on the Health and Survival of Indigenous People (WHO 1999) has not yet been successful in encouraging all countries to address Indigenous inequities. This reflects the failure of non-Indigenous governments to enshrine their obligations to Indigenous people in law or policy. Adequate policy development requires national initiatives around five major areas: evidence-based decision-making on Indigenous health issues; incorporating traditional health knowledge in health promotion systems; improving health systems' capacity to identify, and meet the needs of marginalised, ethnic populations; poverty-reduction strategies, and political will to better meet the health and development needs of all marginalised populations (WHO 1999).

Point to ponder
Both Australia and New Zealand have significant work to do to develop policies that will bring about change in Indigenous health status.

The rhetoric of health policy in Australia and New Zealand reflects a commitment to each of these international recommendations. However, much remains to be done to develop policies that will bring about change. The lack of evidence-based policy-making at either state or Commonwealth levels is a glaring omission from Australian Indigenous policy (Hudson 2009). Linked with this, is the complexity and ineffectiveness of funding for Indigenous health. The Centre for Independent Studies has examined the funding issues, and reported that over the past decade, the Commonwealth government has increased funding for Indigenous health programs by 328%, with no appreciable improvements to Indigenous health, and no clear indication of the level of unmet need (Hudson 2009). Despite funding, the health of Indigenous people is not improving, and in some cases, is deteriorating. Yet, the 2009 Australian National Health and Hospitals Reform Commission (NHHRC) recommended further expenditure on Indigenous health (Hudson 2009). If this recommendation is accepted by the government, the barriers to achieving better health must be addressed.

Barriers to health improvement include a lack of local consultation in implementing many programs for Indigenous people. Some of the worst examples include programs for violence and/or suicide prevention implemented in communities where these have not been problems, but because they are issues associated with Indigenous people, they have attracted government grants. Another barrier lies in the complexity of funding arrangements from different layers of government bureaucracy, and a mixture of private, public and Aboriginal Medical Services (AMS). There is no over-arching policy about the need for accountability, which means that funding is not always linked with health outcomes. Instead, 'bucket

funding', where program money is allocated from specific buckets of money, creates duplication in some places, and service gaps in others (Hudson 2009). As Hudson (2009) reports, one Indigenous health service has received 42 different buckets of money through different applications and reporting mechanisms, while other communities have no funding. Another problem has been that, in trying to be responsive to Indigenous requests, missing reports have often been overlooked, resulting in 'financial mismanagement, insolvency and even fraud' (Hudson 2009:vii).

Despite New Zealand's ongoing commitment to Māori health articulated in policy documents such as the New Zealand Health Strategy (2000), the New Zealand Primary Health Care Strategy (2001), He Korowai Oranga: the Māori Health Strategy (2002), the Māori Mental Health Strategic Framework (2002), and the Māori Health Action Plan (2006), the fact remains that the health status of New Zealand Māori remains poor and ethnic inequalities persist. There have been improvements in some areas: for example Māori are now counted accurately in death registrations, there have been some improvements in morbidity data, and, since 2000, there has been an overall decrease in all-cause mortality rates (Robson & Purdie 2007). There is also increasing documentation and evaluation of the work achieved by Māori Health Service Providers. However, these achievements must be viewed in light of the persisting existence of differential access to health care for Māori, differences in the quality of care that is received by Māori, and increased exposure to health risks as a result of differential access to the determinants of health (Reid & Robson 2007). More intense policy work is required to address these areas based on the knowledge held by Māori, using policy approaches that are culturally embedded.

In Australia, criticisms of the existing arrangements for Indigenous health continue. Some argue that, despite the failures, there are no new policies, simply old policies recycled (Hudson 2009). Most of the old, recycled policies simply thrust money at an undefined target called 'Indigenous health', aimed at 'closing the gap' in life expectancy. Continually highlighting the 'gap' instead of lifestyle factors, or gender issues, perpetuates the notion that every problem is related to race (Hudson 2009). This can be damaging not only as a racist approach, but in developing inappropriate health plans. For example, when maternal smoking and Indigenous status are disentangled and shown as separate risk factors, the difference between non-Indigenous and Indigenous low birth-weight infants disappears (Hudson 2009). Similarly, failing to identify violence against women as a gender issue masks it as an Indigenous problem. The focus of health promotion policies to deal with these issues should therefore be maternal smoking and gender, rather than Indigenous status. Likewise, the appalling state of housing of remote-living Indigenous people should be seen as the main cause of rheumatic fever and infectious diseases, rather than attributing these to Indigenous status (Hudson 2009; McDonald et al 2009). Acknowledging the source of the problems is crucial to developing appropriate solutions.

ACTION POINT
Use tools such as Health Impact Assessment to determine the potential impact of any policy on Indigenous people's health.

Policy responses to the traumas suffered by Indigenous people in Australia have often been tailored to their symptoms, by punitive or legislative responses that respond to the way individuals have reacted to the trauma. Instead, they should be redirected to the root causes, in a holistic and culturally appropriate manner, fostering self-determination, land rights and social justice (Commonwealth of Australia 2009b). Current recommendations for making these a reality include the expansion of healing centres, development of a Healing Foundation, consideration of a treaty such as the Treaty of Waitangi in New Zealand, promoting positive images of Indigenous people in the media, supporting ceremonies, rituals, and traditional ways of healing, including returning to Country, mainstream literacy programs and peer support groups (Commonwealth of Australia 2009b). Policies for community justice are an important part of healing, as well as dealing with current offences. A community justice approach works towards repairing the damage to both victims and the community through restorative justice, prevention and early intervention, and strengthening the community and its self-determination (Ryan et al 2006). This multidimensional strategy includes such things as sentencing circles, which involve

community elders in deciding fair solutions for social development and social sanctions against perpetrators of crime (Ryan et al 2006). Community approaches are inclusive, fostering community engagement instead of the paternalistic law-and-order adversarial approach, which has not succeeded in reducing the over-representation of Indigenous people in prisons in either Australia or New Zealand (Ryan et al 2006).

By far, the most urgent policy area in Australia is related to sovereignty of Indigenous rights, especially land rights. The UN Declaration on Indigenous Rights supports self-determination for all peoples, which means that they have a right to health, and therefore a right to their symbiotic relationship with the land (UN 2007). The role of government in this process is to facilitate, rather than dominate the development of partnerships, and other decision-making processes to help Indigenous communities achieve self-determined goals, cultural protection strategies, health and education (Jackson Pulver & Fitzpatrick 2004). The international policy environment therefore paves the way for stronger policies at the national level. The Australian NHHRC recommended establishment of a National Aboriginal and Torres Strait Islander (ATSI) Health Authority within the Commonwealth government's health portfolio, to commission and broker services for ATSI people and their families, with a view towards promoting better health outcomes and high-quality and timely access to culturally appropriate care (Commonwealth of Australia 2009a). Health promotion policies within such a portfolio should be aimed at developing an integrated strategy to improve the affordability of fresh food, including subsidies, supplementation for school children, infants, pregnant and breastfeeding women, and community nutrition education (Commonwealth of Australia 2009a). Recommendations also redirect policy emphasis on the needs of remote living Indigenous people, to better meet their needs and provide them with a highly trained, Indigenous workforce (Commonwealth of Australia 2009a).

It is vital to recognise the importance of involvement of Indigenous people at all levels of policymaking. Consultation with Indigenous people must occur prior to, during, and after any policy development process. In particular, health impact assessment (HIA) should be undertaken on all new policies, regardless of their perceived relationship with the health sector. HIA has been acknowledged in New Zealand's policy environment, with a tool for health impact assessment developed to specifically examine the impact of any new policy on Māori (MOHNZ 2007). Importantly, there is government recognition that consultation can be a drawn-out process, with some uncertainty about who to consult with. This has led to a government commitment to ensure that consultation time is allowed throughout the policy-making process.

CREATING SUPPORTIVE ENVIRONMENTS

An empowered community has equitable resources, especially in providing the basic hygiene and sanitation to keep people well. Empowered communities also have the capacity to identify and solve problems, participate in community activities, promote self-confidence, and influence social change. This relies on the infrastructure for good health, including housing, transportation, and the facilities that support health and wellbeing. Supportive environments also build human capital through the education, parenting skills and work experience skills that will ensure that those taking care of young people have an understanding of their needs for lifelong sustainable health and development. Importantly, they provide opportunities for capacity building. One of the most important environments for promoting Indigenous health in Australia is 'on Country'. Personal empowerment is more likely to result from grassroots efforts to engage Indigenous people in their homelands where their identity is strong. This is also the setting where birthing on Country can help create a strong bond between family members. It is also an environment where health professionals who are included in conversations or 'yarns' can learn about Indigenous understandings of health, which are more meaningful than those conducted in the somewhat detached environment of traditional health services.

ACTION POINT
Use intersectoral and collaborative strategies to create opportunities for developing environments that will support Indigenous people to achieve good health outcomes.

Interagency, intersectoral collaborative strategies are also more effective in a person's homeland or family context. With a shortage of Indigenous health professionals, strategies are often developed with a mix of Indigenous and non-Indigenous leadership. They should be directed at developing and sharing knowledge, capacity, networks and appropriate resources for change, and guided by Indigenous values and perceptions (Thompson et al 2008). Indigenous people can provide greater expert advice on health issues if their stories are listened to and valued, and their difficulties are acknowledged and acted upon (Thompson et al 2008). Understanding and mobilising Indigenous resources can help foster trust, reciprocity and shared decision-making, thereby helping to overcome the erosion of social capital created by historical disadvantage (Peiris et al 2008). The 'by Māori for Māori' health services discussed earlier, have been developed to build on and use the knowledge held by Māori to address their health needs. In particular, Marae-based health initiatives are being increasingly used to improve access to health services for Māori. Exercise programs, support groups, health clinics, antenatal classes, diabetes education, and cardiovascular rehabilitation are just some of the examples of health care services being offered in the safe environment of the Marae. These Marae-based services improve access to health care for many Māori, who have traditionally been reluctant to access mainstream health services that are perceived to be culturally inappropriate. Attempts are also being made to address the shortage of Indigenous health professionals to lead, manage and provide services in these organisations.

It is a matter of great concern that the very basic necessities, such as food and water, are not secured for a large proportion of Indigenous people. Australia's National Rural Health Alliance (NRHA) has been working relentlessly to advocate for food security and better nutrition for Indigenous people, who constitute a large proportion of Australian remote and rural dwellers. The issue of remoteness from fresh food is only part of the problem, as many people are subjected to outdated and poor-quality food in the only store they have available to them. Those who are poor, are unable to buy even subsistence quantities of food, because of the price, especially when there are differential prices favouring food high in fat, sugar and carbohydrate. Transport of food to the community, and the 'health hardware' that would give them storage and preparation facilities, are often absent. The issues are therefore a combination of cultural, transport, economic and management issues, all of which would be amenable to viable solutions with political will and local advocates.

> ### ACTION POINT
> Strategies that are more likely to improve health for Indigenous people are those developed with Indigenous communities and based in Indigenous communities.

Environments to help build community capacity are strengthened by community justice initiatives for young people who may be at risk of offending, or have already found their way into the criminal justice system. Youth programs, community policing and night patrols can help convey the impression that the community, not the legal or corrections systems, is accountable for behavioural outcomes. When these pro-social reinforcements of community self-determination are established in the community, there is a higher likelihood of developing local leaders and cohesive structures for harmony (Ryan et al 2006). For example, the Māori warden program operating in many towns and cities in New Zealand provides a culturally safe community patrol to assist young Māori who may be on the streets. School-based programs also help strengthen the environment, especially when programs are thoughtfully conceived, and based on in-depth knowledge of the community. The National Children's Nutrition Survey in New Zealand, for example, found that Māori children and Pacific Island children were significantly more likely to skip meals and to purchase food items from school tuckshops than non-Indigenous New Zealand children (Utter et al 2006). Despite the fact that these children were generally physically active, many skipped breakfast and had a low intake of fresh fruits and vegetables, whereas their snack foods contained high sugar and carbohydrate content. Numerous research studies have shown that there is a direct relationship between a diet low in fruit and vegetables and poverty. Therefore programs to improve nutritional health should begin by lobbying for food subsidies in schools to help children in the

setting where they spend the largest part of their day. The New Zealand study showed that obesity among the children was more closely linked to food rather than a lack of exercise, which provides a basis for this type of advocacy (Utter et al 2006).

STRENGTHENING COMMUNITY ACTION

Community action means getting involved in the community's self-defined priorities for health and wellbeing. Our general understandings of Indigenous cultures are often limited due to the widespread confusion over land rights, native title, the various levels of regulation, and how laws are interpreted in various areas. Because of the way these issues are presented in the public media, often with densely worded legal arguments, understandings can be open to misinterpretation. Advocacy is an important role for nurses, midwives and other health professionals working with Indigenous people. To be effective, it is important to maintain current knowledge of the decisions that are being taken at the political level. The most important input to our deliberations will come from seeking the views of local Indigenous people on how that may affect their capacity for self-determination. For example, addressing the social ecology within which cultural traditions are preserved also has the potential to reinvigorate Indigenous authority, and retain the transference of land for the next generations. This can create a self-perpetuating cycle of cultural empowerment.

> ### ACTION POINT
> In order to recognise and preserve the cultural traditions that are vital to Indigenous health, always seek the opinions of Indigenous people on how they would like you to advocate for them.

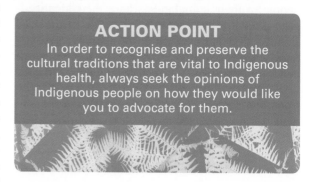

Community action is also locally determined. As the researchers from the Australian Centre for Independent Studies reported, programs such as those targeting family violence, are being developed according to racist policies (Hudson 2009). This is a contradiction of the primary health care (PHC) approach, where community-determined priorities should govern the allocation of resources. A more culturally appropriate program is exemplified by the South Australian Healing program for family violence, which is based on a whole-of-community approach as shown in Box 11.3.

Other strategies to strengthen community action are aimed at developing different types of responses according to self-defined need and preference. Cultural diversity in traditional birthing practices defies making assumptions about preferences. Birthing on Country programs can be developed for those wanting to access midwifery services in a place where they feel supported by family. This is challenging for high-risk pregnancies, but efforts should be made where possible

to try and accommodate cultural needs at the time of childbirth. The most enduring birthing program in the Northern Territory has been the 'Strong Women, Strong Babies, Strong Culture' initiative, which has had a significant effect on improving the birth-weight of Indigenous mothers (D'Espaignet et al 2003).

DEVELOPING PERSONAL SKILLS

Being culturally safe in our approach to helping people develop personal skills begins with self-development. How we personally approach the problems of inequitable ill health for Indigenous people and others disadvantaged by race or ethnicity will be shaped by introspection on our thoughts, feelings and attitudes. For Indigenous communities, health outcomes will only be improved by solutions that are conjointly developed within authentic partnerships between community members and others they choose to include in their decision-making. This will ensure that planning is closely aligned with the culturally embedded knowledge of the community, as transmitted by the guardians of their culture. If our knowledge lies outside the culture of those we seek to assist, our role is to listen, to reflect on both our culture and theirs, then to see whether we can respond to their needs in a way that adds value to their self-determined solutions. This first step is the most important. Each of us needs to build our own personal understanding and tolerance from a studious approach to Indigenous health. Literally, this means that we first assume the role of learner, having the humility to realise that non-Indigenous voices do not speak for Indigenous people. Second, we need to better understand their perspectives and worldviews, through the lens of culturally appropriate ways of knowing. This requires a respectful and receptive attitude, to learn, to build trust, credibility, and ultimately, to share intellectual, cultural and social capital. Once these steps have been taken, personal skills can be developed and strengthened in a spirit of mutual capacity building.

> **BOX 11.3** WHOLE-OF-COMMUNITY HEALING OBJECTIVES: SOUTH AUSTRALIA
>
> 1 Build community capacity to support safe families. This includes physical as well as cultural safety.
>
> 2 Equip Indigenous people with the skills for effective communication and conflict resolution. This includes appropriate counselling and guidance strategies that are aimed at men's and women's styles of communication and confidence building.
>
> 3 Support families in crisis. Multidimensional programs focus on both prevention and interventions, which includes helping women find accommodation, support, legal and financial assistance.
>
> 4 Build capacity of mainstream agencies and services within the region. This requires intersectoral collaboration and partnerships. In the South Australian program women worked with crafts while learning to manage stress and develop new communication skills. A range of programs can be offered that reinforce existing strengths and help build new ones such as anger management or mutual support networks.
>
> 5 Workforce development. Support groups require training programs that help build a healing culture. In many cases, staff members suffer burnout and stress, and they require healing support to help them cope.
>
> 6 Data and evaluation. Systematic evaluation of program effectiveness provides a foundation for change, expansion and sharing knowledge in other programs and centres.
>
> (Kowanko et al 2009)

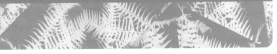

ACTION POINT

In order to work effectively with Indigenous cultures, we must first examine our own personal understandings and attitudes towards Indigenous people and their health status.

In many Indigenous communities, particularly in rural and remote areas, health literacy is the most pressing problem. Education programs in a person's native tongue are helpful in fostering Indigenous identity, but there is also a need to ensure English language comprehension, in order to help Indigenous people develop the ability to read, and understand issues related to health. Some Indigenous adults lack the functional health literacy that would help them read medication labels or understand the instructions given by a medical practitioner, nurse or Aboriginal or Māori Health Worker (Hudson 2009). Aboriginal Health Workers (AHW) practise in stressful conditions, sometimes torn between their obligations as a health service employee and the obligations to their family and community. They are often the only health worker in their remote community, and like the people they are caring for, may also have low literacy and numeracy skills (Hudson 2009). Implementing skills training for health literacy has to be an inclusive strategy, where everyone, including Aboriginal and Māori Health Workers, parents, grandparents, elders, and health professionals working in a particular community, can come together for culturally appropriate planning. In this context, there can be mutual learning opportunities and meaningful input into the best way to change such things as hygiene, child development, education and parenting skills. A further step towards developing health literacy is to ensure that health education materials are framed in culturally appropriate, and symbolic language and images that can be linked to the realities of a person's life. This would help counteract some of the problems that have existed in remote communities to date. In some cases, non-English-speaking Indigenous people have been provided with written materials with no recognisable message in the local language. This is most evident in diabetes self-management programs, some of which have been given to groups with a lack of both literacy and numeracy, and little understanding of terms like 'elevated blood sugar', 'healthy weight range' or the skills to calculate medications (Hudson 2009:14–15).

One of the findings of Zubrick et al's (2005) study of Australian Indigenous children was that there is a 20% loss of Indigenous languages in areas of moderate to extreme geographic isolation. Cultural isolation is also a major problem, often causing emotional difficulties especially for those who have been removed from their natural families in childhood, leaving them unsure of their cultural roots and identities (Eckermann et al 2006; Kickett-Tucker 2009). Continued efforts must therefore be made to preserve, document, teach and encourage identity and the use of local languages and culture. Cultural heritage is also critical to survival of any particular group. Bond (2005) argues that Aboriginality is about pride, strength, determination and survival, not inadequacies, impairment or hopelessness, which can demonise and disconnect people from their cultural identity. Identifying and building on strengths, instead of deficiencies is therefore the appropriate approach for intervention.

ACTION POINT
Implement skills training in health literacy for all people involved in Indigenous health. Practitioners, parents, grandparents, elders, Indigenous health workers and children can then work together to undertake culturally appropriate planning.

Tsey et al (2005) describe a school-based program that responds to the need for empowered leadership, as well as learning. Their program, conducted with the Cape York Partnerships Initiative, and based on a family empowerment program for isolated families, illustrated the positive effect of working to develop personal skills alongside group skills and leadership. They used the school setting with young people living in a remote area, and engaged in a step-by-step development of self-knowledge and understanding, in terms of how they fit into the immediate and broader social environment. The young people had an opportunity to explore relationships, issues typical of school attendance, such as bullying, emotions, beliefs and attitudes, and their own needs and aspirations. They were then offered opportunities to connect these with the needs and aspirations of others. The mutual understanding and self-confidence they gained helped reinforce connections between people, and developed the leadership skills for networking and problem-solving (Tsey et al 2005).

REORIENTING HEALTH SERVICES

Health services for Indigenous people around the world are woefully inadequate. This is an irrefutable fact. As our national and international gaze turns from problems to solutions, another indisputable fact is reiterated over and over. The health of Indigenous people will not be improved until there is culturally appropriate, community-controlled but accountable, community-based health services, supported with adequate financial resources linked to health outcomes. Improving health services also depends on building Indigenous workforce capacity through national training plans and ongoing skills and capacity development. In Australia, the need for Indigenous health professionals is acute. There is also a need to respond to the recommendations of the NHHRC to better manage and coordinate funding for Indigenous programs. Oversight by a national authority that is accountable for funding and administration will help ensure that patient outcomes are linked to the quality, cost and appropriateness of services. Throughout Australia, there is wide variability in models of service delivery, with some areas having small clinics operating out of regional hospitals, others having PHC centres, and others having only intermittent services. As mentioned previously, remoteness can be a health hazard, and this varies depending on which state and under whose control health services are administered. Unless there is transparency and accountability in services, health service–community partnerships pay only lip service to genuine collaboration (Hudson 2009).

ACTION POINT

In order to be able to reorient health services to effectively meet Indigenous health needs, health practitioners must make use of all opportunities for training and education in Indigenous health. If these opportunities do not exist, seek to create them.

Existing health service arrangements for Indigenous people are funded on a basis of per capita allocations, through a number of agencies. This one-size-fits-all model is unfair for those whose communities have few health professionals and many needs. To reduce service inequities it would be necessary to change the funding structure to meet health needs, rather than on the basis of Indigenous status. The other problem with health funding is the fee-for-service model, where wastage occurs because of top-down planning where health services are only considered viable if they stay within budgets. This can lead to over-servicing to meet quotas, and can disadvantage individual patients. Regional allocation of funds for health services with accountable oversight would potentially be more responsive to locally determined needs and result in better coordination of care (Hudson 2009). New Zealand is working towards this approach. A population-based funding model has been introduced with the intention of ensuring equitable funding to address Indigenous health needs, but a fee-for-service model in primary care continues to limit access to PHC for many Indigenous people due to cost (Caccioppoli & Cullen 2005).

One important area requiring attention for health services effectiveness is the training, and continuing education, for health professionals servicing rural and remote areas. The professional, cultural and personal isolation experienced by health professionals in remote areas is profound, and many have little preparation and training for the cultural or geographic context (Kildea et al 2009). Health professionals working in these non-urban areas need an expanded repertoire of skills and attributes, including advocacy skills and in-depth cultural understanding of an Indigenous worldview of health and wellbeing (Durie et al 2008). This includes understanding the relative importance placed on cultural, rather than clinical, proficiency. For those educated in other countries, there may be little understanding of the cultural domains, and layers of identity, that frame Indigenous people's experiences of health and ill health, particularly in their relationship with health and place (Durie et al 2008). To work effectively in diverse areas requires reflexive self-awareness, which is instrumental to culturally safe health care. Reflexive practices can be nurtured in pre-service preparation or as an ongoing expectation of the professional role. Adopting a reflexive approach to community engagement helps connect practice with a more inclusive, culturally competent, caring approach that does not ignore, override, discount, reject or violate the integrity of any group of people (Puzan 2003). The major focus of reflecting on practice is consideration of the notions of 'other' and 'whiteness'; what it is like to feel different, and how those residing at the margins of society must experience their world (Canales & Bowers 2001; Puzan 2003). The nursing profession has yet to achieve cultural representativeness of Indigenous nurses, who would be able to promote culturally appropriate models of care (Puzan 2003; Turale & Miller 2006). In addition to shortages, current programs in Australia have only minimal Indigenous curriculum components, although both curricula and the proportion of Indigenous nurses are improving with the advocacy of organisations like the Congress of Aboriginal and Torres Strait Islander Nurses (CATSIN). In New Zealand, there are two undergraduate nursing degree programs that offer Bachelor degrees designed specifically to focus on the health needs of Māori. These programs are targeted specifically to Māori students and use a kaupapa Māori approach to teaching and learning. The programs aim to produce graduates with both mainstream nursing skills and culturally specific skills.

New Zealand seems to be as far advanced as any country in establishing self-governance for Māori communities. Based on the well-entrenched Treaty of Waitangi, the New Zealand government has adopted a PHC approach to help Māori and non-Māori society have control over the direction and shape of their own institutions, their communities, and their development as people (MOHNZ 2002). The government strategy makes visible its commitment to people accessing support and health care in consideration of their language preference, and participation in decision-making in regards to health and healing. Like Canada and Australia, New Zealand has also built in a plan for workforce development (scholarships and training opportunities) as part of service quality. Coordinated strategies adopted in New Zealand include increasing the number of Māori health care providers and health workers, increasing resources where there are higher levels of deprivation and higher proportions of minority residents, requiring agencies to implement Māori-specific strategies for health, and increasing Māori representation in health sector governance (Bramley et al 2005).

In a socially just, and thus healthy environment, health services would be adequate. They would support dignity and inclusiveness, and recognise the negative effects of racism and discrimination on health (Bramley et al 2005). Solutions need to be empowering, in Indigenous-controlled contexts, from enabling environments (Stanley 2003). As we have reiterated many times, the relationship between health professionals and the community has to be one of mutual respect, partnership and genuine exploration of need. People from all cultures should be free to choose the pathways to health that best suit their needs and customs, and be assured that the over-arching principles of cultural safety pave the way to their self-governance over health (Eckermann et al 2006). This will help ensure system-level cultural competency. When we value diversity, help people develop their capacity for cultural self-assessment, and understand the dynamics of interacting cultures in a health care situation, cultural knowledge becomes institutionalised in service delivery and workforce development (NHMRC 2005).

Case study

Taine (Maria's sister's husband) has come from the rural east coast of New Zealand. There has been a history of intergenerational cycles of abusive behaviour in his family and Taine has struggled to break free from the cycle. The Te Rito New Zealand Family Violence Prevention Strategy has resulted in improved access to family violence prevention services in Taine's hometown and on a trip home to visit his whānau (family), Taine talks to his Kaumatua (chief) about the cycle of violence. The Māori nurse practitioner has been working with Taine's whānau, to address the family violence issues that are present, and welcomes him.

In Sydney, Willie, who is a neighbour of Jim and Maria has become involved in a local 'Strong Families' initiative. He provides support with an interdisciplinary team of health professionals and members of the public working together to preserve culturally safe counselling and support.

REFLECTING ON THE BIG ISSUES

- The reasons for the lower health status and shorter life span of Indigenous people compared with non-Indigenous people include socio-economic disparities, deprivation, unequal treatment, racism and discrimination, and unhealthy environments.
- Societies cannot be inclusive until historical traumas against Indigenous people are dealt with by the wider society.
- Reducing health risk factors for Indigenous people should be planned according to the specific risk rather than Indigenous status.
- Community engagement must be undertaken from a perspective of cultural safety and respect for Indigenous culture.
- Solutions to Indigenous socio-economic disadvantage have to extend beyond increasing funding to long-term capacity building.
- Intersectoral and inter agency collaboration is a major element in ensuring continuity of Indigenous capacity development.
- Developing a base of research evidence is essential to providing a foundation for change in Indigenous communities.

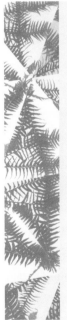

Reflective questions: how would I use this knowledge in practice?

1 Identify the chain of factors related to colonisation that predispose Indigenous people to ill health.

2 Develop a web of causation for the disproportionate burden of chronic illness among Indigenous people.

3 Outline a strategy for promoting health literacy among middle-age Indigenous residents of a rural community with a view towards managing chronic illness.

4 Explain how you would guide Taine in his quest to address problems with family violence.

5 What primary health care initiatives would be included in the program attended by Jim and Maria's neighbour, Willie, to help build family strengths?

6 What steps could be taken to develop a whole-of-community approach to family violence in an Indigenous community?

7 How does a knowledge of cultural safety change the way you work with Taine's or Willie's family?

Research-informed practice

Read Kildea et al's (2009) action research study 'Participative research in a remote Australian Aboriginal setting'.

- In replicating the study in a different community, either urban or rural, what would be the barriers and enabling factors to consider?
- How could the study findings be used as a birthing resource for a wider group of parents?
- What research questions would guide development of such a resource?

References

Aboriginal and Torres Strait Islander Social Justice & Australian Human Rights Commission 2010 Inquiry into the Native Title Amendment Bill (No. 2). Online. Available: www.hreoc.gov.au/Social_Justice/index.html (accessed 14 January 2010)

Adelson N 2005 The embodiment of inequity: health disparities of Aboriginal Canada. Canadian Journal of Public Health 96(S2):S45–S61

Anderson J 2008 Cultural liaison workers. Learnings from the mensline Australia Cultural X Change Project. Australian Institute of Family Studies, Family Relationships Quarterly Issue 12:3–6

Anderson J, Perry J, Blue C, Browne A, Henderson A, Koushambbi B, Reimer Kirkham S, Lynam J, Semiuk P, Smye V 2003 'Rewriting' cultural safety within the postcolonial and postnational feminist project. Advances in Nursing Science 26(3):196–214

Australian Council for Aboriginal Reconciliation (ACAR) 1994 Walking Together: The First Steps. Report of the Australian Council for Aboriginal Reconciliation. AGPS, Canberra.

Australian Institute of Health and Welfare (AIHW) 2008 Australia's Health 2008. AIHW, Cat. No. AUS 99, Canberra

Australian Medical Association (AMA) 2007 Aboriginal and Torres Strait Islander Health: Institutionalised Inequity Not Just a Matter of Money. Report Card Series 2007, AMA, Canberra

Beiser M 2005 The health of immigrants and refugees in Canada. Canadian Journal of Public Health 96(S2):S30–S44

Belfrage M 2007 Why 'culturally safe' health care? Medical Journal of Australia 186(10):537–8

Berry J 1995 Psychology of acculturation. In: Goldberg N, Veroff J (eds) The Culture and Psychology Reader. New York University Press, New York, pp 457–88

Bond C 2005 A culture of ill health: public health or Aboriginality? Dr Ross Ingram Memorial Essay. Medical Journal of Australia 183(10):39–41

Brady M 1995 Culture in treatment, culture as treatment: a critical appraisal of developments in addictions programs for indigenous North Americans and Australians. Social Science and Medicine 41(11):1487–98

Bramley D, Hebert P, Tuzzio L, Chassin M 2005 Disparities in Indigenous health: a cross-country comparison between New Zealand and the United States. American Journal of Public Health 95(5):844–50

Brough M, Bond C, Hunt J 2004 Strong in the city: toward a strength-based approach in Indigenous health promotion. Health Promotion Journal of Australia 15(3):215–20

Browne A 2005 The socio–political context of nurses' encounters with First Nations women in a Canadian health care setting. International Conference on Innovations in Nursing, Keynote Presentation, 12 November, Fremantle, Western Australia

Burgess C, Johnston F, Bowman D, Whitehead P 2005 Healthy Country: Healthy People? Exploring the health benefits of Indigenous natural resource management. Australian and New Zealand Journal of Public Health 29(2):117–22

Caccioppoli P, Cullen R 2005 Māori Health. Kotahitanga Community Trust, Auckland

Callaghan H 2001 Traditional Aboriginal birthing practices in Australia: past and present. Birth Issues 10(3/4):92–9

Canales M, Bowers B 2001 Expanding conceptualizations of culturally competent care. Journal of Advanced Nursing 36(1):102–11

Chandler M, Lalonde C 1998 Cultural continuity as a hedge against suicide in Canada's First Nations communities. Transcultural Psychology 35:191–219

Commonwealth of Australia 2007 National Indigenous Housing Guide. Department of Family and Community Services, Canberra

—— 2009a A Healthier Future For All Australians — Final Report of the National Health and Hospitals Reform Commission. June 2009, Canberra

—— 2009b Voices from the Campfires. Establishing the Aboriginal and Torres Strait Islander Healing Foundation. ATSI Healing Foundation Team, FAHCSIA, Canberra

Couzos S 2004 Practical measures that improve human rights — towards healthy equity for Aboriginal children. Health Promotion Journal of Australia 15(3):186–92

Crengle S 2007 Primary care and Māori: findings from the National Primary Medical Care Survey. In: Robson B, Harris R (eds) Hauora: Māori Standards of Health IV. A study of the Years 2000–2005. Te Ropu Rangahau Hauora a Eru Pomare, Wellington, pp 225–8

Cripps K, McGlade H 2008 Indigenous family violence and sexual abuse: considering pathways forward. Journal of Family Studies 14(2–3):240–53

Culley L 2006 Transcending transculturalism? Race, ethnicity and health-care. Nursing Inquiry 13(2):144–53

D'Espaignet E, Measey M, Carnegie M, Mackerras D 2003 Monitoring the 'Strong Women, Strong Babies, Strong Culture' Program: the first eight years. Journal of Paediatric Child Health, 39:668–72

Draper G, Somerford P, Pilkington A, Thompson S 2009 What is the impact of missing Indigenous status on mortality estimates? An assessment using record linkage in Western Australia. Australian and New Zealand Journal of Public Health 33(4):325–31

Duke J, Connor M, McEldowney R 2009 Becoming a culturally competent health practitioner in the delivery of culturally safe care: a process oriented approach. Journal of Cultural Diversity 16(2):40–9

Durie A, Hill P, Arkles R, Gilles M, Peterson K, Wearne S, Canuto, C Jackson Pulver L 2008 Overseas-trained doctors in Indigenous rural health services: negotiating professional relationships across cultural domains. Australian and New Zealand Journal of Public Health 32(6):512–18

Durie M 1994 Whaiora: Māori Health Development. Oxford University Press, Auckland

—— 2001 Mauri Ora: The Dynamics of Māori Health. Oxford University Press, Auckland

—— 2004 An Indigenous model of health promotion. Health Promotion Journal of Australia 15(3):181–5

Eckermann A, Dowd T, Chong E, Nixon L, Gray R, Johnson S 2006 Binan Goonj: Bridging Cultures in Aboriginal Health (2nd edn). Elsevier, Sydney

Families Commission 2009 Family Violence Statistics Report. Families Commission, Wellington

Fisher R 2006 Congruence and functions of personal and cultural values: do my values reflect my culture's values. Personality and Social Psychology 32(11):1419–31

Fredericks B 2008 Researching with Aboriginal women as an Aboriginal woman researcher. Australian Feminist Studies 23(55):113–29

Harlem Brundtland G 1999 International Consultation on the Health of Indigenous People. WHO, Geneva

Hudson S 2009 Closing the accountability gap: The first step towards better Indigenous health. Centre for Independent Policy Studies CIS Monograph 105, Melbourne

Hull B, McIntyre P, Couzos S 2004 Evaluation of immunisation cover for Aboriginal and Torres Strait Islander children using the Australian childhood immunisation register. Australian and New Zealand Journal of Public Health 28(1):47–52

Human Rights and Equal Opportunity Commission (HREOC) 1997 Bringing Them Home: Report of the National Inquiry into the Separation of Aboriginal and Torres Strait Islander Children from their Families. HREOC, Sydney

Jackson Pulver L, Fitzpatrick S 2004 Sitting 'round the table of rights-based reconciliation: a health perspective. Health Promotion Journal of Australia 15(3):193–9

Janssen J 2009 Meeting the needs of Māori with diabetes: an evaluation of a nurse-led service. Masters thesis. Victoria University, Wellington

Kickett-Tucker C 2009 Moorn [Black]? Djardak [White]? How come I don't fit in Mum? Exploring the racial identity of Australian Aboriginal children and youth. Health Sociology Review 18(1):119–36

Kildea S, Barclay L, Wardaguga M, Dawumal M 2009 Participative research in a remote Australian Aboriginal setting. Action Research 7(2):143–63

King A, Turia T 2002 He Korowai Oranga: Māori Health Strategy. Ministry of Health, Wellington

Kingsley J, Townsend M, Phillips R, Aldous D 2009 'If the land is healthy … it makes the people healthy'. The relationship between caring for Country and health for the Yorta Yorta Nation, Boonwurrung and Bangerang Tribes. Health & Place 15:291–9

Kowanko I, Stewart T, Power C, Fraser R, Love I, Bromley T 2009 An Aboriginal family and community healing program in metropolitan Adelaide: description and evaluation. Australian Indigenous Health Bulletin 9(4):1–12

Kulig J 2000 Culturally diverse communities: the impact on the role of community health nurses. In: Stewart M (ed.) Community Nursing: Promoting Canadians' Health (2nd edn). WB Saunders, Toronto, pp 194–210

Lutschini M 2005 Engaging with holism in Australian Aboriginal health policy — a review. Australia & New Zealand Health Policy 2:15 doi:10.1186/1743-8462-2-15

Māori Health Directorate 2008 Māori Health Providers. Online. Available: www.māorihealth.govt.nz/moh.nsf/menuma/Māori+Health+Providers (accessed 7 October 2009)

Martin-McDonald K, McCarthy A 2007 'Marking' the white terrain in indigenous health research: literature review. Journal of Advanced Nursing 61(2):126–33

Matsumoto D, Juang L 2004 Culture and Psychology (3rd edn). Thomson/Wadsworth, Belmont, Ca

McDonald E, Bailie R, Grace J, Brewster D 2009 A case study of physical and social barriers to hygiene and child growth in Australian Aboriginal communities. BMC Public Health 9:346 doi:1186/1471-2458-9-346

McLennan V, Khavarpour F 2004 Culturally appropriate health promotion: its meaning and application in Aboriginal communities. Health Promotion Journal of Australia 15(3):237–9

McMurray A, Param R 2008 Culture-specific care for Indigenous people: a primary health care approach. Contemporary Nurse 28(1/2):165–72

Menzies P 2008 Developing an Aboriginal healing model for intergenerational trauma. International Journal of Health Promotion and Education 46(2):41–9

Mignone J, O'Neil J 2005 Social capital and youth suicide risk factors in First Nations Communities. Canadian Journal of Public Health 96 (S1):S51–S54

Ministry of Health New Zealand (MOHNZ) 2001 Priorities for Māori and Pacific Health: Evidence from Epidemiology. MOHNZ, Wellington

—— 2002 He Korowai Oranga, Māori Health Strategy. MOHNZ, Wellington

—— 2006a Tatau Kahukura: Māori Health Chart Book. Public Health Intelligence Monitoring Report No. 5. MOHNZ, Wellington

—— 2006b Whakatataka Tuarua: Māori Health Action Plan 2006–2011. MOHNZ, Wellington

—— 2007 Whānau Ora Health Impact Assessment. Ministry of Health, Wellington

—— 2008 A Portrait of Health. Key Results of the 2006/07 New Zealand Health Survey. MOHNZ, Wellington

—— 2009a Mortality and Demographic Data 2006. MOHNZ, Wellington

—— 2009b Mortality and Demographic Data 2005. MOHNZ, Wellington

Ministry of Health New Zealand, Minister of Health 2008 Health and Independence Report 2008. Ministry of Health, Wellington

National Health and Medical Research Council (NHMRC) 2005 Increasing cultural competency for healthier living — a handbook for policy, planning and practice. Consultation Draft Discussion Paper, NHMRC, Canberra

New Zealand in History 2006 Online. Available: www.history-nz.org/māori5.html (accessed 24 June 2006)

New Zealand Statistics 2003 New Zealand Drinking Trends. Wellington, NZ. Online. Available: www.alac.org.nz/NZStatistic.aspx?PostingID=1187 (accessed 16 January 2006)

Nursing Council of New Zealand (NCNZ) 1996 Guidelines for Cultural Safety in Nursing and Midwifery Education. NCNZ, Wellington

—— 1992 Standards for Registration of Comprehensive Nurses from Polytechnic Courses. NCNZ, Wellington

O'Brien A 2006 Moving toward culturally sensitive services for Indigenous people: a non-Indigenous mental health nursing perspective. Contemporary Nurse 21(1):22–31

Pearson N 2004 The Cape York Substance Abuse Strategy. Griffith University Centre for Governance and Public Policy, 3 Sept, Brisbane

Pearson N 2005 The Cape York Agenda. Address to the National Press Club, 30 Nov, Canberra

—— 2009 A people's survival. The Weekend Australian Oct 3–4, Inquirer: 1–2

Peiris D, Brown A, Cass A 2008 Addressing inequities in access to quality health care for indigenous people. Canadian Medical Association Journal 179(10):985–6

Plani F, Carson P 2008 The challenges of developing a trauma system for Indigenous people. Injury. International Journal of Care for the Injured 3955:S43–S53

Pomaika'I Cook, B, Tarallo-Jensen L, Withy K, Berry S 2005 Changes in Kanaka maoli men's roles and health: healing the warrior self. International Journal of Men's Health 4(2):115–30

Puzan E 2003 The unbearable whiteness of being (in nursing). Nursing Inquiry 10(3):193–200

Reading J, Ritchie A, Victor C, Wilson E 2005 Implementing empowering health promotion programs for Aboriginal youth in two distinct communities in British Columbia, Canada. Promotion & Education X11(2):62–5

Reid P, Robson B 2007 Understanding health inequities. In: Robson B, Harris R (eds) Hauora: Māori Standards of Health IV. A Study of the Years 2000–2005. Te Ropu Rangahau Hauora a Eru Pomare, Wellington, pp 3–10

Richmond C, Ross N 2009 The determinants of First Nation and Inuit health: a critical population health approach. Health & Place 15:403–11

Ring I, Brown N, Hunter A 2001 Policy discussion, Indigenous health. Australian Medical Association National Conference, Melbourne

Robson B, Cormack D, Cram F 2007a Social and Economic Indicators. In: Robson B, Harris R (eds) Hauora: Māori Standards of Health IV. A Study of the Years 2000–2005. Te Ropu Rangahau Hauora a Eru Pomare, Wellington, pp 63–102

Robson B, Purdie G 2007 Mortality. In: Robson B, Harris R (eds) Hauora: Māori Standards of Health IV. A Study of the Years 2000–2005. Te Ropu Rangahau Hauora a Eru Pomare, Wellington, pp 33–62

Robson B, Robson C, Harris R, Purdie G 2007b Hospitalisations. In: Robson B, Harris R (eds) Hauora: Māori Standards of Health IV. A Study of the Years 2000–2005. Te Ropu Rangahau Hauora a Eru Pomare, Wellington, pp 63–102

Ryan N, Head B, Keast R, Brown K 2006 Engaging Indigenous communities: towards a policy framework for Indigenous community justice programs. Social Policy & Administration 40(3):304–21

Sen A 1999 Development as Freedom. Alfred A Knopf, New York

Shahid S, Thompson S 2009 An overview of cancer and beliefs about the disease in Indigenous people of Australia, Canada, New Zealand and the US. Australian and New Zealand Journal of Public Health 33(2):109–18

Stanley F 2003 Before the bough breaks. Doing more for our children in the 21st century. Occasional Paper 1/2003, Academy of the Social Sciences in Australia, Canberra

Stewart S 2008 Promoting indigenous mental health: cultural perspectives on healing from Native counsellors in Canada. International Journal of Health Promotion and Education 46(2):49–57

Ten Fingers K 2005 Rejecting, revitalizing, and reclaiming. Canadian Journal of Public Health 96 Supp (1): S60–S63

Thomas D 2009 Smoking prevalence in Indigenous Australians, 1994–2004: a typical rather than an exceptional epidemic. International Journal for Equity in Health 8(37): doi: 10.1186/1475-9276-8-37

Thomas D, Johnston V, Fitz J, McDonnell J 2008 Monitoring local trends in Indigenous tobacco consumption. Australian and New Zealand Journal of Public Health 33(1):64–6

Thompson S, Greville H, Param R 2008 Beyond policy and planning to practice: getting sexual health on the agenda in Aboriginal communities in Western Australia. Australia and New Zealand Health Policy 5(3): doi:10.1186/1743-8462-5-3

Tobias M, Yeh L, Wright C, Riddell T, Chan W, Jackson R, Mann S 2009 The burden of coronary heart disease in Māori: population-based estimates for 2000–02. Australian and New Zealand Journal of Public Health 33(4):384–7

Torzillo P, Pholeros P, Rainow S, Barker G, Sowerbutts T, Short T, Irvine A 2008 The state of health hardware in Aboriginal communities in rural and remote Australia. Australian and New Zealand Journal of Public Health 32(1):7–11

Toussaint S 2003 'Our shame, blacks live poor, die young': Indigenous health practice and ethical possibilities for reform. In: Liamputtong P, Gardner H (eds) Health, Social Change and Communities. Oxford University Press, Melbourne, pp 241–56

Trewin D, Madden R 2005 The Health and Welfare of Australia's Aboriginal and Torres Strait Islander Peoples. ABS Cat. No. 4704.0, AIHW Cat. No. IHW14, Canberra

Tsey K 1997 Aboriginal self-determination, education and health: towards a radical change in attitudes to education. Australian and New Zealand Journal of Public Health 21(1): 77–83

Tsey K, Whiteside M, Daly S, Deemal A, Gibson T, Cadet-James Y, Wilson A, Santhanam R, Hasell-Elkins M 2005 Adapting the 'Family Wellbeing' empowerment program to the needs of remote Indigenous school children. Australian and New Zealand Journal of Public Health 29(2):112–16

Turale S, Miller M 2006 Improving the health of Indigenous Australians: reforms in nursing education. An opinion piece of international interest. International Nursing Review 53:171–7

United Nations (UN) 2007 Report of the Human Rights Council: United Nations Declaration on the Rights of Indigenous Peoples. UN, Geneva

Utter J, Scragg R, Schaaf D, Fitzgerald E 2006 Nutrition and physical activity behaviours among Māori, Pacific and NZ European children: identifying opportunities for population-based interventions. Australian and New Zealand Journal of Public Health 30(1):50–6

Vicary D, Bishop B 2005 Western psychotherapeutic practice: engaging Aboriginal people in culturally appropriate and respectful ways. Australian Psychologist 40(1):8–19

Vincent K, Eveline J 2008 The invisibility of gendered power relations in domestic violence policy. Journal of Family Studies 14(2–3):322–33

Wilding R, Tilbury F 2004 Constructing a changing people. In: Wilding R, Tilbury F (eds). A changing people: diverse contributions to the state of Western Australia. Department of the Premier and Cabinet, Office of Multicultural Interests, Perth, pp 1–7

Wilson D, Neville S 2009 Culturally safe research with vulnerable populations. Contemporary Nurse 33(1):69–79

World Health Organization (WHO) 1999 Indigenous and Tribal Peoples: Legal Frameworks and Indigenous Rights. WHO, Geneva

—— 2007 Media Centre, Health of Indigenous Peoples. Fact Sheet No. 326, WHO, Geneva

—— 2008 World Health Report 2008 Primary Health Care, Now More Than Ever. Online. Available: www.who.int/whr/2008/whr08_en.pdf (accessed 14 July 2009)

Zhao Y, Connors C, Wright J, Guthridge S, Bailie R 2008 Estimating chronic disease prevalence among the remote Aboriginal population of the Northern Territory using multiple data sources. Australian and New Zealand Journal of Public Health 32(4):307–13

Zubrick S, Silburn S, Lawrence D, Mitrou F, Dalby R, Blair E, Griffin J, Milroy H, de Maio J, Cox A, Li J 2005 The Western Australian Aboriginal Child Health Survey: The Social and Emotional Wellbeing of Aboriginal Children and Young People. Curtin University of Technology and Telethon Institute for Child Health Research, Perth

Useful websites

http://www.abs.gov.au — Australian Bureau of Statistics

http://www.aihw.gov.au — Australian Institute of Health and Welfare

http://www.maorihealth.govt.nz — New Zealand Ministry of Health, Māori Health

http://www.health.gov.au/internet/main/publishing.nsf/Content/Aboriginal+and+Torres+Strait+Islander+Health-1lp — Aboriginal and Torres Strait Islander Health

http://www.fahcsia.gov.au/sa/communities/progserv/documents/sfcs_report/sec1.htm — Stronger Families and Communities.

http://www.health.gov.au/mentalhealth — National Mental Health Strategy

http://www.healthyactive.gov.au/internet/main/publishing.nsf/Content/bringing-them-home lpalth — Bringing Them Home Report (Stolen Generations)

http://www.cyi.org.au/ — Cape York Institute for Policy & Leadership (Noel Pearson)

sean@thehealthyaboriginal.net — website for the Healthy Aboriginal Network (creating comic books on Aboriginal youth health issues)

http://www.hreoc.gov.au — Indigenous Native Title, Australian Human Rights website

http://www.reconciliation.org.au/ — Reconciliation Australia

http://nrha.ruralhealth.org.au/?IntCatId=14— National Rural Health Alliance

http://www.waitangi-tribunal.govt.nz — The Waitangi Tribunal

http://www.justice.govt.nz/courts/maori-land-court — The Māori Land Court

Chapter 12

Building the evidence base: research to practice

INTRODUCTION

Rational planning for the health of individuals, families and communities relies on a base of information as to what is effective, efficient in terms of resource use, and appropriate to the people whose lives will be affected. Effectiveness, efficiency and appropriateness are important variables to study in relation to health care systems, national intersectoral initiatives that affect health, and how health services and programs are implemented in communities. What is effective, efficient or appropriate can vary for particular individuals and groups across different settings and circumstances. Because of this variability, and the fact that people's lives are constantly changing, the research agenda is constantly evolving. It will always be necessary to gather information on community needs, strengths and resources to identify what is transferable across settings, and what is unique to a particular community. For example, we know that a multidimensional health promotion strategy to help people quit smoking is more effective than a single factor intervention. However, the way a quit-smoking intervention is introduced, planned, and received by various members of the community can vary widely.

Planning an effective intervention for smoking cessation, or any other initiative, depends not only on aggregated, population-level information from programs that have worked, but on the strengths of the community, and how people view the constraints and/or facilitating factors that affect their health choices. So although the findings from a body of research can be translated into practice across settings, there remains a need for contextual information to study their effectiveness and acceptability at the local level. This is the essence of most community health research. It is often evaluative; focusing on gathering and analysing data, from within and external to the community, to identify what works, for whom, where, why, with what costs and outcomes, including acceptability by local residents. However, research data also needs to develop knowledge, contributing one increment at a time, to the evolving base of knowledge for practice by nurses, midwives and other health professionals.

Primary studies that collect evidence on the effect of certain interventions can be useful in studying population-level outcomes as a basis for benchmarking. This is a process of comparing outcomes across populations to forecast the likelihood of success in other populations. However, research is also needed on the differential effects for various groups, and how certain interventions were experienced by people whose lives were changed. Although scientific evidence is important to indicate what works from a statistical point of view, community health research also requires explanations of why it did, or did not. This type of contextual information can help health planners understand what features of the community contributed to the health outcomes, and whether certain initiatives or processes could be tried in other contexts and with other people.

> **Point to ponder**
> Community health research needs both scientific evidence to support outcomes *and* explanations of why an intervention may or may not have worked.

Besides identifying needs and outcomes, the research agenda also needs to include the type of studies that are aimed at developing conceptual frameworks for community health. These studies advance the field of community health by building a scaffold for knowledge development that can attract scholars and researchers to investigate the broader dimensions of community health. To date, there has been a dearth of studies that provide a framework for researchers to advance knowledge, particularly in the nursing and midwifery evidence base, although this is gradually changing. In addition, there is a need to study examples of good and best practice by nurses, midwives and others who promote the health of a community through health education, advocacy or specific interventions. The research agenda should also include studies that link community health practice outcomes with the level or type of practitioners' educational preparation, experience, expertise and scope of practice. This is a fundamental aspect of informing our professional knowledge development, mapping our progress in developing and adapting new understandings.

The research process is a partnership, where information is seen to be the property of those providing it, often in the spirit of mutual understanding. Despite different methods, designs and philosophical approaches, the common goal of research is to inform improvements to the health of the population or the community itself, either through small incremental contributions to knowledge, or studies of such magnitude as to create system change. This chapter provides an overview of issues and progress related to community health research, and suggests a number of research challenges and strategies that could be used to inform the creation and maintenance of community health.

GLOBAL COMMUNITY HEALTH RESEARCH

Researching community health issues is a challenge throughout the world. This is of concern to all health professionals, as communities throughout the world are part of a global network working towards the common goal of social justice. Ideally, research studies that underpin the social justice agenda would build a body of knowledge to inform health promotion strategies, policies and practices to respond to global problems that also have implications at the local level. These problems include poverty, inequity in resource allocation, disparities in health and education, discrimination and disadvantage on the basis of gender, culture, race, age or geography, infectious diseases among those without access to treatment, and environmental issues such as climate change and its impact on communities. However, the global research agenda continues to be disadvantaged by the lack of large, interlinked databases, inadequate funding and, in some cases, the lack of political will to secure effective mechanisms for research collaborations.

Research studies are expensive. They require funding for researchers, investment in support structures, including the type of databases that could help integrate findings, personnel, and in many cases, specialised equipment. Clinicians, academics, policy-makers, and technical staff with research skills often have work demands other than research, which means that without financial support, their research becomes relegated to a low priority. Funding can help ensure that data are gathered and analysed appropriately, and

Objectives

By the end of this chapter you will be able to:

1 identify the major issues that are critical to translating research evidence into better community health and wellbeing

2 explain the importance of comprehensive risk factor studies

3 explain the relative advantage of mixed-method research studies for researching community health

4 outline the most important ethical issues involved in community-based research

5 develop a research question grounded in the conceptual foundations of primary health care to respond to a specific community health issue

6 identify a set of research questions that correspond to the community health and wellbeing indicators for healthy, safe and inclusive communities.

that researchers have time and resources to promote collegial deliberation and dissemination of findings. Like other activities that have resource implications, research is inherently political. This means that at the national, regional and institutional levels, there are competing agendas for budget allocations. Decisions about funding research can be made on the basis of local issues, researcher interests, or the needs of policy-makers and politicians to demonstrate a short-term impact. When short-term, local goals are the focus, the broader global social justice agenda is likely to be given little attention. As health professionals, it is important to advance local agendas and be responsive to the need for local research, but at the same time, maintain a commitment to the wider agenda of collecting data and translating findings into better health care for the global population.

The most salient community issues are generally those related to the social determinants of health (SDOH). Among the issues that are as yet underresearched are questions that investigate equity of access to health services, models of empowerment for various groups differentiated by gender, culture and ethnicity, mechanisms for education and health literacy, and environmental supports for healthy childhoods, and lifelong wellbeing, including healthy ageing. These are complex issues, and research addressing these social determinants involves long-term, multidisciplinary studies of multiple factors across various settings and groups. The multidimensional nature of community problems is the central reason why so few research studies have been conducted into the SDOH. There are limited opportunities for large-scale studies that would gather data from diverse groups over sufficient time to provide definitive answers to research questions. However, there is an ethical and moral obligation for researchers to conduct studies into the SDOH to motivate social action, and to provide a balanced view of what creates health in society (Venkatapuram & Marmot 2009). Confining research to epidemiological studies of impairments and mortality, without studying the social dimensions, has consequences for health planning that limit the effectiveness of the health system (Venkatapuram & Marmot 2009). When national budgets fail to free up funding or intellectual support for comprehensive, longitudinal and multidimensional research, health care decisions may be made on inadequate or inappropriate information (Gil-Gonzalez et al 2009). This is basically

why there are still so many important research questions left unanswered, including studies of the factors that support or inhibit achievement of the Millennium Development Goals (MDGs) (Gil-Gonzalez et al 2009).

Point to ponder
As health professionals it is vital to advocate for local research but at the same time be committed to translating findings into better health care for the global population.

A further problem is the lack of coherence in the topics studied in different countries. To drive major change, research studies need to be collaborative, right from the stage of establishing the research agenda, to identifying and evaluating solutions. The logistics of international or cross-institutional collaboration is sometimes prohibitive in terms of time or commitment of individual researchers, or when collaborators have different organisational pressures. Another problem is the need for different perspectives in investigating a problem. Funding bodies often favour studies that are highly scientific, such as systematic reviews of existing research or clinical trials, rather than those that may be evaluative, or based on clinical or community perspectives. Research into the issue of accessibility to care illustrates that three systematic reviews of accessibility of care have been conducted, yet all studies were conducted from the perspective of service providers, leaving little understanding of service users' perspectives or needs (Kendall 2008).

Point to ponder
Community-based research studies must be collaborative — locally with community members, and nationally and internationally with those committed to research that advances the global agenda of social equity across nations.

Both the duplication of these studies, and the lack of community input, are problematic. The studies were funded and the research proceeded because expert researchers were able to mount an elegant argument for funding, which was not contested by community members, despite the fact that, as taxpayers, they were actually funding the studies. This holds two lessons. The first is that the art of argument is an essential skill for researchers. The second is that, despite widespread public access to large volumes of information through the internet, most people refrain from questioning its accuracy or seeking information on research, instead being satisfied to devolve responsibility to 'expert' researchers (Buckley 2008). Again, this underlines the emphasis on researchers, rather than the community. To ensure that our research agendas are focused on advancing community health, it is important that researchers work in partnership with community members at every stage of the research.

SOCIAL DETERMINANTS OF HEALTH AND THE RESEARCH AGENDA

Research into the SDOH is fundamental to community health knowledge. The Commission on SDOH, mentioned in previous chapters, conducted a three-year project into the SDOH adopting a multidimensional research approach (Marmot & Friel 2008). Rather than confining their data to scientific evidence, the commissioners adopted 'chains of reasoning' and social epidemiological approaches, to demonstrate the links between interventions and outcomes. For example, they queried whether collective action at the grassroots level was good for health. Their investigation focused on showing that collective action can lead to improved housing and employment conditions, which, in turn, can lead to health equity. Their program of research led the commissioners to argue that researching the SDOH requires many types of evidence. This can be a combination of scientific evidence such as demonstrating through a randomised controlled trial (RCT), that nutritional supplements for young children can improve their cognitive and educational outcomes, and qualitative, descriptive evidence from case studies and action research, as to what is helpful in various communities (Marmot & Friel 2008). Other researchers are now recognising that the current research agendas that focus on population-level effects do not provide a realistic picture of the SDOH, because they fail to analyse differential effects for various sub-groups (Petticrew et al 2009). Rather than confining studies to population-level, causal factors as a basis for decisions about health care, they suggested

the need for schematic descriptions of pathways between interventions and outcomes for different groups (Petticrew et al 2009).

Point to ponder
Current research agendas that focus on population-level effects do not provide a realistic picture of the social determinants of health because they fail to analyse differing impacts on population sub-groups.

The schematic representation of pathways to good health includes information from the policy agendas that help us progress towards equity and social justice. The SDOH commissioners included in their evaluation, an examination of the link between fair policies and greater health equity. For example, when governments invest in skills development there is both an economic and social benefit. So generous social policies that support dual-earner families not only improve the family's economic and social condition, but that of the entire society, which contributes to social justice (Marmot & Friel 2008). These types of policies that support families and communities are a product of political and social trends, which influence what gets researched at the national, regional and local levels and by whom. In Australia, for example, the last decades of the last century saw numerous funding allocations awarded to biomedical research at the expense of public health studies. However, the current health reform agenda has resulted in a subtle shift in research emphasis towards the environment and primary health care (PHC). Examples of recently completed studies include antenatal and postnatal home visiting programs for Indigenous families, strategies for caring for those with depression, diabetes prevention, the effectiveness of practice nurses, health screening and improvements to health information systems (Primary Health Care Research, Evaluation and Development et al 2009). Each of these is invaluable to advancing knowledge for community health practice.

In addition to the political and social agendas, research topics are also selected by researchers on the basis of their responsiveness to professional agendas. For example, Annells et al's (2005) study of the research priorities of district nurses in Victoria sought their views on which practice issues were most important. The study was based on the need to develop a body of knowledge to inform best practice in district nursing, which focuses predominantly on home visiting. A Delphi technique, which seeks a consensus view from the study participants, canvassed the nurses' views, and ultimately generated a list of 10 major practice issues. These issues were then identified as topics for future research, focusing on discharge planning, documentation, retention of home visiting nurses, pain and symptom management for palliative care, protective environments for older people, and nursing assessment (Annells et al 2005). Similarly, a Delphi study was conducted by child health nurses and midwives in Western Australia to identify research priorities for parenting and child health (Hauck et al 2007). The study revealed that the two most important priorities were for infant sleep and settling issues, and postnatal depression. Other important research issues included program evaluation, staffing issues and the need to promote child health services (Hauck et al 2007).

Point to ponder

Recent trends in research show a subtle shift towards agendas that emphasise the environment and primary health care.

Trends within the fields of public and community health also affect topics for research. In the past, studies informing health promotion strategies centred around strategies for influencing individual behaviour change. In the 21st century, health promotion trends indicate a need for studies that include the ecological factors supporting behaviour changes, and how the environments of people's lives can support opportunities to make healthy choices. In addition, there has been a shift away from single factor studies to comprehensive and multifactor studies that investigate the interactive and cumulative effect of proximal (under the control of the individual) and distal (features of the environments of people's lives) factors that contribute to health. To some extent, this multidimensional perspective has rescued the research agenda in community health from its insularity. Recognising the ecological relationships between human behaviour and environmental conditions, researchers today are more inclined to seek input from colleagues from diverse fields. They also tend to adopt varying combinations of approaches

to study health-related questions from multiple perspectives.

As the SDOH Commission revealed, research approaches and techniques have undergone changes that benefit society by including a variety of approaches (Marmot & Friel 2008). The conventions for rigorous and appropriate research methods and designs have remained relatively stable, as have statistical computations, albeit with some changes reflecting more sophistication in analytic techniques. Community health research has shifted from the 'methodological imperialism' or 'methodolatry', which used to privilege certain methods over others, to a more eclectic approach that includes social phenomena. This is also a more ethical approach, in linking scientific evidence with a moral concern for social inequalities in health (Venkatapuram & Marmot 2009). The basis of the ethical and moral obligation of researchers is a shared value system that views the health and wellbeing of the population as an indicator of societal progress (Smith et al 2008). Ethically, this drives a commitment to long-term social change, and the research that will help inform such change (Smith et al 2008). For long-term planning there is a need to adopt multi-method studies, which examine data from more than one perspective, and focus on the real-world context, inclusive of the conditions and outcomes that may not fall within the 'norm' or normal pattern. As a result, research findings will be more dynamic and realistic, eminently better suited to influencing community health. Multi-method, multidimensional approaches provide opportunities to analyse new possibilities in the conception of each new study. Importantly, this allows researchers and those who use their research findings to maintain awareness of the dimensions of social relations that shape people's socio-ecological experience of health. This provides a profusion of opportunities to inform change and to examine responses across time, developments, interventions and contexts.

CONDUCTING RESEARCH FOR POLICY AND PRACTICE

Research and policy development typically occur within a symbiotic relationship. As mentioned above, government policies can dictate research agendas. Reciprocally, research findings can lead to policies for better health. This can occur when there are strong coalitions of health planners, researchers and members of the community. The combination of research evidence, the perspectives and preferences of health service users, and the experience of health practitioners can be invaluable in effecting change. When this type of information is available, research findings can be translated into practice; whether this is clinical or professional practice, education or management practice, or the practice of policy development.

Evidence-based practice

Evidence-based practice (EBP) is generally described in relation to evidence-based medicine (EBM), which was originally devised to inform a medical practitioner's intention to treat or intervene in a person's care. EBP is the integration of three things: the best available research evidence, the clinician's knowledge and expertise, and the individual patient's values. All of these inform decision-making regarding care and treatment (Sackett et al 2000). Evidence-based health care is generally a product of well-conducted, large-scale studies identified in a systematic review (Abbott et al 2008).

Systematic reviews, literature reviews, integrative reviews and meta-analysis

The core focus of EBP is the systematic review, which establishes the parameters for adequate or best available research evidence using preset criteria, derived primarily from RCTs and meta-analyses, to make recommendations for treatment (Bero & Rennie 1995). The advantage of a systematic review is that it uses an explicit and auditable protocol, which is seen to be the most objective type of review (Sandelowski 2008). However, other reviews are informative for nursing and midwifery practice, including literature reviews and integrative reviews. Jackson et al's (2007) literature review on resilience, for example, provides important research findings on how nurses survive and thrive in the face of workplace adversity.

Point to ponder

Evidence-based practice incorporates the best available research evidence, the clinician's knowledge and expertise, and the individual patient's views and preferences.

Integrative reviews also review the literature pertaining to a certain topic, but they are broader reviews of all types of research, including experimental and non-experimental studies (Whittemore & Knafl 2005). An integrative review can also be designed to define concepts, review theories, review evidence, and analyse methodological issues (Whittemore & Knafl 2005). An excellent example of an integrative review is that conducted by Anthony and Jack (2009). Their review was intended to clarify case study methodology as it is being used in nursing research. The main advantage of an integrative review is that, in combining and summarising several types of literature, including theoretical literature, it can provide a more complete picture of a phenomenon or health care problem (Whittemore & Knafl 2005). A meta-analysis is another type of review, which combines, and statistically analyses the evidence from a number of studies on a similar topic to enhance the validity of findings (Whittemore & Knafl 2005).

Systematic review is the method of choice for EBP. Systematic reviews provide a rigorous summary of all existing research evidence related to a specific question, to produce robust evidence for changes in practice and service delivery (Abbott et al 2008). In some cases, a systematic review will include the statistical methods of meta-analysis, but if studies selected cannot be combined statistically, the review can consist of a narrative analysis with other quasi-statistical methods (Whittemore & Knafl 2005). Systematic reviews have been criticised on the basis of restricting intellectual creativity, and excluding alternative ways of understanding health from different perspectives (Mykhalovskiy et al 2008; Sandelowski 2008).

Point to ponder

Although the systematic review is the method of choice for evidence-based practice, it is important to evaluate the effectiveness and appropriateness of health care in the differing contexts in which it is provided.

The systematic review can be useful in community health, but to advance knowledge comprehensively, there is also a need to evaluate the effectiveness and appropriateness of health care in each specific context (Abbott et al 2008; Morrison et al 2008). Another issue concerns the 'disciplined subjectivity' required for analysing data, whether it is from a systematic review or another form of review (Sandelowski 2008:106). All reviews reflect the perspectives and preferences of reviewers, and the different way they conceive problems, pose research questions, and select and compare studies (Sandelowski 2008). Despite these differences the reviews provide an important foundation from which to conduct practice-based research.

One advantage of all of these types of reviews is in identifying gaps in knowledge. Another is that reviews can draw nursing attention to the need for studies; for example, in investigating effectiveness in health promotion, which should be one of the main criteria for interventions (Morrison et al 2008). A literature review by Wilhelmsson and Lindberg (2007) illustrates this. These researchers reviewed a wide range of health promotion and illness prevention research and found that most studies were of little use as a basis for health promotion practice because they were lacking in quality and consistency. This made the findings difficult to translate into practice. They evaluated 40 original articles and 16 literature reviews, but found few studies that were of high enough scientific quality to provide a rational basis for intervention. As nurses, they were intuitively aware that interventions are being based on research evidence, but without publication of existing interventions, or analysis of qualitative accounts of practice change, the studies were clearly not advancing the knowledge base for health promotion practice (Wilhelmsson & Lindberg 2007). This type of information is important in challenging nurses and midwives to further develop the base of professional knowledge that informs practice.

As professional knowledge evolves, new ways of combining data are being developed. One such approach is 'critical interpretive synthesis', which is a method for linking qualitative and quantitative data (Flemming 2010). The method is based on appraising quantitative and qualitative findings from studies addressing a similar topic (such as pain and pain management), translating the qualitative and quantitative findings into each other to study how the concepts and themes interface as a basis for comparison, and developing a synthesis of findings (Flemming 2010). This technique is promising for nursing and midwifery research, and its use in community studies should prove to be informative in advancing the knowledge base.

Point to ponder

Critical interpretive synthesis is a method for linking qualitative and quantitative data from studies addressing similar topics in order to study how the concepts and themes identified interact.

Randomised controlled trials

Randomised controlled trials (RCTs) are described as the 'gold standard' in research, because they use an experimental study design, which allows the researcher the greatest control over the research (Goldenberg 2006). To meet the criteria for the highest level of control, there must be comparison groups with different interventions or manipulation. One of the comparison groups is a control group. All subjects under study are randomly allocated (using precise randomisation techniques) to one of two groups, either the experimental or control group. Muncey (2009) questions whether RCTs are in fact a gold standard, given that they do not consider the context. In fact, they may obscure subjective elements that are important in all forms of human inquiry (Morrison et al 2008). Clearly, RCTs are important for developing well-verified, objective research studies, but in reducing the factors studied within tightly defined criteria they do not reveal the complexity within which people maintain health (Muncey 2009).

Point to ponder

Although RCTs have long been considered the 'gold standard' in research, the method is difficult to implement in community-based studies.

Another criticism of RCTs is that the controlled conditions of a clinical trial are rarely available in communities. It would be unethical and not useful to allocate people to an RCT, giving one group the intervention, and withholding it from the other. On the other hand, a meta-analysis that combines the findings from a group of studies can be useful, especially if the findings and conclusions of the studies are synthesised into new ways of looking at the community or planning for community change. This information would then be combined with people's perspectives on how change can be implemented in their particular community or, where change has occurred, how they perceived the outcome (Morrison et al 2008).

Sources of evidence

The EBP movement is based on the notion that providing research evidence for all activities in the health professions ensures accountability to the population for clinical decision-making and interventions. Most health researchers today are aware of the importance of EBP through the work undertaken by the Cochrane Collaboration, which has maintained a database of systematic reviews of research on health care interventions in a wide range of clinical areas since the 1990s (Bero & Rennie 1995). Because not all community health practitioners have the requisite high-level skills for literature retrieval and appraisal, or the time or management support to develop and use these skills in practice, many access 'predigested' sources of systematic reviews. These include the *Journal of Evidence-based Health Care*, and *Evidence Based Nursing*, and the Joanna Briggs Institute (JBI), which is located at the University of Adelaide in conjunction with Royal Adelaide Hospital, but networked to numerous research groups throughout the world (Joanna Briggs Institute Online. Available: www.joannabriggs. edu.au [accessed 21 January 2010]). A good example of this type of information is provided by JBI in relation to studies on smoking cessation programs. Numerous studies have been combined in systematic reviews that can be used by nurses and midwives working with community groups to help them with smoking cessation. These studies are reported in a 'best practice' information sheet produced by JBI (2008). The information explains the wealth of research findings on this important topic in relation to the effectiveness of self-help treatments, individual and group therapies, including pharmacological and skin patch treatments, and what seems to work for which groups (JBI 2008).

Point to ponder
Tools to support evidence-based practice are readily available from sources such as the Cochrane Collaboration, the Journal of Evidence-based Health Care and the Joanna Briggs Institute.

Evidence-based practice is situated within the paradigm of logical positivism. A paradigm is a set of beliefs or practices that regulates inquiry in a particular discipline (Weaver & Olson 2006). Weaver & Olson's (2006) integrative review of nursing paradigms outlines those most often used in nursing research. The *positivist paradigm* is used in quantitative nursing studies, where the research is based on rigid rules of logic and measurement, truth, absolute principles and prediction (Weaver & Olson 2006). In contrast, the *interpretive paradigm* focuses on the meanings people ascribe to their actions and interactions. Another paradigm used in nursing research is the *critical social theory paradigm*, which addresses social institutions, and issues of power and alienation as well as new opportunities (Weaver & Olson 2006). EBP is predicated on quantifiable data (Mowinski et al 2001), which presents a challenge for researchers who seek to make visible other types of knowing that arise from reflection and intuition, or research knowledge generated within a different paradigm. Many researchers would argue that knowledge of communities must be contextualised and holistic, complete with cultural, spiritual and environmental dimensions. This type of knowing is multifaceted, sometimes superseding that type of knowledge gleaned from systematic assessments or prior research findings. It is often described as *naturalistic inquiry*, as information is gleaned from the natural setting, and interpreted using various *interpretive*, rather than *statistical* techniques. Naturalistic data can include informant interviews, observational data and document analysis (Tripp-Reimer & Doebbeling 2004). The knowledge gained from this type of research is an important element in informing policy and practice changes, especially when more than one type of inquiry is used in combination.

Decision-making for change requires a combination of content and procedural knowledge; what Benner (1984) calls 'knowing that' and 'knowing how'. This 'relational' knowledge (knowing what to do, and knowing how to do it) helps create an understanding of the community through critical reflection, and exploration of practice from performance, quality, and evaluation activities (Rycroft-Malone et al 2004). This in-depth situational knowledge can then be used to identify needs and practice approaches that achieve a good fit with the social and cultural aspects of family and community health (McMurray 2004). When this type of 'internal evidence' is used, any planned changes can be embedded in the local social structure, and based on community ownership of when and how change will occur (Abbott et al 2008; Comino & Kemp 2008). Including relational, situational knowledge is 'evidence-informed' practice (Bowen & Zwi 2005). It represents a pathway to decision-making that involves generating the evidence, understanding how people make sense of their lives, and deciding how this knowledge might assist health promotion efforts (Wainwright et al 2007). This is simplified in a three-step process of 'adopt, adapt, act' (see Box 12.1)

Point to ponder
Naturalistic inquiry allows researchers to make visible other types of knowledge than that found in randomised controlled trials. Naturalistic inquiry is an important source of information for informing policy and making practice changes.

The three-step approach described below can be used as a guide to policy development. This requires the researcher working towards policy change to be engaged with at least the broad contours of government ideas, politics and economics (Labonte et al 2005). For example, Australian researchers need to be aware that Australian public policies are currently following New Zealand's lead in focusing on PHC. Understanding this trend

BOX 12.1 ADOPT, ADAPT, ACT

- Research — from carefully designed studies and comparative trials over time.
- Knowledge and information — results of consultation, networking, internet information and analysis of documents.
- Ideas and interests — expert knowledge shaped by personal and professional experience.
- Politics — information relevant to government agendas, opportunities, crises or challenges.
- Economics — cost-effectiveness or economic evaluation and opportunity cost data, for example, what opportunities are forgone when a program is developed.

(Bowen & Zwi 2005:166)

as a current policy direction can provide leverage for expanding professional and community research goals. When researchers are in tune with government directions and priorities it is easier to construct a rational argument for a research project that is responsive to the policy environment. So, for example, a nurse or midwife would be more likely to secure research funding for a study that corresponds with, or extends one of the areas that have been successful in recent research funding rounds, such as early childhood support, or chronic illness prevention, or improving equity of access to care for older persons, or Indigenous or migrant health. All of these topics resonate with the PHC agenda. They are also in synchrony with another trend, which is called translational research.

LEARNING ACTIVITY
Consider the current political environment, policy development arena and your own clinical interests. Develop a research question that considers these varying contexts, that is applicable to your area of practice, and meets the needs and priorities of the community you work with.

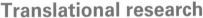

Translational research

Translating research into policy and/or practice typically occurs in two stages: from 'bench to bedside' (clinical laboratory to clinical application) and from clinical application in an ideal setting to real-world practice (Garfield et al 2003). Another use of the term *translational* is in translating knowledge to action or knowledge to practice within the context of theories or models. Although there is some debate about the use of terms, *theories* tend to be used when a set of relationships are explained and there is some predictive capability (Kitson et al 2008). An example of this would be framing a research study within Rogers' (2003) Theory of the Diffusion of Innovations (see Chapter 4), which predicts that community members will be more likely to accept a change if they can see the relative advantage of the change, and its compatibility with their approach or goals. A *model*, on the other hand, is typically more diffuse, and usually refers to a specific way to implement research into practice. A good example of this would be the

Flinders model of chronic illness management, also described in Chapter 4 (Commonwealth of Australia 2009). A *conceptual framework* can also be used as a translational device. Conceptual frameworks present the bigger picture of translating knowledge into practice; often including the paradigm or worldview as well as a set of variables and relationships that should be examined to explain a certain phenomenon (Kitson et al 2008).

To ensure success in translating knowledge into practice, research studies should be inclusive, with input from those who will be affected by the implementation of findings. One area where this has been absent is in occupational health research. To date, most occupational health research has excluded women and their work-related concerns. As a result, exposure data has been standardised to male norms, and the social patterning of risk factors has failed to take into account the occupational and non-occupational stressors that affect women at work (WHO 2006). Translating research findings to the realities of women at work requires consideration of gender-sensitive indicators, and incorporating women's perspectives into reporting systems (WHO 2006). Other examples where community input is important include studies with different cultural groups, or groups defined by place or affiliation, and we will discuss some of this type of research below.

Point to ponder

Translational research translates knowledge to action or practice within the context of theories or models and is integral to quality improvement in health.

Like other research, translational studies should be rigorous and linked to conceptual foundations to advance knowledge (Garfield et al 2003). Multidisciplinary perspectives often increase their applicability, adding the perspectives of a range of practitioners or policy-makers. For example, the social ecological perspective we adopt in writing this text has been used in this way (Richards et al 2008). Conceptual frameworks add value to the rigour of research studies by providing a logical basis for the research, which guides the development of the study and the way findings are analysed and discussed (Fawcett 2008). A good example of this is the framework developed by Duke et al (2009) to guide culturally competent

practice. Their conceptual framework combines Benner's (1984) model of skills acquisition, with the relational inquiry model we outlined in Chapter 5 (Hartrick Doane & Varcoe 2005). It is helpful as a guide to reflective practice focused on cultural safety, but it can also be used to guide culturally oriented research with people from different cultural backgrounds. The major value of using a conceptual framework is to advance knowledge. By reporting the conceptual framework along with study findings, other researchers can see where the findings fit with the body of knowledge, and how the knowledge base can be extended. This is critical in nursing and midwifery research to ensure continued evolution of the disciplines (Fawcett 2008).

Point to ponder

A conceptual framework provides a logical basis for research and when reported with research findings allows other researchers to see where the findings fit with the body of knowledge and how this can be extended.

Translational research is integral to quality improvements in health care, especially in qualitative studies designed to identify what matters to patients, detecting obstacles to changing performance, or explaining why improvement does, or does not, occur (Tripp-Reimer & Doebbeling 2004). Translational research is also useful as a basis for health promotion interventions where the emphasis is on community capacity development. Community capacity is developed from the grassroots level, with the researcher(s) adopting a guiding role in helping frame the way information is generated, shared and used. Where the objective is to study the outcome of nursing or health care interventions, the translational elements can include evaluation of the appropriateness, accessibility, acceptability, effectiveness, efficiency or equity of service improvements that have been implemented elsewhere (Maxwell 1984).

Studies of appropriateness include such things as preferences or satisfaction with services. Accessibility studies could address the services used by different population groups, such as young parents or older persons. Acceptability studies can address community perceptions of health inter-actions. Studies of effectiveness include evaluation of health promotion initiatives, such as antenatal care and its link with birth experiences. Efficiency is typically an examination of the cost–benefit of certain choices; for example, providing community support services for the homeless. Studies of equity generally have a broader reach, such as comparing the impact of affordable food or housing for different populations, including different cultural groups (McMurray 2004). Each of these questions requires a community partnership approach.

Community-based research partnerships

One of the trends guiding research in nursing and other health disciplines is the move towards community-based research partnerships. Community-based research provides an ideal opportunity to inform policies from the ground up. It is also a way of providing feedback to policy-makers of the applicability of policies on the ground, where people live, work, study or play. Funding bodies often support community partners such as government departments, hospitals or health districts, as collaborators in research studies, knowing that the information that will emerge will be more authentic than it would if the researcher was working alone to investigate a community problem. In addition, community-based research partnerships can generate questions of local relevance. This type of participation distinguishes 'community-based' from 'community-placed' research (Minkler 2005).

Community-based participatory research (CBPR) has been described as systematic investigation with the participation of those affected by a certain issue with a view towards education, action or social change. All partners are involved in the research process, and all are valued for their unique strengths. CBPR begins with identifying the topic and designing the study to improve community health, and eliminate health disparities (Minkler 2005). Another strength of this approach is the ability for CBPR studies to foster capacity building, where the partners create something new from examining what is currently occurring in the community (Israel et al 1998). CBPR is also a culturally sensitive method, encompassing a commitment to 'cultural humility', which is intended to redress power imbalances and maintain mutually respectful, dynamic community

partnerships (Minkler 2005). CBPR is often used to uncover sensitive issues that pose questions for certain members of the community, gathering the perspectives of people in their own words, rather than through objective questionnaires. This approach gives voice to the community. The researchers also maintain an attitude of receptivity, locating power issues at every stage of the research process to ensure community empowerment (Minkler 2005). This is also the approach used in action research.

> **Point to ponder**
> Community-based participatory research is research undertaken with the participation of community members affected by an issue with a view towards education, action or social change.

Action research

Action research revolves around flexible planning through iterative (repetitive) cycles, wherein the researchers and their partners in the community consider the research problem, then together engage in cycles of planning, proposed action, evaluation and further cycles of planning and action (Carr & Kemmis 1986). Put simply, action research revolves around cycles of theory, practice and problem-solving (Burgess 2006). Action research takes place in the interpretive paradigm, which is a naturalistic form of inquiry, aimed at engaging with the people and/or issues under study, to understand the multiple dimensions of socially constructed behaviours and processes (Stringer 2004). Like other forms of research, action research has conventions for study design, collecting and analysing data, and presenting and using the findings. One of the most salient issues relevant to community health research is the capacity of action research studies to clarify the meanings and interactions of human behaviours in the cultural contexts of people's lives. When this type of research is planned and executed in partnership with community members, the researchers, and those using their research, are able to see how people make sense of their world, how they see one another, how they engage in resolving issues and problems, and how they draw shared meanings from the processes (Stringer 2004).

Participatory action research

Participatory action research (PAR) is an example of CBPR. The focus of the PAR approach is collective, reflective inquiry aimed at understanding and change (Baum et al 2006). Baum et al (2006) outline a number of antecedents to PAR. These include questioning the nature of knowledge, and how it represents and reinforces the interests of the more powerful people in society; experience as a basis for knowing; and using experiential knowledge to influence practice (Baum et al 2006). The strength of PAR lies in it being a situational, collaborative approach (Carr & Kemmis 1986; Greenwood 1994). As an action research approach, PAR is based on iterative cycles of collaborative decision-making, critical evaluation, action and reflection, which make it an ideal method to evaluate community changes. A fundamental element of the PAR approach is building a trusting relationship between researchers and the community or group (Greenwood 1994).

Point to ponder

Action research and participatory action research involve the researchers and their community partners working together through a cyclical process of planning, action, evaluation and reflection on a chosen topic.

Two features of PAR that distinguish the method from other research are authentic participation and relevancy of actions, both controlled by the community, rather than external researchers (Burgess 2006). The process of PAR includes group reflections designed to identify mutual solutions which are *critical* or *emancipatory* (free from traditional restraints), because they emerge from the community (bottom-up) and not those who seek to study them (top-down). Because PAR engages the community members as partners in the research it is more likely than other methods to facilitate empowerment and sustainable change, especially as the community invests the project with energy and resources. PAR therefore embodies the values and purposes of CBPR. It is aimed at generating mindfulness: relational knowledge that captures the mutual understandings of human beings, connecting problems, critical analysis and values-based actions (Burgess 2006).

PAR studies can be useful in evaluating interventions that have been conducted as a start to a longer-term capacity building project. Within the action research cycle, evaluative information can provide realistic feedback on what worked, and what did not, and the group can decide on any modifications or future plans. Steps are outlined in Box 12.2 (below).

PAR evaluative data can also be used to promote health literacy, identifying each step of the capacity building process, and individual strengths and needs. Collective input can foreground the voices of the community, increasing knowledge of cultural or individual influences on lifestyle behaviours, how people manage their health and risk, or important perspectives on illness or medication management (Tripp-Reimer & Doebbeling 2004). This is particularly helpful in researching with different cultural groups (Foster & Stanek 2007). When individual and collective perspectives are shared, there are often issues of inequities and power imbalances that become visible. Through mutual consciousness raising, the group can become empowered to speak freely and authentically, which ensures that appropriate information is being collected.

BOX 12.2 STEPS IN CONDUCTING PAR EVALUATIONS

- Scoping — establishing what is to be accomplished, how change might occur, what resources are available, which principles underpin the project, and what people's accounts of what is occurring in the community can add to our understanding.
- Focusing — identifying what strategies are effective; what different people believe is working well.
- Gathering information — using different mechanisms to gather data: documents, verbal reports and interviews.
- Making meaning from information — engaging in reflection and group debriefing.
- Communication — drafting a report, discussing ideas with participants and others involved in the evaluation.
- Applying learning — fine tuning, making changes in the report, identifying key strategies and developing participants' skills in shaping the project, to begin the capacity development.

(Haviland 2004)

RESEARCHING THE COMMUNITY: PARADIGMS AND STRATEGIES

One of the greatest challenges for health researchers today lies in the shift from focusing on formulaic ways of investigating community problems and issues, to different paradigms that encourage researchers to articulate the range of problems and solutions in the context of the community or group.

Point to ponder
The importance of multidimensional approaches to research and not simply RCTs is cleverly articulated in examples such as 'the parachute approach'.

A persuasive argument for a multidimensional approach to research is cleverly presented in a study of parachute use to prevent death and major trauma related to gravitational challenge (Smith & Pell 2003). The authors' objective was to determine whether parachutes are effective in preventing major trauma. Predictably, they found no RCTs in their systematic review, and concluded that the effectiveness of parachutes has not been subjected to rigorous evaluation. They suggested that the most radical proponents of EBP, those who criticise observational studies, might want to conduct a double blind, randomised, placebo controlled, crossover trial of the parachute!

Most community health researchers strive to achieve relevance for their communities by using qualitative, interpretive research approaches, or mixed methods that combine both qualitative and quantitative data to capture this breadth of information. This has been called the 'primacy of the practical', where findings are seen to have applicability beyond those of a study that collects only quantitative data (Sandelowski 2004:1367). The research team is then able to interpret the social attributes and meanings held by the members of a group or a community, and examine the surrounding social conditions that shape their lives, all of which is research evidence for change. In some cases, the research question suggests a case study method.

Mixed methods

In today's health care environment, the emphasis in health promotion research is on comprehensive interactions between many factors, particularly those within the social and cultural context of people's lives. Adding qualitative methods that

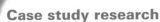

Case study research

Case study has rapidly become a mainstream method for nursing research. It is ideally suited to studies that seek to describe, explore and understand a phenomenon in its real-life context (Yin 2003). Although case studies are not able to be generalised, they do provide important information on community health topics, by integrating multiple sources of evidence that have informational, rather than statistical value (Anthony & Jack 2009; Luck et al 2006). One impediment to case study research is a common misunderstanding of what can be analysed in this methodological approach, particularly case studies that are exclusively interpretive. Although case studies are contextualised to a specific situation or cultural group, if data are carefully interpreted, both unique and common aspects of the case can be illuminated, providing a basis for comparison with other contexts. This is accomplished by taking the analytic data that was used to profile the case and using techniques to 'decontextualise' the information. In interpretive case studies the researcher conducts a thematic analysis to identify themes, or units of meaning (DeSantis & Ugarriza 2000). Once these are identified, theoretical or process relationships can be explored among various clusters of meaning (Ayres et al 2003). These relationships are then studied to create new meanings, by reintegrating themes into larger clusters, across a larger number of cases. Reflecting on themes, and their relationships and implications in different settings, gives a depth of understanding that allows cross-case comparisons (see Figure 12.1). Although a case itself cannot be generalised to other individual cases, comparing elements of the case through a process of pattern matching can provide meaningful information that can be used by others (Yin 2003).

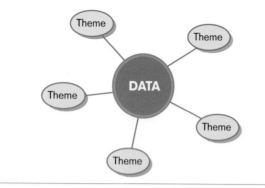

Figure 12.1 Theme cluster

incorporate cultural elements to the traditional designs of RCTs or quasi-experimental studies, can help improve theoretical understanding, develop new knowledge and deepen the understanding of the effects of interventions (Chesla & Rungreangkulkij 2001). Mixed-methods research uses qualitative and quantitative data collection and analysis, either sequentially, or as parallel techniques (Tashakkori & Teddlie 2003). Mixed methods can provide a more complete picture of what is being researched than using only one technique, and can support the analysis of one type of data with another through integration and interpretation (Happ et al 2006).

Questions that require a mixed-method design are those that cannot be explained by only one type of data; issues that require considerable breadth and depth; problems where there is a need to confirm or enhance findings with a second type of data; or studies where a research instrument is being developed from comprehensive information about the topic (Andrew & Halcomb 2009). The findings of a mixed-method study can illuminate different dimensions of a single issue, which can elaborate understandings that come from the analysis. In some cases, a qualitative element can be nested in a quantitative study, or a quantitative element nested in a qualitative study. Important and unique insights can be gained by examining these concurrently (Happ et al 2006). Using mixed methods is not a new technique, but it is growing in popularity for a number of reasons. These include increased reflexivity among nurses and midwives about the relationship between the researcher and the researched; heightened political awareness about the issues surrounding research, increased procedural knowledge about research governance and ethics, and a trend towards international collaboration (Brannen, in Andrew & Halcomb 2009).

Using a variety of research approaches to ascertain the merits of health promotion initiatives helps keep the focus on 'how' and 'why' questions. It also allows the researcher to evaluate many levels of outcomes, and to pose new questions for evaluation as the study progresses, especially if a PAR approach is being used. For example, as a program is being devised, evaluation might emphasise inter-organisational arrangements. The next phase might also include evaluating implementation of the program, and the skills required to deliver various components. A further iteration could add to these components a focus on maintenance and client outcomes (Goodman 2000). At any stage of this process, a comparative study of processes, or outcomes, or both, could be developed. Such a mixed-methods approach would allow the community to be considered a 'case' under study, with multiple dimensions of investigation, multiple methods, and in some cases multiple researchers, some focusing on ascertaining baseline information, some conducting comparative trials of interventions and some evaluating outcomes.

Point to ponder
Mixed-method approaches are increasingly important in obtaining the 'whole picture' about community health.

In an ecologically focused study, for example, the researcher would want to measure community change, and elements of the environment that either support or constrain the desired change, as was used in Richards et al's (2008) study of promoting physical activity and weight management. Using an additional method enhances the validity of the study by 'triangulation'. This involves interrogating the data from different perspectives, as a surveyor would triangulate a point of reference by viewing it from two different perspectives. For example, the study may ask:
• What conditions changed?
• To what extent?
• With what outcomes?
These questions could be answered using a quantitative survey, with responses analysed to judge whether, and to what extent, any responses were significant, or to provide a basis for predicting future initiatives (predictive validity). Following

this phase, or simultaneously, an interpretive, qualitative element could be designed to address the questions:

- What factors support the change?
- Are there cultural barriers to change?
- What other influences affect the change?
- How do local residents believe the physical or social ecology of their community supports or constrains the outcomes?
- Do they perceive any financial, policy or geographic barriers to gaining support for the changes?

The second group of questions requires an interpretive approach, and the methods used to gather data would typically include a combination of observations, interviews, document analysis, and knowledge of policy and social trends. The research team would seek to secure information that is comprehensive, and encompasses the reasons for change, or perceptions about the change. There would also be some detailed analysis of the social ecology or contextual factors involved in the change. To accomplish this, the researchers would likely plan a number of in-depth interviews and conduct a thematic analysis of people's responses to gain insight into the community and its particular areas of need or strength. These data would be analysed in a systematic way to produce new insights (see Figure 12.2).

RESEARCHING CULTURE

Over the past decades, research into cultural issues has grown steadily. As mentioned in previous chapters, this agenda should be extended to provide insights into the features of inclusive societies, intergenerational interactions in different cultures, and how expressions of culture affect health and wellbeing. Investigating cultural issues as a basis for practice is essential to successfully confront the needs of migrant groups during transitions to their new life, to anticipate influences on their health and health service preferences throughout ageing, and to explore how families negotiate, change and work within the context of their cultural and social lives.

Naturalistic research, on its own, or in combination with other methods, is an ideal approach to begin a program of culturally oriented research, especially if the nascent ideas for the study arise from the cultural community itself. This often occurs in a round table or discussion forum, where ideas can evolve into CBPR. One approach that has

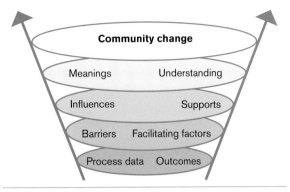

Figure 12.2 Using research information to understand community change

gained popularity with different cultural groups is *appreciative inquiry*, which is conducted within the interpretive, or naturalistic paradigm. An appreciative inquiry is similar to PAR and participatory evaluation in that the objective is to ensure inclusive, empowering research processes that build hope, trust, respect and ultimately, capacity for change. The researcher attempts to bring people together to 'discover, dream, design and deliver' solutions to existing problems and innovations for change (Murphy et al 2004:211). This can begin from a story-telling group, as is often the case in understanding cultural aspects of social life from individuals' oral histories.

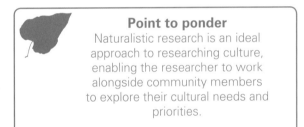

Point to ponder
Naturalistic research is an ideal approach to researching culture, enabling the researcher to work alongside community members to explore their cultural needs and priorities.

In working with a cultural research agenda, researchers should be able to view methodological issues through cultural filters (Foster & Stanek 2007). This means that where quantitative measures are taken, reliability and validity of instruments should be carefully tested with different groups, with special attention to cultural relevance of language and meaning at the individual, group and community level (Chesla & Rungreangkulkij 2001). Research studies that do not attend to these cultural aspects may be well intentioned, but they can potentially negate the socio-cultural reality of a vulnerable population (Wilson & Neville 2009).

BOX 12.3 THE PEEL CHILD HEALTH STUDY

The Peel Child Health Study, called 'Our Children, Our Family, Our Place' is a mixed-method study of child health and development in the context of one regional Australian community. The study was designed to gather scientific knowledge of biological and psychosocial factors, including parenting, within the conceptual framework of the 'enabling community'. This framework proposes that there are features of community life that contribute to child health and wellbeing and to supporting parents.

A central objective of the study is to study the biological and psychosocial dimensions of a child's stress response to his or her environment, first, in the womb, then throughout the pregnancy and for several years after birth. Parental variables are also being studied, to identify characteristics, lifestyle factors and environmental variables that affect children's health. The data for this aspect of the study include behavioural, social, environmental and biological measurements as well as parents' perceptions of raising a child in the Peel region. Analysis of biological, psychosocial and community variables simultaneously is expected to inform strategies for preventing, addressing or overcoming the effects of early adverse experiences or predispositions. Ultimately it is expected that this combination of quantitative and qualitative information will provide the basis for recommendations on how parents and communities can help build resilience and positive developmental outcomes in children.

To gather such widespread data the study is designed as a nested, mixed methods, multi-dimensional study. Biological samples are collected from the pregnant mother, her partner, and the child, and will be analysed using quantitative measurement techniques. Psychosocial data are being collected through questionnaire surveys completed by parents at several time periods. Community data consist of focus groups, individual interviews, and asset mapping, which 'maps' the services and supports available to parents and others, such as grandparents and educators who play a role in supporting child health. Other aspects of the study include a descriptive, qualitative study of Indigenous family members, who are interviewed by Indigenous researchers on their perspectives of parenting and community life. The study has taken several years of meticulous planning, and it is resource intensive, which are typical challenges for mixed-methods studies (Halcomb & Andrew 2009). One of the most important aspects of the study has been the need for ongoing communication and engagement with the community, including local nurses and medical practitioners. Major funding grants have been necessary to begin such a broad, multidimensional and multidisciplinary study, including financial grants for inclusive communication strategies. These strategies include a marketing campaign in the local region to promote the study and recruit participants as well as a website for ongoing community engagement and ultimately, dissemination of findings (www.peelchildhealthstudy.com.au [accessed 7 June 2010]).

Researching with Indigenous people

Indigenous people have been the focus of many studies in Australia and New Zealand, and some of this research has not advanced the type of knowledge that contributes to their empowerment or self-determination. In some cases, researchers have forged relationships that have unearthed important features of Indigenous health, but in other cases, research reports have shown stereotypical perspectives of the researchers, rather than the researched. Some studies have actually damaged relationships, and violated the principles of cultural safety (Wilson & Neville 2009). This has not been an intended goal of the research, but rather, a lack of understanding of the cultural and structural constraints on gathering meaningful data. Fredericks (2008) describes Australian Indigenous people as the most researched in the world, with many Indigenous students now studying research findings from studies that have yet to reflect Indigenous methodologies or knowledge.

In some cases, studies of Indigenous people have presented biased data because of the difficulty of accessing accurate statistics and participants (Couzos et al 2005; Priest et al 2009). As mentioned in Chapter 11, some Indigenous people do not report their Indigenous status or do not wish to provide in-depth information to researchers for personal reasons (Kowanko et al 2009). Many people, both Indigenous and non-Indigenous, prefer not to participate in research, some because they are transient residents of a community, and others because they do not see personal benefits in participating (Buckley 2008; Davies et al 2008). A further issue for Indigenous researchers is the lack

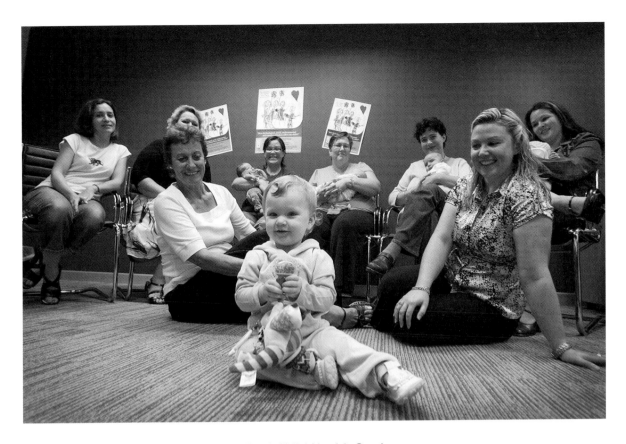

FIGURE 12.3 First babies born in the Peel Child Health Study

of a base of data from methodologically rigorous Indigenous intervention trials, despite a greater burden of disease among Indigenous people (Clifford et al 2009). In some cases, studies have been structured according to Western scientific discourse with inconsistent terminology and culturally insensitive language (Cripps 2008; Priest et al 2009). Dissemination strategies have also been problematic, with passive distribution of clinical guidelines, or resources being used to communicate findings, instead of specific strategies that would help health care providers modify their practice (Clifford et al 2009).

Other problems in Indigenous research include the constraint of small sample sizes, a singular focus on descriptive studies, and a lack of infrastructure for research (Couzos et al 2005). All of these problems indicate a need for researchers to educate themselves about the community and issues related to how members of the community will be affected by the research (Pyett et al 2009).

Point to ponder
Researchers involved in research with Indigenous people must approach any project from a position of humility and cultural safety. Research is never done on people but with people, acknowledging their rights, recognising their sovereignty and respecting their perspective.

Point to ponder
Although comparisons of Indigenous and non-Indigenous health status are useful in identifying areas of need, further research is needed that studies phenomena and events in Indigenous groups over time. This will improve our understanding and knowledge of the strengths that Indigenous people hold and provide guidance in the development of effective health promotion strategies.

Importantly, there is a need for external researchers to eliminate their propensity to draw comparisons between Indigenous and non-Indigenous populations, and instead study phenomena or events in Indigenous groups over time (Cripps 2008; Couzos et al 2005). Longitudinal studies based on a synthesis of traditional and scientific approaches would be more meaningful in terms of capturing the reality of Indigenous communities, and the issues that affect their health and wellbeing (Harvey 2009). Without meaningful and accurate data, it is difficult to monitor changes in health status, evaluate service access, or quantify and evaluate resources spent on Indigenous services (Draper et al 2009). An important gap in the Indigenous research agenda is the life course, social epidemiological approach to studying child health over time in urban environments (Priest et al 2009).

> **ACTION POINT**
> In order to fully hear Indigenous voices, turn down the 'white noise' that represents a researcher's preconceptions, values and conversational habits.

According to Priest et al (2009) the focus on Indigenous rural and remote issues detracts from focusing on the needs of children living in cities, where they also experience disadvantage. Early and genuine collaboration in designing research studies can draw attention to the priorities of community members, help build their research capacities, and demonstrate the researcher's commitment to gather data that will help reduce health inequities (Couzos et al 2005; Priest et al 2009). Developing Indigenous research capacity can also help disseminate findings, which are not always published in the peer-reviewed literature (Clifford et al 2009). Clearly, Indigenous community involvement in each phase of the research agenda is crucial, and is often overlooked by those who seek to address Indigenous health issues, but have not developed the cultural knowledge to do so (Couzos et al 2005; Priest et al 2009).

According to Wilson and Neville (2009:72), studies with Indigenous groups should conform to the principles of the Treaty of Waitangi: 'partnership, participation, protection and power'. When these principles guide the research there is a greater likelihood of maintaining cultural safety. A major task for the researcher is to create safe spaces for dialogue and negotiation, so the group can determine the extent and nature of their involvement. This type of approach is empowering, enabling mutual understanding and the type of cultural humility that characterises CBPR (Minkler 2005; Wilson & Neville 2009). Culturally appropriate dialogue with Indigenous people is described as 'yarning', a process where the researcher interacts with those in the group in a fluid, discursive way, entering a type of 'contact zone' for discussion (Power 2004:40). Power describes the researcher's role as turning down the volume of 'white noise' that represents preconceptions, values and conversational habits, in order to hear the Indigenous voices (Power 2004:40). This can help eliminate the structural disadvantage that often occurs with 'white standpoint', externally imposed research (Martin-McDonald & McCarthy 2007:129).

Confronting the researcher's cultural norms helps create an opportunity for Indigenous perspectives to take priority, helping people feel that the research is connected to the reality of their lives (Belfrage 2007; Couzos et al 2005; Martin-McDonald & McCarthy 2007). Giving voice to Indigenous people is congruent with the critical social theory paradigm, where most research with culturally vulnerable groups is situated. In some cases, there is also a need to ensure the research is gender appropriate; such as in researching Indigenous women's issues. In this type of research it is necessary to plan the study in collaboration with the female custodians of Indigenous culture in the community, to ensure that all sensitivities are considered (Kildea et al 2009).

One of the most important elements of planning Indigenous research is for the researcher to assume a reflexive attitude as a first step in ensuring cultural safety. For a non-Indigenous researcher, this involves reflecting on how her/his worldview might influence the research, and the processes of analysis and dissemination of findings (Wilson & Neville 2009).

> **ACTION POINT**
> The first step in ensuring cultural safety when researching with Indigenous people is to assume a reflexive attitude. Reflect on how your worldview might influence the research, the process of analysis and the dissemination of findings.

Another important element is to actively pursue ethical approval for the research from Indigenous-controlled ethics committees, to ensure that Indigenous interests are represented in all processes (Dunbar & Scrimgeour 2006). These include committees such as the Maori Health Committee of the Health Research Council of New Zealand, the Queensland Aboriginal and Islander Health Forum, and the Western Australian Aboriginal Health Information and Ethics Committee. In other states of Australia besides Western Australia and Queensland, separate arrangements are made for ethical review through Aboriginal peak bodies at state and territory level (Couzos et al 2005). What all have in common, is adherence to the values and principles mandated by the National Health and Medical Research Councils of Australia and New Zealand, to ensure culturally appropriate research. These include *reciprocity* (including the community's perspectives), *respect* (transparent acknowledgement of Indigenous beliefs and practices), *equality* (through authentic research partnership strategies), *responsibility* (developing cultural protocols for all stages of the research), *survival and protection* (promoting the crucial role of culture in the research), and *spirit and integrity* (demonstrating respect for the richness, diversity, and integrity of the Indigenous community) (National Health and Medical Research Council [NHMRC] 2003). This type of approach can be empowering as it helps people feel that the research is connected to the reality of their lives (Belfrage 2007; Couzos et al 2005; Pyett et al 2009). The values and principles for Indigenous research are embedded in the guidelines for researchers as seen in Box 12.4.

RESEARCHING THE FUTURE

Although the research agenda for community health is growing, many areas remain inadequately researched, for a number of reasons. In most cases, the length of time required to investigate a web of factors or situations, is prohibitive. Research may also be hampered by a lack of funding, due to the rigidity of many granting agencies to support broadly based studies. Dilution of interventions in large sites sometimes leads to a lack of clarity in the findings, which can be complicated by time trend effects. This occurs when the circumstances of the community change over time, or where the true costs of engaging with a community at each step of the process are underestimated.

Another difficulty that may arise in community health research, is that there are varying cultural norms and expectations, which makes sharing the experience between different groups somewhat of a challenge. In action research studies, changes in health outcomes as a result of interventions are often not detectable for many years, which may create tensions on those waiting for results, including funding agencies. This is a particular problem if the effect of an intervention falls outside the political planning time frame. A further issue is related to the challenges of measuring place-based improvements at the neighbourhood or community level, especially if the research team has not enlisted the help of someone with statistical expertise. So, although the optimal approach is to investigate multidimensional studies of community health and wellness, the cautionary tale is that current funding agencies tend to seek out and fund research with short, sharp, measurable outcomes, within the parameters of their reporting requirements and political needs.

> ## ACTION POINT
> Challenges to community research are plentiful. Work to develop incremental, expanded programs of community health research that will highlight aspects of community culture and social life in a way that will be useful to funders, providers, managers and community members.

What remains for the future is to develop incremental, expanded programs of community health research that will highlight the aspects of community culture and social life, in a way that can be readily used for policy-makers, health service managers and practitioners, and the community itself. The research to policy agenda will always have gaps to be filled with research into ways of shaping health care systems to provide appropriate, accessible, acceptable, effective, efficient and equitable care. It will also reflect trends and vested interests, particularly with budget constraints on health and research funding bodies. For those who are not working within large networks

BOX 12.4 CHARACTERISTICS OF INDIGENOUS-CONTROLLED HEALTH RESEARCH

Setting the research agenda

- Community-driven research is strategic and based on priority needs.
- Power differentials between community representative bodies and external research bodies are balanced.
- Research focus is holistic, not just biomedical.
- Generalisability of research findings is considered.
- Capacity of community-controlled services is enhanced.
- Multi-centre research involves national community-based leadership.

Research project planning and approval

- Ethical clearance is granted by Indigenous human ethics committees.
- Benefits and risks of the research for individual and community are carefully examined.
- There is valid consent from community representative bodies.
- Support needed by community bodies for research to proceed is appraised.
- Any trial interventions are sustainable.
- Time required for planning and implementation is realistic.
- Cost required for planning and implementation is realistic.

Conduct of research

- There is no withholding of services while the research is being conducted.
- Research coordinators have skills in cross-cultural communication and are respectful of community structures.
- There is appropriate and informed client consent.
- Local community-based leadership and communication networks are harnessed.
- Approaches to data collection and management are flexible.

Analysis, dissemination and application of findings

- Ownership of intellectual property is vested in community-representative bodies.
- There is appropriate early community feedback.
- Communities are enabled to document their experiences.
- Research leads to actions promoting policy changes.

(Couzos et al 2005:94, with permission)

of researchers or organised programs of research, numerous research topics arise out of everyday practice with communities. Many practitioners at the cutting edge of practice have an ideal opportunity through research to make significant inroads into health care improvements, or to manage care and interactions with greater efficiency and effectiveness.

An ideal research agenda could begin with the factors already known to promote healthy, safe and inclusive communities. For example, the Victorian Health Department's (VicHealth) framework for community wellbeing suggests a number of areas for research (Wiseman et al 2007) (see Box 12.5).

Point to ponder

Nurses and midwives at the cutting edge of practice do not have to be involved in organised programs of research to be able to undertake good-quality, appropriate and affordable research with communities.

The areas indicated above are simply suggestions for issues that are important to community health. Others include factors related to employment, work–life balance, housing, air and water quality, and other aspects of the environments

BOX 12.5 WELLBEING INDICATORS FOR HEALTHY, SAFE AND INCLUSIVE COMMUNITIES

Indicator	Potential research
Personal health and wellbeing	Health and quality of life
	Physical activity, weight
	Nutrition
	Alcohol, cigarette, drug use
	Mental health
Community connectedness	Community satisfaction
	Community caring, helping
	Volunteering
	Involvement in school activities
	Cultural inclusion
Early childhood development	Immunisation
	Breastfeeding
	Child health monitoring
Personal and community safety	Public safety, transport
	Crime, violence
	Road trauma, injury
	Occupational health and safety
Lifelong learning	Literacy, numeracy
	School retention
	Pathways to education
	Internet, library use
Service availability	Community perceptions of access, equity, appropriateness

of people's lives (Wiseman et al 2007). On a smaller level, a study of research-related activities by child health nurses in New South Wales indicated that, although participation in research was limited, nurses can make a contribution to the research agenda through reflective practice, quality improvement, and evaluation studies, as well as specific research projects (Comino & Kemp 2008). Although there are few audits of nursing and midwifery research in Australia and New Zealand, a review of published studies in professional journals reveals some interesting trends. The *Journal of Community Health Nursing* publishes a wide range of community research, some of which is focused on behaviour change and chronic illness management, but research reports also include studies that advance knowledge; for example, by framing various interventions within a socio-ecological perspective of community life.

The journal *Family and Community Health* is another journal which reports studies on health promotion interventions for community residents, as well as social and environmental issues. These include studies of community environments that support injury prevention strategies, healthy adolescence and ageing, and reports of various specific nursing interventions. The *Journal of Health and Social Care in the Community* reports numerous studies of home care and other contexts for caregiving. In the past few years, this journal has published widely on service organisation and the needs of carers. Studies also include those addressing the SDOH: housing and homelessness, poverty, health inequalities and social inclusion.

ACTION POINT

There are a range of useful journals that publish good quality community-based research. Access them and use them to support the work you do in your communities.

The *Australian Journal of Rural Health* contains reports of nursing research, but its major focus is on the rural community, so the reports are more interdisciplinary than some of the other nursing and midwifery journals. With workforce shortages, a large proportion of the research concerns recruitment and retention of health professionals, and professional issues related to attracting staff. The *Journal of Advanced Nursing* and the *Journal of Clinical Nursing* publish more frequently than some of the other nursing journals, and these have a strong mix of examples of evidence-based practice and topics addressing community health issues. Some of the more recent studies reported in these journals include research into psychosocial issues in health care, models of service delivery, and approaches for working with vulnerable groups.

Australian journals such as *Contemporary Nurse*, *Collegian* and the *Australian Journal of Advanced Practice* also address a balanced mix of nursing and midwifery research that focuses on interventions, professional development, and the needs of communities. All publish international nursing studies. In some cases, the journals develop special issues dedicated to a certain topic, which can be particularly helpful to nurses and midwives working in the community. For example, the *Journal of Midwifery and Women's Health* has published a special issue on violence against women. *Contemporary Nurse* publishes many special issues, with a strong emphasis on community and family topics, as well as culture and Indigenous health. *Nursing Praxis in New Zealand* publishes a range of nursing research specific to New Zealand and is an excellent source of New Zealand specific studies. A new research journal in New Zealand, *Kai Tiaki Nursing Research,* is also an excellent source of New Zealand specific nursing research.

There are many aspects of community life in Australia and New Zealand that have yet to be sufficiently researched. Our review of journals in which Australian and New Zealand nurses publish their research reveals a dearth of studies that respond to the SDOH, although some of this work is published in the public health and health promotion journals. To advance nursing and midwifery knowledge in the community there remains a need to extend SDOH research, and to continue researching communities themselves as the primary setting within which health and wellbeing can be achieved. This research agenda should make a deliberate attempt to advance knowledge for practice. One of the ways this can be achieved is by basing research studies on existing knowledge, such as that defined in the concept analysis of 'community' developed by Baisch (2009), as we reported in Chapter 1. Following a review of professional literature, and the conventions for concept analysis, Baisch (2009:2472) concluded that community health is achieved through 'participatory, community development processes based upon ecological models that address broad determinants of health'. This suggests study questions such as those found in Box 12.6.

The research questions found in Box 12.6 could be used to guide an entire program of research. However, the most important element in any investigation is the need to pose a manageable question; one that can be addressed in the timeframe allowed, using a defined pool of resources. Although other aspects of the research process are important, the method is ultimately driven by the research question.

BOX 12.6 COMMUNITY HEALTH STUDY QUESTIONS

- What community support mechanisms will create the best opportunities for empowerment and self-determinism among disadvantaged people? Which of these mechanisms are specific to groups differentiated by race, ethnicity, gender, health status, age or geography?

- What policies and practices will create the best opportunities for enriched parenting? What are the barriers to good parenting for different socio-economic groups? How can communities support parenting?

- What are the most helpful strategies in reducing alcohol and tobacco use/overuse? How is this embedded in social and environmental factors?

- Which interventions have shown the most promise in fostering healthy nutrition across the life span? Have they addressed different age groups?

- What is the role of workplace stress in family health and happiness? What community supports can help alleviate stress and promote work–life harmony?

- Are there effective neighbourhood or community-based strategies to counter family disruptions? Where and how are they most effective?

- What is good and best practice, or good and best process in maintaining mental health for different age groups? How are these practices implemented in rural and remote areas?

- How can schools support urban and rural adolescents through the crucial time of emerging identities?

- How can health professionals participate in creating sustainable neighbourhoods to support healthy ageing?

- Are there defensible health benefits for rural communities in emerging technologies, particularly telecommunications?

- What are the barriers and facilitators involved in nurses and midwives becoming active advocates for healthy environments?

GETTING STARTED: FROM RESEARCH QUESTION TO SOLUTION

The basic ingredients for a successful research study are enthusiasm, perseverance and the art of argument. Developing a good research question can sometimes be extremely difficult. One of the best ways of identifying a good question to guide a research study is to contemplate what is already known in the area targeted for study, then to undertake a 'question framing' exercise. The research topic can be developed in consultation with community members, but then the researcher may want to do some further work on refining the topic into a specific question. Often, this can be done away from the research situation, when the researcher is able to think creatively. It also helps to talk to various people, as those with knowledge of the area of study can help to identify strengths and weaknesses in the question. A critical friend with little knowledge of the topic can also be helpful, as they may be able to interrogate ideas objectively and dispassionately in a way that helps the researcher clarify their thoughts.

Once a general topic has been decided, it is helpful to begin thinking of the research process as a strategic plan, as outlined below.

The question

The first step is to fill several pages with questions relating to the topic of study. Often, these questions are ones that a researcher has already thought about. Writing questions in a cohesive and simple manner is a very important step in the planning process. The questions will come from practice, reading, deliberate contemplation, discussion with community members, and reflection on the intention of the study (the purpose). Once the questions have been written and considered, the second stage of the process begins.

The argument

A good argument is a well-substantiated case for the following:

- what we do know about the topic
- what we do not know about it (the gap in knowledge)
- what we should know (how this piece of research can help to fill the knowledge gap)
- the implications of knowing this (i.e. so what?).

The argument has two major elements: the analysis of information, and the crafting of the idea (the proposal). Ultimately, a research study is aimed at generating and analysing data according to the conventions of rigorous research (the method), but all parts of the proposal must reflect precision and clarity, which are considered essential elements of research. The best way to learn to write

in a scholarly style is to read widely from existing research. Although there is some variability in style in the published literature, there is a recognisable style of clear, concise writing. While reading research articles, researchers should attend to the features of style as well as to the mechanisms and findings of the research.

A good argument illustrates two major features: logical thinking and insight. Logical thinking is shown in the use of a disciplined presentation style (precise and clear), and the sequencing of thoughts about the topic from broad contextual issues, to more specific ones. Insight is the ability to clearly analyse the topic and synthesise ideas to create a new coalescence of knowledge.

Conceptual framework

A theoretical framework is a valid theory, used with reliability beyond its original setting. A conceptual framework or model may be a hybrid of one or more theories, or it may simply be an original framework devised from constructs (ideas) generated from the literature review (which should be ongoing throughout the process of writing the research proposal). The researcher's choice of whether to use a conceptual model or theoretical framework is argued briefly in the proposal. An introduction to the framework is given, followed by an explanation of the elements of the framework, and an indication of how the framework is to be used in the research. In quantitative studies, the framework is used to generate and guide the hypotheses, the strategies for testing these, and as a basis for reflecting on the findings. In qualitative (interpretive) studies, it is linked to the philosophical underpinnings of the method, and to the analysis of interpretations.

Method

The 'methods' argument should begin with an introduction to how the study is to be conducted, in what paradigm it is situated (for example, naturalistic or interpretive), and where the methodological approach is derived from. It should include any previous research in the area from which ideas are being extended or challenged. A researcher should then explain the design features of the research, including participants, data collection, and the analytic tests or techniques that will be used.

An explanation is provided of the actual method used, the sample, instruments, and reliability and validity data related to any instruments. If no instrumentation other than the researcher is used, the researcher must argue the data gathering as being justified in terms of the method. For example, in PAR, the process of working with the group is explained. In a case study, the way the case is bounded and what is to be included, is explained. Other interpretive methods have their own conventions for design and analysis, and these should be described. Once the study is explained, the ethical considerations are outlined, including the source of ethical approval.

Research ethics

The major ethical considerations in conducting research studies are universally accepted, and these include ensuring confidentiality and anonymity of research participants, scientific validity and protection of vulnerable people, such as children, and those who become powerless by institutionalisation, or other factors. As mentioned above, where Indigenous people are part of the research, the proposal should be reviewed by the appropriate Indigenous research ethics committee in addition to institutional review by a University or Health service sponsoring or hosting the study. Researchers' accountability to both those being researched and the scientific community holds them responsible to fully explain to research participants any known risks and benefits, regardless of how small, so that participants only consent to their involvement on the basis of being fully informed.

An explanation must be given to assure participants of the right to withdraw from the research at any time without recrimination, and where they will be able to access assistance if the need arises; that is, if they become distressed by the research process. The researcher must also explain how the data will be secured during the research process, and how and when it will be destroyed at the end of the study. It is also helpful to assure participants

of the purpose of the research; whether it is being conducted as part of a work/practice role, as a study for a higher degree, or as commissioned research. Participants should then be reassured that the findings will be published in aggregated form only, with all identifying data removed.

Researchers are also obliged to identify themselves and any others involved in the research (supervisors, co-researchers) and to provide feedback to those supplying information. This helps ensure that the participants are treated as partners, not simply as people supplying information to be taken away from the community. Participants should also be assured that data will be analysed in a culturally sensitive way, with cultural representation from someone who can guide the process if necessary, for cultural safety, and the benefit of the community. This also helps prevent researcher bias from compromising the research rigour and ethical standards. Involving the community should begin prior to the research, as it is helpful in framing the questions appropriately, in establishing the feasibility of the study, guiding the research process, and articulating the findings in language that is meaningful to the community. This creates a greater likelihood that community preferences will find their way into public policies.

Findings/results

Although different methods dictate different conventions for presenting results, it is often useful to organise the findings around the research questions or objectives. The object of presenting the results of research is to clearly demonstrate defensible findings from the evidence collected, and the appropriate use of analytic techniques.

Discussion

This section of the research is found after the presentation of findings, so it is not part of a research proposal. In presenting the findings, the discussion is often the most rewarding, as it revolves around that most important question: 'So what?'. This gives the researcher the opportunity to think creatively while maintaining an academic tone, especially in connecting the findings to the broader body of knowledge and the conceptual framework. A good research study typically moves from the discussion to implications for practice, education, management, system changes and/or policy recommendations and suggests further research, ending with a clear and concise summary of the study.

Case study

Francesca, Maria's cousin, who had previously visited Maria and Jim in Sydney, decides to immigrate from Italy. She arrives with a new resident status and settles in to the family home, offering to babysit the children while she seeks employment. She finds work, moves into a small bed-sitter in Punchbowl, and begins to attend the Migrant Resource Centre. She participates in the language development program, where she meets an Afghanistan refugee, Mahmood. Mahmood spent some time in a refugee camp on the Pakistani border waiting to come to Australia. As a result of his experience, he is receiving counselling for post-traumatic stress disorder. He has had difficulty settling in Australia, as he struggles with English and feels isolated from his culture. Francesca invites him to share her apartment.

Mahmood gets a job as a short order cook in a local restaurant where he encounters racism from co-workers, as well as others while using public transport. His feelings of isolation intensify as time goes on, and he becomes severely depressed. Francesca is unable to console him, and asks him to move out. Shortly after this, Francesca and Mahmood are both invited to take part in a participatory action research project being developed and undertaken with the migrant community through the Migrant Resource Centre. They both agree to take part, and begin attending meetings with the researchers and other community members who have volunteered to participate. Mahmood is hopeful that sharing some of the difficulties he has experienced in settling in Australia with the researchers will help others like him.

REFLECTING ON THE BIG ISSUES

- Research is an important part of nursing and midwifery practice.
- Researching community health issues requires a broader approach than the traditional evidence-based practice methods.
- Mixed-methods research can help provide the community perspective as well as specific investigation of designated variables.
- Research is time and resource intensive.
- Multidisciplinary studies can give a greater breadth to studies of community health.
- Special considerations must be given to researching with Indigenous people, to ensure their cultural safety.
- Community-based participatory research is well suited to studies of the community, particularly those using participatory action research.
- The research questions should dictate the research method, which then follows appropriate conventions for data collection, analysis and dissemination of findings.
- The community research agenda has many gaps that indicate the need for ongoing research, particularly addressing the social determinants of health.

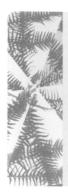

Reflective questions: how would I use this knowledge in practice?

1 Update the genogram you have been developing throughout the text and identify one research question for each family unit involved in the case studies throughout the previous chapters.

2 Explain how you would investigate each of these questions.

3 How would the results of each study inform PHC in nursing and midwifery practice?

Research-informed practice

Read Wilhelmsson and Lindberg's (2007) study 'Prevention and health promotion and evidence-based fields of nursing—a literature review'.

• Can you identify recent studies in health promotion that have broader applicability to community health than those reported by these authors in this 2007 study?
 Or

Read Comino and Kemp's (2008) study 'Research-related activities in community-based child health services'.

• Reflecting on the research activities of this group of nurses, do you think their involvement in research is typical of child and family nurses?

• What constraints do you believe nurses and midwives experience in trying to establish a program of research? How can these be overcome?

• What infrastructure and support would be required to develop a comprehensive agenda for child health research?

References

Abbott S, Bickerton J, Daly M, Procter S 2008 Evidence-based primary health care and local research: a necessary but problematic partnership. Primary Health Care Research & Development 9:191–8

Andrew S, Halcomb E (eds) 2009 Mixed methods research for nursing and health sciences. Wiley-Blackwell, Chichester

Annells M, DeRoche M, Koch T, Lewin G, Lucke J 2005 A Delphi study of district nursing research priorities in Australia. Applied Nursing Research 18:36–43

Anthony S, Jack S 2009 Qualitative case study methodology in nursing research: an integrative review. Journal of Advanced Nursing 65(6):1171–81

Ayres L, Kavanaugh K, Knafl K 2003 Within-case and across-case approaches to qualitative data analysis. Qualitative Health Research 13(6):871–83

Baisch M 2009 Community health: an evolutional concept analysis. Journal of Advanced Nursing 65(11):2464–76

Baum F, MacDougall C, Smith D 2006 Participatory action research. Journal of Epidemiology Community health 60:854–7

Belfrage M 2007 Why 'culturally safe' health care? Medical Journal of Australia 186(10):537–8

Benner P 1984 From Novice to Expert: Power and Expertise in Nursing Practice. Aldine, Chicago

Bero L, Rennie D 1995 The Cochrane Collaboration: preparing, maintaining and disseminating systematic reviews of the effects of health care. Journal of the American Medical Association 274(24):1935–8

Bowen S, Zwi A 2005 Pathways to 'evidence-informed' policy and practice: a framework for action. PLoS Medicine 2(7): E166–E171

Buckley B 2008 The need for wider public understanding of health care research. Primary Health Care Research & Development 9:3–6

Burgess J 2006 Participatory action research. First-person perspectives of a graduate student. Action Research 4(4):419–37

Carr W, Kemmis S 1986 Becoming Critical: Education, Knowledge and Action Research. Falmer Press, London

Chesla C, Rungreangkulkij S 2001 Nursing research on family processes in chronic illness in ethnically diverse families: a decade review. Journal of Family Nursing 7(3):230–43

Clifford A, Jackson Pulver L, Richmond R, Shakeshaft A, Ivers R 2009 Disseminating best-evidence health-care to Indigenous health-care settings and programs in Australia: identifying the gaps. Health Promotion International 24(4):404–15

Comino E, Kemp L 2008 Research-related activities in community-based child health services. Journal of Advanced Nursing 63(3):266–75

Commonwealth of Australia 2009 Capabilities for supporting prevention and chronic condition self-management. DOHA and Flinders University, Canberra

Couzos S, Lea T, Murray R, Culbong M 2005 'We are not just participants — we are in charge': the NACCHO ear trial and the process for Aboriginal community-controlled health research. Ethnicity and Health 10(2):91–111

Cripps K 2008 Indigenous family violence: a statistical challenge. Injury, International Journal of the Care of the Injured 39(S5): S25–S35

Davies G, Boothman N, Duxbury J, Davies R, Blinkhorn A 2008 An investigation of non-participation in health promotion interventions and its impact on population level outcomes. International Journal of Health Promotion & Education 45(3):107–12

DeSantis L, Ugarriza D 2000 The concept of theme as used in qualitative nursing research. Western Journal of Nursing Research 22(3):351–72

Draper G, Somerford P, Pilkington A, Thompson S 2009 What is the impact of missing Indigenous status on mortality estimates? An assessment using record linkage in Western Australia. Australian and New Zealand Journal of Public Health 33(4):325–31

Duke J, Connor M, McEldowney R 2009 Becoming a culturally competent health practitioner in the delivery of culturally safe care: a process oriented approach. Journal of Cultural Diversity 16(2):40–9

Dunbar T, Scrimgeour M 2006 Ethics in Indigenous research — connecting with community. Bioethical Inquiry 3:179–85

Fawcett J 2008 The added value of nursing conceptual model-based research. Journal of Advanced Nursing 61(6):583

Flemming K 2010 Synthesis of quantitative and qualitative research: an example of Critical Interpretive Synthesis. Journal of Advanced Nursing 66(1):201–17

Foster J, Stanek K 2007 Cross-cultural considerations in the conduct of community-based participatory research. Family and Community Health 30(1):42–9

Fredericks B 2008 Researching with Aboriginal women as an Aboriginal woman researcher. Australian Feminist Studies 23(55):113–29

Garfield S, Malozowski S, Chin M, Narayan K, Glasgow R, Green L, Hiss R, Krumholtz H, The Diabetes Mellitus Interagency Coordinating Committee Translation Conference Working Group 2003 Considerations for diabetes translational research in real-world settings. Diabetes Care 26(9):2670–4

Gil-Gonzalez D, Ruiz-Cantero M, Alvarez-Dardet C 2009 How political epidemiology research can address why the millennium development goals have not been achieved: developing a research agenda. Journal of Epidemiology Community Health 63:278–80

Goldenberg M 2006 On evidence and evidence-based medicine. Lessons from the philosophy of science. Social Science & Medicine 62:2621–32

Goodman R 2000 Evaluation of community-based health programs: An alternative perspective. In: Schneiderman N, Speers M, Silva J, Tomes H, Gentry J (eds) Integrating Behavioral and Social Sciences with Public Health. American Psychological Association, Washington, pp 293–304

Greenwood J 1994 Action research and action researchers: some introductory considerations. Contemporary Nurse 3(2):84–92

Halcomb E, Andrew S 2009 Managing mixed methods projects. In: Andrews S, Halcomb E (eds) Mixed Methods Research for Nursing and Health Sciences. Wiley-Blackwell, Chichester, pp 50–64

Happ M, DeVito Dabbs A, Tate J, Hricik A, Erlen J 2006 Exemplars of mixed methods data combination and analysis. Nursing Research 55(2S):S43–S49

Hartrick Doane G, Varcoe C 2005 Family Nursing as Relational Inquiry: Developing Health-Promoting Practice. Lippincott Williams & Wilkins, Philadelphia

Harvey P 2009 Indigenous health — evolving ways of knowing. Australian Health Review 33(4):628–35

Hauck Y, Kelly G, Fenwick J 2007 Research priorities for parenting and child health: a Delphi study. Journal of Advanced Nursing 59(2):129–39

Haviland M 2004 Doing participatory evaluation with community projects. Australian Institute of Family Studies Stronger Families Learning Exchange Bulletin 6(Spring/Summer):10–13

Israel B, Schulz A, Parker E, Becker A 1998 Review of community-based research: assessing partnership approaches to improve public health. Annual Review of Public Health 19:173–202

Jackson D, Firtko A, Edenborough M 2007 Personal resilience as a strategy for surviving and thriving in the face of workplace adversity: a literature review. Journal of Advanced Nursing 60(1):1–9

Joanna Briggs Institute 2008 Smoking cessation interventions and strategies. Best Practice 12(8):1–4

Kendall S 2008 How has primary health care progressed? Some observations since Alma Ata. Primary Health Care Research & Development 9:169–71

Kildea S, Barclay L, Wardaguga M, Dawumal M 2009 Participative research in a remote Australian Aboriginal setting. Action Research 7(2):143–63

Kitson A, Rycroft-Malone J, Harvey G, McCormack B, Seers K, Titchen A 2008 Evaluating the successful implementation of evidence into practice using the PARiHS framework: theoretical and practical challenges. Implementation Science 3(1): doi:10.1186/1748-5908-3-1

Kowanko I, Stewart T, Power C, Fraser R, Love I, Bromley T 2009 An Aboriginal family and community healing program in metropolitan Adelaide: description and evaluation. Australian Indigenous Health Bulletin 9(4):1–12

Labonte R, Polanyi M, Muhajarine N, McIntosh T, Williams A 2005 Beyond the divides: toward critical population health research. Critical Public Health, 15(1):5–17

Luck L, Jackson D, Usher K 2006 Case study: a bridge across paradigms. Nursing Inquiry 13:103–9

Marmot M, Friel S 2008 Global health equity: evidence for action on the social determinants of health. Journal of Epidemiology Community Health 62:1095–7

Martin-McDonald K, McCarthy A 2007 'Marking' the white terrain in indigenous health research: literature review. Journal of Advanced Nursing 61(2):126–33

Maxwell R 1984 Quality assessment in health. British Medical Journal 288:1470–2

McMurray A 2004 Culturally sensitive evidence-based practice. Collegian 11(4):14–18

Minkler M 2005 Community-based research partnerships: challenges and opportunities. Journal of Urban Health: Bulletin of the New York Academy of Medicine 82(2) Suppl 2, doi:10.1093/urban/jti034

Morrison I, Stosz L, Clift S 2008 An evidence base for mental health promotion through supported education: a practical application of Antonovsky's salutogenic model of health. International Journal of Health Promotion & Education 46(1):11–20

Mowinski Jennings B, Loan L 2001 Misconceptions among nurses about evidence-based practice. Journal of Nursing Scholarship 33(2):121–36

Muncey T 2009 Does mixed methods constitute a change in paradigm? In: Andrew S, Halcomb E (eds) Mixed methods research for nursing and the health sciences. Wiley-Blackwell, Chichester,UK, pp 13–30

Murphy L, Kordyl P, Thorne M 2004 Appreciative inquiry: a method for measuring the impact of a project on the wellbeing of an Indigenous community. Health Promotion Journal of Australia 15(30):211–14

Mykhalovskiy E, Armstrong P, Armstrong H, Bourgeault I, Choiniere JU, Lexchin J, Peters S, White J 2008 Qualitative research and the politics of knowledge in an age of evidence: developing a research-based practice of immanent critique. Social Science & Medicine 67:195–203

National Health and Medical Research Council (NHMRC) 2003 Values and Ethics: Guidelines for ethical conduct in Aboriginal and Torres Strait Islander Health Research. Commonwealth of Australia, Canberra

Petticrew M, Tugwell P, Welch V, Ueffing E, Kristjansson E, Armstrong R, Doyle J, Waters E 2009 Better evidence about wicked issues in tackling health inequities. Journal of Public Health 31(3):453–6

Power K 2004 Yarning: a responsive research methodology. Journal of Australian Research in Early Childhood Education 11(1):37–46

Priest N, Mackean T, Waters E, Davis E, Riggs E 2009 Indigenous child health research: a critical analysis of Australian studies. Australian and New Zealand Journal of Public Health 33(1):55–63

Primary Health Care Research, Evaluation and Development in collaboration with Primary Health Care Research & Information Service, Commonwealth Department of Health & Ageing, Australian Association for Academic General Practice, Royal Australian College of General Practitioners 2009 Snapshot of Australian Primary Health Care Research, Canberra. Online. Available: www.phcris.org.au (accessed 10 December 2009)

Pyett P, Waples-Crowe P, van der Sterren A 2009 Engaging with Aboriginal communities in an urban context: some practical suggestions for public health researchers. Australian and New Zealand Journal of Public Health 33(1):51–4

Richards E, Riner M, Prouty Sands L 2008 A social ecological approach of community efforts to promote physical activity and weight management. Journal of Community Health Nursing 25(4):179–92

Rogers E 2003 Diffusion of Innovations (5th edn). The Free Press, New York

Rycroft-Malone J, Seers K, Titchen A, Harvey G, Kitson A, McCormack B 2004 What counts as evidence in evidence-based practice? Journal of Advanced Nursing 47:81–90

Sackett D, Straus S, Richardson W, Rosenberg W, Haynes R 2000 Evidence-Based Medicine: How to Practice and Teach EBM. Churchill Livingstone, London

Sandelowski M 2004 Using qualitative research. Qualitative Health Research 14(10):1366–86

—— 2008 Reading, writing and systematic review. Journal of Advanced Nursing 64(1):104–10

Smith B, Keleher H, Fry C 2008 Developing values, evidence and advocacy to address the social determinants of health. Health Promotion Journal of Australia 19(3):171–2

Smith C, Pell J 2003 Parachute use to prevent death and major trauma related to gravitational challenge: systematic review of randomised controlled trials. British Medical Journal 1459–61

Stringer E 2004 Action Research in Education. Pearson, Upper Saddle River, NJ

Tashakkori A, Teddlie C 2003 Handbook of Mixed Methods in Social and Behavioral Research (2nd edn). Sage, Thousand Oaks, Ca

Tripp-Reimer T, Doebbeling B 2004 Qualitative perspectives in translational research. Worldviews on evidence-based nursing. 1(S1):S65–S72

Venkatapuram S, Marmot M 2009 Epidemiology and social justice in light of social determinants of health research. Bioethics 23(2):79–89

Wainwright N, Surtees P, Welch A, Luben R, Khaw K, Bingham S 2007 Healthy lifestyle choices: could sense of coherence aid health promotion? Journal of Epidemiology and Community Health 61:871–6

Weaver K, Olson J 2006 Understanding paradigms used for nursing research. Journal of Advanced Nursing 53(4):459–69

Whittemore R, Knafl K 2005 The integrative review: updated methodology. Journal of Advanced Nursing 52(5):546–53

Wilhelmsson S, Lindberg M 2007 Prevention and health promotion and evidence-based fields of nursing: a literature review. International Journal of Nursing Practice 13:254–65

Wilson D, Neville S 2009 Culturally safe research with vulnerable populations. Contemporary Nurse 33(1):69–79

Wiseman J, McLeod J, Zubrick S 2007 Promoting mental health and wellbeing: integrating individual, organizational and community-level indicators. Health Promotion Journal of Australia 18(3):198–207

World Health Organization (WHO) 2006 Gender Equality, Work and Health: A Review of the Evidence. WHO, Geneva

Yin R 2003 Case Study Research: Design and Methods (3rd edn). Sage, Thousand Oaks, Ca

Useful websites

http://www.acebcp.org.au — Australian Centre for Evidence Based Clinical Practice

http://www.joannabriggs.edu.au/ — Joanna Briggs Institute and its networks

http://www.cochrane.org — Cochrane Collaboration

http://www.nicsl.com.au — National Institute of Clinical Studies

http://www.phaa@phaa.net.au — Public Health Association of Australia

http://www.ruralhealth.org.au — Australian National Rural Health Alliance

http://www.who.int — World Health Organization (WHO)

http://www.who.int/mental_health/evidence/en/promoting_mhh.pdf — WHO Mental Health Evidence

http://www.who.int/rpc/evipnet/en — WHO Evidence-informed policy network

http://www.icn.ch — International Council of Nurses (ICN)

Chapter 13

Inclusive policies, equitable health care systems

INTRODUCTION

Policy-making for community health is basically a political process in which those in positions of power make decisions on how best to allocate resources. As health professionals, it is our responsibility to become familiar with how these decisions are made, and to advocate for equity in allocations to the communities we assist. This can take us into unfamiliar territory, carefully examining the needs and priorities of the community, while, at the same time, understanding the constraints on services and resources. Policy-making is an important step in health promotion. Without policies, decisions for resource allocation could be made on the basis of the loudest voices, the highest population, or the desires of those best able to articulate their requests. To work towards equitable distribution of resources requires policies that are fair. Fairness means that there is advocacy for those who are most in need, whose voices are often silent. Fairness also means that those born to privilege are not overlooked, but their needs are carefully considered alongside those of the wider population. Guided by the principles of primary health care (PHC), we consider how policies and systems of health service are able to balance needs and services on the basis of social justice at the global, national, regional and local level.

National health policies are usually informed by, and responsive to, global priorities and conditions. Ideally, state/territory or regional priorities would also be designed to follow or complement the directions of national policies. However, where political agendas differ, this may not always be the case. So, for example, it is possible that in one Australian state, policy-makers could place high priority on environmental issues in its health planning, whereas another might see aged care as its greatest priority. Both states would be governed by the goal of better health, but they may change the distribution of resources according to their respective priorities. In countries such as New Zealand, where there is a single health department (the Ministry of Health New Zealand [MOHNZ]), policy-making is more consistent across the country. Yet, even in this environment, there is a need for constant vigilance, to ensure that policy-making is inclusive, and results in all members of the community having equity of access to what they need to maintain good health.

> **Point to ponder**
> Policy development must be fair — that means advocating for those most in need while ensuring the needs of those born to privilege are also not overlooked.

Because of the complexity of health policy-making, it is important to understand how decisions are made. Optimally, decisions would be bi-directional, bottom-up and top-down. Local citizens' groups, health professionals, town councils and city planners would convey the needs of local communities upward, to the regional, state/territory and national levels, where they would participate in informed debates about health and health care. Policy-makers would hear their voices and preferences, and attempt to accommodate multiple perspectives in the way they allocate resources for health. In this context, debates and decisions would be approached on the basis of equal partnerships, and expedient information systems, so that all policy decisions would also be evidence-based; or informed by the latest research and demographic data. Once considerations were aired and consensus was achieved, the policy-making group would communicate with the wider community, gathering further data and/or responses, which would instigate further cycles of input for decision-making. As a result, the policy would achieve three main outcomes. First, it would have a significant effect in improving the health of the population. Second, it would be fair. Third, it would be administered through efficient governance structures, with transparent goals, expectations, financial accountability and evaluation strategies. Yet, impediments to achieving this type of system remain for reasons that are political and financial. Too often, political positions dictate the terms or targets of health decisions, especially if there are vested interests involved. The discussion to follow outlines some of the most important issues in policy-making in the 21st century, with implications for the sustained involvement of all health professionals.

Point to ponder

Optimal policy-making would ensure decisions are made in a bi-directional manner — from ensuring that consumer group input at the local level is heard at the national level, and that their input is accommodated in policy, and then fed back to the local level.

POLITICS, POLICY-MAKING AND HEALTH CARE

The main goal of health policy-making should be to improve and enhance health. This requires a strong health care system, and decisive leadership to guide the way policies are developed. The ideal health care system is ethical, fair, strategic in its endeavour to meet the needs of current and future communities; transparent in communicating its goals and capabilities; oriented towards

community empowerment for informed choices, and resourced to the extent that it can support those choices. But the health care system alone cannot create or sustain health. This is why there has been an urgent call from global health policy-makers to incorporate health in all policies. If health was included in all policies our governments would ensure health and safety in education, transportation, media advertising, food services and the environment. Community planning would include health considerations in their plans for housing, infrastructure and public works. Health planners would participate in policies for safe neighbourhoods, community policing and disaster planning. There would be health considerations in decisions made by departments of immigration and multicultural affairs, and health plans for primary industry development and innovation, and workplace and industrial relations. Health issues are embedded in each of these aspects of daily life, and affect people at all stages of the life course from family planning, safe maternity care, illness management, injury prevention to healthy ageing and end-of-life care.

Point to ponder

The health care system alone cannot create or sustain health. Health must be considered in *all* policy development activities.

As mentioned previously, the defining purpose of a health care system lies in the provision of accessible, appropriate, equitable health care that is responsive to people's expectations. When equity is achieved, the health care system,

Objectives

By the end of this chapter you will be able to:

1 identify the factors influencing the development of policies that affect the health of the population

2 explain the global issues that have an impact on national and regional policy development

3 explain the importance of community health literacy in all policy-making

4 discuss the issues that must be considered in planning health services to be responsive to the needs of different population groups

5 describe the features of a PHC system that contribute to better health and wellbeing

6 discuss the role of nurses and midwives in policy planning and implementation.

its policies, and the policies of other government departments are inclusive, and aligned with the social determinants of health (SDOH). The fact that we live in conditions of inequity indicates that this continues to be an elusive, yet worthy goal for our actions. To some extent, this may be due to the complexity of policy-making and all the competing interests that influence the outcome. However, some inequities persist because of events in the global and/or local environment. The global financial crisis of 2008–09 interrupted progress in achieving equity. This occurred partly because policy decisions distributed many of the scarce resources that remained after the financial meltdown, to prop up financial institutions. Deploying resources to financial institutions was criticised as governments catering to the wealthy, yet it was seen as a necessary policy decision to ensure affordable mortgages, and retention of employment opportunities. Financial institutions hold vested interests in the allocation of government funding, yet their viability is crucial to many people's lives, and therefore their health. This illustrates the complexity and ecological perspective of policy-making. Everything is connected to everything else.

Politics was once defined by Sax (1978) as the art of the possible in satisfying a 'strife of interests' (in Kamien 2009:65). In health policy-making there has always been a strife of interests, between rich and poor, urban and rural, young and old, sick and well, and those with competing biomedical or health promotion needs. Health care decisions revolve around distributive justice: who gets what. Ethically, the poor should receive the lion's share of resources, as this would bring them up to the same level of opportunity as the rest of the population. However, no country in the world has achieved equity in resource allocation, leaving many people living impoverished lives. At the global level, the United Nation's Report on the World Social Situation 2010 indicates a need to 'Rethink Poverty' (Online. Available: www. un.org/esa/socdec/rwss/2010_media.html [accessed 29 January 2010]). The report argues that poverty remains the central issue for global policy-makers, which should inspire governments to work towards equality and social justice throughout all countries in the world.

The global financial crisis, and the neoliberal policies that led up to the crisis, represented the global trend of over-reliance on market forces, where government efforts were focused on economic development, to the detriment of health and social services for the world's poor. The United Nations (UN) suggests that the most important policy implication for the future is for governments to play a developmental role, integrating economic and social policies to support productivity and employment growth, while attacking inequality and promoting social justice. This is a more balanced approach to alleviating poverty, and it urges governments to work towards equitable, sustainable employment opportunities and public social expenditures on PHC, universal education and the provision of social security. The latter includes insurance, pensions, disability and child benefits (UN 2010).

Point to ponder

At the global level, poverty remains the central issue for policy-makers with an urgent need to integrate economic and social policies to achieve health.

The UN focus on employment policies is shared by others, including researchers who have developed a database of studies demonstrating how working conditions affect national competitiveness and unemployment throughout the world (Online. Available: www.RaisingtheGlobalFloor.org [accessed 5 December 2009]). This work, and that of other large research groups, is intended to draw global attention to the link between the SDOH and global inequalities (Bambra et al 2008). Bambra et al's (2008) analysis of systematic reviews of health inequalities in relation to the SDOH, situates the workplace as one of the most significant settings for policy development. Where workplace policies are unfair or insufficient to support the labour force, there are implications across all of the SDOH. Parents are unable to care for their children. Maternal health suffers. Family relationships can be eroded. The lack of financial resources can prohibit children's educational opportunities. Cultural and family connections can be disrupted. People may have to work into older age and consequently suffer illness and injury. These are only a few of the factors that cascade through family life from one type of policy. Together, these factors reinforce the primary role of employment policies in global and national policy-making.

HEALTH SERVICES POLICIES AND THE SOCIAL DETERMINANTS OF HEALTH

No one would doubt that health service policies are also fundamental to improving the SDOH. However, there is a gap in our research knowledge of the policies that would be most responsive to the SDOH, and how these are linked to health services (Bambra et al 2008). Baum et al (2009) argue that this will only occur with a complete reorientation of health care systems. To date, health service policies continue to reflect the biomedical approach, and, because the political power rests with the medical, technological and pharmaceutical industries, this is where the greatest level of funding is allocated. Public demand for these services also plays a role in maintaining the dominance of biomedical, technological and pharmaceutical services. Politicians and decision-makers find it easier to provide expensive clinical care in urban environments, where it is most cost-effective. However, privileging hospital services, and concentrating health care in urban environments, deprives many rural areas of services such as obstetric care, care for older people and adequate distribution of health professionals (Farmer & Currie 2009; Kamien 2009).

Point to ponder
There is a significant gap in our understanding of the type of policies that will be most responsive to addressing the SDOH.

Rural health policies

Rural health is therefore an important area for policy development. Policies to address the needs of those disadvantaged by distance would include a national e-health strategy, patient-assisted travel, community support systems for oral and mental health, and an adequate workforce (National Rural Health Alliance [NRHA] 2009). To advance the rural health agenda, there is a need for policymakers to collect evaluative data on current issues and needs, and then to support evidence-informed practice and services that are framed in conjunction with other health policies (Farmer & Currie 2009; Wakerman 2009). However, after nearly a decade of development, Australia's rural health policy discussions remain focused on health services and workforce issues, rather than the SDOH or proximal risk factors (Wakerman 2008). A similar situation exists in New Zealand. A recent health workforce policy has seen the introduction of bonding for health professionals who choose to work in areas difficult to staff, including some rural locations. As an incentive to work there, medical doctors and midwives who stay in a rural location for three to five years, can have up to $10 000 per year written off their student loans (Online. Available: www.moh.govt.nz/moh.nsf/indexmh/bonding [accessed 8 February 2010]). Interestingly nurses who are in an ideal position to provide essential PHC to rural communities, are not eligible for bonding.

Health promotion policies

Health policies oriented towards hospital care are only part of the problem creating inequities. For many years, health promotion policies have been developed on the basis of exhorting individuals to change their behaviour, rather than focus on the upstream causes of ill health, or the needs of the poor or those with disabling conditions. As a result, those with the worst health status, many of whom cannot afford health care, receive the fewest health services, and the cycle of inequities continues (Baum et al 2009). This does not mean that policies focusing on behaviours have been entirely ineffective, because there have been some remarkable successes. These include policies that have guided programs aimed at reducing injuries from road traffic accidents, preventing deaths from tobacco smoking and sudden infant death syndrome (SIDS) (now often referred to in New Zealand as sudden unexpected death in infancy, or SUDI), those focusing on screening for breast and cervical cancer, and early detection of cardiovascular disease, public awareness programs cautioning against behaviours that would spread HIV/AIDS or other communicable diseases, and initiatives to prevent suicide by creating public awareness of the warning signs (Wise 2008). But there remains a need for policies recognising the

Point to ponder
Health policies in Australia and New Zealand continue to focus on hospital care and behaviour change rather than on the causes of ill health or needs of the poor.

pivotal role of community life in creating and sustaining health. These should be focused on community capacity development.

Community development policies

The absence of community development and community self-determinism in policies adds an additional layer to inequitable health systems. The lack of such policies runs counter to the need for community empowerment as a principle of PHC, which would foster full participation by community members in determining the direction and priorities for their health services (DeVos et al 2009). Community participation would help identify the need for services for the disadvantaged and vulnerable; those with the best understanding of the most urgent needs. Community input could also provide a basis for developing realistic policies for children's health, adolescent health, men's health, women's health, migrant health, disabilities services, aged care, Indigenous health, rural health, mental health and other areas of policy development. If these groups participated in policy-making there would not only be greater inclusiveness, but better guidance on appropriate implementation strategies.

POLICY-MAKING AND PRIMARY HEALTH CARE

An inclusive approach to policy development resonates with a careful balance of comprehensive and selective PHC, as we discussed in Chapter 2. Equitable services can be provided from comprehensive PHC systems that also accommodate selective care based on prioritised needs (Birn 2009; DeVos et al 2009). Yet the logic of this type of policy environment has yet to be acknowledged by those competing for limited resources. Marginalised communities remain unable to control key processes that control their lives and their health or to select what they need. They are subjected to inadequate services, and difficult living conditions that prevent them from being able to challenge power brokers, or work towards building local capacity (DeVos et al 2009; WHO 2008).

When people live in disadvantaged situations, their predominant focus is on day-to-day survival, which not only causes substandard health, but erodes social capital. Without political leadership

that is committed to addressing the inequities of disadvantage, this situation will remain unchanged. The policy 'problem' is that, rather than try to mitigate the consequences of powerless groups, policy-makers tend to shy away from redefining labour relations or unemployment arrangements, or imposing regulations on environmental pollution, or taxes on alcohol that affect the poor disproportionately (WHO 2008). Instead, spurred on by economic goals, social and health policies have continued to concentrate wealth in the hands of the powerful, which has left the poor and voiceless with a disproportionate amount of health-damaging experiences (Commission on the Social Determinants of Health [CSDH] 2008).

Clearly, change is necessary, but it does not occur spontaneously. What is needed is an overt process of inviting community input, then an ongoing level of support. This would produce a combination of perspectives from the public, health professionals, health planners, and intersectoral policy-makers to encourage multilevel, multidimensional approaches for better health. The key to success in accommodating such a breadth of opinions is authentic communication between all participants (Hawe 2009). But first, those in charge of health care have to extend the invitations. Then practitioners need to advocate for communities, engaging with people to gain their support and input.

Point to ponder

In order to achieve health equity based on the principles of primary health care, health policy-makers must initiate and maintain authentic communication with community members.

Globally, changing policies, and changing health care systems to be more equitable, is based on the notion that redistributive justice is not only humanitarian, but an investment in the health of each country's population (Smith & MacKellar 2007). This situates health as a public good, not a commodity (Baum 2009; Labonte 2008). In each country, inclusive policies for better health must be aimed at improving daily living conditions. They should tackle the inequitable distribution of power, money and other resources, and then they should measure and understand local problems in the context of global issues (CSDH 2008; WHO

2008). From this foundation, policy-makers can then assess the impact of action and inaction on community health in terms of the principles of PHC: accessible health care, appropriate technology, health promotion and health education, cultural sensitivity and cultural safety, intersectoral collaboration, and community participation.

POLICY ACTION AT THE NATIONAL LEVEL: THINK GLOBAL, ACT LOCAL

As health professionals, we can be conscious and concerned about global issues and the failure of the global community to create equity. But this can also add to the 'change fatigue' that plagues many of us who are concerned about communities throughout the world. What we can do, is act on a local level to encourage community participation in the policy arena, and ensure that our knowledge and skills are used to the community's advantage. As nurses and midwives, our participation in all policy areas is invaluable. In Australia, the National Review of Maternity Services mentioned in Chapter 6 (Commonwealth of Australia 2009a) is a good example of a national policy development that has relied heavily on input from nurses and midwives. The Australian Research Alliance for Children & Youth Declaration and Call to Action (see Appendix F) has had significant input from many nurses and midwives throughout the country (Australian Research Alliance for Children and Youth [ARACY] 2009). The Te Rito Family Violence Intervention Strategy in New Zealand relied heavily on input from nurses and other health professionals prior to, and during development. Wide consultation was also undertaken with Maori and Pacific Island people to ensure development of the policy was culturally safe.

Policies governing adult health such as the anti-tobacco strategies, national chronic disease strategies, falls prevention, healthy ageing, rural health, social inclusion and mental health have also been developed with input from nurses in Australia and New Zealand (Australian Nursing Federation [ANF] 2009; Francis et al 2008). Although each of these policy initiatives has invited comment from members of the public, in some cases, a lack of health literacy has prevented people from responding. Some people may be reluctant to participate in technical policy discussions, or they may have felt that their views have not been considered in the past, or that an invitation is simply tokenism

(Bruni et al 2008). This suggests an important role for nurses and midwives in helping community members become aware of the issues involved, and assisting them in putting forward their views.

A number of national policy areas currently under review would be incomplete without the perspectives of the nursing and midwifery professions. These include: the proposed Australian Women's Health Policy and the Male Health Policy; Indigenous Health Policy; the Intergenerational Strategy to address workplace and investment strategies for younger and older workers; Education policies; Healthy Ageing Policy; the National Drug Strategy; Quality Use of Medicines; and the National Mental Health Strategy. Each of these offers important opportunities to participate in policy development, which is integral to the role of nurses and midwives as part of our social contract with society to promote health and social justice (Fawcett & Russell 2001). Equally as important is the need for nurses and midwives to ensure that policies are framed within a caring discourse, especially those that have been developed with an emphasis on economics and the market.

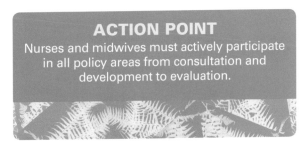

ACTION POINT
Nurses and midwives must actively participate in all policy areas from consultation and development to evaluation.

THE NEED FOR POLICY INTEGRATION: LESSONS FROM MENTAL HEALTH

Mental health is among the most significant policy areas for all countries of the world. In most countries, the incidence of mental illness has steadily increased over the past 30 years, while government funding has continued to decline (WHO 2008; 2010). In 2008, the WHO launched a global action program, the 'Mental Health Gap Action Program' (mhGAP) to forge strategic partnerships that would enhance countries' efforts to combat stigma, reduce the burden of mental disorders, and promote mental health (WHO 2010). The mhGAP program and other WHO initiatives are based on the notion that 'there is no health without mental health' (WHO 2010).

The policy change that has had the most powerful effect on mental health is that of deinstitutionalisation, wherein from the 1970s, mentally ill patients were shifted from psychiatric hospitals to be treated in their communities. Since this change occurred, the onus has been placed on families and community support systems to care for those with mental illness. However, without the provision of sufficient support services, many families caring for their loved ones have experienced enormous difficulties in the burden of care. In Australia and New Zealand, mental health support services are provided by a range of agencies, with heavy reliance on community mental health nurses or psychiatric nurses working as part of a team (see Chapter 4). This system is intended to provide families with specialist services and emergency responses when there are mental health crises, but major shortages of mental health specialists have meant that these services are unreliable, especially in rural areas. Even those without the need for crisis care suffer from a lack of guidance and support services in the community.

Point to ponder

Mental health is one of the most significant health policy areas. There is a growing need for new emphasis on mental health prevention strategies to guide health professionals to work effectively with those experiencing mental health issues.

Another important aspect of mental health policy is the need for guidance on preventative strategies. The mental health policy environment has thus far been directed towards mental illness, but the need for health promotion policies that respond to the SDOH is acute. Raphael (2009) explains that, compared with other kinds of health promotion, there is less infiltration of mental health promotion into government and public health-related documents. Although his comments refer to the Canadian situation, it is similar to the policy environments of Australia and New Zealand. The omission of mental health in the SDOH discourse is important, as mental health is seen as a mediating force between the SDOH and physical health. This primarily involves mental states associated with exposure to adverse living conditions and psychosocial stress, which can cause maladaptive

biological responses, weaken immune systems, and create a greater likelihood of metabolic disorders (Raphael 2009). Responses to inequalities, such as feelings of shame, worthlessness, and envy, also have psycho–biological effects on health, precipitating coping behaviours such as over-spending, over-eating, use of alcohol and tobacco, or a range of other social behaviours that threaten health (Raphael 2009).

Good mental health policies should guide appropriate service provision for those needing help, but they should also work toward decreasing vulnerability by helping people develop coping skills. In response to the SDOH, such policies attempt to reduce people's exposure to negative conditions; for example, by providing educational and recreational opportunities as community entitlements. Mental health policies should also provide employment and job security, social assistance for those in need, and balance universal and identified needs, again, through comprehensive and selective PHC (Raphael 2009). This illustrates the integrated nature of mental health and other policies.

Social policies and family life

Many policies have a cascade effect that can permeate family and community life; for example, policies governing child care. For parents who are both in the workplace, child care is a major source of stress. Family leave policies that provide income replacement and incentives for parents to take leave can help alleviate the stress of parenting. Although New Zealand has provision for 14 weeks of paid parental leave, Australia, like the United States, does not have a paid leave policy for parents (Brennan 2007). Instead, current policies see the male partner spending longer hours at work to cover family expenses when a mother chooses to stay at home. This leaves the child deprived of the father's time, and the mother having to be the constant parent. For some women, the lack of respite can undermine their mental health, adding to the vulnerability of new parenthood. For both parents, economic hardship also compromises their mental health, and sometimes has an effect on physical health. In combination, these factors can also be a

Point to ponder

It is vital to maintain a 'big picture', intergenerational, ecological perspective in policy-making.

difficult challenge for the relationship, especially when parents are also physically tired from caring for the child and/or other children.

The policy on paid leave for child care is only one example of how important it is to maintain a big picture, intergenerational, ecological perspective in policy-making. Another example lies in the inter-relatedness of government policies to encourage child bearing, fair employment, productivity, retirement and superannuation. In 2010, Australian policy-makers realised that, after a decade of policy-driven cash incentives for young Australian couples to boost the fertility rate, there is a virtual baby boom occurring throughout the country. It was expected that providing cash grants to young couples to have a child would result in a modest change to the fertility rate. The idea was that by increasing the fertility rate, the children would become active in the workplace just when their tax contributions were most needed; that is, when they could support the growing number of retirees, who would be withdrawing their superannuation investments.

In Australia, the intergenerational view of family leave policies was seen as appropriate to solve the dual problems of declining infertility and population ageing, while maintaining productivity. However, so many couples have taken advantage of the scheme, that there is a drain on government funds (to pay the child bonus). One option being considered by the government to rebalance the situation, is a policy to encourage older people not to retire, but to undertake part-time employment, so they can continue to contribute to the government superannuation scheme, rather than drain existing resources. Retirees are naturally concerned, and plan on watching the policy debate closely. Others are concerned at moves towards increasing the population, and therefore productivity, either through further incentives to lift the fertility rate, or by increasing the number of migrants. On the other side of these arguments, is the need for sustainability of the environment and its infrastructure. This is a classic policy debate illustrating the fact that everything is indeed, connected to everything else.

What's your opinion?
Will increasing the fertility rate now have the intended consequences? What are some of the advantages and disadvantages of this policy?

BOX 13.1 AUSTRALIAN AND NEW ZEALAND MENTAL HEALTH POLICY

Australian mental health policy

Australia's Mental Health Strategy has undergone numerous transformations from its inception in the 1970s. At that time, government authorities had assumed responsibility for those with mental illness, but with deinstitutionalisation, this responsibility was devolved to families (Henderson 2005). The expectation of deinstitutionalisation was, that by integrating those with mental illness into the community, they would receive more humane, individualised and culturally appropriate care. This was seen to be more empowering, and equated mental ill health with physical ill health in terms of treatment options. However, the lack of a national approach to mental health care and prevention inspired a second Mental Health Strategy in 1992 (Department of Health and Ageing [DoHA] 2010a). This was aimed at strengthening mental health reform, and developing a national approach that would include input by the states and territories to prioritise mental health issues. Importantly, a centrepiece of the strategy was to establish advisory committees throughout the country, to foster community input on mental health.

The goals of the Mental Health Strategy were admirable, but one of the problems was that it was written in the language of the market, and, typical of the 1980s thinking on health, polarised people as 'consumers' or 'providers' of health care. This type of language illustrated how commodified health had become, with policy-makers valuing the input of market forces and competition for services. Like many other commodities, services became fragmented, and dominated by medical specialists. The policy also created a moral imperative for families to care for the mentally ill in this context, which undermined their autonomy in planning care (Henderson 2005).

Despite its shortcomings, the emphasis of the 1992 strategy on cooperation between different government levels has been widely accepted. The newer policy has aimed to increase health literacy, including the development of programs to promote mental health in schools. It is also intended to address the stigma of mental health, by reversing negative media images and reports of those with mental illness, developing community advocacy for those with mental illness, supporting global initiatives such as World Mental Health Day, and enhancing relationships between mental health professionals, carers, and those with mental health needs (DoHA 2010a). It is an imperfect system, but working towards a slightly more preventative orientation than in the past.

Point to ponder
Australian mental health policy is slowly moving towards a preventative orientation.

New Zealand mental health policy

New Zealand's history of mental health policy is not dissimilar to that of Australia. Deinstitutionalisation, responsibility for care placed on family members, and commodification of health care with business models and language, have all been similar features. In 1994, the first New Zealand Mental Health Strategy was released. This was followed in 1998, by publication of the *Blueprint for Mental Health Services in New Zealand* (Mental Health Commission 1998). The Blueprint described the mental health service developments required for implementation of the 1994 Mental Health Strategy, setting the scene for incorporation of mental health as a priority area in health policy. Mental health as a priority health area for the government was subsequently reflected in the New Zealand Health Strategy (Minister of Health 2000), New Zealand Disability Strategy (MOHNZ 2001b) and the New Zealand Primary Health Care Strategy (King 2001). Although a number of areas for development outlined in the Mental Health Strategy and subsequent blueprint are still to be implemented, progress has been made in many areas — in particular, a focus on models of recovery has been a defining feature of current New Zealand mental health services.

In 2005, *Te Tahuhu — Improving Mental Health 2005–2015: The Second New Zealand Mental Health and Addiction Plan* (Minister of Health 2005) was published. This was followed in 2006, by *Te Kōkiri: The Mental Health and Addiction Action Plan 2006–2015* (Minister of Health 2006). Building on many of the achievements in mental health since publication of the first Mental Health Strategy and the Blueprint, the new plan set goals that have extended the previous policy focus from care for those most seriously affected by mental illness, to promoting the mental health of all New Zealanders. Of particular importance has been a specific focus on PHC. There are three areas of immediate emphasis in the plan. The first focuses on building workforce capability in the PHC sector to assess the mental health and addiction needs of people in the community, and treat them as appropriate. The second is on building and strengthening linkages between primary and secondary services, and the third focuses on strengthening the role of primary health care organisations in promoting mental health and wellbeing and preventing mental ill health.

Point to ponder
Mental health policy in New Zealand now focuses on promoting the mental health of all New Zealanders, not just those experiencing severe illness.

The broadening of focus from identifying and treating more serious mental ill health to promoting mental wellbeing in PHC is intended to promote social equity. Care, and access to care, has already been improved for those experiencing lifestyle-related stress and anxiety (Dowell et al 2009). It is also expected to improve access to appropriate care for those who currently experience more severe mental illness, but who also experience co-morbidities such as cardiovascular disease and diabetes (Minister of Health 2005). The onus is now on health professionals to work closely with their communities to ensure that primary mental health care is provided in an appropriate, accessible, affordable and culturally safe manner.

THE NEW ZEALAND HEALTH CARE SYSTEM

Health and disability services in New Zealand are delivered by a complex network of people and organisations. Overall responsibility for the delivery of health services lies with the Minister of Health, who is elected through the democratic process to government, and appointed to the role of Minister. The Minister of Health, in conjunction with the Ministry of Health, provides overall leadership and direction for the numerous providers of health care in New Zealand. The New Zealand Health Strategy (Minister of Health 2000) provided the direction for the current system of health care in New Zealand. The strategy identified seven fundamental principles that were to be reflected across the health sector. These were:

1 Acknowledgement of the special relationship that exists between the Crown and Maori under the Treaty of Waitangi

2 Good health and wellbeing for all New Zealanders throughout their lives

3 An improvement in health status of those currently disadvantaged

4 Collaborative health promotion and disease and injury prevention by all sectors

5 Timely and equitable access for all New Zealanders to a comprehensive range of health and disability services, regardless of ability to pay

6 A high-performing system in which people have confidence

7 Active involvement of consumers and communities at all levels.

(Minister of Health 2000)

For the first time, the New Zealand Health Strategy signalled the importance of health inequalities, the SDOH, and active participation by communities as key contributors to the health of the New Zealand population. The Strategy provided a framework and context for District Health Boards (DHBs) as the majority providers of public health services to develop services for their identified populations.

There are currently 21 DHBs in New Zealand. DHBs plan, manage, provide and purchase services for the population of their district. This includes funding for public health services, aged care, and services provided by other non-government health providers including Maori and Pacific Island providers (Online. Available: www.moh.govt.nz/moh .nsf/indexmh/healthsystem-overview [accessed 10 February 2010]). DHBs employ a range of health professionals to provide services including medical doctors, nurses and allied health staff, such as physiotherapists and occupational therapists. However, long waiting lists to receive care from public health services has seen the development of a robust private health care sector in New Zealand, particularly for the provision of surgical care. Many individual New Zealanders who can afford it, choose to purchase their own health insurance policies, in order to ensure they have access to surgical care quickly if they need it. However, for those people who cannot afford health insurance, poor access to surgical care can mean prolonged suffering and disability that is easily preventable. Many medical specialists work in both private and public health systems, potentially increasing the risk of long public health waiting lists and the inequities this creates. DHBs also have responsibility for funding PHC, and this is done primarily through primary health organisations (PHOs).

Point to ponder
District Health Boards (DHBs) have responsibility for planning, managing, providing and purchasing health services for New Zealanders.

The Primary Health Care Strategy (King 2001) provided a framework for the development of PHC services in New Zealand. Primary health organisations were mooted as the vehicles through which services would be funded and provided. As of January 2010 there were 81 PHOs throughout New Zealand, funded by DHBs to provide PHC services to an enrolled population. PHOs vary in size and structure, are not-for-profit, and either provide services directly by employing staff or through provider members. Most general practices are members of PHOs and provide the bulk of PHC services in New Zealand (Online. Available: www.moh.govt.nz/moh.nsf/indexmh/phcs-pho [accessed 10 February 2010]).

General practices charge a fee-for-service on top of the funding they receive through the PHO. Most general practices are run as businesses by the general practitioner, who then employs staff, such as nurses, within the business. This business model creates difficulties for practice nurses seeking to extend their practice, due to power imbalances inherent in employee and employer relationships, and traditional models of practice. It was hoped that population-based funding and the advent of PHOs would go some way towards addressing this issue, but to date there has been little progress. With the business model being the predominant model of care in PHC settings, nurses have been

Point to ponder
Primary health organisations (PHOs) are funded by DHBs to provide primary health care services to New Zealanders.

unable to develop more effective models of care for patients.

A unique feature of the New Zealand health system is the Accident Compensation Corporation (ACC). The ACC was established in 1974 and is in effect an insurance scheme that provides personal injury cover for all New Zealanders and some visitors. The ACC is funded through a mixture of levies from people's earnings, businesses, petrol and vehicle licensing fees, and government funding. This means that if a person has an accident in New Zealand, the majority of costs associated with this will be covered by the ACC at no cost to the person. In return for this injury cover, an individual is unable to sue another person or company for personal injury except for exemplary damages (Online. Available: www.acc.co.nz/about-acc/overview-of-acc/introduction-to-acc/index.htm [accessed 10 February 2010]). There are inequities associated with ACC funding. For example, if an accident results in a person becoming permanently disabled, the ACC will fund all the care and equipment that person requires on an ongoing basis. On the other hand, if a person is permanently disabled due to a congenital abnormality or a medical condition, all costs associated with the disability are borne by the individual with limited financial support.

Paramedic care is provided largely by the St John Ambulance Service. Exceptions include the Wellington Free Ambulance Service covering the greater Wellington area, and air ambulance and rescue helicopter services, which are provided privately through a mix of government funding and corporate sponsorship. The St John Ambulance Service has a significant volunteer base with volunteers providing the majority of paramedic services in rural areas. This has both advantages and disadvantages. Volunteerism is known to increase social capital in a community, however increasing demands on volunteer ambulance officers and limited funding to employ full-time officers is increasing health risks for rural populations.

Point to ponder
Lead Maternity Carers (LMCs) are funded to provide maternity care in New Zealand. Most LMCs are midwives.

As we mentioned in Chapter 4, primary maternity care in New Zealand is provided by Lead Maternity Carers (LMCs). A woman selects an LMC to provide her maternity care throughout the duration of the pregnancy, birth and first weeks following birth. An LMC may be a general practitioner with a Diploma in Obstetrics, an obstetrician or a midwife. Midwifery as a profession in New Zealand has its own distinct body of knowledge, scope of practice, standards of practice and code of ethics. The *Nurses Amendment Act 1990* enabled a registered midwife to undertake full responsibility for the care of women throughout their pregnancy. It also made provision for direct-entry midwifery education. Where previously, nurses would complete a year-long post-graduate education program to become a midwife, now midwifery qualifications are only offered through a three-year Bachelor of Midwifery program.

Health Professionals in New Zealand are regulated by the *Health Practitioners Competency Assurance Act (HPCAA) 2003*. The HPCAA is designed to protect public safety, by providing mechanisms to ensure the lifelong competency of health practitioners. A number of titles are protected under the HPCAA, and only health practitioners who are registered under the Act are entitled to use such titles. Professions regulated include nursing, midwifery, medicine, pharmacy, physiotherapy, and a range of other allied health professions. The HPCAA separates health practitioner registration activities from competence and disciplinary processes. Registration activities are undertaken by the respective health profession's council or board. For example, the Nursing Council of New Zealand is the statutory body that governs the practice of nurses, monitors and sets standards for practice, and maintains the register of nurses. The Health Practitioner Disciplinary Tribunal, however, is responsible for hearing and determining disciplinary proceedings brought against registered nurses under the HPCAA.

Point to ponder
The *Health Practitioner Competency Assurance Act* governs the competency of health professionals to practise in New Zealand.

Despite a number of inequities in the system, at present all New Zealanders have access to universal health care. New Zealand spends approximately $12 billion dollars on health every year, representing approximately 7% of GDP (New Zealand Treasury 2009). Current thinking suggests that this expenditure is unsustainable, and that consolidation of spending and new models of health care provision need to be considered. The election of a National conservative government in 2008 has seen a dramatic shift in thinking around health expenditure, as well as a reconsideration of the priorities around PHC and social equity. Although the New Zealand Health Strategy and Primary Health Care Strategy have not been superseded, there has been a clear refocusing on efficiencies in provision of care and more emphasis on acute care. The 'Better, Sooner, More Convenient Primary Health Care' document (Ryall 2009) calls for the development of a 'single system personalised care' approach to PHC along with the development of Integrated Family Health Centres — clinics that provide a full range of medical, nursing and allied health services including minor surgery, chronic care and walk-in access. Many of the current government goals for PHC revolve around devolution of secondary services to PHC as a means to achieve cost savings. However, there is still significant work to be done in terms of up-skilling the PHC workforce to take on devolving services.

Also in 2009, a Ministerial Review Group led by Murray Horn was established to consider the challenges faced by the New Zealand health care sector, and to develop recommendations to help meet these challenges (Ministerial Review Group 2009). Recommendations in the 'Horn Report' are structured around nine key themes:

1 new models of care which see the patient rather than the institution at the centre of service delivery

2 stronger clinical and management partnerships

3 a sharper focus on patient safety and quality of care

4 identifying the services people need

5 putting the right services in the right place

6 ensuring the right capacity is in place

7 building a sustainable workforce

8 shifting resources to the front-line, and

9 improving hospital productivity.

(Ministerial Review Group 2009)

The New Zealand government has already begun enacting a number of strategies designed to meet the recommendations of the 'Horn Report', and for the most part, these are focused specifically on the need for fiscal restraint. For example, a National Health Board was established in early 2010 to

Point to ponder
The 'Horn Report' provides a new direction for New Zealand health care focusing on sustainability.

provide a better national focus on health spending, and PHOs with a population of less than 40 000 are no longer funded, and will be required to merge with larger PHOs. The goal is to cut the number of PHOs from 81 to 40. The risk of focusing on fiscal savings, however, is that those most disadvantaged are likely to continue to miss out on vital health care. It will be imperative that health professionals advocate for a continued focus on social equity, the impact of the SDOH, and community participation in future policy — aspects that are noticeably missing from the 'Horn Report'. At real risk is the progress the New Zealand Ministry of Health had made in recognising the importance of PHC as a means of improving the health of populations. Previous health policy documents have focused closely on improving outcomes for some of the most disadvantaged groups in New Zealand, and have provided direction for health professionals as they seek to address some of the glaring inequities in health. In particular, He Korowai Oranga: Maori Health Strategy (MOHNZ 2001a), and the Pacific Health and Disability Action Plan (MOHNZ 2002) both provide strategic direction and actions to improve health outcomes for Maori and Pacific people in New Zealand (see Box 13.2). Maori health has been covered in detail in previous chapters, but we reiterate that significant disparities exist in the health of Pacific people in New Zealand compared with non-Pacific people, despite the fact that New Zealand has demonstrated its commitment to Pacific health in a number of ways. It can only be hoped that the progress thus far achieved will continue.

THE AUSTRALIAN HEALTH CARE SYSTEM

The system of health care in Australia is built on the principle of universal care for all citizens paid for by their taxes. This is funded through Medicare, the national insurance scheme that provides each member of society with the ability to attend any one of a number of services at no cost, or, where the service provider charges an extra fee, at an affordable cost. Most Australians use the services of medical practitioners, who charge a

BOX 13.2 NEW ZEALAND'S COMMITMENT TO PACIFIC HEALTH

Pacific people in New Zealand experience poorer health outcomes than other New Zealanders across a range of health and disability indicators. Life expectancy for Pacific people is lower than all other groups except Maori, and Pacific people have higher rates of morbidity and mortality in a range of chronic diseases. For example, Pacific men and women have three times the prevalence of diagnosed diabetes than other New Zealanders (MOHNZ 2008a). Pacific children also experience poorer health outcomes than non-Pacific children and are more likely to live in areas of higher neighbourhood deprivation (MOHNZ 2009), placing them at even greater risk of poor health outcomes than their non-Pacific counterparts.

New Zealand has made a significant commitment to addressing the inequities experienced by Pacific people, working closely with the Pacific community to develop a range of policies designed to improve health. The Pacific Health and Disability Action Plan (MOHNZ 2002) provided the initial framework and strategic direction for improving Pacific people's health and participation, and reducing inequalities. This was followed up in 2004 by release of the Pacific Health and Disability Workforce Development Plan (MOHNZ 2004) that provided a framework for health and education organisations to positively influence pathways for participation by Pacific people in the health workforce.

Significant work has been done more recently into Pacific people and disability (MOHNZ 2008b), mental health (MOHNZ 2008c), youth health (MOHNZ 2008d), and Pacific children's health (MOHNZ 2009). These more recent documents are part of the Pacific Health and Disability Plan Review series, providing the most up-to-date data on the health of Pacific people and their experiences with health services. Wide consultation with Pacific communities has been a feature of all policy development activities, ensuring social equity and participation goals remain at the forefront of policy development.

their family, for a wider range of services than are paid for by Medicare, including dental health care, massage, optometry and other services. Nurse practitioners also charge a fee-for-service, but only for a small number of tightly controlled services, under the supervision of a medical practitioner.

Point to ponder
Medicare is Australia's national insurance scheme that provides all Australians with the ability to attend many health care services at no cost or at an affordable cost.

The Commonwealth Department of Health and Ageing (DoHA) has the overall responsibility for quality and safety in health care, working through a number of statutory agencies and Commissions, such as the Australian Safety and Quality Commission. The Department oversees the National Aged and Community Care Program, which includes care and support for those with a disability; the National Mental Health Program, Aboriginal and Torres Strait Islander Health, primary and ambulatory care, and health protection. Health protection includes public health surveillance, emergency preparedness and responses, food policy, chronic and communicable disease control, health promotion, and harm reduction related to substance abuse (Francis et al 2008). The DoHA also governs the Medical Benefits Scheme and the Pharmaceutical Benefits Scheme, which subsidise reimbursements to people for medical services, and medications, respectively, and the Therapeutic Goods Administration, which monitors and regulates medicines, blood and tissue (Francis et al 2008).

State and territory governments are responsible for hospital and community care, including private hospitals, even though the funding for these services is provided jointly, through cooperative arrangements between Commonwealth, state and territory governments. In some state- and territory-based health and hospital services, restructuring is a regular occurrence. Various administrative bodies take responsibility for individual hospitals, or district level services. In most cases, a health service district will include both general and specialist hospitals, some specialising in certain populations (women and children) and others specialising in certain types of treatment (cancer care,

fee-for-services provided, and then are subsidised through the Medicare system to a standard rate. Most medical specialists, and a large number of general practitioners charge their patients a fee above the subsidised rate. Many people also have private health insurance, which covers them, and various surgical specialties). Certain hospitals are designated as state or territory trauma centres, able to accommodate a wide range of emergencies, while others have the capacity for only minor emergency treatments, and are usually bypassed in emergencies of any substance. In addition to hospital services, patients in most health service districts have access to specialised drug and alcohol treatment services, territory- and state-based ambulance services, aged care, mental health hostels, the Australian Red Cross Blood service and the Royal Flying Doctor Service, which provides air transportation for health professionals to attend to people in remote areas.

Point to ponder
In 2010 a national regulatory body and National Registration and Accreditation Scheme was established to oversee accreditation, regulation and monitoring of all health professionals in Australia.

Until recently, state and territory governments had responsibility for the regulation of health professionals, but in 2010 this changed to a national regulatory body, and a National Registration and Accreditation Scheme, which has oversight for accreditation, regulation, and monitoring of all health professionals. Although many health professions continue to have their own accrediting body, such as the Australian Nursing and Midwifery Council, they will be expected to meet the governance standards of the national system. Professions included in the scheme include chiropractors, dental practitioners, medical practitioners, nurses and midwives, optometrists, osteopaths, pharmacists, physiotherapists, podiatrists and psychologists. In 2011, Aboriginal and Torres Strait Islander health practitioners, Chinese medicine practitioners and medical radiation practitioners will also be regulated under the scheme (DoHA 2010c).

In the Australian system, most medical practitioners are self-employed general practitioners (GPs) or consultants, who practise on a contractual basis in public, and sometimes, private hospitals. Allied health professionals and paramedics are typically employed by hospitals or health districts, and some can charge a fee-for-service, including acupuncturists, podiatrists and naturopaths (Francis

et al 2008). Nurses and midwives can be employed in hospitals or health agencies, with many being appointed to government agencies either at the state, territory, regional or local level. As we mentioned in Chapter 4, some nurse practitioners have established public clinics, and there are also midwives who work privately to provide home birthing services, or other consultations. However, with the hospital and health system undergoing major reforms, their legal position is unclear, particularly in relation to the need for malpractice insurance. Initial policy discussions at the Commonwealth level led to a recommendation that midwives have subsidised insurance, but that was quickly followed by a retraction, because of opposition by the Australian Medical Association. It is an issue yet to be decided in the context of ongoing reform.

Point to ponder
The Commonwealth Government of Australia is responsible for establishing national health priorities for the people of Australia.

The Commonwealth government establishes national health priorities for the people of Australia, and these are based on data provided by the Australian Institute of Health and Welfare (AIHW). Although priorities can change according to a particular political agenda, the priorities for population health are generally non-partisan, and based on strong research evidence. Priorities for the public's health have been relatively stable throughout the past decade, and include cancer control, injury prevention and control, cardiovascular health, diabetes mellitus, mental health, asthma, and arthritis and musculoskeletal conditions (DoHA 2010b).

Health sector reform in Australia

In 2009 the Commonwealth government embarked on a program of dramatic reform for the health system. The strength of their approach was the widespread consultation with stakeholders throughout the country. The weaknesses included the fact that various aspects of the health system were discussed separately, with three separate reviews that included health and hospitals, PHC, and preventative health strategies. Despite these difficulties, and the complexities of consulting across so many different health authorities and geographic areas, some common issues emerged from all discussions. One of the most significant of these was the view that separate state, territory and Commonwealth health services have provided a complex and fragmented system of funding responsibilities and performance accountabilities, under growing pressure to respond to diverse and changing health needs (Commonwealth of Australia 2009b).

The challenges of the Australian health care system have also been recognised in comparison with the health systems of other countries. International comparisons measure health systems in terms of quality care, efficiency, equity, healthy lives and health expenditure per capita. Quality care and efficiency have been found to be relatively high, less than that of the Canadian or American systems, but considerably higher than New Zealand. Health expenditure per capita is on a par with most other OECD countries, at around 9% of GDP.

However, the area of poorest performance in the Australian health system is in healthy lives, which is one-third of the score for Canada, one-sixth of the score for the US, and less than one-quarter of that of the New Zealand system (Commonwealth of Australia 2009b). The National Health and Hospitals Reform Commission (NHHRC) report (Commonwealth of Australia 2009b:51) declared the system 'out of balance', with a focus on illness, at the expense of wellness. This includes a failure to consider the workplace as an opportunity for health promotion, which is one of the recommendations of the United Nations (UN 2010) and international researchers (Bambra et al 2008). Other failures include favouring 'providers' rather than patients, especially those who could be better served by a range of health professionals, if the system allowed them access to the Pharmaceutical Benefits Scheme (PBS) and Medical Benefits Scheme (MBS). The review also found a disjunction between service provision, teaching and research, and a number of population groups

Point to ponder
Fragmentation of state, territory and Commonwealth health services has seen the development of a complex and unresponsive health sector in Australia.

who are not well served by acute or community care systems. As in other countries, there are also safety and quality issues, and workforce shortages (Commonwealth of Australia 2009b).

Recommendations for change

The NHHRC (Commonwealth of Australia 2009b) strongly recommended three immediate and crucial responses:

1 tackling major access and equity issues that affect health outcomes
2 redesigning the health system to better respond to emerging challenges
3 creating an agile and self-improving health system for long-term sustainability.

The major access and equity issues revolve around improving outcomes for Indigenous people, those with serious mental illness, people living in rural and remote areas, those without access to dental care, or timely care in public hospitals. Emerging challenges include embedding prevention and early intervention for a healthy start to life, and the need to create youth friendly community-based services, to promote adolescent mental health. These would be expedited through establishing a National Health Promotion and Prevention Agency.

Point to ponder
Strengthening Australian PHC services is a key recommendation of the National Health and Hospitals Reform Committee (NHHRC) report in 2009.

In addition to services for young people, a redesigned health system would see better integration of health and aged care services, so that many older persons presenting to hospitals for acute or sub-acute care, could be treated in their home or community through programs such as Hospital in the Home (HITH), or designated palliative care services. Of course, these changes would have to be structured so that family caregivers and community-based health professionals would have extra support and infrastructure to meet their needs. The NHHRC also recommended reshaping hospitals to separate elective and emergency care, with outpatient services organised around the needs of patients and their communities. One of the most important recommendations of the NHHRC is for strengthened PHC services. This would involve integration of PHC services so that they would be multidisciplinary, and provided in comprehensive centres and PHC organisations, which would rely on input from the community and make better use of community specialists.

Creating an agile and self-improving system would be achieved with a stronger voice from the community, and would focus on building health literacy, fostering community participation, and empowering people to make fully informed health care decisions. In addition, the new system would foster clinical leadership and governance, new frameworks for education, and training for health professionals, governed by the National Clinical Education and Training Agency. The expected outcome would be a modern learning and supported health workforce. Other recommendations include the smart use of data, information and communication, well designed funding and strategic purchasing models, and knowledge-led, continuous improvement, innovation and research. The reforms shift arrangements to a single health system, markedly changing existing funding arrangements, which is possibly the most contentious issue for debate in 2010 (Commonwealth of Australia 2009b).

Point to ponder

NHHRC recommendations should see the development of a more equitable and effective approach to the provision of health care in Australia.

If the recommendations were adopted, the changes would move the Australian system of health care from one skewed towards managing sickness, and an emphasis on the providers, to a wellness orientation, and a focus on patients and communities, especially vulnerable groups. At the same time, there would be support for new technologies to tailor treatments to individual needs rather than a one-size-fits-all model of care. These new developments would include rational drug design, pharmacogenomics, imaging and diagnostic advances, telemedicine, robotics and virtual surgery, gene therapies, new vaccines, bioengineering for joint or tissue replacement, stem cell therapies, and nanotechnologies for accurate

delivery of medication dosages (Commonwealth of Australia 2009b).

These recommendations, like those of the discussion document 'Towards a National Primary Health Care Strategy' (Commonwealth of Australia 2008), acknowledge the problems in the current health system. Both have elicited numerous responses from around the country that converge on the need for a system of PHC, for equity, client-centredness, simplified systems of community-based care, and more resources for health promotion and illness prevention. These issues were even further reinforced by the responses to the National Prevention Strategy document, which was also circulated in 2009. In 2010 the Commonwealth government will deliberate on these recommendations, with a view towards examining the feasibility of such wide-sweeping changes. The main objective will be to work towards continuous improvement and a fair, accessible, democratic health system. It will require greater vertical and horizontal integration, where primary care providers (mainly GPs) change from operating relatively independently of the rest of the health system, to becoming more collaborative (Wakerman 2009). These recommendations resonate with international trends, which include a move away from the fee-for-service model which relies on referral to specialists, to one that brings primary care closer to other services, and encourages interdisciplinary collaboration and community participation (Wakerman 2009; WHO 2004). The PHC model has been found to produce better population outcomes, at lower cost with greater user satisfaction (WHO 2004).

HEALTH CARE: BUILDING A BETTER SYSTEM

Three decades ago, few health care planners were concerned with the SDOH. Yet, gradually, as more evidence came to light, policy-makers throughout the world came to realise that good health evolves from equity, and the social aspects of people's lives, supported by an accessible health care system. Resources and good management practices play an important role, but there are other critical elements of a health system that contribute to the health of any given population. These are listed as health system features in Box 13.3.

- Health care systems should be fair, not focused on privileging hospital care in its funding at the expense of prevention or community care.
- Universal care, along with universal systems of health insurance can help reduce the disadvantage experienced by those already disadvantaged by socio-economic status and health status.
- A health system should provide appropriate, adequate and culturally acceptable care for the most vulnerable.
- The majority of health care needs are in chronic disease and disability management and these must be met with continuity of care between acute and home and community settings.
- Service decisions should be made in partnership with the end users of the system.
- Efficiencies in the system should carefully balance technological and biomedical care as well as community care.
- Health information systems are integral to efficient and effective services.
- Effective systems are client-oriented, so they deal with waiting lists and the patient journey through hospital to home and community from a client, rather than a service provider, perspective.
- A self-regulating system monitors and addresses threats to patient quality and safety.
- Adequate service provision relies on sufficient health professionals, educated appropriately for their scope of practice.
- A robust health care system is based on research evidence as a basis for good and best practice.
- A health care system should include best practice in health promotion, including capacity building based on health literacy.

BEST PRACTICE IN HEALTH CARE SYSTEMS

The Scandinavian countries are often held up as exemplars of best practice in health care systems. Although each country's political and economic context differs, each of their health care systems continue to work towards equity, and equalising the social gradient. There is much to be learned from the way Sweden, Norway, Denmark and Finland have adopted systemic approaches to meet these goals, by prioritising social policies for their citizens, and by regulating the private sector (Birn 2009). Private sector involvement can be an advantage in helping a health system benchmark services for greater efficiency, effectiveness and consistency. However, privately owned health services can also be exclusive because of their focus on profit-taking, which prevents access to health care for those who cannot afford it (Baum et al 2009; Bayoumi 2009). They often have the financial resources to attract the best health professionals, which can further drain the public system.

Point to ponder

Scandinavian health care systems are considered some of the best in the world, particularly in their approach towards equity and equalising the social gradient in society.

The Scandinavian health systems monitor private providers, and establish goals on the basis of the SDOH: gender, class, sexual orientation, socio-economic status, ethnicity, disability, education, parenting, employment, health care and the environments for health (Raphael & Bryant 2006). They also have very high reports of patient satisfaction with care, and higher life expectancy than in many other countries (Bambra et al 2007; WHO 2004). The Nordic systems, designed to be socially democratic, are well positioned for capacity building, improving health through a 'nuanced balance of leadership', and by facilitating intersectoral collaborations for health promoting environments, which include education, infrastructure, urban planning and trade (Baum et al 2009:1967). This is described as good stewardship in health care.

The commitment to health and social justice in these countries is matched by distributive justice in government funding, which is aimed at creating a more equal society (Raphael et al 2008). For example, Sweden commits 31% of its GDP on social spending. Compared with other OECD countries, Sweden has lower levels of socio-economic inequalities than most other countries, and the lowest levels of infant mortality, child injury deaths and child poverty (Raphael & Bryant 2005). The country also has the lowest levels of paid employment, yet it maintains one of the highest levels of women in the paid workforce (Raphael & Bryant 2005). Similarly, in Norway, child poverty is 10 times less among the population than it is in the US (Schrecker 2008). This poses the question of why some governments seem to resist looking after their citizenry, while others see it as a matter of moral principle.

At the societal level, redistributive justice is the main driver of health promoting change. Although it seems an elusive goal, at the global level, the 6 million impoverished children throughout the world could be provided with safe drinking water, sanitation and protection from diarrhoea and parasitic diseases with the amount of money spent by the US military in 4 days (Schrecker 2008). To date, there has been only modest success in meeting the Millennium Development Goals to act on global inequities. However, in each nation's political system there are actions that would help equalise access and equity with a view towards better health. These should be aimed at achieving the goals for a healthy society as listed in Box 13.4.

CONCLUDING COMMENTS

Since the health communities of the world began to focus on the SDOH, we have had a closer global connection to those things that help, and those that hinder our quest for health and wellness. Rapid communication brings into our consciousness the cold, hard reality of health inequalities. We are responding to a wider breadth of knowledge on the quality, as well as the quantity of life, and a backlash against the failures of the market to improve health in the population. As Katz (2009) suggests, we need to work towards replacing the invisible hand of the market with the visible hand of social justice. To foster vibrant, cohesive, healthy and safe communities requires leadership and advocacy (Ridde 2007). Given the financial, demographic, environmental and epidemiological threats of modern society, it will take great leadership to nurture our communities and render our health care systems safe, effective and efficient. The challenge lies in strengthening individuals, strengthening communities, improving living and working conditions, and promoting health-giving policies and practices (Whitehead 2007).

As health professionals, we must remain in our imperfect health care systems to improve, rather than abandon, our roles as purveyors of health. Every nurse, every midwife has a certain sphere

BOX 13.4 GOALS FOR HEALTHY SOCIETIES

1 Inclusivity and fairness — through a values-based commitment to equity, freedom, social inclusion and capacity development.

2 Equality — where men and women and members of minority groups are treated equally for common needs.

3 Cultural safety — through culturally competent management and clinical systems to ensure that all care processes acknowledge diversity, difference and ability, with an ultimate aim of empowerment.

4 Responsive health systems — with timely, affordable, safe, coordinated care.

5 Support for healthy behaviours — by arranging structural features of the environment to support people in achieving and maintaining health.

6 Sustainable ecosystems — through public awareness and action on preserving the environment.

7 Evidence-based, evidence-informed management of health and health care, where research, interventions and policy analysis are interlinked and translated into better health.

8 Democratic citizen participation — where all voices are heard.

9 Social capital is valued — human, spiritual, cultural and social capital is seen as equal to economic capital.

10 Resources are adequate and appropriate — there is congruence between needs and resources.

11 Well managed for best processes, best practices — good stewardship and strong community leadership is rewarded and supported.

12 Goals and strategies are developed on the basis of multiple levels of influence by an appropriate, well-educated and satisfied workforce.

of influence, which can be used to build the capacity of a human community to shape its culture and its future (Gray 2009). This is leadership. It grows from a dialogue between people, between those of us in the health care professions, and those who need us. We must use this to advance the goals of PHC with a common language and the wisdom gleaned from community engagement.

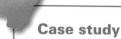

Case study

Susie (Taine and Deirdre's eldest daughter who is living with Maria and is 15) and Francesca are pregnant in Sydney. Maria had her third child, Luke, as a home birth. Susie has decided she'll also have a home birth. Francesca has booked into her local hospital where she is having antenatal care. While Taine is visiting his family on the east coast of New Zealand he is pleased to learn that his sister, Denise, is also pregnant. She has a Lead Maternity Carer who is a midwife and plans to deliver her baby at the local birthing unit.

REFLECTING ON THE BIG ISSUES

- Policy-making is a political process of deciding how resources are allocated.
- Many local policies are linked to global and regional goals.
- All policies influence health, and most policies are linked with one another, which means there is a need for health to be considered in all policy-making.
- Community members should have a voice in policy-making.
- Nurses and midwives can help communities develop a level of health literacy that would facilitate their participation in policy development.
- Health care systems continue to privilege hospital and high-tech care over community care.
- Some inequities persist in access to care, with the most disadvantaged often excluded from the services they need.
- Primary health care can provide the fairest systems of health care.
- An ideal health care system is based on the social determinants of health.

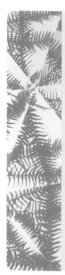

Reflective questions: how would I use this knowledge in practice?

1 Identify the factors influencing policy development in your health service district or primary health organisation.

2 Explain why policy development is guided by the mantra 'think global, act local'.

3 What strategies would you use to ensure Susie's level of health literacy for her home birth is adequate?

4 How does the New Zealand PHC system promote access and equity in services?

5 What steps could you take to support the proposals to develop a primary health care system in Australia?

6 Update the family genogram for the Miller family.

Research-informed practice

Read the article by Boucher et al 2009 'Staying home to give birth: why women in the United States choose to home birth'.

- Do you think women in Australia and New Zealand base their decision for a home birth on similar reasons to those given by women in the US?

- What policies act as facilitating factors and barriers to home birth in Australia and New Zealand?

- Is there a role for nurses and midwives to advocate for home births?

- If so, how would you go about promoting home births in your community?

References

Australian Nursing Federation (ANF) 2009 Primary health care in Australia. A nursing and midwifery consensus view. ANF, Canberra

Australian Research Alliance for Children and Youth (ARACY) 2009 Transforming Australia for our children's future. ARACY National Conference, 4 September, Melbourne

Bambra C, Fox D, Scott-Samuel A 2007 A politics of health glossary. Journal of Epidemiology and Community Health 61:571–4

Bambra C, Gibson M, Petticrew M, Sowden A, Whitehead M, Wright K 2008 Tackling the wider social determinants of health and health inequalities: evidence from systematic reviews. The Public Health Research Consortium funded by the UK Department of Health Policy Research Program, University of York. Online. Available: www.york.ac.uk/phrc/D2-06%20Final%20Report.pdf (accessed 13 August 2009)

Baum F 2009 Envisioning a healthy and sustainable future: essential to closing the gap in a generation. Global Health Promotion 1757–9759 Supp (1):72–80

Baum F, Begin M, Houweling T, Taylor S 2009 Changes not for the fainthearted: reorienting health care systems toward health equity through action on the social determinants of health. American Journal of Public Health 99(11):1967–74

Bayoumi A 2009 Equity and health services. Journal of Public Health Policy 30:176–82

Birn A 2009 Making it politic(al): Closing the gap in a generation: health equity through action on the social determinants of health. Social Medicine 4(3):166–82

Boucher D, Bennett C, McFarlin B, Freeze R 2009 Staying home to give birth: why women in the United States choose to home birth. Journal of Midwifery & Women's Health 54(2):119–26

Brennan D 2007 Babies, Budgets, and Birthrates: Work/family Policy in Australia 1996–2006. Oxford University Press, 31–57 doi: 10.1093/sp/jxm003

Bruni R, Laupacis A, Martin D 2008 Public engagement in setting priorities in health care. Canadian Medical Association Journal 179(1):15–18

Commission on the Social Determinants of Health (CSDH) 2008 Closing the gap in a generation. Health equity through action on the social determinants of health. Final report of the Commission on the Social Determinants of Health. WHO, Geneva

Commonwealth of Australia 2008 Towards a National Primary Health Care Strategy: a Discussion Paper from the Australian Government, Canberra

—— 2009a Report of the maternity services review. Online. Available: www.health.gov.au/maternityservicesreview (accessed 19 October 2009)

—— 2009b A healthier future for all Australians. Final Report of the National Health and Hospitals Reform Commission. AGPS P3-5499, Canberra

—— 2010 Department of Health and Ageing Mental Health Information Development: National Information Priorities and strategies under the Second Mental Health Plan 1998–2003. Online. Available: www.health.gov.au (accessed 1 February 2010)

Department of Health and Ageing (DoHA) 2010a The National Mental Health Policy and Plan. Online. Available: www.health.gov.au/internet/main/publishing.nsf/Content/mental_pubs-k-kit-toc (accessed 1 February 2010)

—— 2010b The National Health Priority Areas. Online. Available: www.safetyandquality.gov.au/internet/safety/publishing.nsf/Content/strategies (accessed 1 February 2010)

—— 2010c Design of new national registration and accreditation scheme. Online. Available: www.health.gov.au/internet/main/publishing.nsf/Content/mr-yr09-dept-dept0805 (accessed 1 February 2010)

DeVos P, Malaise G, De Ceukelaire W, Perez D, Lefevre P, Van der Stuyft P 2009 Participation and empowerment in primary health care: from Alma Ata to the era of globalization. Social Medicine 4(2):121–7

Dowell AC, Garrett S, Collings S, McBain L, McKinlay E, Stanley J 2009 Evaluation of the Primary Mental Health Initiatives: Summary report 2008. University of Otago and Ministry of Health, Wellington

Farmer J, Currie M 2009 Evaluating the outcomes of rural health policy. Australian Journal of Rural Health 17:53–7

Fawcett J, Russell G 2001 A conceptual model of nursing and health policy. Policy, Politics, & Nursing Practice 2(2):108–16

Francis K, Chapman Y, Hoare K, Mills J 2008 Australia and New Zealand community as partner: theory and practice in nursing. Wolters Kluwer/Lippincott Williams & Wilkins, Philadelphia

Gray M 2009 Public health leadership: creating the culture for the twenty-first century. Journal of Public Health 31(2):208–9

Hawe P 2009 The social determinants of health: how can a radical idea be mainstreamed? Canadian Journal of Public Health 100(4):291–3

Henderson J 2005 Neo-liberalism, community care and Australian mental health policy. Health Sociology Review 14(3:242–54

Kamien M 2009 Evidence-based policy versus evidence-based rural health care reality checks. Australian Journal of Rural Health 17:65–7

Katz A 2009 Prospects for a genuine revival of primary health care — through the visible hand of social justice rather than the invisible hand of the market: Part 1. International Journal of Health Services 39(3):567–85

King A 2001 Primary Health Care Strategy. Ministry of Health, Wellington

Labonte R 2008 Global health in public policy: finding the right frame? Critical Public Health 18(4):467–82

Mental Health Commission 1998 Blueprint for Mental Health Services in New Zealand: How Things Need To Be. Mental Health Commission, Wellington

Minister of Health 2000 New Zealand Health Strategy. Ministry of Health, Wellington

—— 2005 Te Tahuhu — Improving Mental Health 2005–2015: The Second New Zealand Mental Health and Addiction Plan. Ministry of Health, Wellington

—— 2006 Te Kōkiri: The Mental Health and Addiction Action Plan 2006–2015. Ministry of Health, Wellington

Ministerial Review Group 2009 Meeting the Challenge: Enhancing Sustainability and the Patient and Consumer Experience within the Current Legislative Framework for Health and Disability Services in New Zealand. Report of the Ministerial Review Group. New Zealand Government, Wellington

Ministry of Health New Zealand (MOHNZ) 2001a He Korowai Oranga, Maori Health Strategy. MOHNZ, Wellington

—— 2001b New Zealand Disability Strategy: Making a World of Difference Whakanui Oranga. MOHNZ, Wellington

—— 2002 Pacific Health and Disability Action Plan. MOHNZ, Wellington

—— 2004 Pacific Health and Workforce Development Plan. MOHNZ, Wellington

—— 2008a A Portrait of Health. Key Results of the 2006–07 New Zealand Health Survey. MOHNZ, Wellington

—— 2008b Pacific Peoples' Experience of Disability: A paper for the Pacific Health and Disability Action Plan review. MOHNZ, Wellington

—— 2008c Pacific Peoples and Mental Health: A paper for the Pacific Health and Disability Action Plan review. MOHNZ, Wellington

—— 2008d Pacific Youth Health: A paper for the Pacific Health and Disability Action Plan Review. MOHNZ, Wellington

—— 2009 A Focus on the Health of Māori and Pacific Children: Key findings of the 2006–07 New Zealand Health Survey. MOHNZ, Wellington

National Rural Health Alliance (NRHA) 2009 Partyline. Online. Available: www.nrha.org.au (accessed 1 December 2009)

New Zealand Treasury 2009 Financial Statements of the Government of New Zealand. New Zealand Treasury, Wellington

Raphael D 2009 Restructuring society in the service of mental health promotion: are we willing to address the social determinants of mental health? International Journal of Mental Health Promotion 11(3):18–31

Raphael D, Bryant T 2005 The state's role in promoting population health: public health concerns in Canada, USA, United Kingdom, and Sweden. Health Policy 78:39–55

—— 2006 Maintaining population health in a period of welfare state decline: political economy as the missing dimension in health promotion theory and practice. Promotion and Education 13(4):236–42

Raphael D, Curry-Stevens A, Bryant T 2008 Barriers to addressing the social determinants of health: insights from the Canadian experience. Health Policy 88(2–3):222–35

Ridde V 2007 Reducing social inequalities in health: public health, community health or health promotion? Promotion & Education 2:63–7

Ryall T 2009 Better, Sooner, More Convenient: Health Discussion Paper. National Party, Wellington

Schrecker T 2008 Denaturalizing scarcity: a strategy of enquiry for public health ethics. Bulletin of the World Health Organization 86(8):600–5

Smith R, MacKellar L 2007 Global public goods and the global health agenda: problems, priorities and potential. Globalization and Health 3(9): doi:10.1186/1744-8603-3-9

United Nations 2010 Rethinking poverty. Report on the World Social Situation 2010. Online. Available: www.un.org/esa/socdec/rwss/2010_media.html (accessed 29 January 2010)

Wakerman J 2008 Rural and remote public health in Australia: building on our strengths. Editorial, Australian Journal of Rural Health 16:52–5

—— 2009 Innovative rural and remote primary health care models: What do we know and what are the research priorities? Australian Journal of Rural Health 17:21–6

Whitehead M 2007 A typology of actions to tackle social inequalities in health. Journal of Epidemiology and Community Health 61:473–8

Wise M 2008 Health promotion in Australia: reviewing the past and looking to the future. Critical Public Health 18(4):497–508

World Health Organization 2004 What are the advantages and disadvantages of restructuring a health care system to be more focused on primary care services? Health Evidence Network, WHO Europe, Copenhagen

—— 2008 World Health Report 2008 Primary Health Care, Now More Than Ever. Online. Available: www. who.int/whr/2008/whr08_en.pdf (accessed 14 July 2009)

—— 2010 Mental health. Online. Available: www.who.int/mental_health/en (accessed 1 February 2010)

Useful websites

http://www.who.int/social_determinants/knowledge_networks/en/ — WHO SDOH network

http://www.who.int/social_determinants/knowledge_networks/en/ — WHO SDOH advocacy network

http://www.who.int/social_determinants/knowledge_networks/en/ — WHO social exclusion network

http://www.who.int/whosis/whostat/EN_WHS09_Full.pdf — WHO statistics reports

http://www.who.int/social_determinants/knowledge_networks/en/ — WHO priority public health conditions

http://www.sweden.gov.se/content/1/c6/05/13/34/4eb4fe08.pdf — Sweden's report on measures to prevent poverty and social exclusion

http://www.sweden.gov.se/sb/d/6570/a/51334 — Sweden's commitment to social determinants of health

http://www.eurohealthnet.eu — European health network

http://www.health-inequalities.com/health-inequalities/Welcome.html — European inequalities network

http://www.equitychannel.net — European health equity network

http://www.health-gradient.eu — European health gradients

http://www.RaisingtheGlobalFloor.org — Global policy discussions on SDOH as a gateway to international labour and work policy data

http://www.health.vic.gov.au/healthstatus/inequalities.htm — Fair health facts 2009: report on inequalities in health, A Fairer Victoria

http://www.health.gov.au — Australian health policies

http://www.fahcsia.gov.au — Australian family policies, including disabilities

http://www.safetyandquality.org — Safety and Quality in Health Care

http://nrha.ruralhealth.org.au/cms/uploads/publications/hh_2003_03.pdf — National Rural Health Alliance: Healthy Horizons rural health policy 2000–2007

http://www.deewr.gov.au/Schooling/Programs/REDI/readingroom/profile/Pages/nat_school_drug_ed_strat.aspx — National School Drug Education Strategy

http://www.health.gov.au/internet/main/publishing.nsf/Content/health-budget2000-fact-acfact1.htm — National Strategy for an Ageing Australia

http://www.health.gov.au/internet/main/publishing.nsf/content/mental-pubs-f-plan09 — National Mental Health Plan 2003–2008

http://www.health.gov.au/mentalhealth — National Mental Health Strategy

http://www.healthinsite.gov.au/topics/Living_with_a_Disability — Australian Government Health Insite page on disabilities

http://www.health.gov.au — Department of Health & Ageing

http://www.aihw.gov.au — Australian Institute of Health and Welfare

http://www.foodstandards.gov.au — Food standards, Australia and New Zealand

http://www.mhca.org.au — Mental Health Council of Australia

http://www.nhmrc.gov.au — National Health and Medical Research Council

http://www.midwives.org.au — Australian College of Midwives

http://www.anmc.org.au — Australian Nursing and Midwifery Council

http://www.indiginet.com.au/catsin/ — Congress of Aboriginal and Torres Strait Islander Nurses

http://www.rcna.org.au — Royal College of Nursing Australia

http://www.health.act.gov.au/c/health — ACT Health

http://www.health.nt.gov.au — Department of Health and Human Services Northern Territory

http://www.dhhs.tas.gov.au — Department of Health and Human Services Tasmania

http://www.health.sa.gov.au — Department of Health South Australia

http://www.health.wa.gov.au/home — Department of Health Western Australia

http://www.dhs.vic.gov.au/home — Department of Human Services Victoria

http://www.health.nsw.gov.au — New South Wales Health

http://www.health.qld.gov.au — Queensland Health

Appendices

Appendix A   **Symbols used in a genogram**

Appendix B   **Jakarta Declaration on Leading Health Promotion into the 21st Century**

Appendix C   **People's Health Charter**

Appendix D   **The Bangkok Charter for Health Promotion in a Globalised World**

Appendix E   **Chart for community assessment**

Appendix F   **Transforming Australia for our children's future: making prevention work**

Appendix G   **HEEADSSS assessment tool for use with adolescents**

Appendix H   **Ecomap**

SYMBOLS USED IN A GENOGRAM

A genogram is a graphic representation of a family tree that displays the interaction of generations within a family. It goes beyond a traditional family tree by allowing the user to analyse family, emotional and social relationships within a group. It is used to identify repetitive patterns of behaviour and to recognise hereditary tendencies. Here are some of the basic components of a genogram.

Genogram symbols

In a genogram, males are represented by a square and females by a circle. If you are unsure of how to place individuals in complex family situations, such as reconstituted families, please visit the rules to build a genogram. GenoPro also has two other *gender symbols*, the diamond for a pet and the question mark for unknown gender.

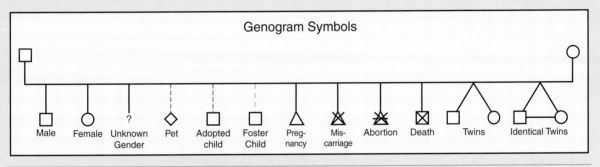

Standard gender symbols for a genogram

In a standard genogram, there are three different types of child: biological/natural child, adopted child and foster child. A triangle is used to represent a pregnancy, a miscarriage or an abortion. In the case of a miscarriage, there is a diagonal cross drawn on top of the triangle to indicate death. Abortions have a similar display to miscarriages, only they have an additional horizontal line. A still-birth is displayed by the gender symbol; the diagonal cross remains the same size, but the gender symbol is twice as small.

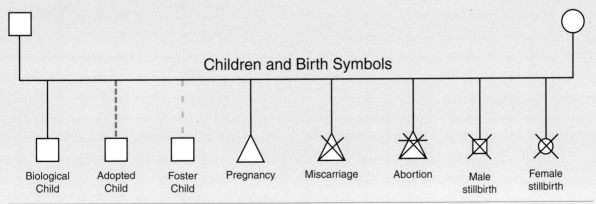

Genogram symbols for children's links and pregnancy terminations

In the case of multiple births such as twins, triplets, quadruplets, quintuplets, sextuplets, septuplets, octuplets, or more, the child links are joined together. GenoPro uses the term **twin** to describe any type of multiple birth. With GenoPro, creating twins is as simple as a single click on the toolbar button 'New Twins'. GenoPro take cares of all the drawing, including joining the lines together. Identical twins (or triplets …) are displayed by a horizontal line between the siblings. In the example below, the mother gave birth to fraternal twin brothers, identical twin sisters and triplets, one of whom died at birth.

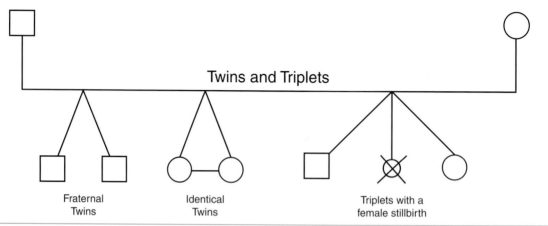

Child links are joined for multiple births such as twins and triplets

In addition to this, GenoPro supports medical genograms by using colour codes and special drawing in the gender symbol. To learn more, please visit medical genograms (http://www.genopro.com/genogram/symbols).

Genogram legend

At any time you can add a genogram legend by right-clicking on your mouse and selecting a new legend. The legend symbols have already been marked to be excluded from the report, so they will not appear when you generate a report.

(Source: Genopro, with permission)

JAKARTA DECLARATION ON LEADING HEALTH PROMOTION INTO THE 21ST CENTURY

1 Promote social responsibility for health

Decision-makers must be firmly committed to social responsibility. Both the public and private sectors should promote health by pursuing policies and practices that:

- avoid harming the health of other individuals
- protect the environment and ensure sustainable use of resources
- restrict production and trade in inherently harmful goods and substances such as tobacco and armaments, as well as unhealthy marketing practices
- safeguard both the citizen in the marketplace and the individual in the workplace
- include equity-focused health impact assessments as an integral part of policy development.

2 Increase investments for health development

In many countries, current investment in health is inadequate and often ineffective. Increasing investment for health development requires a truly multi-sectoral approach, including additional resources to education, housing and the health sector. Greater investment for health, and reorientation of existing investments — both within and between countries — has the potential to significantly advance human development, health and quality of life.

Investments in health should reflect the needs of certain groups such as women, children, older people, indigenous, poor and marginalised populations.

3 Consolidate and expand partnerships for health

Health promotion requires partnerships for health and social development between the different sectors at all levels of governance and society. Existing partnerships need to be strengthened and the potential for new partnerships must be explored.

Partnerships offer mutual benefit for health through the sharing of expertise, skills and resources. Each partnership must be transparent and accountable and be based on agreed ethical principles, mutual understanding and respect. WHO guidelines should be adhered to.

4 Increase community capacity and empower the individual

Health promotion is carried out *by* and *with* people, not on or to people. It improves the ability of individuals to take action, and the capacity of groups, organisations or communities to influence the determinants of health.

Improving the capacity of communities for health promotion requires practical education, leadership training and access to resources. Empowering individuals demands more consistent, reliable access to the decision-making process and the skills and knowledge essential to effect change.

Both traditional communication and the new information media support this process. Social, cultural and spiritual resources need to be harnessed in innovative ways.

5 Secure an infrastructure for health promotion

To secure an infrastructure for health promotion, new mechanisms of funding it locally, nationally and globally must be found. Incentives should be developed to influence the actions of governments, non-government organisations (NGOs) educational institutions and the private sector to make sure that resource mobilisation for health promotion is maximised.

'Settings for health' represent the organisational base of the infrastructure required for health promotion. New health challenges mean that new and diverse networks need to be created to achieve intersectoral collaboration. Such networks should provide mutual assistance within and between countries and facilitate exchange of information on which strategies are effective in which settings.

Training and practice of local leadership skills should be encouraged to support health promotion activities. Documentation of experiences in health promotion through research and project reporting should be enhanced to improve planning, implementation and evaluation.

All countries should develop the appropriate political, legal, educational, social and economic environments required to support health promotion.

PEOPLE'S HEALTH CHARTER

Introduction

In 1978, at the Alma-Ata Conference, ministers from 134 member countries in association with WHO and UNICEF declared 'Health for All by the Year 2000' selecting Primary Health Care as the best tool to achieve it.

Unfortunately, that dream never came true. The health status of third world populations has not improved. In many cases it has deteriorated further. Currently we are facing a global health crisis, characterized by growing inequalities within and between countries. New threats to health are continually emerging. This is compounded by negative forces of globalization which prevent the equitable distribution of resources with regard to the health of people and especially that of the poor.

Within the health sector, failure to implement the principles of primary health care, as originally conceived in Alma-Ata has significantly aggravated the global health crisis.

Governments and the international bodies are fully responsible for this failure.

It has now become essential to build up a concerted international effort to put the goals of health for all to its rightful place on the development agenda. Genuine, people-centered initiatives must therefore be strengthened in order to increase pressure on decision-makers, governments and the private sector to ensure that the vision of Alma-Ata becomes a reality.

Several international organizations and civil society movements, NGOs and women's groups decided to work together towards this objective. This group together with others committed to the principles of primary health care and people's perspectives organized the 'People's Health Assembly' which took place from 4–8 December 2000 in Bangladesh, at Savar, on the campus of the Gonoshasthasthaya Kendra or GK (People's Health Centre).

1453 participants from 92 countries came to the Assembly which was the culmination of eighteen months of preparatory action around the globe. The preparatory process elicited unprecedented enthusiasm and participation of a broad cross section of people who have been involved in thousands of village meetings, district level workshops and national gatherings.

The plenary sessions at the Assembly covered five main themes: Health, Life and Well-Being; Inequality, Poverty and Health; Health Care and Health Services; Environment and Survival; and The Ways Forward. People from all over the world presented testimonies of deprivation and service failure as well as those of successful people's initiatives and organization. Over a hundred concurrent sessions made it possible for participants to share and discuss in greater detail different aspects of the major themes and give voice to their specific experiences and concerns. The five-day event gave participants the space to express themselves in their own idiom. They put forward the failures of their respective governments and international organizations and decided to fight together so that health and equitable development become top priorities in the policy-makers agendas at the local, national and international levels.

Having reviewed their problems and difficulties and shared their experiences, they have formulated and finally endorsed the People's Charter for Health. The charter from now on will be the common tool of a worldwide citizens' movement committed to make the Alma-Ata dream a reality.

We encourage and invite everyone who shares our concerns and aims to join us by endorsing the charter.

Preamble

Health is a social, economic and political issue and above all a fundamental human right. Inequality, poverty, exploitation, violence and injustice are at the root of ill-health and the deaths of poor and marginalised people. Health for all means that powerful interests have to be challenged, that globalisation has to be opposed, and that political and economic priorities have to be drastically changed. This Charter builds on perspectives of people whose voices have rarely been heard before, if at all. It encourages people to develop their own solutions and to hold accountable local authorities, national governments, international organisations and corporations.

Vision

Equity, ecologically-sustainable development and peace are at the heart of our vision of a better world — a world in which a healthy life for all is a reality; a world that respects, appreciates and celebrates all life and diversity; a world that enables the flowering of people's talents and abilities to enrich each other; a world in which people's voices guide the decisions that shape our lives. There are more than enough resources to achieve this vision.

The health crisis

'Illness and death every day anger us. Not because there are people who get sick or because there are people who die. We are angry because many illnesses and deaths have their roots in the economic and social policies that are imposed on us.'

(A voice from Central America)

In recent decades, economic changes world-wide have profoundly affected people's health and their access to health care and other social services.

Despite unprecedented levels of wealth in the world, poverty and hunger are increasing. The gap between rich and poor nations has widened, as have inequalities within countries, between social classes, between men and women and between young and old.

A large proportion of the world's population still lacks access to food, education, safe drinking water, sanitation, shelter, land and its resources, employment and health care services. Discrimination continues to prevail. It affects both the occurrence of disease and access to health care.

The planet's natural resources are being depleted at an alarming rate. The resulting degradation of the environment threatens everyone's health, especially the health of the poor. There has been an upsurge of new conflicts while weapons of mass destruction still pose a grave threat.

The world's resources are increasingly concentrated in the hands of a few who strive to maximise their private profit. Neoliberal political and economic policies are made by a small group of powerful governments, and by international institutions such as the World Bank, the International Monetary Fund and the World Trade Organization. These policies, together with the unregulated activities of transnational corporations, have had severe effects on the lives and livelihoods, health and well-being of people in both North and South.

Public services are not fulfilling people's needs, not least because they have deteriorated as a result of cuts in governments' social budgets. Health services have become less accessible, more unevenly distributed and more inappropriate.

Privatisation threatens to undermine access to health care still further and to compromise the essential principle of equity. The persistence of preventable ill-health, the resurgence of diseases such as tuberculosis and malaria, and the emergence and spread of new diseases such as HIV/AIDS are a stark reminder of our world's lack of commitment to principles of equity and justice.

Principles of the People's Charter for Health

- The attainment of the highest possible level of health and well-being is a fundamental human right, regardless of a person's colour, ethnic background, religion, gender, age, abilities, sexual orientation or class.
- The principles of universal, comprehensive Primary Health Care (PHC), envisioned in the 1978 Alma-Ata Declaration, should be the basis for formulating policies related to health. Now more than ever an equitable, participatory and intersectoral approach to health and health care is needed.

- Governments have a fundamental responsibility to ensure universal access to quality health care, education and other social services according to people's needs, not according to their ability to pay.
- The participation of people and people's organisations is essential to the formulation, implementation and evaluation of all health and social policies and programmes.
- Health is primarily determined by the political, economic, social and physical environment and should, along with equity and sustainable development, be a top priority in local, national and international policy-making.

A call for action

To combat the global health crisis, we need to take action at all levels — individual, community, national, regional and global — and in all sectors. The demands presented below provide a basis for action.

Health as a human right

Health is a reflection of a society's commitment to equity and justice. Health and human rights should prevail over economic and political concerns.

This Charter calls on people of the world to:
- Support all attempts to implement the right to health.
- Demand that governments and international organisations reformulate, implement and enforce policies and practices which respect the right to health.
- Build broad-based popular movements to pressure governments to incorporate health and human rights into national constitutions and legislation.
- Fight the exploitation of people's health needs for purposes of profit.

Tackling the broader determinants of health

Economic challenges

The economy has a profound influence on people's health. Economic policies that prioritise equity, health and social well-being can improve the health of the people as well as the economy.

Political, financial, agricultural and industrial policies which respond primarily to capitalist needs, imposed by national governments and international organisations, alienate people from their lives and livelihoods. The processes of economic globalisation and liberalisation have increased inequalities between and within nations. Many countries of the world and especially the most powerful ones are using their resources, including economic sanctions and military interventions, to consolidate and expand their positions, with devastating effects on people's lives.

This Charter calls on people of the world to:
- Demand transformation of the World Trade Organization and the global trading system so that it ceases to violate social, environmental, economic and health rights of people and begins to discriminate positively in favour of countries of the South. In order to protect public health, such transformation must include intellectual property regimes such as patents and the Trade Related aspects of Intellectual Property Rights (TRIPS) agreement.
- Demand the cancellation of Third World debt.
- Demand radical transformation of the World Bank and International Monetary Fund so that these institutions reflect and actively promote the rights and interests of developing countries.
- Demand effective regulation to ensure that TNCs do not have negative effects on people's health, exploit their workforce, degrade the environment or impinge on national sovereignty.
- Ensure that governments implement agricultural policies attuned to people's needs and not to the demands of the market, thereby guaranteeing food security and equitable access to food.
- Demand that national governments act to protect public health rights in intellectual property laws.
- Demand the control and taxation of speculative international capital flows.
- Insist that all economic policies be subject to health, equity, gender and environmental impact assessments and include enforceable regulatory measures to ensure compliance.

- Challenge growth-centred economic theories and replace them with alternatives that create humane and sustainable societies. Economic theories should recognise environmental constraints, the fundamental importance of equity and health, and the contribution of unpaid labour, especially the unrecognised work of women.

Social and political challenges

Comprehensive social policies have positive effects on people's lives and livelihoods. Economic globalisation and privatisation have profoundly disrupted communities, families and cultures. Women are essential to sustaining the social fabric of societies everywhere, yet their basic needs are often ignored or denied, and their rights and persons violated.

Public institutions have been undermined and weakened. Many of their responsibilities have been transferred to the private sector, particularly corporations, or to other national and international institutions, which are rarely accountable to the people. Furthermore, the power of political parties and trade unions has been severely curtailed, while conservative and fundamentalist forces are on the rise. Participatory democracy in political organisations and civic structures should thrive. There is an urgent need to foster and ensure transparency and accountability.

This Charter calls on people of the world to:
- Demand and support the development and implementation of comprehensive social policies with full participation of people.
- Ensure that all women and all men have equal rights to work, livelihoods, to freedom of expression, to political participation, to exercise religious choice, to education and to freedom from violence.
- Pressure governments to introduce and enforce legislation to protect and promote the physical, mental and spiritual health and human rights of marginalised groups.
- Demand that education and health are placed at the top of the political agenda. This calls for free and compulsory quality education for all children and adults, particularly girl children and women, and for quality early childhood education and care.
- Demand that the activities of public institutions, such as child care services, food distribution systems, and housing provisions, benefit the health of individuals and communities.
- Condemn and seek the reversal of any policies, which result in the forced displacement of people from their lands, homes or jobs.
- Oppose fundamentalist forces that threaten the rights and liberties of individuals, particularly the lives of women, children and minorities.
- Oppose sex tourism and the global traffic of women and children.

Environmental challenges

Water and air pollution, rapid climate change, ozone layer depletion, nuclear energy and waste, toxic chemicals and pesticides, loss of biodiversity, deforestation and soil erosion have far-reaching effects on people's health. The root causes of this destruction include the unsustainable exploitation of natural resources, the absence of a long-term holistic vision, the spread of individualistic and profit-maximising behaviours, and over-consumption by the rich. This destruction must be confronted and reversed immediately and effectively.

This Charter calls on people of the world to:
- Hold transnational and national corporations, public institutions and the military accountable for their destructive and hazardous activities that impact on the environment and people's health.
- Demand that all development projects be evaluated against health and environmental criteria and that caution and restraint be applied whenever technologies or policies pose potential threats to health and the environment (the precautionary principle).
- Demand that governments rapidly commit themselves to reductions of greenhouse gases from their own territories far stricter than those set out in the international climate change agreement, without resorting to hazardous or inappropriate technologies and practices.
- Oppose the shifting of hazardous industries and toxic and radioactive waste to poorer countries and marginalised communities and encourage solutions that minimise waste production.

- Reduce over-consumption and non-sustainable lifestyles — both in the North and the South. Pressure wealthy industrialised countries to reduce their consumption and pollution by 90 per cent.
- Demand measures to ensure occupational health and safety, including worker-centred monitoring of working conditions.
- Demand measures to prevent accidents and injuries in the workplace, the community and in homes.
- Reject patents on life and oppose bio-piracy of traditional and indigenous knowledge and resources.
- Develop people-centred, community-based indicators of environmental and social progress, and press for the development and adoption of regular audits that measure environmental degradation and the health status of the population.

War, violence, conflict and natural disasters

War, violence, conflict and natural disasters devastate communities and destroy human dignity. They have a severe impact on the physical and mental health of their members, especially women and children. Increased arms procurement and an aggressive and corrupt international arms trade undermine social, political and economic stability and the allocation of resources to the social sector.

This Charter calls on people of the world to:
- Support campaigns and movements for peace and disarmament.
- Support campaigns against aggression, and the research, production, testing and use of weapons of mass destruction and other arms, including all types of landmines.
- Support people's initiatives to achieve a just and lasting peace, especially in countries with experiences of civil war and genocide.
- Condemn the use of child soldiers, and the abuse and rape, torture and killing of women and children.
- Demand the end of occupation as one of the most destructive tools to human dignity.
- Oppose the militarisation of humanitarian relief interventions.
- Demand the radical transformation of the UN Security Council so that it functions democratically.
- Demand that the United Nations and individual states end all kinds of sanctions used as an instrument of aggression which can damage the health of civilian populations.
- Encourage independent, people-based initiatives to declare neighbourhoods, communities and cities areas of peace and zones free of weapons.
- Support actions and campaigns for the prevention and reduction of aggressive and violent behaviour, especially in men, and the fostering of peaceful coexistence.
- Support actions and campaigns for the prevention of natural disasters and the reduction of subsequent human suffering.

A people-centred health sector

This Charter calls for the provision of universal and comprehensive Primary Health Care, irrespective of people's ability to pay. Health services must be democratic and accountable with sufficient resources to achieve this.

This Charter calls on people of the world to:
- Oppose international and national policies that privatise health care and turn it into a commodity.
- Demand that governments promote, finance and provide comprehensive Primary Health Care as the most effective way of addressing health problems and organising public health services so as to ensure free and universal access.
- Pressure governments to adopt, implement and enforce national health and drugs policies.
- Demand that governments oppose the privatisation of public health services and ensure effective regulation of the private medical sector, including charitable and NGO medical services.
- Demand a radical transformation of the World Health Organization (WHO) so that it responds to health challenges in a manner which benefits the poor, avoids vertical approaches, ensures intersectoral work, involves people's organisations in the World Health Assembly, and ensures independence from corporate interests.
- Promote, support and engage in actions that encourage people's power and control in decision-making in health at all levels, including patient and consumer rights.

- Support, recognise and promote traditional and holistic healing systems and practitioners and their integration into Primary Health Care.
- Demand changes in the training of health personnel so that they become more problem-oriented and practice based, understand better the impact of global issues in their communities, and are encouraged to work with and respect the community and its diversities.
- Demystify medical and health technologies (including medicines) and demand that they be subordinated to the health needs of the people.
- Demand that research in health, including genetic research and the development of medicines and reproductive technologies, is carried out in a participatory, needs-based manner by accountable institutions. It should be people- and public health-oriented, respecting universal ethical principles.
- Support people's rights to reproductive and sexual self-determination and oppose all coercive measures in population and family planning policies. This support includes the right to the full range of safe and effective methods of fertility regulation.

People's participation for a healthy world

Strong people's organisations and movements are fundamental to more democratic, transparent and accountable decision-making processes. It is essential that people's civil, political, economic, social and cultural rights are ensured. While governments have the primary responsibility for promoting a more equitable approach to health and human rights, a wide range of civil society groups and movements, and the media have an important role to play in ensuring people's power and control in policy development and in the monitoring of its implementation.

This Charter calls on people of the world to:

- Build and strengthen people's organisations to create a basis for analysis and action.
- Promote, support and engage in actions that encourage people's involvement in decision-making in public services at all levels.
- Demand that people's organisations be represented in local, national and international fora that are relevant to health.
- Support local initiatives towards participatory democracy through the establishment of people-centred solidarity networks across the world.

Amendment

After the endorsement of the PCH on December 8, 2000, it was called to the attention of the drafting group that action points number 1 and 2 under Economic Challenges could be interpreted as supporting the social clause proposed by the WTO, which actually serves to strengthen the WTO and its neoliberal agenda. Given that this countervails the PHA demands for change of the WTO and the global trading system, the two paragraphs were merged and amended.

The section of War, Violence and Conflict has been amended to include natural disasters. A new action point, number 5 in this version, was added to demand the end of occupation. Furthermore, action point number 7, now number 8, was amended to read to end all kinds of sanctions. An additional action point number 11 was added concerning natural disasters.

The People's Health Assembly and the Charter

The idea of a People's Health Assembly (PHA) has been discussed for more than a decade. In 1998 a number of organisations launched the PHA process and started to plan a large international Assembly meeting, held in Bangladesh at the end of 2000. A range of pre- and post-Assembly activities were initiated including regional workshops, the collection of people's health-related stories and the drafting of a People's Charter for Health. The present Charter builds upon the views of citizens and people's organisations from around the world, and was first approved and opened for endorsement at the Assembly meeting in Savar, Bangladesh, in December 2000. The Charter is an expression of our common concerns, our vision of a better and healthier world, and of our calls for radical action. It is a tool for advocacy and a rallying point around which a global health movement can gather and other networks and coalitions can be formed.

Join Us — Endorse the Charter

We call upon all individuals and organisations to join this global movement and invite you to endorse and help implement the People's Charter for Health.

PHM Global Secretariat

Email: secretariat@phmovement.org
Web: www.phmovement.org

Endorse the People's Charter for Health

Personal information

Name

First: ....

Last: ....

Mailing Address

Street and No.: ....

City: ....

State: ....

Zip Code: ....

Country: ....

Email: ....

Organization

Name: ....

Website: ....

Comments on the Charter

....

....

....

....

....

....

....

....

....

....

Any Suggestions for the PHM?

....

....

....

....

....

....

....

....

....

....

....

....

....

....

....

....
....
....
....
....
....
....
....
....
....
....
....
....

Don't be hesitant to add any further suggestions in separate papers.
Please fill -in & send to: secretariat@phmovement.org

The People's Health Charter was produced by the People's Health Movement and endorsed at the first People's Health Assembly held in Savar Bangladesh in December 2000. It resulted from a consultation process with grassroots communities across the globe about the health issues that most concerned them.

THE BANGKOK CHARTER FOR HEALTH PROMOTION IN A GLOBALIZED WORLD
Introduction

Scope
The Bangkok Charter identifies actions, commitments and pledges required to address the determinants of health in a globalized world through health promotion.

Purpose
The Bangkok Charter affirms that policies and partnerships to empower communities, and to improve health and health equality, should be at the centre of global and national development.

The Bangkok Charter complements and builds upon the values, principles and action strategies of health promotion established by the *Ottawa Charter for Health Promotion* and the recommendations of the subsequent global health promotion conferences which have been confirmed by Member States through the World Health Assembly.

Audience
The Bangkok Charter reaches out to people, groups and organizations that are critical to the achievement of health, including:
- governments and politicians at all levels
- civil society
- the private sector
- international organizations, and
- the public health community.

Health promotion
The United Nations recognizes that the enjoyment of the highest attainable standard of health is one of the fundamental rights of every human being without discrimination.

Health promotion is based on this critical human right and offers a positive and inclusive concept of health as a determinant of the quality of life and encompassing mental and spiritual wellbeing.

Health promotion is the process of enabling people to increase control over their health and its determinants, and thereby improve their health. It is a core function of public health and contributes to the work of tackling communicable and non-communicable diseases and other threats to health.

Addressing the determinants of health

Changing context
The global context for health promotion has changed markedly since the development of the *Ottawa Charter.*

Critical factors
Some of the critical factors that now influence health include:
- increasing inequalities within and between countries
- new patterns of consumption and communication
- commercialization

- global environmental change, and
- urbanization.

Further challenges

Other factors that influence health include rapid and often adverse social, economic and demographic changes that affect working conditions, learning environments, family patterns, and the culture and social fabric of communities.

Women and men are affected differently and the vulnerability of children and exclusion of marginalized, disabled and indigenous peoples have increased.

New opportunities

Globalization opens up new opportunities for cooperation to improve health and reduce transnational health risks; these opportunities include:

- enhanced information and communications technology, and
- improved mechanisms for global governance and the sharing of experiences.

Policy coherence

To manage the challenges of globalization, policy must be coherent across all:

- levels of governments
- United Nations bodies, and
- other organizations, including the private sector.

This coherence will strengthen compliance, transparency and accountability with international agreements and treaties that affect health.

Progress made

Progress has been made in placing health at the centre of development, for example through the Millennium Development Goals, but much more remains to be achieved; the active participation of civil society is crucial in this process.

Strategies for health promotion in a globalized world

Effective interventions

Progress towards a healthier world requires strong political action, broad participation and sustained advocacy.

Health promotion has an established repertoire of proven effective strategies which need to be fully utilized.

Required actions

To make further advances in implementing these strategies, all sectors and settings must act to:

- **advocate** for health based on human rights and solidarity
- **invest** in sustainable policies, actions and infrastructure to address the determinants of health
- **build capacity** for policy development, leadership, health promotion practice, knowledge transfer and research, and health literacy
- **regulate and legislate** to ensure a high level of protection from harm and enable equal opportunity for health and wellbeing for all people
- **partner and build alliances** with public, private, non-governmental and international organizations and civil society to create sustainable actions.

Commitments to health for all

Rationale
The health sector has a key role to provide leadership in building policies and partnerships for health promotion.

An integrated policy approach within government and international organizations, and a commitment to working with civil society and the private sector and across settings, are essential to make progress in addressing the determinants of health.

Key commitments
The four key commitments are to make the promotion of health:
1 central to the global development agenda
2 a core responsibility for all of government
3 a key focus of communities and civil society
4 a requirement for good corporate practice.

1 Make the promotion of health central to the global development agenda
Strong intergovernmental agreements that increase health and collective health security are needed. Government and international bodies must act to close the health gap between rich and poor. Effective mechanisms for global governance for health are required to address all the harmful effects of:

- trade
- products
- services, and
- marketing strategies.

Health promotion must become an integral part of domestic and foreign policy and international relations, including in situations of war and conflict.

This requires actions to promote dialogue and cooperation among nation states, civil society, and the private sector. These efforts can build on the example of existing treaties such as the World Health Organization Framework Convention for Tobacco Control.

2 Make the promotion of health a core responsibility for all of government
All governments at all levels must tackle poor health and inequalities as a matter of urgency because health determines socio-economic and political development. Local, regional and national governments must:

- give priority to investments in health, within and outside the health sector
- provide sustainable financing for health promotion.

To ensure this, all levels of government should make the health consequences of policies and legislation explicit, using tools such as equity-focused health impact assessment.

3 Make the promotion of health a key focus of communities and civil society
Communities and civil society often lead in initiating, shaping and undertaking health promotion. They need to have the rights, resources and opportunities so that their contributions are amplified and sustained. In less developed communities, support for capacity building is particularly important.

Well organized and empowered communities are highly effective in determining their own health, and are capable of making governments and the private sector accountable for the health consequences of their policies and practices.

Civil society needs to exercise its power in the marketplace by giving preference to the goods, services and shares of companies that exemplify corporate social responsibility.

Grass-roots community projects, civil society groups, and women's organizations have demonstrated their effectiveness in health promotion, and provide models of practice for others to follow.

Health professional associations have a special contribution to make.

4 Make the promotion of health a requirement for good corporate practice

The corporate sector has a direct impact on the health of people and on the determinants of health through its influence on:

- local settings
- national cultures
- environments, and
- wealth distribution.

The private sector, like other employers and the informal sector, has a responsibility to ensure health and safety in the workplace, and to promote the health and wellbeing of their employees, their families and communities.

The private sector can also contribute to lessening wider global health impacts, such as those associated with global environmental change by complying with local national and international regulations and agreements that promote and protect health. Ethical and responsible business practices and fair trade exemplify the type of business practice that should be supported by consumers and civil society, and by government incentives and regulations.

A global pledge to make it happen

All for health

Meeting these commitments requires better application of proven strategies, as well as the use of new entry points and innovative responses.

Partnerships, alliances, networks and collaborations provide exciting and rewarding ways of bringing people and organizations together around common goals and joint actions to improve the health of populations.

Each sector — intergovernmental, government, civil society and private — has a unique role and responsibility.

Closing the implementation gap

Since the adoption of the *Ottawa Charter,* a significant number of resolutions at national and global level have been signed in support of health promotion, but these have not always been followed by action. The participants of this Bangkok Conference forcefully call on Member States of the World Health Organization to close this implementation gap and move to policies and partnerships for action.

Call for action

Conference participants request the World Health Organization, in collaboration with others, and its Member States, to allocate resources for health promotion, initiate plans of action and monitor performance through appropriate indicators and targets, and to report on progress at regular intervals. United Nations organizations are asked to explore the benefits of developing a Global Treaty for Health.

Worldwide partnership

This Bangkok Charter urges all stakeholders to join in a worldwide partnership to promote health, with both global and local engagement and action.

Commitment to improve health

We, the participants of the 6th Global Conference on Health Promotion in Bangkok, Thailand, pledge to advance these actions and commitments to improve health.

11 August 2005

Note: This charter contains the collective views of an international group of experts, participants to the 6th Global Conference on Health Promotion, Bangkok, Thailand, August 2005, and does not necessarily represent the decisions or the stated policy of the World Health Organization.

CHART FOR COMMUNITY ASSESSMENT

People	**Data**

1 People–place relationship

2 Networks for communication, volunteerism support systems, family and professional caregivers

3 Community leadership

4 Psychosocial factors

5 Cultural factors, ethnic mix

6 Demographic characteristics

Place	**Data**

1 Geographic area

2 Natural resources

3 Development base, including taxation

4 Other structural features

5 Access to welfare, housing, transportation, schools

6 Land owners, non-land owners

7 Urban–rural–regional–remote

Health patterns	**Data**

1 Local burden of disease and disability

2 Social determinants of health

3 Access, availability, affordability of health and disability services

4 Local patterns of service utilisation

Gatekeepers	**Data**

1 Intersectoral coalitions

2 Local, state/provincial, national health policies and priorities

3 Financial resources

4 Competing political, development goals

5 Health professionals

6 Global factors

TRANSFORMING AUSTRALIA FOR OUR CHILDREN'S FUTURE: MAKING PREVENTION WORK

ARACY 2009 Conference declaration and call to action

From 2 to 4 September 2009 more than 560 delegates joined the Australian Research Alliance for Children and Youth in Melbourne to examine the theme 'Transforming Australia for our children's future: making prevention work'.

Eminent speakers at the ARACY conference discussed the urgent need to transform Australia into a society that truly nurtures and respects children and young people, to improve their wellbeing and prevent the problems that are increasingly affecting them.

The conference concluded with delegates showing overwhelming support for the following Declaration and call to action to the entire Australian community — to the Australian Government; to state, territory and local governments; and to community and business leaders.

ARACY is taking the Declaration to federal, state and territory governments, local governments and community leaders and organisations around the country. We welcome the use of the Declaration by community organisations, governments and business committed to improve the wellbeing of children and young people. If you are using the Declaration or would like more information, please contact ARACY.

We, the delegates to the national conference of the Australian Research Alliance for Children and Youth held in Melbourne from 2 to 4 September 2009,

- representing a wide range of research, policy and community interests and perspectives
- believing that Australia must raise its international standing on child and youth wellbeing to match the best of the Organisation for Economic Co-operation and Development (OECD) countries
- confident that by working together to transform Australia into a society that truly values, nurtures and respects children and young people, we can create a community with a greater sense of wellbeing where all children and young people can thrive and achieve their potential

have agreed on the following Declaration as a call to the entire Australian community and to all levels of government, to take action to change Australia to improve the wellbeing of our children and young people.

Principles for action

Action to improve the wellbeing of Australia's children and young people must be firmly guided by the following principles:

1. All Australian children and young people have a right to the care, conditions and opportunities they need for their wellbeing and to achieve their potential.
2. Nurturing and trusting relationships with parents and carers are essential for the long-term wellbeing of children and young people.
3. The physical, social, cultural and economic environments in which children and young people live play a key role in their wellbeing.
4. Australia must urgently lower the levels of poverty and inequality to improve the wellbeing of all children and young people.
5. Children and young people have the right to be respected and heard in matters affecting their wellbeing.
6. All Australians share responsibility for the wellbeing of children and young people, and need to value the role of parents, carers, families and people who work with them.

7 Empowered, active communities working in partnership with active governments play a critical part in enhancing the wellbeing of children and young people.

8 What is good for children and young people is good for all of us. The entire Australian community bears the social and economic cost caused by preventable problems.

9 Australia must learn from cultures with a positive attitude to children and young people. We must also learn from public policies that achieve high levels of child wellbeing; adequate support for parents, carers and families; and low levels of child poverty (for example, policies in the Nordic countries).

10 Effective prevention requires a strong theoretical framework; a sound evidence base; and effective design, implementation and evaluation.

Critical issues and challenges facing Australia today

1 Relative to Organisation for Economic Co-operation and Development (OECD) standards, Australian children and young people are not faring well. This is particularly so for Indigenous children.

2 The link between poverty, inequality and poor outcomes for children is clear. One in seven Australian children live in poverty, including 50 percent of all Indigenous children.

3 Problems that are mostly preventable compromise the wellbeing of many young Australians.

4 Preventing problems is more ethical than a focus on treatment. Prevention delivers improved health and wellbeing to individuals, and social and economic benefits to the community. However funding for prevention remains only a fraction of recurrent funding for treatment.

5 A strong and effective preventive approach requires a major change in the way we operate. Practice, policy and research, and also governments and non-government funders, need to adopt preventive approaches and longer timeframes to achieve sustainable outcomes.

6 Many initiatives by the Australian Government, states and territories and not-for-profits are building blocks contributing to the wellbeing of children and young people. We will be successful if we sustain the current momentum towards change over the long term, with better integration of initiatives and effective collaboration across sectors and disciplines.

Four key strategies for action

Four key strategies will address these challenges and improve the wellbeing of Australia's children and young people.

Strategy 1: Make the wellbeing of children and young people a national priority.

- Critical elements — whole-of-nation social change is the key to advancing the prevention agenda to reduce the level of problems affecting children and young people.

The critical elements of a social change strategy are:

(a) achieving widespread public agreement that the entire community shares responsibility for the wellbeing of children and young people

(b) increasing the value Australians place on children, young people and those who care for them

(c) empowering and supporting parents and carers, increasing their confidence and competence

(d) empowering communities to form local partnerships to improve the wellbeing of children and young people

(e) ensuring that every government department, every organisation, every profession, every business, and every local community group thinks about and acts with the wellbeing of children in mind, and

(f) listening to the voices of children and young people.

- Who should take action? — The Australian community, in partnership with business, non-government organisations and all levels of government. ARACY is asking the Australian Government to take leadership by supporting ARACY's national strategy for social change. This comprehensive strategy involves all sections of the community. It promotes a long-term, integrated program of public information; coordination of existing and new initiatives; and partnerships (national and local) between communities, non-government organisations, business and government to increase the wellbeing of children and young people.

- Timeframe — Action must start immediately and will need to be sustained over at least 10 to 15 years to achieve lasting social change.

Strategy 2: Set internationally comparable health and wellbeing targets for children and young people for the next 20 years.

Critical elements of this strategy are:

(a) adopting international indicators and gathering the data required to ensure Australia can fully participate in international comparisons of child wellbeing

(b) raising Australia's international standing to high levels of child and youth wellbeing, to match the levels achieved by the Nordic countries (as determined by the OECD report Doing better for children or similar indicators), and

(c) listening to the voices of children and young people.

- Who should take action? — The Australian Government and its statutory agencies such as the Australian Institute for Health and Welfare and the Australian Bureau of Statistics, in consultation with relevant non-government organisations.
- Timeframe — From September 2009.

Strategy 3: Agree on a national child and youth development agenda integrating existing early years, middle years and youth agendas.

Critical elements of this strategy are:

(a) ensuring a whole-of-government approach to children and young people

(b) integrating child-focused programs

(c) supporting parents, carers and families, and promoting their key role for the wellbeing of children and young people

(d) achieving an effective balance between targeted prevention (focused on single issues or risk groups) and holistic (primary prevention) approaches

(e) developing, supporting and retaining workers to enable them to deliver the national agenda

(f) assessing all government policies for 'child and youth impact' before implementing, and

(g) listening to the voices of children and young people.

- Who should take action? — Collaboration between the Australian and state/territory governments, Council of Australian Governments (COAG), and non-government organisations, building on and integrating existing government initiatives such as COAG's National Early Childhood Development Strategy — Investing in the Early Years, the Office for Youth's Work and the Social Inclusion Agenda.
- Timeframe — A meeting should be convened in March 2010 to discuss broad parameters with government, non-government and business; and the aim should be to finalise the national agenda by the end of 2010.

Strategy 4: Develop a collaborative research plan on the prevention of problems affecting children and young people, linked with the child and youth development agenda.

Critical elements of this strategy are:

(a) achieving a better understanding of causal pathways to problem outcomes and developing effective preventive interventions to tackle them

(b) increasing our knowledge on dissemination, implementation and evaluation of preventive strategies in 'real world' situations

(c) building the evidence base on what works for priority areas (eg Aboriginal populations), and

(d) listening to the voices of children and young people.

- Who should take action? — Collaborations of researchers, practitioners and policy-makers; for example, ARACY's Prevention Science Network.
- Timeframes — The research plan should be finalised by the end of 2010.

For more information, contact ARACY:

Email: enquiries@aracy.org.au

Phone:

Canberra	Melbourne	Sydney	Perth
02 6232 4503	03 9345 5145	02 9085 7247	08 9476 7800

September 2009

HEEADSSS ASSESSMENT TOOL FOR USE WITH ADOLESCENTS

A psychosocial assessment of young people is equally as important as a physical assessment. The following tool is based on Goldenring & Cohen's (1988), Goldenring's (2004), and the Ministry of Health New Zealand (2002) HEEADSSS method of interviewing. HEEADSSS stands for **H**ome, **E**ducation/employment, **E**ating, peer group **A**ctivities, **D**rugs, **S**exuality, **S**uicide/depression, and **S**afety. We suggest that you also consider exploring the adolescent's level of community involvement as this may be an area of strength for the individual or an area where support can be found.

We recommend you undertake formal training in the use of the HEEADSSS assessment tool prior to use.
Goldenring J 2004 Getting inside adolescents heads: an essential update. Contemporary Pediatrics
Goldenring J, Cohen E 1988 Getting into adolescents' heads. Contemporary Paediatrics: 75–90
Ministry of Health New Zealand 2002 Family Violence Intervention Guidelines: Child and Partner Abuse. Ministry of Health, Wellington

Home
In home we cover family, culture and connections, looking for both resiliency and risk issues.
- Where do you live? Who do you live with?
- Ask about extended family links and culture — iwi, hapu, whanau, tribe.
- Where were you born? How long have you been here?
- Do you belong to a church? What activities and length of time have you been involved with the church?
- Do you have jobs or responsibilities at your place?
- Who makes the rules? What happens if rules are broken?
- What happens when you fight at your house?
- Is there any violence occurring at your house?
- Who in your family do you get along well with? Not so well?
- Who is the person who you talk to most?

Education
- Do you go to school/training course/work?
- If no — how long have you been out of school/work? Why? Plans? What do you do with your time now?
- If yes — which school? What is good about school? Not so good?
- Do you have friends at school? Is there a teacher you get along well with?
- How do you do in your school work and classes?
- Do you have ideas about what you might like to do when you leave school?
- Do you miss much school? Why?
- Are you bullied at school?

Eating
- What do you like and not like about your body?
- Have there been any recent changes in your diet?
- Have you dieted in the last year? How? How often?
- Have you done anything else to try to manage your weight?
- How much exercise do you get in an average day? Week?
- What do you think would be a healthy diet? How does that compare to your current eating patterns?

Activities

Here we cover what you do; for example, with your friends, with your family and in your community.
- What do you and your friends do for fun? (With whom, where and when?)
- What do you and your family do for fun? (With whom, where and when?)
- Do you participate in any sports or other activities?
- Do you regularly attend a church group, club or other organised activity?
- Are you involved in any community activities?
- How do you get money?
- How do you get around? Do you drive sometimes?
- What about sleeping? Do you sleep well?

Drugs/Alcohol

Introduce, for example, 'We know that many young people try alcohol and drugs; is it all right if I ask you some questions about that now?'
- Do young people at your school smoke? Do your friends smoke? Do you smoke?
- Do your friends/parents ever drink alcohol? Do you?
- Have you ever used marijuana? What other drugs/solvents are young people using these days?
- What do you think about that? What have you tried?
- If the young person is using:
  - How much are you using? In what circumstances? What do you like and not like about using?
  - What risks do you take when using? Have you ever considered using less?

Sexuality

Introduce, for example, 'We ask everyone about sexuality because that is a very important aspect of young people's lives and can affect their health so much. Is that OK with you? You can "pass" on questions if you want to.'
- Have you had any sexuality education at school? What was that like?
- Do your friends have sexual relationships? Do you?
- Are any of them wondering about sexual orientation — liking girls or boys? Are you?
- What do you know about safe sex?
- What do you do (in terms of keeping sexually safe)? Do you use condoms? How much of the time (every time, just when you can get them, sometimes)?
- What could you do if you thought you might be pregnant?
- Has anybody ever touched you in a way that you don't like?
- If you ever felt uncomfortable or something unpleasant happened to you, is there anyone that you could tell?
- Are there adults you can go to for advice/help about sex and relationships?
- Do you want to talk about anything else about relationships or sex?

Suicide and Depression

In this we cover issues of mental health and self-harm.
- How would you describe your mood/feelings most of the time? (Scale 1–10)
- Do you have really good/bad times?

If low mood is an issue, review sleeping, eating, energy, concentration, feelings of guilt/worthlessness and safety.
- Do you ever have worries or hassles that bother you?

If yes:
  - Do they keep you awake at night?
  - Do you have to do anything to keep them under control?
  - Do you sometimes feel that life is not worth it?
  - Have you ever harmed yourself deliberately?

If no, you may not need to continue this line of questioning.
- Have you ever thought of ending your pain once and for all?
- Do you know anyone who has died from suicide? Who? When?
- How often do you think about doing it? How did you think you would do it?
- How strong are these feelings for you at the moment?
- Do you think you might try?
- What if something went wrong for you? (Relationship break-up, etc.)
- Who could you tell about feeling suicidal?

Regarding previous suicidal behaviour:
- What did they do? How many times? How long ago? What happened?
- How do they feel about the fact that they did not die?
- Do they wish they had died?
- Have things changed since then? What?
- Do they think that they might try again?

Safety

- Have you ever been seriously injured? How? How about anyone else you know?
- Do you always wear a seatbelt in the car?
- Have you ever ridden with a driver who was drunk or high? When? How often?
- Do you use safety equipment for sports and/or other physical activities (e.g. helmets for biking or skateboarding)?
- Is there any violence in your home?
- Does the violence ever get physical?
- Is there a lot of violence at your school? In your neighbourhood? Among your friends?
- Have you ever been physically or sexually abused? Have you ever been raped on a date or at any other time?
- Have you ever been in a car or motorbike accident? (What happened?)
- Have you ever been picked on or bullied? Is that still a problem?
- Have you gotten into any physical fights in school or in your neighbourhood? Do you still feel that way?
- Have you ever felt like you needed to carry a knife, gun or other weapon to protect yourself? Do you still feel that way?

ECOMAP

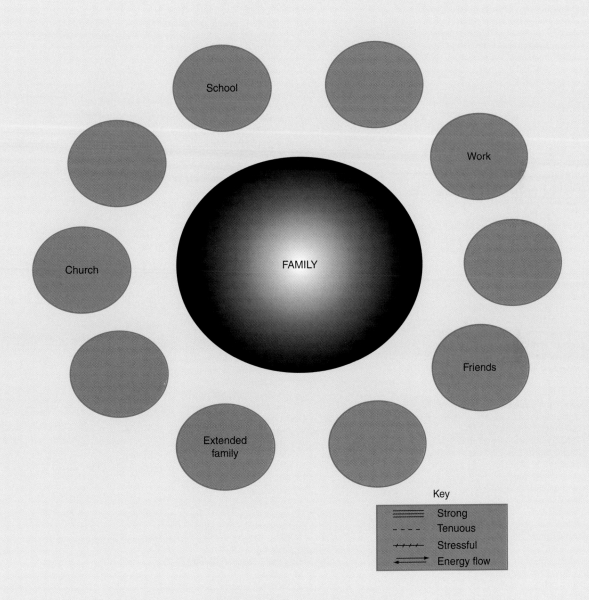

Key

═══════	Strong
‒ ‒ ‒ ‒	Tenuous
┼┼┼┼┼	Stressful
←————→	Energy flow

Index

Aboriginality, culture and health 335
    colonisation and disconnection 336–8
    culture blindness and the Stolen Generations 338
    relationships between health and place 335–6
    see also Indigenous health
Accident Compensation Corporation (NZ) 252
action research 373
    see also research
adolescent
    decision-making 220
    hope and self-esteem 220–2
    mothers 186, 212
    networking 218–20
    pregnancy 180, 212
adolescent health 207–8, 222
    alcohol, drug use, smoking 213–14
    community action 226
    community life 216–18
    cyber-bullying 219
    depression, self-harm, suicide 214–15
    eating disorders 210
    eating disorders and family life 211
    electronic information risk 230
    Eyes Wide Open (EWO) project 228–9
    goals for 222
    harm minimisation policies 223
    identity and body image 209–10
    media and health education 229
    peer contagion 218
    personal skill development for 227–8
    public policy for 222–3
    reorienting health services for 228–32
    risky sexual behaviours 211–12
    school life 218
    social competence development 208–9
    social determinants of 209
    supporting parenting for 225–6
    supportive environments for 223–5
    weight control 219–20
adult health 239–40, 255
    community action for 258–9
    environmental factors affecting 254–5
    family stress 249
    goals for 255
    lifestyle and chronic disease 242–5
    mental health 246–7
    morbidities 241–2
    obesity 243–4
    positive mental health 247–8
    public policy for 256–7
    reorienting health services for 260–1
    risk factors 240–1
    rural lifestyle risks 245–6
    skill development for 259–60
    social determinants of 246–7
    social exclusion and mental ill health 248–9

    stress 241, 246
    stress in the workplace 249–51
    stressful working conditions 252–4
    supportive environments for 257–8
    workplace health and safety 251–2
advanced practice nurses 85
    see also nursing
ageing 269
    and society 269–71
    chronic disease 274
    community action for 299
    critical pathways to 282–3
    dignity in coping 281–2
    elder abuse 280
    end of life transitions 285–6
    global perspectives 271–3
    goals for 287
    health and place in older age 277–8
    intimacy and sexuality transitions 284–5
    mental health issues 276–7
    physical activity and 275–6
    population 271
    public policy for 287–8
    reorienting health services for 290–2
    resilience and health 286–7
    risk and potential in older persons 273–5
    safe environments for 279–80
    single ageing or widowhood transitions 283–4
    skill development for 300
    social and spiritual support 280–1
    social disadvantage 274
    supportive environments for 288–9
    transitions 283
    weight and mobility 275
    workplace and retirement transitions 283
alcohol consumption
    adolescent 213–14
    Indigenous 342, 347
AMA *see* Australian Medical Association
ANMC *see* Australian Nursing and Midwifery Council
Annan, Kofi 58
anorexia nervosa 210–11
    see also adolescent health
antenatal care 180
    see also child health
ARACY *see* Australian Research Alliance for Children & Youth
Australia
    adolescent pregnancy 212
    aid policy 61
    alcohol consumption 213, 342
    child health indicators 175–6
    child obesity 177
    Health Literacy Alliance 19
    health promotion programs 72
    Indigenous health 339–40, 342, 349–50
    Medicare reimbursement 43

nurse practitioner role 86–7
paramedic practice 103
practice nursing 90–1
Australian health care system 403–5
mental health policy 399–400
mental health policy integration 397–8
recommendations for change 406–7
reform 405–6
Australian Medical Association (AMA) 43
Australian Nurses Federation 90–1
Australian Nursing and Midwifery Council (ANMC) 87
Australian Research Alliance for Children & Youth (ARACY) 192
declaration 435–8

balance and potential 7–8
Bangkok Charter for Health Promotion in a Globalized World 429–32
behavioural risk factors 342–3
best practice in health care systems 408–9
binge eating 210–11
see also adolescent health
biological embedding and childhood stress 172
Black Report on Inequalities in Health 34
body image 209–10, 219
breastfeeding 178–9
see also child health
building healthy public policy
see public policy
bulimia 210–11
see also adolescent health

CALD see culturally and linguistically diverse
Canada
advanced practice nurses 85
community healing process 346
Inclusive Cities Canada (ICC) Initiative 320
Index of Wellbeing 8
national multiculturalism law 333
nurse practitioners 87
Public Health Agency 85
caregiver stress 150–1
caregiving issues 149–50
caring for children with disabilities 150
case study research 375
see also research
casualisation or work 132
see also workforce transformation
CBPR see community-based participatory research
CDSMP see Chronic Disease Self-Management Program
change, community 76–8
child health 170–2
antenatal care 180
biological embedding and stress 172
breastfeeding 178–9
childbirth 180–1
chronic illnesses 176–7
collaborative policy development 192–3
community action 196–7
critical pathways to 189–90
developing personal skills for 197
divorce and the rights of the child 143–4
family lifestyle practices 186–8
global picture, disadvantage and poverty 173–4
goals 190–1
homelessness 175
indicators for Indigenous children 176
indicators in Australia and New Zealand 175–6
learning readiness and social development 183–4
nutrition and physical activity 177–8

obesogenic environments 187–8
parenting patterns and 185–6
postnatal depression 181–2
pregnancy health 179–80
psychosocial wellbeing 182
public policy for 191–2
reorienting health services for 197–9
resilience 184–5
socio-economic factors and stress 172–3
supportive environments 194–6
child health nursing 94–5
see also nursing
child poverty 173–4
child safety 188–9
childbirth 180–1
see also child health
children and homelessness 175
children with disabilities 150
children's rights policies 154
Chlamydia 211–12
Chronic Disease Self-Management Program (CDSMP) 93
chronic illnesses in childhood 176–7
citizenship 47–8
civic participation 159
Clinical Excellence Commission NSW 20
CMHNs see community mental health nurses
collaboration
child health policy 192–3
intersectoral 42–3
models of nursing and midwifery 108–10
Commission on Social Determinants of Health (CSDH) 12
communication within families 138–40
see also families
community 5
change 76–8
defined 9
development 16–20
development policies 396–7
empowerment 2, 28–9, 41–2, 46–7, 63, 71
health and wellness 9–11
health capacity 14
health sustainability 15–16
protection policies 156
role in intergenerational health 13
community action
for adult health 258–9
for gender issues 319–20
for healthy adolescents 226
for healthy ageing 299
for healthy children 196–7
for healthy families 157–9
for Indigenous health 352–3
community assessment 72–4
chart 433
Phase five: strengths, weaknesses, threats, opportunities 75–6
Phase four: people, place, health and gatekeepers 75
Phase one: the lay of the land 74–5
Phase three: who will help? 75
Phase two: mapping resource 75
tree 74
wellbeing indicators 383
community-based participatory research (CBPR) 373–4, 377
community-based research partnerships 373
see also research
community health promotion see health promotion
community mental health nurses (CMHNs) 103–5
see also nursing
community supports for women 307

comprehensive primary health care 2, 29–30
    see also primary health care
contraception 212–13
couple relationships 136–8
    see also families
critical pathways to ageing 282–3
critical pathways to child health 189–90
critical social theory paradigm 370
CSDH *see* Commission on Social Determinants of Health
cultural
    inclusiveness 329
    literacy 41–2
    norms and social exclusion 302–3
    safety 41–2, 84, 332–3
    sensitivity 41–2
culturally and linguistically diverse (CALD)
        families 195–6
culturally inclusive support 157
culture
    and health 330–1
    blindness 338
    conflict 331–2
    researching 377–81
    see also Indigenous health
cyber-bullying 219
    see also adolescent health

Declaration of Alma Ata 33–4
Declaration on the Rights of Indigenous Peoples 339
definitions
    community 9
    community health 9
    families 125
    health 5, 7, 33–4
    PHC nurses 91
    politics 394
    population health 32
    practice nurse 90
    primary health care 30, 33
    public health 33
    sexuality 285
    violence 144
Department of Health and Ageing (DoHA) 404
depression 214
DIDO *see* drive-in drive-out
dignity in coping with ageing 281–2
disparity between rich and poor 36–7
divorce 129–30
    and parenting 141
    and the blended family 142
    impact on parents 142
    non-resident parenting 142–3
    parenting and child support 143
    rights of the child 143–4
    see also families
DoHA *see* Department of Health and Ageing
drive-in drive-out (DIDO) worker 134
    see also workforce transformation
drug use 213–14

EBP *see* evidence-based practice
ecomap 158, 443
education 40–1
    women and 305
elder abuse 280
    see also ageing
embryonic stem cell research 38–9
empowerment 2, 28–9, 41–2, 46–7, 63, 71, 303–4
    intimate partner violence and empowerment 308–10

empowerment for Indigenous health 346
    see also Indigenous health
environmental factors affecting adult
        health 254–5
    see also adult health
environmental research 16
environments for ageing safely 279–80
    see also ageing
epidemiology
    and health promotion 63
    health and place 66–8
    of health and ill health 64–6
    social 66
equal opportunity for women 128
equity and social justice 36–7
equity as a human right 53
ethics in research 386
ethics of technology 38–9
ethnic cleansing 334
ethnocentrism to racism 333–5
evidence-based practice (EBP) 20, 108, 300
    for healthy families 161
    paradigms and 370
    research and 368
    sources of evidence 370–1
    see also research
Eyes Wide Open (EWO) project 228–9

falls prevention programs 291
    see also ageing
families 123
    adaptation and resilience 140
    caregiving issues 149–50
    changing 127–30, 139–40
    communication 138–9
    couple relationships 136–7
    defined 125
    developmental pathways 126–7
    fertility and child bearing 130–1
    functions of 125–6
    goals for healthy 153
    illness in 148–51
    marriage 140–1
    migrant 147–8
    place in communities 123–5
    power and communication 139
    public policy for 153–6
    relationship satisfaction 137–8
    rural 151–2
    skill development for 159–60
    social influences on couple relationships 137
    social policies and family life 398–9
    supportive environments for 156–7
    violence in 144–7
    see also divorce; workforce transformation
family
    advocacy 158–9
    life 152–3
    lifestyle practices 186–8
    relationship skills 159–60
    stress 249
family-centred care 161
family structure and adolescent health 208–9
    see also adolescent health
feminist movement 29
fertility and child bearing 130–1
FIFO *see* fly-in fly-out
fly-in fly-out (FIFO) employment 134–6
food policy from the school 194

GBD *see* global burden of disease
gender issues 301–2
    community action for 319–20
    empowerment 303–4
    expectations of life experiences 303
    goals for 316–17
    health policies 314
    inequality and social exclusion 302–3
    intimacy 314–15
    intimate partner violence and empowerment 308–10
    life experience expectations 303
    public policy for 317–18
    reorienting health services for 321–3
    sexually diverse populations 302, 315–16
    skill development for 320–1
    supportive environments for 318–19
    workplace 133–4
    see also men's health issues; women's health issues; workforce
        transformation
general practice 31–2
genogram symbols 417–18
global
    ageing perspectives 271–3
    child health, disadvantage and poverty 173–4
    community health research 364–6
    health conferences 34–5
    Indigenous health 338–9
    warming 254–5
global burden of disease (GBD) study 63–4
Global Humanitarian Forum 58
Global Peace Index 72
globalisation 53–5
    as a health promotion variable 57–8
    changes to social determinants of health 57, 65–6
    health promotion planning 69–70
    health promotion strategies for 58–63
    impact on family functions 128
    Millennium Development Goals (MDG) 59–60
    pros and cons 55–7
GNH *see* gross national happiness
goals
    for adult health 255
    for child health 190–1
    for gender issues 316–17
    for healthy adolescents 222
    for healthy ageing 287
    for healthy families 153
    for Indigenous health 348
gross national happiness (GNH) index 8

happiness 8
Happy Planet Index 8
harm minimisation policies for adolescents 223
    see also adolescent health
Harvard School of Public Health 63
health
    and place 66–8
    and place in older age 277–8
    and wellness 7–8
    as a global public good 61–2
    as a human right 62
    as development 59–61
    as security 59
    costs 37
    defining 5, 7
    education 40–1, 70–2
    Lalonde Report definition 33–4
    lifelong 121–2
    poverty linked to 36

socio-ecological concept of 5–6
    see also social determinants of health
health care systems
    Australia and New Zealand mental health policy 399–400
    Australian 403–5
    best practice 408–9
    features 408
    National Health and Medical Research Council's
        recommendations 406–7
    New Zealand 400–3
    reform in Australia 405–7
    Scandinavian 408
health care workplace stress 253
health–illness carrying capacity 15
health literacy 2, 17–18, 71
    conceptual model 45
    Indigenous community 354
    interventions 19–20
    levels 18–19
    strategies for promoting 21
Health Literacy Alliance, South Australia 19
health professional reorientation 161
Health Promoting Schools (HPS) framework 96–7
health promotion 39–40, 46, 53, 63–4
    as a global public good 61–2
    as a human right 62
    as development 59–61
    as security 59
    charters and PHC 34–6
    community assessment 72–6
    community-wide 70–2
    epidemiology 63
    focus of PHC 39–40
    globalisation and 53–7
    leadership, professionalism and citizenship 47–8
    Millennium Development Goals (MDG) 59–60
    Ottawa Charter 44–6, 71
    planning 69–70
    policies 395–6
    questions 62
    strategies for globalisation 58–9
    see also primary health care
health service
    assessment and screening 160–1
    policies and the social determinants of health 395–6
    problems 38
healthy cities 68–9
Healthy Cities Movement 69
healthy communities 2
healthy families *see* families
Healthy Workplace movement 108
HEEADSSS assessment tool for use with adolescents 217, 439–41
HITH *see* Hospital in the Home
HIV/AIDS 42, 72, 395
    adolescents and 211
    globalisation and 56
    LGBT groups and 316
    web of causation for 65
holistic practice 5, 83
homelessness 68
    for children 175
    for women 398
homosexual couples 127
    see also families
hospital care spending 37
Hospital in the Home (HITH) 406
HPS *see* Health Promoting Schools
human right to health 62
human rights policies 154–5

illness in families 148–51
see also families
inclusive communities 2
inclusive policies 155
Independent Life Expectancy (NZ) 241
Index of Wellbeing, Canada 8
Indigenous children health indicators 176
Indigenous health 329–30
alcohol abuse 342, 347
Australian 339–40
behavioural risk factors 342–3
capacity building for 346–8
child abuse 345
colonisation and disconnection 336–8
community action 352–3
cultural safety 41–2, 84, 332–3
culture blindness and the Stolen
Generations 338
culture conflict 331–2
globally 338–9
goals for 348
healing and empowerment 346
injury and family violence 345
mental health 343–5
multiculturalism 333
New Zealand 341–2, 349, 356
overcoming oppression 346–7
public policy 348–51
relationships between health and place 335–6
reorienting health services for 355–6
skill development 353–4
social capital for 346–8
supportive environments 351–2
violence 345–6
inequality and social exclusion 302–3
inequities in health 36–7
information technology's impact on families 128
see also families
injury and family violence 345
integrative reviews 368–9
see also research
intergenerational families 127
see also families
intergenerational health and communities 13
interpretive paradigm 370
intersectoral collaboration 42–3
intimacy 314–15
intimacy for older people 284–5
see also ageing
intimate partner violence (IPV) 145–7
and empowerment 308–10
IPV *see* intimate partner violence

Jakarta Declaration on Leading Health Promotion into the
21st Century 419–20
Japanese health care expenditure 37–8

Lalonde Report 34
Lead Maternity Carer (LMC) 109, 402
leadership 47–8
learning readiness of children 183–4
see also child health
lesbian, gay, bisexual, transgender 302, 315–16
LGBT *see* lesbian, gay, bisexual, transgender
life experience expectations 303
lifestyle and chronic disease 242–5
literature reviews 368–9
see also research
LMC *see* Lead Maternity Carer

marital law liberalisation 129
marriage policies 153–4
masculinity and behaviour 313–14
MDG *see* Millennium Development Goals
Medicare 404
men's health issues 310–11
health risks 312–13
intimacy 314–15
lifestyles and health 311–12
masculinity and behaviour 313–14
risk of abusing partner 309
see also gender issues
mental health 246–7
ageing and 276–7
Australian policy 399–400
New Zealand policy 400
of Indigenous peoples 343–5
policy integration 397–8
positive 247–8
social exclusion and 248–9
Mental Health Gap Action Program (mhGAP) 397
mental ill health in children 183
see also child health
mental illness anti-discrimination 249
meta-analyses 368–9
see also research
mhGAP *see* Mental Health Gap Action Program
midwives promoting social justice 83–5
migrant families and health 147–8
see also families
migrant women's health 306
Millennium Development Goals (MDG) 59–60, 409
Ministry of Health, New Zealand 43
mixed methods research 375–6
morbidities, adult 241–2
multiculturalism 333

National Health and Medical Research Council's recommendations
406–7
National Rural Health Alliance (NRHA) 351
NCNZ *see* Nursing Council of New Zealand
New South Wales Clinical Excellence Commission 20
New Zealand
alcohol consumption 213
child health indicators 175–6
child health nursing 94–5
child obesity 177
commitment to Pacific health 404
community mental health nursing 105
community representation 67
disparity with health resources 37
general practice 32
Global Peace Index ranking 72
globalisation of milk production 57
ground contamination 58
health care system 400–3
Indigenous health 341–2, 349, 356
intersectoral collaboration 43
intimate partner violence screening 308–9
Kaupapa Māori Health Services 342
mental health policy 400
mental illness anti-discrimination campaign 249
nurse practitioner role 86–7
paramedic practice 102
population health 241
practice and PHC nursing 91–2
primary health care 32
Primary Health Care Strategy 86, 91, 401
primary maternity care 109, 402

re-orientation of aid policy 61
rural and remote area nursing 102
school nursing 99
smoking prevalence 72
Treaty of Waitangi 72, 329, 341
New Zealand Ministry of Health 43
non-resident parenting 142–3
see also divorce
non-violence policies 154–5
NPs *see* nurse practitioners
NRHA *see* National Rural Health Alliance
NSW Pitstop program 322
nurse practitioners (NPs) 85–7
nurses promoting social justice 83–5
nursing
chronic condition management 92–3
collaborative models 108–10
community mental health 103–5
core skills to promote capabilities 93
models of NPs and advanced practice 85–7
occupational health 105–8
paramedic practice 102–3
practice and PHC nursing in New Zealand 91–2
practice nurses in Australia 90–1
rural and remote area 99–102
school health 95–9
nursing and midwifery goals for supporting parents 191
Nursing Council of New Zealand (NCNZ) 87

obesity 243–4
in children 177–8
obesogenic environments 187–8
objective information 22
occupational health nurses (OHNs) 105–8
see also nursing
OHNs *see* occupational health nurses
other workplace health and safety issues
Ottawa Charter for Health Promotion 44–6, 53, 71

PAR *see* participatory action research
paramedic practice 102–3
see also nursing
parent groups 156–7
parental leave 132
see also workforce transformation
parental rights policies 154
parenting and child support 143
see also divorce
parenting patterns and children's health outcomes 185–6
parenting support for healthy adolescents 225–6
see also adolescent health
part-time work 132
see also workforce transformation
participatory action research (PAR) 374
see also research
Peel Child Health Study 378
peer contagion 218
see also adolescent health
pelvic inflammatory disease (PID) 212
People's Health Charter 421–8
personal skills *see* skill development
pharmaceutical industry expenditure 38
PHC *see* primary health care
physical activity and ageing 275–6
see also ageing
PID *see* pelvic inflammatory disease
Pitstop program 322
Plunket nurses 95
PNs *see* practice nurses

policies *see* public policy
policy action at the national level 397
policy-making 392–3
community development policies 396–7
health promotion policies 395–6
integration 397–8
mental health policy 399–400
politics 393–4
primary health care and 397
social determinants of health and 395–6, 407
population ageing 271
population health 32
population trends 130–1
positivist paradigm 370
postnatal depression 181–2
see also child health
poverty and health 36
poverty and women 304–5
practice and PHC nursing in New Zealand 91–2
practice nurses (PNs) 90–1
see also nursing
pregnancy 179–80
teenage 180, 186, 212
see also child health
primary care 30–2
primary health care (PHC) 28–9
caravan park example 88
core skills to promote capabilities 93
Declaration of Alma Ata 33
health promotion charters 34–6
history 32–4
prevention 30
roles 89–90
social gradient and 34
primary health care principles
accessibility 36–7
appropriate technologies 37–9
cultural sensitivity, cultural safety 41–2
emphasis on health promotion 39–40
health education 40–1
intersectoral collaboration 42–3
public participation 43–4
primary prevention 107
professionalism 47–8
psychosocial wellbeing of children 182–4
see also child health
public health 33–4
see also health care systems; policy-making; public policy
public participation 43–4
see also community action
public policy
children's rights 154
gender issues 317–18
harm minimisation for adolescents 223
healthy adolescents 222–3
healthy adults 256–7
healthy ageing 287–8
healthy children 191–2
healthy families 153
inclusive 155
Indigenous health 348–51
marriage 153–4
non-violence 154–5
parental rights 154
protecting human rights 154–5
protecting the community 156
vulnerable families 155–6
see also policy-making
pursuit of happiness 8

racism 334
randomised controlled trials (RCTs) 369–70
    see also research
RCTs see randomised controlled trials
reciprocal determinism 10
refugee health 147–8
refugee women's health 306
relationship satisfaction 137–8
    see also families
remote area nursing see rural and remote area nursing
reorienting health services 160–2
    for adult health 260–1
    for gender issues 321–3
    for healthy adolescents 228–32
    for healthy ageing 290–2
    for healthy children 197–9
    for healthy families 160–1
    for Indigenous health 355–6
research 20, 22, 300, 363–4
    action research 373
    arguments 385
    case study 375
    community-based research partnerships 373
    conceptual framework 385
    discussion 386
    ethics 386
    evidence-based practice 368
    findings/results 386
    for policy and practice 367–8
    global community health 364–6
    integrative reviews 368–9
    literature reviews 368–9
    meta-analyses 368–9
    method 385–6
    mixed methods 375–6
    participatory action research 374
    Peel Child Health Study 378
    question to solution 384–5
    questions 385
    randomised controlled trials 369–70
    social determinants of health and 366–7
    sources of evidence 370–1
    stem cell 38–9
    systematic reviews 368–9
    translational 371–3
researching
    community supports for women 307
    culture 377
    the community 375–7
    the future 381–84
    with Indigenous people 378–82
resilience and health
    in adolescence 220
    in adulthood 140
    in childhood 184–5
    in older people 286–7
risk and potential in older persons 273–5
    see also ageing
RNZPS see Royal New Zealand Plunket Society
road traffic accidents 241
Royal New Zealand Plunket Society (RNZPS) 94–5
rural and remote area Indigenous health 340
    see also Indigenous health
rural and remote area nursing 99–102
    see also nursing
rural families 151–2
    social determinants of health 152
rural health policies 395
rural lifestyle risks 245–6

Scandinavian health care system 408
    see also health care systems
school nurses (SNs) 95–9
    see also nursing
School Nursing Professional Practice
        Standards 97
SDOH see social determinants of health
secondary prevention 107
selective primary health care 2, 29
    see also primary health care
self-esteem 220–2
self-harm 215–16
sexuality for older people 284–5
    see also ageing
sexually diverse populations 302, 315–16
sexually transmitted infections (STIs) 211–12
skill development
    for adult health 259–60
    for families 159–60
    for gender issues 320–1
    for healthy adolescents 227–8
    for healthy ageing 300
    for healthy children 197
    for Indigenous health 353–4
smoking see tobacco smoking
Snow, John 63, 69
SNs see school nurses
social and spiritual support for older persons 280–1
    see also ageing
social capital 14, 331–2
social determinants of adolescent health 209
    alcohol, drug use, tobacco smoking 213–14
    depression, self-harm, suicide 214–15
    eating disorders 210–11
    identity and body image 209–10
    risky sexual behaviours 211–12
social determinants of health (SDOH) 5, 11
    child health 177–82
    commission 12
    community role in 13–14
    gender and 301
    globalisation impact 57–8, 65–6
    health services policies and 395–6
    research agenda and 366–7
    rural families 152
    social capital 14
    socio-economic status 13
    stress, mental health and 246–7
    see also health
social development of children 183–4
    see also child health
social epidemiology 66
social exclusion and mental ill health 248–9
social inclusion and exclusion 299
social influences on couple relationships 137
social justice 2, 36–7
    core competencies for public health 85
    nurses and midwives promoting 83–5
social policies and family life 398–9
socio-ecological concept of health 5–6
socio-economic factors and childhood stress 172–3
sources of evidence 370–1
    see also research
South Australian Health Literacy Alliance 19
stem cell research 38–9
stereotypes of older persons 271
    see also ageing
stereotypical pattern of systemic racism 334
STIs see sexually transmitted infections 211–12

Stolen Generations 338
  see also Indigenous health
strengths, weaknesses, opportunities, threats (SWOT) analysis 75–6
stress 241, 246
  childhood 172–3
  environmental factors affecting 254–5
  family 249
  workplace 132–3, 249–51
  working condition 252–4
substantive freedom 347
suicide 215–17, 395
supportive environments
  for adolescent parenting 225–6
  for adult health 257–8
  for families 156–7
  for gender issues 318–19
  for healthy adolescents 223–5
  for healthy ageing 288–9
  for healthy children 194–6
  for Indigenous health 351–2
sustainable community health 15–16
SWOT see strengths, weaknesses, opportunities, threats
systematic reviews 368–9
  see also research
systemic bias and racism 334

Tamarika Ora nurses 94–5
teenage pregnancy and motherhood 180, 186, 212
  see also adolescent health
tertiary prevention 108
tobacco smoking, adolescents 214
tobacco smoking, adults 243–4
Transforming Australia for our Children's Future:
    Making Prevention Work 435–8
transitions in ageing 283
  end of life 285–6
  intimacy and sexuality 284–5
  single ageing or widowhood 283–4
  workplace and retirement 283
  see also ageing
translational research 371–3
  see also research
Treaty of Waitangi 72, 329, 341

UN see United Nations
UNICEF Child Friendly Cities 195
United Kingdom
  Black Report on Inequalities in Health 34
  child poverty study 174
  Happy Planet Index 8
  practice roles and models of care 87–9
  primary care system 32
United Nations (UN) 36
  Declaration on the Rights of Indigenous Peoples 339
  identifying violence against women 145
  Millennium Development Goals (MDG) 59–60
  policy implications for the future 394
  United Nations Development Programme 64
United States
  health and productivity management (HPM) model 106
  health care expenditure 37–8
  health literacy strategies 20–1
  national health education campaign 70

nurse home visiting for low SES mothers 197–8
  special needs students 98
United States Department of Health and Human Services
unprotected sexual activity 211–12

victim blaming 70
Victorian RANs 103
  see also nursing
violence
  children and 146–7
  empowerment and 308–10
  family 144–5
  Indigenous community 345–6
  intimate partner 145–6
Vision of Humanity 72
Vital@Work 252
VITAL@WORK 252
vulnerable families policies 155–6

weight and mobility in older age 275
  see also ageing
weight control 219–20
  see also adolescent health
Well Child nurses 94
Wellbeing Index, Canada 8
wellbeing indicators for healthy communities 383
WHO see World Health Organization
Whole-of-Community Healing Objectives 353
women and social disadvantage 307–8
women's health issues 304–7
  homelessness 308
  intimate partner violence and empowerment 308–10
  social disadvantage 307–8
  see also gender issues
women's movement 127
work and stress 132–3
workforce changes 128
workforce transformation 131–2
  casualisation 132
  fly-in fly-out employment 134–6
  gender issues 133–4
  parental leave 132
  part-time work 132
  stress 132–3
workplace
  bullying 251
  health and safety 251–2
  stress 249–51
  support for families 158
World Bank 63–4
World Health Organization (WHO)
  definition of health 5
  domestic violence declaration 145
  Geneva Declaration of the Health and Survival of Indigenous
      People 348
  global violence against women campaign 308
  Health Promoting Schools (HPS) framework 96–7
  Healthy Cities Movement 69
  Healthy Workplace movement 108
  Mental Health Gap Action Program (mhGAP) 397
  supporting healthy workplaces 253–4

xenophobia 334